a LANGE medical book

CURRENT
Guidelines in
Primary Care
2020

Jacob A. David, MD, FAAFP
Associate Program Director
Family Medicine Residency Program
Ventura County Medical Center
Clinical Instructor
UCLA School of Medicine
Los Angeles, California

New York   Chicago   San Francisco   Athens   London   Madrid
Mexico City   Milan   New Delhi   Singapore   Sydney   Toronto

CURRENT Practice Guidelines in Primary Care, 2020

Copyright © 2020, 2019, 2018, 2017, 2016, 2015 by McGraw Hill. All rights reserved. Printed in the United States of America. Except as permitted under the United States Copyright Act of 1976, no part of this publication may be reproduced or distributed in any form or by any means, or stored in a data base or retrieval system, without the prior written permission of the publisher. Copyright © 2000 through 2013 by the McGraw-Hill Companies, Inc.

1 2 3 4 5 6 7 8 9   LCR   24 23 22 21 20

ISBN 978-1-260-46984-4
MHID 1-260-46984-0
ISSN 1528-1612

Notice

Medicine is an ever-changing science. As new research and clinical experience broaden our knowledge, changes in treatment and drug therapy are required. The authors and the publisher of this work have checked with sources believed to be reliable in their efforts to provide information that is complete and generally in accord with the standards accepted at the time of publication. However, in view of the possibility of human error or changes in medical sciences, neither the authors nor the publisher nor any other party who has been involved in the preparation or publication of this work warrants that the information contained herein is in every respect accurate or complete, and they disclaim all responsibility for any errors or omissions or for the results obtained from use of the information contained in this work. Readers are encouraged to confirm the information contained herein with other sources. For example and in particular, readers are advised to check the product information sheet included in the package of each drug they plan to administer to be certain that the information contained in this work is accurate and that changes have not been made in the recommended dose or in the contraindications for administration. This recommendation is of particular importance in connection with new or infrequently used drugs.

This book was set in Minion Pro by MPS Limited.
The editor was Kay Conerly.
The production supervisor was Jeffrey Herzich.
Project management was provided by Ishan Chaudhary, MPS Limited.

This book is printed on acid-free paper.

McGraw Hill books are available at special quantity discounts to use as premiums and sales promotions, or for use in corporate training programs. To contact a representative please visit the Contact Us pages at www.mhprofessional.com.

This book is dedicated to all of our current and former residents at the Ventura County Medical Center.

Contents

Contributors

David Araujo, MD, FAAFP
Program Director, Family Medicine Residency Program, Ventura County Medical Center, Associate Clinical Professor, David Geffen School of Medicine at UCLA, Los Angeles, California
[Chapters 6, 9, 18, 20, 32, 38]

Wallace Baker, MD, MS
Family Medicine Residency Program, Ventura County Medical Center, Ventura, California
[Chapters 8, 28, 37]

Dorothy DeGuzman, MD, MPH, FAAFP
Core Faculty, Family Medicine Residency Program, Ventura County Medical Center, Ventura, California
[Chapters 10, 11, 21, 22]

Gabrielle Flamm, MD
Family Medicine Residency Program, Ventura County Medical Center, Ventura, California
[Chapters 1, 13, 24, 25, 36]

Audrey Gray, MD
Faculty, Sea Mar Marysville Family Medicine Residency Program, Marysville, Washington
[Chapters 1, 13, 24, 25, 36]

James Helmer, Jr., MD, FAAFP
Core Faculty, Family Medicine Residency Program, Ventura County Medical Center, Ventura, California
[Chapters 26, 35]

Neil Jorgensen, MD
Faculty, Ventura Family Medicine Residency, Ventura County Medical Center, Ventura, California
[Chapters 2, 3, 5, 14, 15, 17]

Shadia Karim, MD
Family Medicine, Ravenswood Family Health Center, East Palo Alto, California
[Chapters 4, 7, 16, 19]

Tipu V. Khan, MD, FAAFP, FASAM

Program Director, Primary Care Addiction Medicine Fellowship; Core Faculty, Family Medicine Residency Program, Ventura County Medical Center; Assistant Clinical Professor, UCLA School of Medicine, Los Angeles, California
[Chapters 1, 13, 24, 25, 36]

Cheryl Lambing, MD, FAAFP

Core Faculty, Family Medicine Residency Program, Ventura County Medical Center, Assistant Clinical Professor, UCLA David Geffen School of Medicine, Los Angeles, California
[Chapters 12, 23, 27, 29]

Luyang Liu, MD

Family Medicine Residency Program, Ventura County Medical Center, Ventura, California
[Chapters 2, 3, 5, 14, 15, 17]

Eric Monaco, MD

Family Medicine Residency Program, Ventura County Medical Center, Ventura, California
[Chapters 30, 31]

Marina Morie, MD

Family Medicine Residency Program, Ventura County Medical Center, Ventura, California
[Chapters 12, 23, 27, 29]

John Nuhn, MD

Family Medicine Residency Program, Ventura County Medical Center, Ventura, California
[Chapters 8, 28, 37]

Carolyn Pearce, MD

Family Medicine Residency Program, Ventura County Medical Center, Ventura, California
[Chapters 10, 11, 21, 22]

Magdalena Reinsvold, MD

Family Medicine Residency Program, Ventura County Medical Center, Ventura, California
[Chapters 6, 9, 18, 20, 32, 38]

James Rohlfing, MD
Family Medicine Residency Program, Ventura County Medical Center, Ventura, California
[Chapters 33, 34]

Kristi M. Schoeld, MD
Family Medicine Residency Program, Ventura County Medical Center, Ventura, California
[Chapters 4, 7, 16, 19]

Tanya Shah, MD
Family Medicine Residency Program, Ventura County Medical Center, Ventura, California
[Chapters 26, 35]

Ian Wallace, MD
Family Medicine Residency Program, Ventura County Medical Center, Ventura, California
[Chapters 30, 31]

Zachary M. Zwolak, DO, FAAFP
Core Faculty, Family Medicine Residency Program, Ventura Country Medical Center, Assistant Clinical Professor of Medicine, UCLA School of Medicine, Los Angeles, California
[Chapters 33, 34]

Preface

Current Practice Guidelines in Primary Care 2020 is intended for all clinicians interested in updated, evidence-based guidelines for primary care topics in both the ambulatory and hospital settings. This handy reference consolidates information from nationally recognized medical associations and government agencies into concise recommendations and guidelines of virtually all ambulatory care topics. This book is organized into topics related to disease screening, disease prevention, and disease management, and further subdivided into organ systems, for quick reference to the evaluation and treatment of the most common primary care disorders.

The 2020 edition of *Current Practice Guidelines in Primary Care* contains updates reflecting more than 150 new guidelines, and nearly 30 new sections on topics including transgender health, opiate use disorder, systemic lupus erythematosus, rotator cuff injury, and abortion. It is a great resource for residents, medical students, midlevel providers, and practicing physicians in family medicine, internal medicine, pediatrics, and obstetrics and gynecology.

Although painstaking efforts have been made to find all errors and omissions, some errors may remain. If you find an error or wish to make a suggestion, please e-mail us at EditorialServices@mheducation.com.

Jacob A. David, MD, FAAFP

Screening

Behavioral Health Disorders

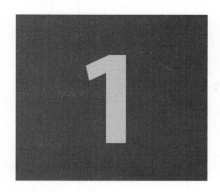

ALCOHOL ABUSE AND DEPENDENCE

Population
–Adults older than 18 y of age.

Recommendations

▶ CDC 2018, USPSTF 2018, ASAM 1997
–Screen all adults in primary care settings, including pregnant women, for alcohol misuse.
–If positive screen for risky or hazardous drinking, provide brief behavioral counseling interventions to reduce alcohol misuse.

Sources
–CDC. *Alcohol Screening and Brief Intervention for People Who Consume Alcohol and Use Opioids.* 2018.
–USPSTF. *JAMA.* 2018;320(18):1899-1909.
–ASAM. *Public Policy Statement on Screening for Addiction in Primary Care Settings.* 1997.

Comments
1. Screen regularly using a validated tool such as the AUDIT, CAGE, or MAST questionnaires.
2. The TWEAK and the T-ACE are designed to screen pregnant women for alcohol misuse.

Population
–Children and adolescents.

Recommendation

▶ USPSTF 2018

–Insufficient evidence to recommend for or against screening or counseling interventions to prevent or reduce alcohol misuse by adolescents.

Source

–USPSTF. *JAMA*. 2018;320(18):1899-1909.

Comments

1. Screen using a tool designed for adolescents, such as the CRAFFT, BSTAD, or S2BI.
2. Reinforce not drinking and driving or riding with any driver under the influence.
3. While behavioral counseling has been proven to be beneficial in adults, data do not support its benefit in adolescents.

DEPRESSION

Population

–Children aged 11 y and younger.

Recommendation

▶ USPSTF 2016

–Insufficient evidence to recommend for or against routine screening.

Source

–USPSTF. *Depression in Children and Adolescents: Screening*. 2016.

Population

–Adolescents.

Recommendation

▶ USPSTF 2016

–Screen all adolescents age 12–18 y for major depressive disorder (MDD). Systems should be in place to ensure accurate diagnosis, effective treatment, and adequate follow-up.

Source

–USPSTF. *Depression in Children and Adolescents: Screening*. 2016.

Comments

1. Screen in primary care clinics with the Patient Health Questionnaire for Adolescents (PHQ-A) (73% sensitivity; 94% specificity) or the Beck Depression Inventory-Primary Care (BDI-PC) (91% sensitivity; 91% specificity). See Chapter 39.

2. Treatment options include pharmacotherapy (fluoxetine and escitalopram have FDA approval for this age group), psychotherapy, collaborative care, psychosocial support interventions, and CAM approaches.
3. SSRI may increase suicidality in some adolescents, emphasizing the need for close follow-up.

Population
–Adults.

Recommendation
▶ USPSTF 2016

–Recommend screening adults for depression, including pregnant and postpartum women. Have staff-assisted support systems in place for accurate diagnosis, effective treatment, and follow-up.

Source
–USPSTF. *Depression in Adults: Screening*. 2016.

Comments
1. PHQ-2 is as sensitive (96%) as longer screening tools:
   a. "Over the past 2 wk, have you felt down, depressed, or hopeless?"
   b. "Over the past 2 wk, have you felt little interest or pleasure in doing things?"
2. Optimal screening interval is unknown.

ILLICIT DRUG USE

Population
–Adults, adolescents, and pregnant women.

Recommendation
▶ USPSTF 2008

–Insufficient evidence to recommend for or against routine screening for illicit drug use.

Source
–USPSTF. *Drug Use, Illicit: Screening*. 2008.

TOBACCO USE

Population
–Adults including pregnant women.

Recommendation
▶ AAFP 2015, USPSTF 2015
–Recommend screening all adults for tobacco use and provide tobacco cessation interventions for those who use tobacco products.

Source
–USPSTF. *Tobacco Smoking Cessation in Adults, Including Pregnant Women: Behavioral and Pharmacotherapy Interventions.* 2015.

Comment
1. Provide some type of SBIRT (Screening, Brief Intervention, and Referral to Treatment) such as:
   a. The "5-A" framework is helpful for smoking cessation counseling:
      i. Ask about tobacco use.
      ii. Advise to quit through clear, individualized messages.
      iii. Assess willingness to quit.
      iv. Assist in quitting.
      v. Arrange follow-up and support sessions.

Population
–School-aged children and adolescents.

Recommendation
▶ USPSTF 2013
–Recommends that primary care clinicians provide interventions including education or brief counseling to prevent the initiation of tobacco use.

Comment
1. The efficacy of counseling to prevent tobacco use in children and adolescents is uncertain.

Source
–USPSTF. *Tobacco Use in Children and Adolescents: Primary Care Interventions.* 2013.

Cardiovascular Disorders

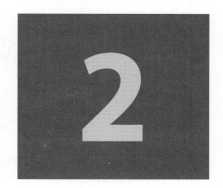

ABDOMINAL AORTIC ANEURYSM

Population
- Men age ≥65y.

Recommendations

▶ USPSTF 2014, ACC/AHA 2006, Canadian Society for Vascular Surgery 2006, Society for Vascular Surgery 2018
- Screen once before age 75, with ultrasound, if they have ever smoked.

▶ Canadian Society for Vascular Surgery 2018
- Screen once between age 65 and 80 y with ultrasound, regardless of smoking history.

▶ ESVS 2011
- Screen once with ultrasound at age 65 y if have smoked >100 cigarettes lifetime or have a family history of AAA.

▶ ESVS 2014
- Screen with ultrasound all men >65 y of age.

▶ ACRa/AIUM/SRU 2014
- Screen with ultrasound all men ≥65 y (or ≥50 y with family history of aneurysmal disease) and women ≥65 y with cardiovascular risk factors.
- Patients ≥50 y with a family history of aortic and/or peripheral vascular aneurysmal disease.
- Patients with a personal history of peripheral vascular aneurysmal disease.
- Groups with additional risk include patients with a history of smoking, hypertension, or certain connective tissue diseases (eg, Marfan syndrome).

–ACR-AIUM-SRU Practice Parameter for the Performance of Diagnostic and Screening Ultrasound of the Abdominal Aorta in Adults. 2014.

▶ Society for Vascular Surgery 2018

–Screen once with ultrasound between age 65 and 75 if ever smoked, or after 75 if in "good health" and never screened previously.

Sources

–*Ann Intern Med.* 2014;161(4):281-290.

–*J Vasc Surg.* 2007;45:1268-1276.

–Moll FL, Powell JT, Fraedrich G, et al. Management of abdominal aortic aneurysms clinical practice guidelines of the European Society for Vascular Surgery. *Eur J Vasc Endovasc Surg.* 2011;(41):S1-S58.

–Erbel R, Aboyans V, Boileau C, et al. 2014 ESC guidelines on the diagnosis and treatment of aortic diseases. *Eur Heart J.* doi:10.1093/eurheartj/ehu281

–*ACR-AIUM-SRU Practice Parameter for the Performance of Diagnostic and Screening Ultrasound of the Abdominal Aorta in Adults.* 2014.

–*J Vasc Surg.* 2018;67(1):2-77.

–https://canadianvascular.ca/Clinical-Guidelines

Population

–Women age ≥65 y.

Recommendation

▶ Canadian Society for Vascular Surgery 2018

–Consider screening once between age 65 and 80 y if history of smoking or cardiovascular disease.

Source

–https://canadianvascular.ca/Clinical-Guidelines

ATRIAL FIBRILLATION

Population

–Asymptomatic adults over age 65.

Recommendation

▶ USPSTF 2018

–Insufficient evidence to recommend routine ECG screening for atrial fibrillation to impact risk of stroke from untreated atrial fibrillation.

Source

–*JAMA.* 2018;320(5):478-484.

CAROTID ARTERY STENOSIS (CAS) (ASYMPTOMATIC)

Population
–Asymptomatic adults.

Recommendations

▶ ASN 2007, USPSTF 2014, AHA/ASA 2011, ACCF/ACR/AIUM/ ASE/ASN/ICAVL/SCAI/SCCT/SIR/SVM/SVS 2011, AAFP 2013

–Do not screen the general population or a selected population based on age, gender, or any other variable alone.
–Do not screen asymptomatic adults.

Sources
–*J Neuroimaging.* 2007;17:19-47.
–USPSTF. *Carotid Artery Stenosis: Screening.* 2014.
–*J Am Coll Cardiol.* 2012;60(3):242-276.
–Choosing Wisely: American Academy of Family Physicians. 2013.
–*Stroke.* 2011;42(2):e26.

Recommendation

▶ ACR–AIUM–SRU 2016, ACC/AHA/ASA/ACR/SVS 2011

–Indications for carotid ultrasound: evaluation of patients with a cervical bruit, not routine screening.

Sources
–*Stroke.* 2011;42(8):e464-e540.
–*ACR–AIUM–SPR–SRU Practice Parameter for the Performance of an Ultrasound Examination of the Extracranial Cerebrovascular System.* 2016. http://www.acr.org/~/media/ACR/Documents/PGTS/guidelines/ US_Extracranial_Cerebro.pdf

Recommendation

▶ Society of Thoracic Surgeons 2013

–Do not routinely evaluate for carotid artery disease prior to cardiac surgery in the absence of symptoms or other high-risk criteria.

Source
–Choosing Wisely: Society of Thoracic Surgeons. 2013.

Comments
1. The prevalence of internal CAS of $\geq$70% varies from 0.5% to 8% based on population-based cohort utilizing carotid duplex ultrasound. For population age >65 y, estimated prevalence is 1%. No risk stratification tool further distinguishes the importance of CAS. No evidence suggests that screening for asymptomatic CAS reduces fatal or nonfatal strokes.

2. Carotid duplex ultrasonography to detect CAS ≥60%; sensitivity, 94%; specificity, 92%. (*Ann Intern Med.* 2007;147(12):860)
3. If true prevalence of CAS is 1%, number needed to screen to prevent 1 stroke over 5 y = 4368; to prevent 1 disabling stroke over 5 y = 8696. (*Ann Intern Med.* 2007;147(12):860)

CHOLESTEROL AND LIPID DISORDERS

Population
  –Asymptomatic adults 40–79 y.

Recommendations
▶ ACC/AHA 2013
  –Perform 10-y ASCVD Risk Score.
  –High-risk categories include:
   • Primary elevation of LDL-C ≥190 mg/dL.
   • Diabetes (type 1 or 2) with LDL-C 70–189 mg/dL and without clinical ASCVD.
   • Without clinical ASCVD or diabetes with LDL-C 70–189 mg/dL and estimated 10-y ASCVD Risk Score ≥7.5%.

▶ ESC 2016
  –Perform SCORE risk assessment tool available at: www.heartscore.org
  –Secondary hyperlipidemia should be ruled out.
  –Total cholesterol and LDL-C primary target: goal LDL ≤70 mg/dL in patients with very high CV risk, LDL ≤100 mg/dL in patients with high CV risk.
  –Secondary targets are non-HDL-C and ApoB.
  –HDL is not recommended as a target for treatment.

▶ Canadian Cardiovascular Society 2016
  –Screen all men/women over age 40, or those of any age at high risk (clinical evidence of atherosclerosis, AAA, DM, HTN, cigarette smoking, stigmata of dyslipidemia, family history of early CVD or dyslipidemia, CKD, BMI >30, inflammatory bowel disease, HIV, erectile dysfunction, COPD, hypertensive diseases of pregnancy).
  –Nonfasting lipid tests are acceptable.
  –Repeat a risk assessment using Framingham or Cardiovascular Life Expectancy Model every 5 y or as clinical circumstances dictate.

Sources
  –*Circulation.* 2013;2013;01.cir.0000437738.63853.7a.

–European Society of Cardiology. Dyslipidaemias 2016.
–*Canadian Journal of Cardiology.* 2016;32(11):1263-1282.

Comment

1. Prior to initiating statin therapy, perform lipid panel, ALT, HgbA1c to R/O DM, and baseline CK (if patient is at increased risk for muscle events based on personal or family history of statin intolerance).

Population

–Adults with diabetes.

Recommendations

▶ ADA 2013

–Measure fasting lipids at least annually in adults with diabetes.
–Every 2 y for adults with low-risk lipid values (LDL-C <100 mg/dL, HDL-C >50 mg/dL, TG <150 mg/dL).

Source
–*Diabetes Care.* 2013;36(suppl 1):S11-S66.

Population

–Adults >20 y.

Recommendations

▶ NLA 2014

–Fasting lipid profile (LDL-C and TG) or nonfasting lipid panel (non-HDL-C and HDL-C) should be measured at least every 5 y.
–Also assess ASCVD risk.
–Non-HDL-C (primary target), ApoB (secondary target) have more predictive power than LDL-C.
–Apolipoprotein B (ApoB) is considered an optional, secondary target for therapy. More predictive power than LDL-C, but not consistently superior to non-HDL-C.
–HDL-C is not recommended as a target therapy.

Source
–*J Clin Lipidol.* 2014;8:473-488.

Comment

1. Non-HDL-C values:
   a. Desirable <130 mg/dL.
   b. Above desirable 130–159.
   c. Borderline high 160–189.
   d. High 190–219.
   e. Very high ≥220.

CHOLESTEROL GUIDELINES

Source	Recommended Lipoprotein Measurements for Risk Assessment	Recommended Lipoprotein Targets of Therapy	Recommended Risk Assessment Algorithm
National Cholesterol Education Program Adult Treatment Panel III	Fasting lipid panel Calculation of non-HDL-C when TG >200 mg/dL	Primary target: LDL-C Secondary target: non-HDL-C	Identify number of CHD risk factors Framingham 10-y absolute CHD risk
International Atherosclerosis Society	Fasting lipid panel with calculation of non-HDL-C	Non-HDL-C LDL-C is considered alternative target of therapy	Lifetime risk of total ASCVD morbidity/ mortality (by Framingham, CV Lifetime Risk pooling project, or QRisk)
European Society of Cardiology/European Atherosclerosis Society	Fasting lipid panel with calculation of non-HDL-C and TC/HDL-C ratio ApoB or ApoB/ apoA1 ratio are considered alternative risk markers	Primary target: LDL-C Secondary targets: non-HDL or ApoB in patients with cardiometabolic risk	10-y risk of total fatal ASCVD by the Systematic Coronary Risk Evaluation (SCORE) system
Canadian Cardiovascular Society	European Society of Cardiology/ European Atherosclerosis Society	Primary target: LDL-C Secondary targets: non-HDL-C and ApoB	10-y risk of total ASCVD events by the Framingham Risk Score
American Association of Clinical Endocrinologists	Fasting lipid panel Calculation of non-HDL-C is a more accurate risk assessment if TG is between 200 and 500 mg/dL, diabetes, insulin resistance, or established CAD	Primary targets: LDL-C Secondary targets: non-HDL-C in patients with cardiometabolic risk or established CAD ApoB recommended to assess success of LDL-C-lowering therapy	Men: Framingham Risk Score (10-y risk of coronary event) Women: Reynolds Risk Score (10-y risk of coronary event, stroke, or other major heart disease)

American Diabetes Association/ American Heart Association Statement on Cardiometabolic Risk	Stronger risk discrimination provided by non-HDL-C, ApoB, LDL-P	Strong recommendation for ApoB and non-HDL-C as secondary targets	30-y/lifetime global ASCVD risk
American Diabetes Association: Standards of Medical Care in Diabetes	Fasting lipid panel	LDL-C	Not applicable in setting of diabetes (CHD risk equivalent)
Kidney Disease: Improving Global Outcomes: Clinical Practice Guideline for Lipid Management in Chronic Kidney Disease	Fasting lipid panel to screen for more severe forms of dyslipidemia and secondary causes of dyslipidemia	None: therapy guided by absolute risk of coronary event based on age, and stage of CKD or eGFR	CKD considered CHD risk equivalent Treatment with evidence-based statins/statin doses based on age, and stage of CKD or eGFR
Secondary Prevention of Atherosclerotic Cardiovascular Disease in Older Adults: A Scientific Statement from the American Heart Association	Fasting lipid panel Calculation of non-HDL-C when TG >200 mg/dL	Primary target: LDL-CSecondary target: non-HDL-C	N/A
National Lipid Association: Familial Hypercholesterolemia	Fasting lipid panel	LDL-C	Not applicable due to extremely high lifetime risk
Expert Panel on Integrated Guidelines for Cardiovascular Health and Risk Reduction in Children and Adolescents	Fasting lipid panel with calculation of non-HDL-C	Primary target: LDL-C Secondary target: non-HDL-C	No risk algorithm, treatment based on the number of ASCVD risk factors

CHOLESTEROL GUIDELINES (Continued)

Source	Recommended Lipoprotein Measurements for Risk Assessment	Recommended Lipoprotein Targets of Therapy	Recommended Risk Assessment Algorithm
AHA Women's Cardiovascular Disease Prevention Guidelines	Fasting lipid panel Consider hs-CRP in women >60 y and CHD risk >10%	LDL-C	Updated Framingham risk profile (coronary, cerebrovascular, and peripheral arterial disease and heart failure events)
			Reynolds Risk Score (10-y risk of coronary event, stroke, or other major heart disease)
2013 American College of Cardiology/American Heart Association: Blood Cholesterol Guidelines for ASCVD Prevention	Fasting lipid panel to screen for more severe forms of dyslipidemia and secondary causes of dyslipidemia	LDL-C measured for assessment of therapeutic response and compliance Therapy guided by identification of 40 categories of patients who benefit from high- or moderate-dose statin therapy	CV Risk Calculator based on Pooled Risk Equations (10-y risk of total ASCVD events) Lifetime risk provided for individuals 20–59 y of age

apoA1, apolipoprotein A1; ApoB, apolipoprotein B; ASCVD, atherosclerotic cardiovascular disease; CAD, coronary artery disease; CHD, coronary heart disease; CKD, chronic kidney disease; CV, cardiovascular; eGFR, estimated glomerular filtration rate; HDL-C, high-density lipoprotein cholesterol; hs-CRP, high-sensitivity C-reactive protein; LDL-C, low-density lipoprotein-cholesterol; LDL-P, low-density lipoprotein particle; TC, total cholesterol; TG, triglycerides.

Source: Morris PB, Ballantyne CM, et al. Review of clinical practice guidelines for the management of LDL-related risk. *JACC.* 2014;64(2):196-206.

CORONARY ARTERY DISEASE

Population
–Adults at low risk of CHD events.[a]

Recommendations

▶ AAFP 2012, USPSTF 2018, American College of Physicians 2012, American Society of Echocardiography 2013, American College of Cardiology 2013

–Do not routinely screen men and women at low risk for CHD risk[b] with resting electrocardiogram (ECG), exercise treadmill test (ETT), stress echocardiogram, or electron-beam CT for coronary calcium.

–Do not screen with stress cardiac imaging or advanced non-invasive imaging in the initial evaluation of patients without cardiac symptoms, unless high-risk markers are present.

–Do not perform annual stress cardiac imaging or advanced non-invasive imaging as part of routine follow-up in asymptomatic patients.

Sources

–*AAFP Clinical Recommendation: Coronary Heart Disease.* 2012.
–Choosing Wisely: American College of Physicians. 2012. http://www.choosingwisely.org/societies/american-college-of-physicians/
–Choosing Wisely: American Academy of Family Physicians. 2013. http://www.choosingwisely.org/societies/american-academy-of-family-physicians/
–Choosing Wisely. American Society of Echocardiography. 2012. http://www.choosingwisely.org/societies/american-society-of-echocardiography/
–Choosing Wisely: American College of Cardiology. 2014. http://www.choosingwisely.org/societies/american-college-of-cardiology/
–*Ann Intern Med.* 2012;157:512-518.
–*JAMA.* 2018;319(22):2308-2314.

[a]Increased risk for CHD events: older age, male gender, high BP, smoking, elevated lipid levels, diabetes, obesity, sedentary lifestyle. Risk assessment tool for estimating 10-y risk of developing CHD events available online, http://cvdrisk.nhlbi.nih.gov/calculator.asp, or see Appendices VI and VII.
[b]AHA scientific statement (2006): Asymptomatic persons should be assessed for CHD risk. Individuals found to be at low risk (<10% 10-y risk) or at high risk (>20% 10-y risk) do not benefit from coronary calcium assessment. High-risk individuals are already candidates for intensive risk-reducing therapies. In clinically selected, intermediate-risk patients, it may be reasonable to use electron-beam CT or multidetector computed tomography (MDCT) to refine clinical risk prediction and select patients for more aggressive target values for lipid-lowering therapies (*Circulation.* 2006;114:1761-1791).

Comment

1. USPSTF recommends against screening asymptomatic individuals because of the high false-positive results, the low mortality with asymptomatic disease, and the iatrogenic diagnostic and treatment risks.

Population

–All asymptomatic adults age ≥20 y.
–Risk score assessment.

Recommendations

▶ ACC/AHA 2013, ESC 2012

–ASCVD Risk Score has replaced the FRS in the United States for patients age 40–79 y.
–Assess 10-y ASCVD Risk Score every 4–6 y.
–Framingham Risk Score (FRS), including blood pressure (BP) and cholesterol level, should be obtained in asymptomatic adults age ≥20 y.
–The SCORE Risk Score remains the screening choice in Europe.
–No benefit in genetic testing, advanced lipid testing, natriuretic peptide testing, high-sensitivity C-reactive protein (CRP), ankle-brachial index, carotid intima-medial thickness, coronary artery score on electron-beam CT, homocysteine level, lipoprotein (a) level, CT angiogram, MRI, or stress echocardiography regardless of CHD risk.

Sources
–*Circulation.* 2007;115:402-426.
–*J Am Coll Cardiol.* 2010;56(25):2182-2199.

Population

–Adults at intermediate risk of CHD events.

Recommendations

▶ ACC/AHA 2013, ESC 2012

–May be reasonable to consider use of coronary artery calcium and high-sensitivity CRP (hs-CRP) measurements in patients at intermediate risk.
–hs-CRP is not recommended in low- or high-risk individuals.

Sources
–*Eur Heart J.* 2007;28(19):2375-2414.
–*Eur Heart J.* 2012;33:1635-1701.
–*J Am Coll Cardiol.* 2007;49:378-402.
–*Circulation.* 2013;2014;129(25 Suppl 2):S49-S73.

Comment

1. 10-y ASCVD risk calculator (The Pooled Cohort Equation) can be found at: http://tools.acc.org/ASCVD-Risk-Estimator/

Population

–Adults at high risk of CHD events.

Recommendations

▶ AAFP 2012, AHA 2007, USPSTF 2012

–Insufficient evidence to recommend for or against routine screening with ECG, ETT.

–In addition, there is insufficient evidence to recommend routine MRI.

Sources

–*Arch Intern Med.* 2011;171(11):977-982.

–*AAFP Clinical Recommendations: Coronary Heart Disease.* 2012.

–*Ann Intern Med.* 2012;157:512-518.

Population

–Men and women with no history of CHD.

Recommendation

▶ USPSTF 2009

–Insufficient evidence to assess the balance of benefits and harms of using the nontraditional risk factors to prevent CHD events (hs-CRP, ankle-brachial index [ABI], leukocyte count, fasting blood glucose level, periodontal disease, carotid intima-media thickness, coronary artery calcification [CAC] score on electron-beam computed tomography, homocysteine level, and lipoprotein [a] level).

Source

–USPSTF. *Coronary Heart Disease: Screening Using Non-Traditional Risk Factors.* 2009.

Comment

1. 10-y ASCVD risk calculator (The Pooled Cohort Equation) can be found at: http://tools.acc.org/ASCVD-Risk-Estimator/

Population

–Women.

Recommendations

▶ ACCF/AHA 2011

–Cardiac risk stratification by the Framingham Risk Score should be used. High risk in women should be considered when the risk is ≥10% rather than ≥20%.

–An alternative 10-y risk score to consider is the Reynolds Risk Score, although it requires measurement of hs-CRP.

Source

–J Am Coll Cardiol. 2011;57(12):1404-1423.

Population

–Adults with stable CAD.

Recommendation

▶ CCS 2013

–Risk assessment by Framingham Risk Score should be completed every 3–5 y for men age 40–75 y and women age 50–75 y. Frequency of measurement should increase if history of premature cardiovascular disease (CVD) is present. Calculate and discuss a patient's "cardiovascular age" to improve the likelihood that the patient will reach lipid targets and that poorly controlled hypertension will be treated.

Source

–Can J Cardiol. 2013;29:151-167.

Recommendation

▶ AAFP 2009, AHA/APA 2008

–All patients with acute myocardial infarction (MI) to be screened for depression at regular intervals during and post hospitalization.

Sources

–Circulation. 2008;118:1768-1775.

–Ann Fam Med. 2009;7(1):71-79.

HYPERTENSION (HTN), ADULTS

Population

–Adults age >18 y.

Recommendations

▶ USPSTF 2015, AAFP 2009, CHEP 2015, ESH/ESC 2013, Canadian Task Force on Preventive Health Care 2013

–Screen for HTN.

–HTN is >140/90 mm Hg on two or more BP readings.

–All adults should have their BP assessed at all appropriate clinical visits.

–Ambulatory BP monitoring (ABPM) is the standard to confirm diagnosis.

–Annual F/U of patients with high-normal BP (2-y risk of developing HTN is 40%).

Sources
–*Am Fam Physician*. 2009;79(12):1087-1088.
–http://www.aafp.org/online/en/home/clinical/exam.html
–USPSTF. *High Blood Pressure in Adults: Screening*. 2015.
–Hypertension Canada: http://www.hypertension.ca/en/chep
–*Can Fam Physician*. 2013;59(9):927-933.
–*J Hypertens*. 2007;25:1105.
–*Eur Heart J*. 2013;34:2159-2219.

Recommendations

▶ ESH/ESC 2013

–In cases of severe BP elevation, especially if associated with end-organ damage, the diagnosis can be based on measurements taken at a single visit.
–In asymptomatic subjects with hypertension but free of CVD, chronic kidney disease (CKD), and diabetes, total cardiovascular risk stratification using the SCORE model is recommended as a minimal requirement.

Sources
–*J Hypertens*. 2007;25:1105.
–*Eur Heart J*. 2013;34:2159-2219.

Comments

1. Electronic (oscillometric) measurement methods are preferred to manual measurements. Routine auscultatory Office BP Measurements (OBPMs) are 9/6 mm Hg higher than standardized research BPs (primarily using oscillometric devices). (CHEP, 2015)
2. Confirm diagnosis out-of-office before starting treatment.
3. ABPM has better predictive ability than OBPM.
4. Home BP Measurement (HBPM) is recommended if ABPM is not tolerated, not readily available, or due to patient preference; 15%–30% of elevations by OBPM will have lower BP at home. (USPSTF, 2015)
5. Assess global cardiovascular risk in all hypertensive patients. Informing patients of their global risk ("vascular age") improves the effectiveness of risk factor modification.

Population

–Age >18 y.

Recommendation

▶ JNC 8 2014

–Treatment thresholds:
- Age ≥60: 150/90.
- Age <60: 140/90.
- DM or CKD: 140/90.

Source

–*JAMA*. 2014;311(5):507-520.

Comment

1. "Hypertension" and "pre-hypertension" are no longer defined.

Population

–Age >65 y.

Recommendation

▶ ACCF/AHA 2011

–Identification and treatment of systolic and diastolic HTN in the very elderly are beneficial in the reduction of all-cause mortality and stroke death.

Source

–*J Am Coll Cardiol*. 2011;57(20):2037-2110.

Comments

1. Increased frequency of systolic HTN compared with younger patients.
2. HTN is more likely associated with end-organ damage and more often associated with other risk factors.

PERIPHERAL ARTERY DISEASE

Population

–Asymptomatic adults.

Recommendation

▶ USPSTF 2018

–Insufficient evidence to recommend for or against routine screening with Ankle-Brachial Index.

Source

–*JAMA*. 2018;320(2):177-183.

SLEEP APNEA

Population
–Asymptomatic adults.

Recommendation

▶ USPSTF 2017, AAFP 2017
–Insufficient evidence to recommend for or against routine screening.

Sources
–AAFP. *Obstructive Sleep Apnea in Adults: Screening.* 2017.
–*JAMA.* 2017;317(4):407-414.

TOBACCO USE

Population
–Adults.

Recommendation

▶ AAFP 2015, USPSTF 2015, ICSI 2014
–Recommend screening all adults for tobacco use and provide tobacco cessation interventions for those who use tobacco products.

Sources
–*AAFP Clinical Preventive Service Recommendation: Tobacco Use.* 2015.
–USPSTF. *Tobacco Smoking Cessation in Adults, Including Pregnant Women: Behavioral and Pharmacotherapy Interventions.* 2015.
–ICSI. *Preventive Services for Adults.* 20th ed. 2014.

Comment
1. The "5-A" framework is helpful for smoking cessation counseling:
   a. Ask about tobacco use.
   b. Advise to quit through clear, individualized messages.
   c. Assess willingness to quit.
   d. Assist in quitting.
   e. Arrange follow-up and support sessions.

Disorders of the Skin, Breast, and Musculoskeletal System

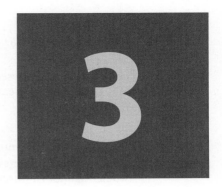

3

BREAST CANCER

Population
–Women.

Recommendations

▶ **USPSTF 2016**

–Age 40–49 y: Individualize assessment of breast cancer risk; incorporate woman's preference and cancer risk profile to determine whether to screen.

–Age ≥50–75 y: Mammography every 2 y, with or without clinical breast exam.

–Age >75 y: Inconclusive data for screening.

▶ **ACS 2016**

–Age 20–40 y: Advise women to report lumps or breast symptoms.

–Age 40–44 y: Allow women to begin annual screening if desired.

–Age 45–54 y: Mammography every year.

–Age ≥55 y: Mammography every 1–2 y as long as overall health is good and life expectancy is ≥10 y.

–Do not use clinical breast examination for screening.

▶ **NCCN 2018**

–Age 25–40 y: Teach breast awareness.

–Age 40–80 y: Mammography and clinical encounter annually.

–Age >80 y: Do not screen.

Sources
–http://www.cancer.org
–*Ann Intern Med.* 2012;156:609.
–*Ann Intern Med.* 2014;160:864.

–*CA Cancer J Clin.* 2016;66:95.

–*JAMA.* 2015;314:1599.

–https://www.uspreventiveservicestaskforce.org/Page/Document/ UpdateSummaryFinal/breast-cancer-screening1

–http://www.nccn.org

Comments

1. Harm and benefit of mammography screening
   a. *Benefits:* Based on fair evidence, screening mammography in women age 40–70 y decreases breast cancer mortality. The benefit is higher in older women (reduction in risk of death in women age 40–49 y = 15%–20%, 25%–30% in women age ≥50 y) but still remains controversial. (*BMJ.* 2014;348:366) (*Ann Intern Med.* 2009;151:727)
   b. *Harms:* Based on solid evidence, screening mammography may lead to potential harm by overdiagnosis (indolent tumors that are not life threatening) and unnecessary biopsies for benign disease. It is estimated that 20%–25% of diagnosed breast cancers are indolent and unlikely to be clinically significant. (*CA Cancer J Clin.* 2012;62:5) (*Ann Intern Med.* 2012;156:491)
   c. BSE does not improve breast cancer mortality (*Br J Cancer.* 2003;88:1047) and increases the rate of false-positive biopsies. (*J Natl Cancer Inst.* 2002;94:1445)
   d. Twenty-five percent of breast cancers diagnosed before age 40 y are attributable to *BRCA1* or *2* mutations.
   e. The sensitivity of annual screening of young (age 30–49 y) high-risk women with magnetic resonance imaging (MRI) and mammography is superior to either alone, but MRI is associated with a significant increase in false positives. (*Lancet.* 2005;365:1769) (*Lancet Oncol.* 2011;378:1804)
   f. Computer-aided detection in screening mammography appears to reduce overall accuracy (by increasing false-positive rate), although it is more sensitive in women age <50 y with dense breasts. (*N Engl J Med.* 2007;356:1399)
   g. Digital mammography and film screen mammography have equal accuracy in women 50- to 79-y-old, but digital is more accurate in women 40- to 49-y-old. (*Ann Intern Med.* 2011;155:493)
   h. Estimated 252,710 new cases of invasive breast cancer (63,400 with DCIS) are expected in 2017, with 40,600 expected deaths. (NCI. 2017)
   i. Future cancer screening: circulating tumor DNA mutations have been identified that correlate with specific underlying malignancy. Promising preliminary data exists for detection. (*Nat Med.* 2014;20:548) (*J Clin Oncol.* 2014;82:5)

j. In 2016, 246,000 new invasive breast cancer cases per year and 40,500 deaths were recorded. Mortality rates have declined by 1.9%/y from 1998 to 2012, with widespread annual screening.

k. It is estimated that 1.6 million breast biopsies are performed each year in the United States with the overwhelming majority having benign disease. (*JAMA.* 2015;313:1122)

2. Continued controversy over screening

a. The Canadian National Breast Screening study that began in 1980 found no survival benefit for mammography in 40- to 59-y-old women, but most experts in the United States consider the study to be flawed because of its design. (*BMJ.* 2014;348:g366) (*N Engl J Med.* 2014;370:1965)

b. A recent meta-analysis (*JAMA.* 2014;311:1327) from Harvard found an overall reduction of 19% in breast cancer mortality (15% for women in their forties and 32% for women in their sixties). They were concerned about overdiagnosis and other potential harms of screening including false-positive findings and unnecessary biopsies. (*N Engl J Med.* 2016;375:1438)

c. Recent trials have led to an increase in further screening studies based on the predicted individual risk of breast cancer occurrence. These also include a history of lobular carcinoma in situ, atypical hyperplasia, or history of breast cancer (invasive and DCIS). (*Ann Intern Med.* 2016;165:700, 737)

Population

– Patients who receive thoracic radiation therapy between ages 10 and 30 y.

Recommendations

▶ NCCN 2018

– For women younger than 25 y, recommend annual clinical encounter starting 10 y after radiation therapy.

– For women 25 y or greater; recommend annual clinical encounter starting 10 y after radiation therapy; annual mammography to begin 10 y after RT but not prior to age 30 y; annual breast MRI to begin 10 y after RT but not prior to age 25 y.

Source

– www.nccn.org

BREAST CANCER—*BRCA1* AND *2* MUTATIONS

▶ **Population**
  –Women age <60 y.

Recommendations

▶ **NCCN 2018**

  –Who to screen: patients without cancer.
  - Individual from a family with known deleterious *BRCA1* and *2* gene mutation.
  - Test only for the known mutation, not a full genetic evaluation.
  - If strong family history (FH) but unable to test family member with cancer (not alive or unavailable to be tested) then do full genetic evaluation. A strong FH includes:
    ◦ Two primary breast cancers in a single close relative (first-, second-, and third-degree relatives).
    ◦ Two breast cancer primaries on same side of family with at least one diagnosis occurring in a patient <50 y.
    ◦ Ovarian cancer or male breast cancer at any age.
  - Start screening 10 y prior to diagnosis of youngest family member but not before age 30.

  –Who to screen: patients with breast, ovarian, pancreas, and prostate cancer.
  - A known mutation in a cancer susceptibility gene within a family.
  - Early age onset of breast cancer (<50 y).
  - Triple negative (ER-PR-, Her2-) breast cancer diagnosed in <60-y-old.
  - An individual of Ashkenazi Jewish descent with breast, ovarian, or pancreatic cancer at any age.
  - All women with ovarian cancer (epithelial and non-mucinous) at any age should be tested for *BRCA1* and *2* mutations.

Recommendations

▶ **ACS 2017**

  –Women who are at high risk for breast cancer based on certain factors should get an MRI and a mammogram every year, typically starting at age 30.
  –High risk includes:
  - Lifetime risk of breast cancer 20%–25% or greater (according to risk assessment tools).
  - Known *BRCA1* and *2* mutation-positive women should begin MRI and mammogram screening at age 30 y or younger.

- Have a first-degree relative (parent, brother, sister, or child) with a *BRCA1* or *BRCA2* gene mutation, and have not had genetic testing themselves.
- Had radiation therapy to the chest when they were between the ages of 10 and 30 y.
- Have Li–Fraumeni syndrome, Cowden syndrome, or Bannayan–Riley–Ruvalcaba syndrome, or have first-degree relatives with one of these syndromes.

Population

–Lifetime risk of breast cancer >20% based on personal and family history (utilize Gail model, BRCAPRO model, or Tyrer–Cuzick model) and genetic predisposition (*BRCA1* or *2*), PALB 2, CHEK 2 (http://www.cancer.gov/bcrisktool/).

Recommendations

▶ NCCN 2018

–Clinical encounter every 6–12 mo to begin when identified as being at increased risk; referral to genetic counseling if not already done.

–Annual screening mammogram: to begin 10 y prior to the youngest family member but not prior to age 30 y.

–Recommend annual breast MRI: to begin 10 y prior to youngest family member but not prior to age 25 y.

Sources

–*CA Cancer J Clin.* 2015;65:30.
–*N Engl J Med.* 2015;372:2353.
–*J Clin Oncol.* 2016;34:1882.
–*JAMA.* 2012;307:1394.
–*J Clin Oncol.* 2016;34:1840.

Comments

1. *BRCA2*-related breast cancer is more like sporadic BC with 75% of patients with hormonal receptor positivity and significant decrease in aggressive growth. Only 15% of *BRCA2* patients will develop ovarian cancer with the average time of onset being in the mid-fifties.
2. One in forty Ashkenazi Jewish men and women carry a deleterious *BRCA1* or *2* gene (BRCA1 185del AG, 5382inse mutations, and BRCA2 6174delT mutation).
3. Some experts believe all men and women of Ashkenazi descent should be tested for these three genes, even with no personal or family history of malignancy. (*N Engl J Med.* 2016;374:454)

4. Tamoxifen or raloxifene has not been studied as de novo chemo prevention in *BRCA1* or *2* patients, but tamoxifen will decrease risk of contralateral breast cancer by 50% in *BRCA*-mutated breast cancer patients. (*Int J Cancer*. 2006;118:2281)
5. Risk-reducing bilateral mastectomy in *BRCA1* and *2* mutation carriers results in a 90% risk reduction in incidence of breast cancer and a 90% rate of satisfaction among patients who underwent risk-reducing surgery at 10-y follow-up. (*N Engl J Med*. 2001;345:159) (*JAMA*. 2010;304:967)

ORAL CANCER

Population
   –Asymptomatic persons.

Recommendations

▶ **AAFP 2015, USPSTF 2013**
   –Insufficient evidence to recommend for or against routinely screening adults for oral asymptomatic cancer.

▶ **NCCN 2018**
   –For women younger than 25 y, recommend annual clinical encounter starting 10 y after radiation therapy.
   –For women 25 y or greater, recommend annual clinical encounter starting 10 y after radiation therapy; annual mammography to begin 10 y after RT but not prior to age 30 y; annual breast MRI to begin 10 y after RT but not prior to age 25 y.

Sources
   –http://www.aafp.org/online/en/home/clinical/exam.html
   –http://www.ahrq.gov/clinic/uspstf/uspsoral.htm
   –www.nccn.org

Comment
1. Primary risk factors for oral cancer are tobacco and alcohol use. Additional risk factors include male sex, older age, use of betel quid, ultraviolet light exposure, infection with Candida or bacterial flora, and a compromised immune system. Recently, sexually transmitted oral human papillomavirus infection has been recognized as an increasing risk factor for oropharyngeal cancer, another subset of head and neck cancer.

SKIN CANCER (MELANOMA)

Recommendations

▶ USPSTF 2016

–Insufficient evidence to assess the balance of benefits and harms of visual skin examination by a clinician to screen for skin cancer in adults.[a,b]

–Recommends counseling of children, adolescents, and young adults age 10–24 y who have fair skin, to minimize exposure to ultraviolet radiation to reduce the risk of skin cancer.

Sources

–*JAMA.* 2016;316:429.

–http://www.ahrq.gov/clinic/uspstf/uspsskca.htm

Comments

1. Benefits and harms

   a. *Benefits:* Basal and squamous cell carcinoma are the most common types of cancer in the United States and represent the vast majority of all cases of skin cancer; however, they rarely result in death or substantial morbidity, whereas melanoma skin cancer has notably higher mortality rates. In 2016, an estimated 76,400 US men and women will develop melanoma and 10,100 will die from the disease.

   b. *Harms:* Potential for harm clearly exists, including a high rate of unnecessary biopsies, possibly resulting in cosmetic or, more rarely, functional adverse effects, and the risk of overdiagnosis and overtreatment.

   c. Direct evidence on the effectiveness of screening in reducing melanoma morbidity and mortality is limited to a single fair-quality ecologic study with important methodological limitations.

   d. Twenty-eight million people in the United States use UV indoor tanning salons, increasing risk of squamous, basal cell cancer, and malignant melanoma. (*J Clin Oncol.* 2012;30:1588)

   e. Clinical features of increased risk of melanoma (family history, multiple nevi previous melanoma) are linked to sites of subsequent

---

[a]Clinicians should remain alert for skin lesions with malignant features when examining patients for other reasons, particularly patients with established risk factors. Risk factors for skin cancer include evidence of melanocytic precursors (atypical moles), large numbers of common moles (>50), immunosuppression, any history of radiation, family or personal history of skin cancer, substantial cumulative lifetime sun exposure, intermittent intense sun exposure or severe sunburns in childhood, freckles, poor tanning ability, and light skin, hair, and eye color.

[b]Consider educating patients with established risk factors for skin cancer (see above) about signs and symptoms suggesting skin cancer and the possible benefits of periodic self-examination. Alert at-risk patients to significance of asymmetry, border irregularity, color variability, diameter >6 mm, and evolving change in previous stable mole. All suspicious lesions should be biopsied (excisional or punch, not a shave biopsy) (*Ann Intern Med.* 2009;150:188) (USPSTF; ACS; COG).

malignant melanoma, which may be helpful in surveillance. (*JAMA Dermatol.* 2017;153:23)

f. There are no guidelines for patients with familial syndromes (familial atypical mole and melanoma [FAM-M]), although systematic surveillance is warranted.[a]

SKIN CANCER

▶ Minimize Risk Factor Exposure

−Based on solid evidence, sun and UV radiation exposure are associated with an increased risk of squamous cell carcinoma (SCC) and basal cell carcinoma (BCC).

▶ Therapeutic Approaches

−Sunscreen, protective clothing, limited time in the sun, avoiding blistering sunburn in adolescence and young adults.

−Self-exam of skin, looking for changes that could possibly be cancer; higher risk patients need to be examined by dermatologist every 6–12 mo.

Source

−http://www.cancer.gov/types/skin/hp/skin-prevention-pdq

VITAMIN D DEFICIENCY

Population

−Nonpregnant adults age 18 y or older.

Recommendations

▶ USPSTF 2015, Endocrine Society 2011

−Insufficient evidence to screen for vitamin D deficiency in asymptomatic adults.

−Screen with serum 25-hydroxyvitamin D level in patients at risk[b] for deficiency.

Sources

−*J Clin Endocrinol Metab.* 2011;96(7):1911-1930.
−*Ann Intern Med.* 2015;162(2):133-140.

---

[a]Consider dermatologic risk assessment if family history of melanoma in ≥2 blood relatives, presence of multiple atypical moles, or presence of numerous actinic keratoses.
[b]Indications for screening include rickets, osteomalacia, osteoporosis, CKD, hepatic failure, malabsorption syndromes, hyperparathyroidism, certain medications (anticonvulsants, glucocorticoids, AIDS drugs, antifungals, cholestyramine), African-American and Hispanic race, pregnancy and lactation, older adults with history of falls or nontraumatic fractures, BMI >30, and granulomatous diseases.

Endocrine and Metabolic Disorders

4

DIABETES MELLITUS (DM), TYPE 2 AND PREDIABETES

Population
–Nonpregnant adults, children, adolescents.

Recommendations
▶ USPSTF 2015, ADA 2019, IDF 2017

–Screen as part of cardiovascular risk assessment if age 40–70 y and BMI >25.

–Screen asymptomatic adults of any age with BMI ≥25 and risk factor(s). Screen asymptomatic Asian-American adults of any age with BMI ≥23 and risk factor(s).

–Screen children and adolescents who are overweight (BMI ≥85th percentile) or obese (BMI ≥95th percentile) with additional risk factor(s) after the onset of puberty or after 10 y of age, whichever occurs first.

–Screen women who were diagnosed with gestational diabetes (GDM) every 3 y.

–Screen patients with prediabetes annually for the development of diabetes.

–Use a validated screening test such as the FINDRISC score.[a] If unavailable, use fasting plasma glucose (FPG) as a screening test. If negative, the screening test should be repeated at least every 3 y. If positive, proceed to a diagnostic test. Confirmatory diagnostic tests include FPG, random blood glucose (RPG), 2-hour plasma

[a]FINDRISC score incorporates age, BMI, waist circumference, history of medication use, history of hyperglycemia, and family history to predict risk of type 2 diabetes. Janghorbani et al, *Rev Diabet Stud* 2013;10(4). https://www.ncbi.nlm.nih.gov/pmc/articles/PMC4160014/

glucose during a 75-g oral glucose tolerance test (OGTT), or HgbA1C. If diagnostic test is normal, repeat the diagnostic test every year.

Sources

–USPSTF. *Abnormal Blood Glucose and Type 2 Diabetes Mellitus: Screening.* 2015.

–ADA. *Standards in Medical Care in Diabetes—2019, Abridged for Primary Care Providers.* 2019;37(1):11-34.

–International Diabetes Federation. *IDF Clinical Practice Recommendations for Managing Type 2 Diabetes in Primary Care.* 2017. www.idf.org/managing-type2-diabetes

Comments

1. Repeat screening at least every 3 y in asymptomatic adults above the age of 40.
2. Screen and treat patients with prediabetes for modifiable cardiovascular risk factors such as hypertension and dyslipidemia.
3. Risk factors for diabetes and prediabetes in asymptomatic adults:
   a. First-degree relative with diabetes
   b. High-risk race/ethnicity (eg, African-American, Latino, Native American, Asian-American, Pacific Islander)
   c. History of CVD
   d. Hypertension
   e. HDL <35 and/or triglycerides >250
   f. Women with polycystic ovary syndrome (PCOS)
   g. Physical inactivity
   h. Increased abdominal waist circumference
   i. Clinical conditions associated with insulin resistance (eg, severe obesity, acanthosis nigricans)
4. Risk factors for diabetes and prediabetes in asymptomatic children:
   a. Maternal history of diabetes or GDM during the child's gestation
   b. Family history of type 2 diabetes in first- or second-degree relatives
   c. High-risk race/ethnicity (eg, African-American, Latino, Native American, Asian-American, Pacific Islander)
   d. Clinical conditions associated with insulin resistance (eg, acanthosis nigricans, hypertension, dyslipidemia, PCOS, small-for-gestational-age birth weight)
5. Overweight or obese children and adolescents in whom type 2 diabetes is being considered should be tested for pancreatic autoantibodies to exclude the possibility of autoimmune type 1 diabetes.

OBESITY

Population
–All adults, children >6-y-old, and adolescents.

Recommendations
▶ **AAFP 2012, USPSTF 2018, USPSTF 2017, VA/DoD 2014**
–Screen all adults using body mass index (BMI) and offer intensive counseling and behavioral interventions to promote sustained weight loss in obese adults with BMI ≥30 kg/m².
–Consider annual measurement of waist circumference.
–Screen for obesity in children aged 6 y and older and adolescents using BMI and refer patients with age- and sex-specific BMI ≥95th percentile to comprehensive, intensive behavioral interventions to promote weight loss.

Sources
–USPSTF. *Obesity in Adults: Screening and Management.* 2018.
–USPSTF. *Obesity in Children and Adolescents: Screening.* 2017.
–VA/DoD Clinical Practice Guideline for Screening and Management of Overweight and Obesity, Version 2.0. 2014.

Comments
1. Intensive counseling involves more than one session per month for at least 3 mo.
2. Offer intensive intervention to promote weight loss in
   a. Obese adults (BMI ≥30 or waist circumference ≥40 in. [men] or ≥35 in. [women]).
   b. Overweight adults (BMI 25–29.9) with an obesity-associated condition.[a]

THYROID CANCER

Population
–Asymptomatic persons.

Recommendations
▶ **USPSTF 2017, American Cancer Society, NIH/National Cancer Institute 2019**
–Do not screen asymptomatic people with ultrasound.

---

[a]HTN, DM type 2, dyslipidemia, obstructive sleep apnea, degenerative joint disease, or metabolic syndrome.

–Genetic testing is recommended for patients with a family history of medullary thyroid cancer (MTC), with or without multiple endocrine neoplasia type 2 (MEN2).

–Be aware of higher risk patients: head-and-neck radiation administered in infancy and childhood for benign (thymus enlargement, acne) or malignant conditions, which results in an increased risk beginning 5 y after radiation and continuing until >20 y later; nuclear fallout exposure (eg, Japanese survivors of atomic bombing); history of goiter; family history of thyroid disease or thyroid cancer; MEN2; female gender; Asian race.

Sources

–*JAMA.* 2017;317(18):1882-1887.

–*N Engl J Med.* 2015;373:2347.

–PDQ® Screening and Prevention Editorial Board. *PDQ Thyroid Cancer Screening.* Bethesda, MD: National Cancer Institute. https://www. cancer.gov/types/thyroid/hp/thryoid-screening-pdq. Accessed April 16, 2019.

Comments

1. Neck palpation for nodules in asymptomatic individuals has sensitivity of 15%–38% and specificity of 93%–100%. Only a small proportion of nodular thyroid glands are neoplastic, resulting in a high false-positive rate.

2. Fine-needle aspiration (FNA) is the procedure of choice for evaluation of thyroid nodules. (*Otolaryngol Clin North Am.* 2010;43:229-238; *N Engl J Med.* 2012;367:705)

THYROID DYSFUNCTION

Population

–Asymptomatic nonpregnant adults.

–Newborns.

Recommendations

▶ AAFP 2015, USPSTF 2015, ATA 2012, AACE 2012, ASRM 2015

–Insufficient evidence to recommend for or against routine screening for thyroid disease in asymptomatic adults without risk factors.

- ATA/AACE: consider screening patients older than 60, those with risk factors, and women planning pregnancy.

–Screen all newborns for congenital hypothyroidism.

–Screen adults with risk factors for hypothyroidism.

–Screen adults with laboratory or radiologic abnormalities that could be caused by thyroid disease.

–Use serum TSH to screen for thyroid disease.

–Do not test for thyroid disease in hospitalized patients unless thyroid disease is strongly suspected.

Sources

–*Am Fam Phys.* 2015;91(11).

–*Endocr Pract.* 2012;18(6):988.

–*Ann Intern Med.* 2015;162(9):641-650.

–*ASRM.* 2015;104(3):545-553.

Comments

1. Individuals with symptoms and signs potentially attributable to thyroid dysfunction require TSH testing.
2. Less than 1% of adults have subclinical hypothyroidism; outcomes data to support treatment are lacking. Subclinical hyperthyroidism detected during routine screening may be treated in select patients at high risk of cardiovascular or skeletal complications.
3. Higher risk individuals are those with autoimmune disorders (eg, type 1 diabetes), pernicious anemia, goiter, previous radioactive iodine therapy and/or head-and-neck irradiation or surgery, pituitary or hypothalamic disorders, first-degree relative with a thyroid disorder, use of medications that may impair thyroid function, and those with psychiatric disorders.
4. Thyroid function should be measured in patients with the following: substantial hyperlipidemia, hyponatremia, high-serum muscle enzymes, macrocytic anemia, pericardial or pleural effusions.
5. Consider TSH screening in infertile women attempting pregnancy.

Gastrointestinal Disorders

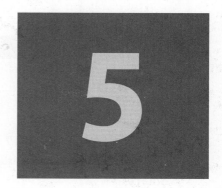

BARRETT ESOPHAGUS (BE)

Population
- Lower risk: General population with gastroesophageal reflux disease (GERD).
- Moderate risk: GERD and ≥1 other risk factor: age >50 y, male sex, white, obesity (BMI ≥30), central adiposity, tobacco use.
- High risk: Family history of esophageal adenocarcinoma or BE.

Recommendations
▶ ASGE 2019
- Do not screen lower risk general population with GERD.
- Screen moderate- to high-risk individuals using upper endoscopy (EGD) and biopsy.

Sources
- *Gastrointest Endosc.* 2019;90(3):335-359.
- *Am J Gastroenterol.* 2016;111(1):30-50.

Comments
1. **Forty percent of persons** with BE and esophageal cancer have no preceding GERD symptoms.
2. Treat all persons with biopsy-proven BE with proton pump inhibitor (PPI) therapy, including asymptomatic individuals.

CELIAC DISEASE

Population
–Children and adults.

Recommendations

▶ USPSTF 2017, AAFP 2017

–Insufficient evidence regarding screening of asymptomatic individuals.

Sources

–USPSTF. *JAMA*. 2017;317(12):1252.

–AAFP. *Clinical Recommendations: Screening for Celiac Disease*. 2017.

▶ ACG 2013

–Consider serologic testing with IgA tissue transglutaminase antibody and total IgA level, in asymptomatic persons with type 1 diabetes mellitus (3%–10% concurrent celiac disease) every 1–2 y.

Source

–*Am J Gastroenterol*. 2013;108(5):656-676.

▶ NICE 2015

–Do not screen the general population.

–Screen first-degree relatives of individuals with celiac disease.

–Offer testing to persons with persistent unexplained abdominal or gastrointestinal symptoms, faltering growth, prolonged fatigue, unexpected weight loss, severe or persistent mouth ulcers; unexplained iron, vitamin B12 or folate deficiency; type 1 diabetes, autoimmune thyroid disease, adult irritable bowel syndrome.

–Consider testing individuals with metabolic bone disease, unexplained neurological symptoms (particularly peripheral neuropathy or ataxia), unexplained subfertility or recurrent miscarriage, persistently raised liver enzymes with unknown cause, dental enamel defects, Down syndrome, Turner syndrome.

Source

–NICE. *Coeliac Disease: Recognition, Assessment and Management*. 2015.

Comments

1. Serologic testing and biopsy must be performed while on gluten-containing diet.
2. IgA tissue transglutaminase (TTG) antibody is the test of choice (>90% sensitivity and specificity), along with total IgA level. If equivocal TTG, perform IgA endomysial antibody test.

COLORECTAL CANCER

Population
–Average-risk adults.[a]

Recommendations

▶ AAFP 2018, USPSTF 2017

–Age 50–75 y: Screen all patients.
–Age 76–85 y: Individualize screening decision.
–Age >85 y: Do not screen.
–No preferred screening modality.

▶ ACS 2018

–Age 45–75 y: Screen all patients.
–Age 76–85 y: Individualize screening decision.
–Age >85 y: Do not screen.
–No preferred screening modality.

▶ American College of Gastroenterology 2009

–Age 50–75 y: Screen all patients (start at age 45 in African-Americans).
–Colonoscopy is the preferred test; fecal immunohistochemistry if colonoscopy is declined.

▶ US Multi-Society Task Force 2017

–Age 50–75 y: Screen all patients (consider starting at age 45 in African-Americans).
–Age >75 y: Do not screen.
–Prefer colonoscopy or fecal immunohistochemistry test.

▶ Canadian Task Force 2016

–Age 50–74 y: Screen all patients.
–Screen with stool-based test or flexible sigmoidoscopy, not colonoscopy.

▶ NCCN 2018

–Age 50–75 y: Screen all patients.
–Age 76–85 y: Individualize screening decisions.

[a]Risk factors indicating need for earlier/more frequent screening: personal history of CRC or adenomatous polyps or hepatoblastoma, CRC or polyps in a first-degree relative age <60 y or in 2 first-degree relatives of any age, personal history of chronic inflammatory bowel disease, and family with hereditary CRC syndromes (*Ann Intern Med.* 1998;128(1):900; *Am J Gastroenterol.* 2009;104:739; *N Engl J Med.* 1994;331(25):1669; 1995;332(13):861). Additional high-risk group: history of ≥30 Gy radiation to whole abdomen; all upper abdominal fields; pelvic, thoracic, lumbar, or sacral spine. Begin monitoring 10 y after radiation or at age 35 y, whichever occurs last (http://www.survivorshipguidelines.org). Screening colonoscopy in those age ≥80 y results in only 15% of the expected gain in life expectancy seen in younger patients (*JAMA.* 2006;295:2357).

Sources

–ACS: *CA Cancer J Clin.* 2018;68:250-281.

–USPSTF: https://www.uspreventiveservicestaskforce.org/Page/
Document/UpdateSummaryFinal/colorectal-cancer-screening2

–AAFP: https://www.aafp.org/patient-care/clinical-recommendations/
all/colorectal-cancer.html

–ACG: *Am J Gastroenterol.* 2009;104(6):1613.

–CTF: *CMAJ.* 2016;188(5):340-348.

–USMSTF: *Am J Gastroenterol.* 2017;112(7):1016-1030.

–NCCN: http://www.nccn.org

Comments

1. Acceptable screening methods:[a,b,c]
   a. Guaiac fecal occult blood test (gFOBT-guaiac based or FIT = fecal immunochemical test) annually.[d]
   b. Flexible sigmoidoscopy every 5 y with reflex colonoscopy if abnormal.
   c. FIT[e] annually plus flexible sigmoidoscopy every 10 y.
   d. Colonoscopy every 10 y.
   e. CT colonoscopy every 5 y.
2. Follow-up colonoscopy according to findings:
   a. Normal or small, distal hyperplastic polyps—10 y.
   b. 1 or 2 small (<10 mm) tubular adenomas—5–10 y.
   c. Small (<10 mm) serrated polyps without dysplasia—5 y.
   d. Three to ten tubular adenomas, a tubular adenoma, or serrated polyp ≥10 mm, adenoma with villous features or high-grade dysplasia, a sessile serrated polyp with cytologic dysplasia, traditional serrated adenoma—3 y.
3. FOBT alone decreased CRC mortality by 33% compared with those who were not screened. (*Gastroenterology.* 2004;126:1674)
4. Accuracy of colonoscopy is operator dependent—rapid withdrawal time, poor prep, and lack of experience will increase false-negatives. (*N Engl J Med.* 2006;355:2533) (*Ann Intern Med.* 2012;156:692) (*Gastroenterology* 2015;110:72)

---

[a]A positive result on an FOBT should be followed by colonoscopy. An alternative is flexible sigmoidoscopy and air-contrast barium enema.
[b]FOBT should be performed on 2 samples from 3 consecutive specimens obtained at home. A single stool guaiac during annual physical examination is not adequate.
[c]USPSTF did not find direct evidence that a screening colonoscopy is effective in reducing CRC mortality rates.
[d]Use the guaiac-based test with dietary restriction, or an immunochemical test without dietary restriction. Two samples from each of 3 consecutive stools should be examined without rehydration. Rehydration increases the false-positive rate.
[e]Population-based retrospective analysis: risk of developing CRC remains decreased for >10 y following negative colonoscopy findings (*JAMA.* 2006;295:2366).

5. Multitargeted DNA stool testing vs. iFOBT with more cancers detected (92.3% vs. 73.8%) but more false-positives with DNA test. (*N Engl J Med.* 2014;370:1287-1306)
6. Percentage of US adults receiving some form of CRC screening increased from 44% in 1999 to 63% in 2008. The goal is 80% by 2018. (*CA Cancer J Clin.* 2015;65:30) (*Arch Intern Med.* 2011;171:647; 2012;172:575) In 2016, an estimated 134,000 new cases of CRC were diagnosed and 49,000 Americans died from CRC. Median age of diagnosis is 68. (*CA Cancer J Clin.* 2016;66:7)
7. Colonoscopy vs. iFOBT testing in CRC with similar detection of cancer, but more adenomas identified in the colonoscopy group. (*N Engl J Med.* 2012;366:687, 697)

COLORECTAL CANCER

The following options are acceptable choices for CRC screening in average-risk adults beginning at age 45 y. As each test has inherent characteristics related to prevention potential, accuracy, costs, and potential harms, individuals should have an opportunity to make an informed decision when choosing one of the following options.

For all positive non-colonoscopy tests, follow up with a timely colonoscopy to continue screening/diagnostic process. These follow-up colonoscopies may be subject to decreased insurance reimbursement or increased out-of-pocket costs.

In the opinion of the guidelines development committee, *colon cancer (CA) prevention* should be the primary goal of CRC screening. Tests that are designed to detect both early CA and adenomatous polyps should be encouraged if resources are available and patients are willing to undergo an invasive test.

Structural/Visual Screening Tests (for Cancer and Adenomatous Polyps)

Test	Interval	Key Issues for Informed Decisions
Colonoscopy—gold standard	Every 10 y	Complete bowel prep is required. Procedural sedation often required, necessitating time off work and chaperone for transport from facility. Advantages: Early detection and prevention through polypectomy. Disadvantages: Need for thorough bowel cleansing, high risk of bowel perforation (4 in 10,000) relative to other screening tests, risk of aspiration pneumonitis if deep sedation is used; small risk of splenic injury, greater risk of post-procedural bleeding (8 in 10,000). (*Am J Gastroenterol.* 2017;112:1016-1030)

COLORECTAL CANCER (*Continued*)

Structural/Visual Screening Tests (for Cancer and Adenomatous Polyps)

Test	Interval	Key Issues for Informed Decisions
Flexible sigmoidoscopy (FSIG)	Every 5 y	Complete or partial bowel prep with enema is required. Advantages: Lower cost and risk compared with colonoscopy. Decreased bowel prep. No need for sedation. Disadvantages: Does not assess proximal colon (which disproportionately affects women >60 y and certain high-risk familial groups), lower benefit in protection against right-sided colon cancer. (*Am J Gastroenterol.* 2017;112:1016-1030)
CT colonography (CTC)	Every 5 y	Complete bowel prep is required. Advantages: Comparable sensitivity/specificity to colonoscopy for adenomas ≥1 cm in size. Lower risk of bowel perforation. Disadvantage: Complete bowel prep required in most centers. Radiation exposure. (*Am J Gastroenterol.* 2017;112:1016-1030)

STOOL-BASED SCREENING TESTS (FOR CANCER, LESS EFFECTIVE FOR ADENOMATOUS POLYPS)

All positive test results require follow-up with colonoscopy, subject to additional out-of-pocket costs.

Test	Interval	Key Issues for Informed Decisions
Fecal immuno-chemical test (FIT)	Annual	Single stool sample collected at home. No diet or medication restrictions. More specific (and expensive) than gFOBT. High nonadherence rate to annual testing.
High-sensitivity guaiac-based fecal occult blood test (HSgFOBT)	Annual	Two to three stool samples collected at home. A single stool gathered during office digital rectal examination is not sufficient. Diet and medication restriction required. Higher false-positive rate than FIT. High nonadherence rate to annual testing.

Multitarget stool DNA (mt-sDNA)	Every 3 y per manufacturer	Single stool sample collected at home, then packaged with appropriate preservatives. New test, with limited data on screening outcomes. Higher false-positive rate than FIT. Insufficient evidence regarding management of positive results followed by negative diagnostic colonoscopy; may lead to overly intensive surveillance.

Population

–Adults with family history of CRC or advanced adenoma (AA).

Recommendations

▶ **USMSTF on CRC 2017**

–For persons with 1 first-degree relative with CRC or documented AA diagnosed at age <60 y, or 2 first-degree relatives with CRC and/or documented AA diagnosed at any age, obtain screening colonoscopy every 5 y starting at age 40 y or 10 y before the age at diagnosis of the youngest affected relative, whichever is earlier.

–For persons with 1 first-degree relative with CRC, AA, or advanced serrated lesion diagnosed at age ≥60 y, start routine screening at age 40 y.

▶ **ACG 2014, USMSTF on CRC 2017**

–Use Amsterdam I and II criteria to diagnose hereditary nonpolyposis CRC (HNPCC), with subsequent genetic screen for Lynch syndrome (LS).

- Amsterdam I criteria:
  ◦ ≥3 relatives with histologically verified CRC, one of which is a first-degree relative of the other two. Diagnosis of familial adenomatous polyposis (FAP) excluded.
  ◦ ≥2 generations with CRC.
  ◦ ≥1 CRC diagnosis before age 50 y.
- Amsterdam II criteria:
  ◦ ≥3 relatives with histologically verified HNPCC-associated cancer (colorectal, endometrial, small bowel, ureter, renal pelvis), one of which is a first-degree relative of the other two. Diagnosis of FAP excluded.
  ◦ ≥2 generations with CRC.
  ◦ ≥1 CRC diagnosis before age 50 y.

–Lynch syndrome (LS): Screening colonoscopy every 1–2 y for persons with LS or at-risk (first-degree relatives of those affected), starting at age 20–25 y, or 2–5 y before youngest age of family CRC diagnosis if diagnosed before age 25 y.

–Family CRC Type X syndrome: Screening colonoscopy every 3–5 y beginning 10 y before the age at diagnosis of the youngest affected relative.

Sources
–*Am J Gastroenterol.* 2017;112(7):1016-1030.
–*Am J Gastroenterol.* 2014;109(8):1159-1179.

Population
–Individuals at risk for or affected by adenomatous polyposis (AP) syndromes:
- FAP: 100% lifetime risk of CRC.
- Attenuated FAP (AFAP): 69% lifetime risk of CRC.
- MUTYH-associated polyposis (MAP): 60% lifetime risk of CRC.

Recommendations
▶ ACS 2015
–In individuals at risk for or affected by FAP, screen for CRC by annual colonoscopy or flexible sigmoidoscopy beginning at puberty.
–In individuals at risk for or affected by AFAP or MAP, screen by colonoscopy every 1–2 y beginning in late teens to early 20s.

Source
–*Am J Gastroenterol.* 2015;110(2):223-263.

Comment
1. Start EGD screening for gastric and proximal small bowel tumors starting at age 25–30 y, with follow-up depending on stage of duodenal polyposis.

ESOPHAGEAL ADENOCARCINOMA

Population
–Individuals with biopsy-proven BE.

Recommendations
▶ ASGE 2017
–Follow-up intervals:
- No dysplasia: Follow-up EGD with biopsy every 3–5 y.
- Indeterminate dysplasia: Repeat EGD with biopsy in 3–6 mo after optimizing PPI therapy.

- Low-grade dysplasia: Endoscopic eradication therapy or ongoing annual endoscopic surveillance.
- High-grade dysplasia: Endoscopic eradication therapy.

Source
   –*Gastrointest Endosc.* 2017;85(5):889-903.

Comments

1. In 2017, 16,940 new cases of esophageal cancer were diagnosed in the United States; 15,690 persons died from esophageal cancer.
2. There is a 4-fold incidence of esophageal adenocarcinoma compared to squamous cell carcinoma.

GASTRIC CANCER

Population
   –Adults.

Recommendations

▶ **ACG 2015**

   –Do not routinely screen average-risk adults, given low incidence in the United States.
   –Screen with EGD for specific high-risk subgroups.[a] For AP syndromes, start EGD screening for gastric and proximal small bowel tumors starting at age 25–30 y, with follow-up depending on stage of duodenal polyposis.

Sources
   –*Gastrointest Endosc.* 2016;84(1):18-28.
   –*Am J Gastroenterol.* 2015;110(2):223-262.

HEPATOCELLULAR CARCINOMA (HCC)

Population
   –Adults with cirrhosis.
   –Adults with risk factors[b] for cirrhosis.

---

[a]High-risk groups include those with gastric adenomas, pernicious anemia, gastric intestinal metaplasia, Lynch syndrome, familial adenomatous polyposis, and family history of gastric cancer.
[b]Risk factors include chronic Hepatitis B virus (HBV), hepatitis C virus (HCV), alcohol, nonalcoholic steatohepatitis, hereditary hemochromatosis, primary biliary cholangitis, and Wilson's disease.

Recommendations

▶ **AASLD 2018**

  –For adults with cirrhosis, screen using ultrasound with or without alfa-fetoprotein (AFP) every 6 mo to improve overall survival.
  –For Child's class C cirrhosis, do not screen unless they are on a transplant waiting list, given the low anticipated survival associated with Child's class C.
  –For individuals with risk factors without cirrhosis, do not screen, given significantly lower risk of HCC.

Source

  –AASLD. *Hepatology*. 2018;68(2):723-750.

Comments

1. In 2016, there were an estimated 39,230 new diagnoses of HCC and 27,170 deaths due to this disease in the United States; 80% of HCC cases occur in persons with cirrhosis.
2. Due to low-level evidence, HCC screening is considered controversial.
3. Due to low sensitivity, AFP alone should not be used for screening unless ultrasound is not available.

HEREDITARY HEMOCHROMATOSIS (HH)

Population

  –Adults.

Recommendations

▶ **AASLD 2011, AAFP 2013**

  –Obtain iron studies (particularly ferritin, transferrin saturation) in persons with evidence of active liver disease.
  –Evaluate for HH in individuals with abnormal iron studies.
  –Screen with iron studies and serum HFE mutation analysis in first-degree relatives of patients with classic HFE mutation–related HH.

Sources

  –AASLD. *Hepatology*. 2011;54(1):328-343.
  –*Am Fam Physician*. 2013;87(3):183-190.

▶ **ACP 2005**

  –Insufficient evidence to recommend for or against screening.[a]

---

[a]Discuss the risks, benefits, and limitations of genetic testing in patients with a positive FH of hereditary hemochromatosis, or those with elevated serum ferritin levels or transferrin saturation.

–In case-finding for hereditary hemochromatosis, serum ferritin and transferrin saturation tests should be performed initially. (*Ann Int Med.* 2006;145:200; 2008;149:270)

Sources

–*Ann Intern Med.* 2005;143:517-521.
–http://www.acponline.org/clinical/guidelines/
–*N Engl J Med.* 2004;350:2383.

Comments

1. There is no established consensus regarding elevated ferritin or transferrin saturation threshold levels that would warrant further evaluation for HH. Possible threshold values are serum ferritin >200 µg/L in women and >300 µg/L in men, and transferrin saturation >45%.
2. There is fair evidence that clinically significant disease caused by hereditary hemochromatosis is uncommon in the general population. Male homozygotes for *C282Y* gene mutation have a 2-fold increase in the incidence of iron overload–related symptoms, compared with females.
3. There is poor evidence that early therapeutic phlebotomy improves morbidity and mortality in screening-detected vs. clinically detected individuals.
4. Both men and women who have a heterozygote *C282Y* gene mutation rarely develop iron overload.
5. For clinicians who choose to screen, one-time screening of non-Hispanic white men with serum ferritin level and transferrin saturation has highest yield.

HEPATITIS B VIRUS (HBV) INFECTION

Population

–Adults and children.

Recommendations

▶ USPSTF 2014, CDC 2008

–Screen high-risk individuals using HBV surface antigen (HBsAg):
  • Foreign-born persons from countries where HBV prevalence ≥2%.[a]
  • US-born persons not vaccinated at birth whose parents were born in countries where HBV prevalence ≥8%.

[a]HBV prevalence ≥2% in Africa, Asia, South Pacific, Middle East (except Cyprus and Israel), Eastern Europe (except Hungary), Malta, Spain, indigenous populations of Greenland, Alaska natives, indigenous populations of Canada, Caribbean, Guatemala, Honduras, and South America.

- HIV-positive individuals.
- Household contacts or sexual partners of HBV-positive individuals.
- Men who have sex with men.
- Hemodialysis patients.
- Individuals who are immunosuppressed or receiving cytotoxic therapy.
- Intravenous illicit drug users.
- Blood, organ, or tissue donors.
- Individuals with occupational or other exposures to infectious blood or body fluids.

Sources
-USPSTF. *Hepatitis B Virus Infection: Screening.* 2014.
-CDC. *MMWR.* 2008;57(RR-8).

Population
-Pregnant women.

Recommendations

▶ **USPSTF 2019, CDC 2015, ACOG 2015, AAP 2017**
-Screen all pregnant women using HBsAg at their first prenatal visit.

Sources
-USPSTF. *JAMA.* 2019;322(4):349-354.
-CDC/ACOG. *Screening and Referral Algorithm for Hepatitis B Virus (HBV) Infection among Pregnant Women.* 2015.
-AAP/ACOG. *Guidelines for Perinatal Care.* 8th ed. 2017.

HEPATITIS C VIRUS (HCV) INFECTION

Population
-Adults born between 1945 and 1965.
-Individuals at increased risk:
- Intravenous or intranasal illicit drug users.
- Recipients of blood transfusions before 1992.
- Long-term hemodialysis patients.
- Children of HCV-infected mothers.
- Incarcerated persons.
- Recipients of unregulated tattoos.
- Hemophiliacs.
- Health care providers who have sustained needlestick injury.

Recommendations

▶ AASLD 2014, USPSTF 2013

–Screen using anti-HCV antibody testing for individuals at increased risk or who were born between 1945 and 1965 regardless of other risk factors.

Sources

–AASLD. *Hepatology.* 2015;62(3):932.
–USPSTF. *Hepatitis C: Screening.* 2013.

Comments

1. Anti-HCV antibodies typically develop 2–6 mo after exposure. In patients with negative anti-HCV antibody testing, perform HCV RNA testing for suspicion of acute HCV infection, or for unexplained liver disease in an immunocompromised patient.
2. Of persons with acute hepatitis C, 15%–25% resolve their infection; of the remaining, 10%–20% develop cirrhosis within 20–30 y after infection, and 1%–5% develop hepatocellular carcinoma.

Population

–Pregnant women at increased risk.[a]

Recommendations

▶ SMFM/ACOG 2017, CDC 2015

–Screen using anti-HCV antibody testing at first prenatal visit.
–If initial result is negative, repeat testing for persistent or new risk factors such as new or ongoing intravenous illicit drug use.

Sources

–SMFM/ACOG. *AJOG.* 2017;217(5):B2-B12.
–CDC. *Sexually Transmitted Diseases Treatment Guidelines.* 2015.

PANCREATIC CANCER

Population

–Adults.

Recommendations

▶ USPSTF 2019

–Do not screen asymptomatic adults.

---

[a]Risk factors, as in the general population, include intravenous or intranasal illicit drug use, recipients of blood transfusions before 1992, long-term hemodialysis patients, children of HCV-infected mothers, incarcerated persons, recipients of unregulated tattoos, hemophiliacs, and health care providers who have sustained needlestick injury.

–No established screening guidelines in individuals with inherited genetic cancer syndromes or familial pancreatic cancer.

Sources
–USPSTF. *JAMA.* 2019;322(5):438-444.
–*Gastroenterology.* 2019;156(7):2024-2040.

Comments

1. Cigarette smoking has consistently been associated with increased risk of pancreatic cancer. BRCA2 mutation is associated with a 5% lifetime risk of pancreatic cancer. Blood group O with lower risk and diabetes with a 2-fold higher risk of pancreatic cancer. (*J Natl Cancer Inst.* 2009;101:424) (*J Clin Oncol.* 2009;27:433)

2. Patients with a strong family history (≥2 first-degree relatives with pancreatic cancer) should undergo genetic counseling and may benefit from interval screening with CA 19-9, CT scan, and magnetic resonance cholangiopancreatography (MRCP). (*Nat Rev Gastroenterol Hepatol.* 2012;9:445-453)

Genitourinary Disorders

BLADDER CANCER

Population
–Asymptomatic persons.

Recommendation
▶ AAFP 2011, USPSTF 2016
–Do not screen routinely for bladder cancer (CA) in adults.

Sources
–http://www.aafp.org/online/en/home/clinical/exam.html
–http://www.ahrq.gov/clinic/uspstf/uspsblad.htm
–http://www.cancer.gov

Comments
1. There is inadequate evidence to determine whether screening for bladder CA would have any impact on mortality. Based on fair evidence, screening for bladder CA would result in unnecessary diagnostic procedures and overdiagnosis (70% of bladder CA is in situ) with attendant morbidity. (NCI, 2017)
2. Urinary biomarkers (nuclear matrix protein 22, tumor-associated antigen p300, presence of DNA ploidy) do not have significant sensitivity or specificity to be utilized in clinical practice. Microscopic hematuria leads to a diagnosis of bladder CA in only 5% of patients.
3. Seventy-nine thousand cases of bladder CA are expected in 2017 in the United States, with the majority being noninvasive (70%), but still 16,900 Americans are expected to die of bladder CA in 2017. (*Ann Inter Med.* 2010;153:461) (*Eur Urol.* 2013;63:4)

4. Maintain a high index of suspicion in anyone with a history of smoking (4- to 7-fold increased risk[a]), an exposure to industrial toxins (aromatic amines, benzene), therapeutic pelvic radiation, cyclophosphamide chemotherapy, a history of *Schistosoma haematobium* cystitis, hereditary nonpolyposis colon CA (Lynch syndrome), and history of transitional cell carcinoma of ureter (50% risk of subsequent bladder CA). Large screening studies in these high-risk populations have not been performed.

5. Voided urine cytology with sensitivity of 40% but only 10% positive predictive value, urinary biomarkers (nuclear matrix protein 22, telomerase) with suboptimal sensitivity and specificity. Screening for microscopic hematuria has <10% positive predictive value.

CERVICAL CANCER

Population
–Women age <21 y.

Recommendation
▶ ACS 2017, USPSTF 2015, ACOG 2016

–Do not screen for cervical cancer.

Population
–Women age 21–29 y.

Recommendations
▶ ACS 2017, USPSTF 2018, ACOG 2016

–Cytology alone (PAP smear) every 3 y until age 30 y.
–Do not use human papillomavirus (HPV) DNA testing in this age group—the majority of young patients will clear the infection.

Population
–Women age 30–65 y at average risk.

Recommendations
▶ ACS 2017, ACOG 2016

–Screen with HPV and cytology "co-testing" every 5 y (preferred) or cytology alone every 3 y (acceptable).

---

[a]Individuals who smoke are 4–7 times more likely to develop bladder CA than individuals who have never smoked. Additional environmental risk factors: exposure to aminobiphenyls; aromatic amines; azo dyes; combustion gases and soot from coal; chlorination by-products in heated water; aldehydes used in chemical dyes and in the rubber and textile industries; organic chemicals used in dry cleaning, paper manufacturing, rope and twine making, and apparel manufacturing; contaminated Chinese herbs; arsenic in well water. Additional risk factors: prolonged exposure to urinary *S. haematobium* bladder infections, cyclophosphamide, or pelvic radiation therapy for other malignancies.

–If HPV positive/cytology negative—either follow up in 12 mo with co-testing or test for HPV 16 or 18 genotypes and proceed to colposcopy if positive.

–Continue to screen more frequently if high-risk factors are present.[a,b,c,d]

▶ USPSTF 2018

–Screen with cytology every 3 y.

–If a woman wants to extend her screening interval, perform co-testing (cytology + HPV testing) every 5 y.

–Primary hrHPV testing every 5 y is a valid alternative to co-testing or cytology alone.

Population

–Age >65 y or after hysterectomy.

Recommendation

▶ ACS 2017, ACOG 2016, USPSTF 2015

–Do not screen if the patient has had adequate prior screening with negative results (no history of CIN2, CIN3, or adenocarcinoma in situ in the past 20 y or in the history of cervical cancer ever).

Sources

–http://www.cancer.org

–http://www.survivorshipguidelines.org

–*CA Cancer J Clin.* 2012;62:147-172.

–*N Engl Med.* 2013;369:2324.

–https://www.uspreventiveservicestaskforce.org/Page/Document/RecommendationStatementFinal/cervical-cancer-screening2

–*Ann Intern Med.* 2012;156:880.

Comments

1. Ten percent of women age 30–34 y will have normal cytology but a positive HPV test and will need more frequent testing. In women 60–65 y only 2.5% will have negative cytology but positive HPV testing.

2. Clinical concerns: It is estimated that 12,820 cases of invasive cervical CA will be diagnosed in the United States in 2017, and 4210 women will die of this disease (American Cancer Society: facts and figures 2017).

[a]Sexual history in patients <21 y is not considered in beginning cytologic screening, which should start at age 21.
[b]New tests to improve CA detection include liquid-based/thin-layer preparations, computer-assisted screening methods, and HPV testing. (*Am Fam Physician.* 2001;64:729. *N Engl J Med.* 2007;357:1579. *JAMA.* 2009;302:1757)
[c]High-risk factors include DES exposure before birth, HIV infection, or other forms of immunosuppression, including chronic steroid use.
[d]Women with a history of cervical CA, DES exposure, HIV infection, or a weakened immune system should continue to have screenings as long as they are in >5-y life expectancy.

3. Cervical CA is causally related to infection with HPV (>70% associated with either HPV-18 or HPV-16 genotype).

4. Immunocompromised women (organ transplantation, chemotherapy, chronic steroid therapy, or human immunodeficiency virus [HIV]) should be tested twice during the first year after initiating screening and annually thereafter. (*CA Cancer J Clin.* 2011;61:8) (*Ann Intern Med.* 2011;155:698)

5. Women with a history of cervical CA or in utero exposure to diethylstilbestrol (DES) should indefinitely continue average-risk protocol for women age <30 y.

6. HPV vaccination of young women is now recommended by ACIP, UK-NHS, and others. Cervical CA screening recommendations have not changed for women receiving the vaccine because the vaccine covers only 70% of HPV serotypes that cause cervical CA. (*MMWR.* 2007;56(RR-2):1-24) (*CA cancer J Clin.* 2014;64:30) (*N Engl J Med.* 2015;372:711)

7. Long-term use of oral contraceptives may increase risk of cervical CA in women who test positive for cervical HPV DNA. (*Lancet.* 2002;359:1085)

8. Smoking increases risk of cervical CA 4-fold. (*Am J Epidemiol.* 1990;131:945)

9. A vaccine against HPV-16 and HPV-18 significantly reduces the risk of acquiring transient and persistent infection. (*N Engl J Med.* 2002;347:1645) (*Obstet Gynecol.* 2006;107(1):4)

10. New dosing schedule for HPV vaccinations: 2 doses for girls and boys who initiate vaccination series at age 9–14; 3 doses are recommended for ages 15–26 y and for immunosuppressed persons. (*CA Cancer J Clin.* 2017;67:100)

11. *Benefits:* Based on solid evidence, regular screening of appropriate women with the Pap test reduces mortality from cervical CA. Screening is effective when started at age 21. *Harms:* Based on solid evidence, regular screening with the Pap test leads to additional diagnostic procedures and treatment for low-grade squamous intraepithelial lesions (LSILs), with uncertain long-term consequences on fertility and pregnancy. Harms are greatest for younger women, who have a higher prevalence of LSILs. LSILs often regress without treatment. False positives in postmenopausal women are a result of mucosal atrophy. (NCI, 2008)

12. A study with 43,000 women ages 29–61 with both HPV DNA and cervical cytology co-testing every 5 y found that the cumulative incidence of cervical cancer in women negative for both tests at baseline was 0.01% at 9 y and 0.07% after 14 y. (*BMJ.* 2016;355:4924)

13. The risk of developing invasive cervical CA is 3–10 times greater in women who have not been screened. (*CA Cancer J Clin.* 2017;67:106)

CERVICAL CANCER SCREENING GUIDELINES FOR AVERAGE-RISK WOMEN[a]

	American Cancer Society (ACS), American Society for Colposcopy and Cervical Pathology (ASCCP), and American Society for Clinical Pathology (ASCP) 2012	US Preventive Services Task Force (USPSTF) 2018	American College of Obstetricians and Gynecologists (ACOG) 2016	Society of Gynecologic Oncology (SGO) and the American Society for Colposcopy and Cervical Pathology (ASCCP): Interim clinical guidance for primary hrHPV testing 2015
When to start screening[b]	Age 21. Women aged <21 y should not be screened regardless of the age of sexual initiation or other risk factors.	Age 21 (A recommendation). Recommend against screening women aged <21 y (D recommendation).	Age 21 regardless of the age of onset of sexual activity. Women aged <21 y should not be screened regardless of age at sexual initiation and other behavior-related risk factors (Level A evidence).	Refer to major guidelines.
Statement about annual screening	Women of any age should not be screened annually by any screening method.	Individuals and clinicians can use the annual Pap test screening visit as an opportunity to discuss other health problems and preventive measures. Individuals, clinicians, and health systems should seek effective ways to facilitate the receipt of recommended preventive services at intervals that are beneficial to the patient. Efforts also should be made to ensure that individuals are able to seek care for additional health concerns as they present.	In women aged 30–65 y annual cervical cancer screening should not be performed. (Level A evidence) Patients should be counseled that annual well-woman visits are recommended even if cervical cancer screening is not performed at each visit.	Not addressed.

CERVICAL CANCER SCREENING GUIDELINES FOR AVERAGE-RISK WOMEN[a]   (Continued)

	American Cancer Society (ACS), American Society for Colposcopy and Cervical Pathology (ASCCP), and American Society for Clinical Pathology (ASCP) 2012	US Preventive Services Task Force (USPSTF) 2018	American College of Obstetricians and Gynecologists (ACOG) 2016	Society of Gynecologic Oncology (SGO) and the American Society for Colposcopy and Cervical Pathology (ASCCP): Interim clinical guidance for primary hrHPV testing 2015
Screening method and intervals				
Cytology (conventional or liquid-based)[c]				
21–29 y of age	Every 3 y.[d]	Every 3 y (A recommendation).	Every 3 y (Level A evidence).	Not addressed.
30–65 y of age	Every 3 y.[d]	Every 3 y (A recommendation).	Every 3 y (Level A evidence).	Not addressed.
HPV co-test (cytology + HPV test administered together)				
21–29 y of age	HPV co-testing should not be used for women aged <30 y.	Recommend against HPV co-testing in women aged <30 y (D recommendation).	HPV co-testing[e] should not be performed in women aged <30 y (Level A evidence).	Not addressed.

30–65 y of age	Every 5 y; this is the preferred method.	For women who want to extend their screening interval, HPV co-testing every 5 y is an option (*A recommendation*).	Every 5 y; this is the preferred method (*Level A evidence*).	Not addressed.
Primary hrHPV testing[f] (as an alternative to co-testing or cytology alone)[g]	For women aged 30–65 y, screening by HPV testing alone is not recommended in most clinical settings.[h]	Every 5 y for women 30–65 y of age (*A recommendation*).	Alternative screening every 3 y for women ≥ 25 y as per SGO and ASCCP interim guidance (*Level B evidence*).	Every 3 y. Recommend against primary hrHPV screening in women aged <25 y of age.[i]
When to stop screening	Aged >65 y with adequate negative prior screening* and no history of CIN2 or higher within the last 20 y.[j] *Adequate negative prior screening results are defined as 3 consecutive negative cytology results or 2 consecutive negative co-test results within the previous 10 y, with the most recent test performed within the past 5 y.	Aged >65 y with adequate screening history* and are not otherwise at high risk for cervical cancer[j] (*D recommendation*).	Aged >65 y with adequate negative prior screening* results and no history of CIN2 or higher[j] (*Level A evidence*).	Not addressed.

CERVICAL CANCER SCREENING GUIDELINES FOR AVERAGE-RISK WOMEN[a] (Continued)	American Cancer Society (ACS), American Society for Colposcopy and Cervical Pathology (ASCCP), and American Society for Clinical Pathology (ASCP) 2012	US Preventive Services Task Force (USPSTF) 2018	American College of Obstetricians and Gynecologists (ACOG) 2016	Society of Gynecologic Oncology (SGO) and the American Society for Colposcopy and Cervical Pathology (ASCCP): Interim clinical guidance for primary hrHPV testing 2015
When to screen after age 65 y	Aged >65 y with a history of CIN2 CIN3, or adenocarcinoma in situ, routine screening[j] should continue for at least 20 y.	Women aged >65 y who have never been screened, do not meet the criteria for adequate prior screening, or for whom the adequacy of prior screening cannot be accurately accessed or documented.[k] Routine screening[j] should continue for at least 20 y after spontaneous regression or appropriate management of a high-grade precancerous lesion, even if this extends screening past age 65 y. Certain considerations may support screening in women aged >65 y who are otherwise considered high risk (such as women with a high-grade precancerous lesion or cervical cancer, women with in utero exposure to diethylstilbestrol, or women who are immunocompromised).	Women aged >65 y with a history of CIN2, CIN3, or AIS should continue routine age-based screening[j] for at least 20 y (Level B evidence).	Not addressed.

Screening post-hysterectomy	Women who have had a total hysterectomy (removal of the uterus and cervix) should stop screening.[m] Women who have had a supra-cervical hysterectomy (cervix intact) should continue screening according to guidelines.	Recommend against screening in women who have had a hysterectomy (removal of the cervix)[n] (D recommendation).	Women who have had a hysterectomy (removal of the cervix) should stop screening and not restart for any reason[n,o] (Level A evidence).	Not addressed.
The need for a bimanual pelvic exam	Not addressed in 2012 guidelines but was addressed in 2002 ACS guidelines.[p]	Addressed in USPSTF ovarian cancer screening recommendations (draft).[q]	Addressed in 2012 well-woman visit recommendations.[r] **Aged <21 y,** no evidence supports the routine internal examination of the healthy, asymptomatic patient. An "external-only" genital examination is acceptable. **Aged ≥21 y,** no evidence supports or refutes the annual pelvic examination or speculum and bimanual examination. The decision whether or not to perform a complete pelvic examination should be a shared decision after a discussion between the patient and her health care provider. Annual examination of the external genitalia should continue.[s]	Not addressed.

CERVICAL CANCER SCREENING GUIDELINES FOR AVERAGE-RISK WOMEN[a] (Continued)

	American Cancer Society (ACS), American Society for Colposcopy and Cervical Pathology (ASCCP), and American Society for Clinical Pathology (ASCP) 2012	US Preventive Services Task Force (USPSTF) 2018	American College of Obstetricians and Gynecologists (ACOG) 2016	Society of Gynecologic Oncology (SGO) and the American Society for Colposcopy and Cervical Pathology (ASCCP): Interim clinical guidance for primary hrHPV testing 2015
Screening among those immunized with HPV vaccine	Women at any age with a history of HPV vaccination should be screened according to the age-specific recommendations for the general population.	The possibility that vaccination might reduce the need for screening with cytology alone or in combination with HPV testing is not established. Given these uncertainties, women who have been vaccinated should continue to be screened.	Women who have received the HPV vaccine should be screened according to the same guidelines as women who have not been vaccinated (Level C evidence).	Not addressed.

HPV = human papillomavirus; CIN = cervical intraepithelial neoplasia; AIS=adenocarcinoma in situ; hrHPV = high-risk HPV.

[a]These recommendations do not address special, high-risk populations who may need more intensive or alternative screening. These special populations include women with a history of CIN2, CIN3, or cervical cancer, women who were exposed in utero to diethylstilbestrol, women who are infected with HIV, or women who are immunocompromised (such as those who have received solid organ transplants).

[b]Since cervical cancer is believed to be caused by sexually transmissible human papillomavirus infections, women who have not had sexual exposures (eg, virgins) are likely at low risk. Women aged >21 y who have not engaged in sexual intercourse may not need a Pap test depending on circumstances. The decision should be made at the discretion of the women and her physician. Women who have had sex with women are still at risk of cervical cancer. Ten to fifteen percent of women aged 21–24 y in the United States report no vaginal intercourse (Saraiya M, Martinez G, Glaser K, et al. Obstet Gynecol. 2009;114(6):1213–1219. doi: 10.1097/AOG.0b013e3181be3db4.). Providers should also be aware of instances of non-consensual sex among their patients.

[c]Conventional cytology and liquid-based cytology are equivalent regarding screening guidelines, and no distinction should be made by test when recommending next screening.

[d]There is insufficient evidence to support longer intervals in women aged 30–65 y, even with a screening history of negative cytology results.

[e]All ACOG references to HPV testing are for high-risk HPV testing only. Tests for low-risk HPV should not be performed.

[f]Primary hrHPV testing is defined as a stand-alone test for cervical cancer screening without concomitant cytology testing. It may be followed by other tests (like a Pap) for triage. This test specifically identifies HPV 16 and HPV 18, while concurrently detecting 12 other types of high-risk HPVs.

[g]Because of equivalent or superior effectiveness, primary hrHPV screening can be considered as an alternative to current US cytology-based cervical cancer screening methods. Cytology alone and co-testing remain the screening options specifically recommended in major guidelines.

[h]More experience and data analysis pertaining to the primary hrHPV screening will permit a more formal ACS evaluation.

[i]Primary hrHPV screening should begin 3 y after the last negative cytology and should not be performed only 1 or 2 y after a negative cytology result at 23–24 y of age.

[j]Once screening is discontinued it should not resume for any reason, even if a woman reports having a new sexual partner.

[k]Women older than age 65 y who have never been screened, women with limited access to care, minority women, and women from countries where screening is not available may be less likely to meet the criteria for adequate prior screening.

[l]Routine screening is defined as screening every 5 y using co-testing (preferred) or every 3 y using cytology alone (acceptable).

[m]Unless the hysterectomy was done as a treatment for cervical pre-cancer or cancer.

[n]And no history of CIN2 or higher in the past 20 y.

[o]Women should continue to be screened if they have had a total hysterectomy and have a history of CIN2 or higher in the past 20 y or cervical cancer ever. Continued screening for 20 y is recommended in women who still have a cervix and a history of CIN2 or higher. Therefore, screening with cytology alone every 3 y for 20 y after the initial post-treatment surveillance for women with a hysterectomy is reasonable (Level B evidence).

[p]2002 guidelines statement: The ACS and others should educate women, particularly teens and young women, that a pelvic exam does not equate to a cytology test and that women who may not need a cytology test still need regular health care visits including gynecologic care. Women should discuss the need for pelvic exams with their providers. Saslow D, Runowicz CD, Solomon D, et al. American Cancer Society Guideline for the Early Detection of Cervical Neoplasia and Cancer. CA Cancer J Clin 2002;52:342–362.

[q]The bimanual pelvic examination is usually conducted annually in part to screen for ovarian cancer, although its effectiveness and harms are not well known and were not a focus of this review. No randomized trial has assessed the role of the bimanual pelvic examination for cancer screening. In the PLCO Trial, bimanual examination was discontinued as a screening strategy in the intervention arm because no cases of ovarian cancer were detected solely by this method and a high proportion of women underwent bimanual examination with ovarian palpation in the usual care arm.

[r]ACOG Committee Opinion No. 534: Well-Woman Visit. Committee on Gynecologic Practice. Obstet Gynecol. 2012;120(2)1:421–24. doi: 10.1097/AOG.0b013e3182680517.

[s]For women aged ≥21 y, annual pelvic examination is a routine part of preventive care even if they do not need cervical cytology screening, but also lacks data to support a specific time frame or frequency of such examinations. The decision to receive an internal examination can be left to the patient if she is asymptomatic and has undergone a total hysterectomy and bilateral salpingo-oophorectomy for benign indications, and is of average risk.

ENDOMETRIAL CANCER

Population
–Postmenopausal women.

Recommendations

▶ ACS 2008

–Do not screen routinely.

–Inform women about risks and symptoms of endometrial CA and strongly encourage them to report any unexpected bleeding or spotting. This is especially important for women with an increased risk of endometrial CA (history of unopposed estrogen therapy, tamoxifen therapy, late menopause, nulliparity, infertility or failure to ovulate, obesity, diabetes, or hypertension).

Source
–http://www.cancer.org

Comments

1. *Benefits:* There is inadequate evidence that screening with endometrial sampling or transvaginal ultrasound (TVU) decreases mortality. *Harms:* Based on solid evidence, screening with TVU will result in unnecessary additional exams because of low specificity. Based on solid evidence, endometrial biopsy may result in discomfort, bleeding, infection, and, rarely, uterine perforation. (NCI, 2008)

2. Presence of atypical glandular cells on Pap test from postmenopausal (age >40 y) women not taking exogenous hormones is abnormal and requires further evaluation (TVU and endometrial biopsy). Pap test is not sensitive for endometrial screening.

3. Endometrial thickness of <4 mm on TVU is associated with low risk of endometrial CA. (*Am J Obstet Gynecol.* 2001;184:70)

4. Most cases of endometrial CA are diagnosed as a result of symptoms reported by patients (uterine bleeding), and a high proportion of these cases are diagnosed at an early stage and have high rates of cure. Type II endometrial CA accounts for 15% of patients. Histology is serous or clear cell. Five year survival is 55% vs. 85% for endometrial Type I cancer. (NCI, 2008) (*Lancet.* 2016;387:1094)

5. Tamoxifen use for 5 y raises the risk of endometrial CA 2- to 3-fold, but CAs are low stage, low grade, with high cure rates. (*J Natl Cancer Inst.* 1998;90:1371)

6. In 2016, there were 60,050 new cases of endometrial cancer with 10,170 deaths. The mean age at diagnosis is 60 y.

Population

–Women at highest risk for endometrial CA.[a]

Recommendations

▶ ACS 2016

–Annual screening beginning at age 35 y with endometrial biopsy.

–International guidelines advise transvaginal ultrasound and annual endometrial biopsy beginning at 25 y old.

Sources

–*CA Cancer J Clin.* 2005;55:31.

–*JAMA.* 1997;277:915.

–http://www.cancer.org

Comments

1. High-risk women: Lynch syndrome carries a lifetime risk of 60%.
   a. Variable screening with ultrasound among women (age 25–65 y; $n =$ 292) at high risk for HNPCC mutation detected no CAs from ultrasound. Two endometrial cancers occurred in the cohort that presented with symptoms. (*Cancer.* 2002;94:1708) (*Gynecol Oncol.* 2007;107:159)
   b. The death rate from sporadic endometrial cancer and Lynch syndrome–related uterine cancer is the same.
   c. The Women's Health Initiative (WHI) demonstrated that combined estrogen and progestin did not increase the risk of endometrial CA but did increase the rate of endometrial biopsies and ultrasound exams prompted by abnormal uterine bleeding. (*JAMA.* 2003;290(13):1739-1748)

OVARIAN CANCER

Population

–Asymptomatic women at average risk.[b]

Recommendations

▶ USPSTF 2018, ACOG 2017, ACS 2017, ACR 2010, AAFP 2017

–Do not screen routinely.

---

[a]High-risk women are those known to carry HNPCC-associated genetic mutations, or at high risk to carry a mutation, or who are from families with a suspected autosomal dominant predisposition to colon CA (45%–50% lifetime risk of endometrial CA).

[b]Lifetime risk of ovarian CA in a woman with no affected relatives is 1 in 70. If 1 first-degree relative has ovarian CA, lifetime risk is 5%. If 2 or more first-degree relatives have ovarian CA, lifetime risk is 7%. Women with 2 or more family members affected by ovarian cancer have a 3% chance of having a hereditary ovarian CA syndrome. If BRCA1 mutation, lifetime risk of ovarian CA is 45%–50%; if BRCA2 mutation, lifetime risk is 15%–20%. Lynch syndrome = 8%–10% lifetime risk of ovarian CA.

–Beware of symptoms of ovarian CA that can be present in early-stage disease (abdominal, pelvic, and back pain; bloating and change in bowel habits; urinary symptoms). (*Ann Intern Med.* 2012;157:900-904) (*J Clin Oncol.* 2005;23:7919) (*Ann Intern Med.* 2012;156:182)

Sources
–*JAMA.* 2018;319(6);588-594.
–*Obstet Gynecol.* 2017;130(3):e146-149.
–*CA Cancer J Clin.* 2017;67(2):100-121.
–*Ultrasound Q.* 2010;26(4):219-223.
–https://www.aafp.org/patient-care/clinical-recommendations/all/ovarian-cancer.html

Population

–Women whose family history is associated with an increased risk for deleterious mutations in *BRCA1* or *2* genes.[a]

Recommendations

▶ USPSTF 2013, NCCN 2017, ACOG 2017

–Refer for genetic counseling and evaluation for *BRCA* testing. Do not routinely screen.
–Consider screening with CA-125, transvaginal ultrasound, and pelvic exam, though they have not been shown to improve survival rate.
–Test for BRCA1 and 2 mutations in any woman with ovarian cancer at any age.

Sources
–NCCN guideline version 2;2017. https://www.nccn.org
–*Obstet Gynecol.* 2017;130:e110-126.
–http://www.ahrq.gov/clinic/uspstf/uspsbrgen.htm

Population

–High-risk patients with known or suspected BRCA1 or 2 mutations.

Recommendations

▶ ACOG 2009, NCCN 2011

–Screen with CA-125 and TVU at age 30–35 y or 5–10 y earlier than earliest onset of ovarian CA in family members.
–Risk-reducing salpingo-oophorectomy should be strongly considered. (*JAMA.* 2010;304:967)

Source
–http://www.ahrq.gov/clinic/uspstf/uspsbrgen.htm

---

[a]USPSTF recommends against routine referral for genetic counseling or routine BRCA testing of women whose family history is not associated with increased risk for deleterious mutation in *BRCA1* or *2* genes.

Comments

1. Transvaginal ultrasound and CA-125 are useful to evaluate signs and symptoms of ovarian cancer.
2. Risk factors: age >60 y; low parity; personal history of endometrial, colon, or breast CA; family history of ovarian CA; and hereditary breast/ovarian CA syndrome. Use of oral contraceptives for 5 y decreases the risk of ovarian CA by 50%. (*JAMA.* 2004;291:2705)
3. *Benefit:* There is inadequate evidence to determine whether routine screening for ovarian CA with serum markers such as CA-125 levels, TVU, or pelvic examinations would result in a decrease in mortality from ovarian CA. *Harm:* Problems have been lack of specificity (positive predictive value) and need for invasive procedures to make a diagnosis. Based on solid evidence, routine screening for ovarian CA would result in many diagnostic laparoscopies and laparotomies for each ovarian CA found. (NCI, 2008) (*JAMA.* 2011;305:2295)
4. Additionally, cancers found by screening have not consistently been found to be lower stage. (*Lancet Oncol.* 2009;10:327)
5. Preliminary results from the Prostate, Lung, Colorectal and Ovarian (PLCO) Cancer Screening Trial: At the time of baseline examination, positive predictive value for invasive cancer was 3.7% for abnormal CA-125 levels, 1% for abnormal TVU results, and 23.5% if both tests showed abnormal results. (*Am J Obstet Gynecol.* 2005;193:1630)
6. Large United Kingdom trial assessing multimodal screening strategy (annual CA-125, risk of ovarian CA algorithm [ROLA], transvaginal ultrasound) vs. usual care: 202,639 women recruited (age 50–74) found nonsignificant mortality reduction up to 14 y F/U. (*J Natl Compr Cancer Netw.* 2016;14:1143) (*Lancet.* 2016;387:945)

PELVIC EXAMINATIONS

Population

–Asymptomatic, nonpregnant women.

Recommendation

▶ AAFP 2017, ACP 2014

–Do not perform routine screening pelvic examinations.

Sources

–AAFP. *Clinical Recommendation: Screening Pelvic Exam.* 2017.
–*Ann Intern Med.* 2014;161(1):67-72.

Recommendation

▶ USPSTF 2017

　　–Insufficient evidence to recommend for or against screening pelvic
　　examinations.

Source
　　–*JAMA*. 2017;317(9):947-953.

Recommendation

▶ ACOG 2012

　　–Screen all women age 21+ with annual pelvic exam.

Source
　　–*Obstet Gynecol*. 2012;120:421-424.

Comments

1. Pelvic examination remains a necessary component of evaluation for many complaints.
2. While tradition and patient or physician experience may support an annual exam, outcome data does not (nor does the data clearly refute the exam).
3. Potential harms associated with screening include overdiagnosis, fear/anxiety/embarrassment, discomfort, and additional diagnostic procedures.

PROSTATE CANCER

Population

　　–Asymptomatic men.

Recommendations

▶ USPSTF 2018, AUA 2018

　　–Do not screen men younger than 55 y or older than 70 y. (AUA: consider screening age 40–55 if elevated risk.)

　　–For men age 55–69 y, discuss potential benefits and harms of PSA screening (false-positive results) overdiagnosis and overtreatment and treatment complications vs. small potential benefit of reducing the chance of dying of prostate cancer. Individualize decision making so that each man can understand the potential benefits and harms of screening and make his decision.

　　–In high-risk patients (African-Americans, first-degree family members with prostate cancer and BRCA 1 and 2), help the patient weigh benefits and risks of screening.

-Consider screening q2 years to preserve benefits of screening but reduce false-positives.

▶ ACS 2016

-For men age 50 y and older, discuss annual prostate-specific antigen (PSA) and digital rectal exam (DRE) if $\geq$10-y life expectancy.[a]

-Discuss risks and benefits of screening strategy to enable an informed decision.

-Follow up annually if PSA level is $\geq$2.5 ng/mL, or q2 years if <2.5 ng/mL.

▶ EAU 2017

-There is a lack of evidence to support or disregard widely adopted, population-based screening programs for early detection of prostate CA. Consider individual risk and offer screening if risk elevated or if patient prefers and has 10–15 y life expectancy.

▶ NCCN 2019

-Employ informed decision making. NCCN could not reach consensus on screening age and intervals based on available data.

-For men age 45–75 who elect screening:

- PSA <1 ng/mL—DRE normal—repeat testing @ 2–4 y intervals.
- PSA 1–3 ng/mL—DRE normal—repeat testing @ 1–2 y intervals.
- PSA >3 ng/mL or suspicious DRE—consider biopsy and workup for benign disease. (*J Natl Compr Canc Netw.* 2015;13:570) (*Mayo Clin Proc.* 2016;91:17)

-After age 75, PSA testing should be individualized and indications for biopsy carefully evaluated.

-Refer patients for prostate biopsy if serum PSA rises >0.9 ng/mL in 1 y.

Sources

-USPSTF. 2018. https://www.uspreventiveservicestaskforce.org/Page/Document/UpdateSummaryFinal/prostate-cancer-screening1

-*JAMA.* 2018;319(18):1901-1913.

-*Eur. Urol.* 2017;71:618-629.

-https://www.auanet.org/guidelines/prostate-cancer-early-detection-guideline

-*NCCN Guidelines.* Version 1.2019. NCCN.org.

-http://www.cancer.org

---

[a]Men in high-risk groups (1 or more first-degree relatives diagnosed before age 65 y, African-Americans) should begin screening at age 45 y. Men at higher risk because of multiple first-degree relatives affected at an early age could begin testing at age 40 y (http://www.cancer.org/).

Comments

1. Prevalence: there are 220,800 new cases of prostate cancer and 27,500 deaths expected in 2017.

2. 75% of men with PSA >3 ng/mL will have no cancer on subsequent biopsy. More than 10% of men screened will have a false-positive PSA elevation if tested annually for 4 y and >5% will undergo a negative biopsy. (AUA 2018)

3. There is good evidence that PSA can detect early-stage prostate CA (2-fold increase in organ-confined disease at presentation with PSA screening), but mixed and inconclusive evidence that early detection improves health outcomes or mortality. Two long-awaited studies add to the confusion. A US study of 76,000 men showed increased prostate CA in screened group, but no reduction in risk of death from prostate CA. A European study of 80,000 men showed a decreased rate of death from prostate CA by 20% but significant overdiagnosis (there was no difference in overall death rate). To prevent 1 death from prostate CA, 1410 men needed to be screened, and 48 cases of prostate CA were found. Patients older than age 70 y had an increased death rate in the screened group. (*N Engl J Med.* 2009;360:1310,1320) (*N Engl J Med.* 2012;366:981, 1047) These 2 very large studies set the framework for new PC guidelines. The US study (prostate, lung, colorectal, and ovarian cancer screening trial) showed no evidence for overall survival benefit from PSA screening and postulated that many patients with low-grade cancers were treated aggressively, leading to morbidity and mortality. Subsequent evaluation found that approximately 90% of patients in the control arm had undergone PSA testing during the course of the trial. This fact makes the trial result uninterpretable. The European study found that PSA screening did reduce prostate-specific mortality by 20%. In this trial 781 men needed to be invited to screening to prevent 1 death. What should be the response to this new data? First, we can improve survival by recognizing low-risk patients to be followed by active surveillance and not exposed to treatment until evidence of disease progression. Recognized high-risk patients (African-Americans and men with first-degree relatives with prostate cancer) should be screened early and frequently. Average-risk men can be screened by PSA twice between the ages of 45 and 55 and if the PSA is 0.70 ng/mL, their risk of lethal prostate cancer is quite low. Guideline groups are presently working on new guidelines for PC screening to minimize overtreatment of this disease but at the same time screening a higher risk population for aggressive prostate cancer at a stage that can be treated with conservative intent. (*N Engl J Med.* 2017;376:1285) (*J Clin Oncol.* 2016;34:2705-2711, 3481-3491, 3499-3501)

4. *Benefit:* Insufficient evidence to establish whether a decrease in mortality from prostate CA occurs with screening by DRE or serum PSA. *Harm:* Based on solid evidence, screening with PSA and/or DRE detects some prostate CAs that would never have caused important clinical problems. Based on solid evidence, current prostate CA treatments result in permanent side effects in many men, including erectile dysfunction and urinary incontinence. (NCI, 2008)

5. Men with localized, low-grade prostate CAs (Gleason score 2–4) have a minimal risk of dying from prostate CA during 20 y of follow-up (6 deaths per 1000 person-years) (*JAMA.* 2005;293:2095) (*N Engl J Med.* 2014;370:932)

6. Many physicians continue to screen African-American men and men with a strong FH of prostate cancer despite the guidelines. (*J Urol.* 2002;168:483) (*J Natl Cancer Inst.* 2000;92:2009) (*JAMA.* 2014; 311:1143) African-American men have double risk of prostate cancer and a >2-fold risk of prostate cancer–specific death. These patients and those with first-degree relatives <65 y with prostate cancer are at high enough risk to justify PSA screening until a definitive study of this population is available. (*JAMA.* 2014;311:1143)

7. Increase in prostate cancer distant metastases at diagnosis in the United States over the last 3 y. (*JAMA Oncol.* 2016;2:1657)

8. Radical prostatectomy (vs. watchful waiting) reduces disease-specific and overall mortality in patients with early stage prostate CA. (*N Engl J Med.* 2011;364:1708) This benefit was seen only in men age >65 y. Active surveillance for low-risk patients is safe and increasingly used as an alternative to radical prostatectomy. (*J Clin Oncol.* 2010;28:126) (*Ann Intern Med.* 2012;156:582) A gene signature profile reflecting virulence and treatment responsiveness in prostate CA is now available. (*J Clin Oncol.* 2008;26:3930) (*J Natl Compr NNetr.* 2016;14:659)

9. PSA velocity (>0.5–0.75 ng/y rise) is predictive for the presence of prostate CA, especially with a PSA of 4–10. (*Eur Urol.* 2009;56:573)

10. Multi-parametric MRI scanning is emerging as a tool for more accurate detection of early prostate cancer as well as distinguishing indolent from high-grade cancers. (*J Urol.* 2011;185:815) (*Nat Rev Clin Oncol.* 2014;11:346)

11. PSA screening is confounded by the morbidity and mortality associated with the treatment of prostate cancer. Molecular profiling that can stratify patients into high-risk and low-risk groups is a critical need for individualized adaptive therapies, which could minimize toxicity and maximize benefit from there in many patients (oncotype, Decipher, and Polaris are now available to look at molecular profiling).

12. The NCCN recommendation aims to strike a balance between testing too seldom and testing too often to "maximize benefit and minimize harm."

TESTICULAR CANCER

Population
–Asymptomatic adolescent and adult males.[a]

Recommendations
▶ AAFP 2008, USPSTF 2011
–Do not screen routinely. Be aware of risk factors for testicular CA—previous testis CA (2%–3% risk of second cancer), cryptorchid testis, family history of testis CA, HIV (increased risk of seminoma), and Klinefelter syndrome.
–There is a 3- to 5-fold increase in testis cancer in white men vs. other ethnicity. (*N Engl J Med.* 2014;371:2005) (*N Engl J Med.* 2007;356:1835)

Sources
–http://www.aafp.org/online/en/home/clinical/exam.html
–http://www.ahrq.gov/clinic/uspstf/uspstest.htm

Population
–Asymptomatic men.
–High-risk males.[a]

Recommendation
EAU 2008
–Self-physical exam is advisable.

Source
–www.uroweb.org

Comments
1. Benefits and Harms:
    a. Benefits: Based on fair evidence, screening would not result in appreciable decrease in mortality, in part because therapy at each stage is so effective.
    b. Harms: Based on fair evidence, screening would result in unnecessary diagnostic procedures and occasional removal of a noncancerous testis. (NCI, 2011)
    c. In 2016 approximately 8850 men in the United States were diagnosed with testicular cancer but only 400 men died of this disease. Worldwide there are approximately 72,000 cases and 9000 deaths annually. (*CA Caner J Clin.* 2017;67:7)

[a]Patients with history of cryptorchidism, orchiopexy, family history of testicular CA, or testicular atrophy should be informed of their increased risk for developing testicular CA and counseled about screening. Such patients may then elect to be screened or to perform testicular self-examination. Adolescent and young adult males should be advised to seek prompt medical attention if they notice a scrotal abnormality. (USPSTF, 2011)

Infectious Diseases

GONORRHEA AND CHLAMYDIA

Population
–Women <25 y who are sexually active.
–Women ≥25 y if at increased risk.[a]

Recommendations

▶ CDC 2015, AAP 2014

–Screen annually.

Sources
–CDC. *Sexually Transmitted Diseases Guidelines*. 2015.
–*Pediatrics*. 2014;134(1):e302.

▶ USPSTF 2014

–Screen interval to be determined by patient's sexual practices.

Source
–USPSTF. *Chlamydia and Gonorrhea: Screening*. 2014.

Population
–Young heterosexual men; nonpregnant women >25 y without risk factors.

Recommendations

▶ CDC 2015, USPSTF 2014

–Insufficient evidence for or against routine screening.
–Consider screening in high prevalence clinical settings.

---

[a]Women age <25 y are at highest risk for gonorrhea infection. Other risk factors that place women at increased risk include a previous gonorrhea infection, the presence of other sexually transmitted diseases (STDs), new or multiple sex partners, inconsistent condom use, commercial sex work, and drug use.

Sources
  –USPSTF. *Chlamydia and Gonorrhea: Screening.* 2014.
  –CDC. *Sexually Transmitted Diseases Guidelines.* 2015.

Comment

1. *Chlamydia* and *Gonorrhea* are a reportable infection to the Public Health Department in every state.

Population

  –Men who have sex with men.

Recommendations

▶ CDC 2015

  –Annual testing, regardless of condom use.
  –Frequency of q 3–6 mo for high-risk activity.

Source
  –CDC. *Sexually Transmitted Diseases Treatment Guidelines.* 2015.

Comments

1. Urine nucleic amplification acid test (NAAT) for *Chlamydia* and/or *Gonorrhea* for men who have had insertive intercourse and women with vaginal/penile intercourse.
2. NAAT of rectal swab for persons who have had receptive anal intercourse.
3. NAAT of oropharyngeal swab for persons engaged in oral sexual intercourse.

HERPES SIMPLEX VIRUS (HSV), GENITAL

Population

  –Adolescents, adults.

Recommendation

▶ CDC 2015, USPSTF 2016

  –Do not screen routinely for HSV with serologies.

Sources
  –*JAMA.* 2016;316(23):2525-2530.
  –CDC. *Sexually Transmitted Diseases Treatment Guidelines.* 2015.

Comment

1. In women with a history of genital herpes, routine serial cultures for HSV are not indicated in the absence of active lesions.

HUMAN IMMUNODEFICIENCY VIRUS (HIV)

Population
–Adolescents, adults.

Recommendations

▶ **AAFP 2013**

–Screen everyone age 18–65 y. Consider screening high-risk individuals[a] of other ages.

▶ **USPSTF 2019**

–Screen everyone age 15–65 y. Consider screening high-risk individuals of other ages.

▶ **CDC 2015**

–Screen everyone age 13–64 y. Consider screening high-risk individuals of other ages.

Sources

–AAFP. *Clinical Recommendations: HIV Infection, Adolescents and Adults*. 2013.
–CDC. *Sexually Transmitted Diseases Treatment Guidelines*. 2015.
–USPSTF. *HIV Infection: Screening*. 2013.

Comments

1. Educate and counsel all high-risk patients regarding HIV testing, transmission, risk-reduction behaviors, and implications of infection.
2. If acute HIV is suspected, use plasma RNA test also.
3. False-positive results with electroimmunoassay (EIA): nonspecific reactions in persons with immunologic disturbances (eg, systemic lupus erythematosus or rheumatoid arthritis), multiple transfusions, recent influenza, or rabies vaccination.
4. Confirmatory testing is necessary using Western blot or indirect immunofluorescence assay.
5. Awareness of HIV positively reduces secondary HIV transmission risk and high-risk behavior and viral load if on highly active antiretroviral therapy (HAART). (CDC, 2006)

---

[a]Risk factors for HIV: men who have had sex with men after 1975; multiple sexual partners; history of intravenous drug use; prostitution; history of sex with an HIV-infected person; history of sexually transmitted disease; history of blood transfusion between 1978 and 1985; or persons requesting an HIV test.

SYPHILIS

Population

–Persons at increased risk.[a]

Recommendation

▶ **USPSTF 2016, AAFP 2016, CDC 2015**

–Screen high-risk persons.

Sources

–*JAMA.* 2016;315(21):2321-2327
–AAFP. *Clinical Recommendations: Syphilis.* 2016.
–CDC. *Sexually Transmitted Diseases Treatment Guidelines.* 2015.

Comments

1. A nontreponemal test (Venereal Disease Research Laboratory [VDRL] test or rapid plasma reagent [RPR] test) should be used for initial screening.
2. All reactive nontreponemal tests should be confirmed with a fluorescent treponemal antibody absorption (FTA-ABS) test.
3. Syphilis is a reportable disease in every state.

TRICHOMONAS

Population

–Women.

Recommendation

▶ **CDC 2015**

–Consider for women in high-prevalence settings (STD clinics, correctional facilities) and at increased risk (multiple sex partners, commercial sex, illicit drug use, history of STD).

Population

–Persons with HIV.

---

[a]High risk includes commercial sex workers, persons who exchange sex for money or drugs, persons with other STDs (including HIV), sexually active homosexual men, and sexual contacts of persons with syphilis, gonorrhea, *Chlamydia*, or HIV infection.

▶ CDC 2015
–Screen sexually active women at first visit and at least annually thereafter.

Source
–CDC. *Sexually Transmitted Diseases Treatment Guidelines.* 2015. https://www.cdc.gov/std/tg2015/trichomoniasis.htm

Pulmonary Disorders

CHRONIC OBSTRUCTIVE PULMONARY DISEASE

Population
–Adults, asymptomatic.

Recommendation

▶ USPSTF 2016
–Do not screen asymptomatic adults for COPD.

Source
–*JAMA.* 2016;315(13):1372-1377.

Comments

1. Detection while asymptomatic doesn't alter disease course or improve outcomes.
2. Several symptom-based questionnaires have high sensitivity for COPD.
3. In symptomatic patients (ie, dyspnea, chronic cough, or sputum production with a history of exposure to cigarette smoke or other toxic fumes), diagnostic spirometry to measure FEV1/FVC ratio is indicated.

LUNG CANCER

Population
–Asymptomatic persons with smoking history.

Recommendations

▶ USPSTF 2013, ACCP 2018, NCCN 2019
–Screen for lung cancer annually with low-dose chest CT in older adults who have at least a 30 pack-year smoking history.

- USPSTF: age 55–80 y.
- ACCP: age 55–77 y.
- NCCN: 55–74 y, or age $\geq$50 with $\geq$20 pack-year smoking history and other cancer risk factors.[a]

–Stop screening if a person has not smoked for 15 y, or if they develop a significant medical problem that would limit ability to receive treatment for an early stage lung cancer.

–Do not screen routinely with chest x-ray and/or sputum cytology.

–Only screen if a highly skilled support team is available to evaluate CT scans, schedule appropriate follow-up, and perform lung biopsies safely when indicated.

Sources

–https://www.uspreventiveservicestaskforce.org/Page/Document/UpdateSummaryFinal/lung-cancer-screening

–*J Natl Compr Canc Netw.* 2018;16:412-441.

–https://www.cancer.org/health-care-professionals/american-cancer-society-prevention-early-detection-guidelines/lung-cancer-screening-guidelines.html

–*CHEST.* 2018;153(4):954-985. https://www.ncbi.nlm.nih.gov/pubmed/29374513

–National Comprehensive Cancer Network Guidelines Version 2.2019, Lung Cancer Screening. https://www.nccn.org/professionals/physician_gls/

Comments

1. Less than 1 in 1000 patients with a false-positive result experience a major complication resulting from diagnostic workup.

   a. Counsel all patients against tobacco use, no matter their age. Smokers who quit gain ~10 y of increased life expectancy and have maximum reduction in risk of lung cancer after 15 y of no tobacco use. (*Br Med J.* 2004:328)

   b. Spiral CT screening can detect greater number of lung cancers in smokers with a >10-pack-year exposure. (*N Engl J Med.* 2006;355:1763-1771)

   c. The NCI has reported data from the National Lung Screening Trial (NLST), a randomized controlled trial comparing LDCT and CXR yearly × 3 with 8-y follow-up. A total of 53,500 men and women age 50–74 y, 30 pack-year smokers were randomized. A 20.3% reduction in deaths from lung cancer was reported for the LDCT group (estimated that 10,000–15,000 lives could be saved per year).

---

[a]The Tammemagi lung cancer risk calculator (https://brocku.ca/lung-cancer-risk-calculator) score of >1.3% 6-year risk is considered sufficient risk to pursue screening. (*PLOS Med.* 2014;11:1-13).

Problems with false-positives (25% have lung nodules <1 cm that are not cancer) and cost of workup were noted, but benefits have led to a change in guidelines.

d. The ACCP, ACS, NCCN, and ASCO formally recommend LDCT screening for patients who meet the criteria of the NLST study. (It is estimated that 8.6 million Americans meet NLST criteria for screening, which would save 12,000 lives annually.)

e. There is increasing concern regarding the cost of lung cancer screening. Twenty-five percent of patients screened have indeterminate abnormal findings requiring repeat imaging at intervals, and a significant number of patients who are biopsied show benign disease. Also, many patients are screened yearly instead of just 3 consecutive years of screening that was done in the randomized trials. (*Ann Intern Med.* 2011;155:540) (*N Engl J Med.* 2011;365:395) (*CA Cancer J Clin.* 2013;63:87) (*N Engl J Med.* 2013;368:1980-1991) (*N Engl J Med.* 2014;369:910) (*N Engl J Med.* 2015;372:387, 2083) (*Ann Intern Med.* 2014;160:330) (*Lancet Oncol.* 2016;17:543, 590)

f. Problem with overdiagnosis and potential harm in surgical resection of small slow growing cancers. (*JAMA Intern Med.* published online 1/30/2017) (*JAMA Intern Med.* 2014;174:269)

g. Lung cancer prediction models will help designate who needs to be screened and how often. (*J Clin Oncol.* 2017;35:861)

h. Risk Factors for Lung Cancer:

    i. Cigarette smoking (20-fold increased risk) and second-hand exposure to tobacco smoke (20% increased risk). Medication and counseling together are better than either alone in increasing cessation rates.

    ii. Beta-carotene, in pharmacologic doses, actually increases the risk of lung cancer, especially in high-intensity smokers.

    iii. Radon gas exposure, severe air pollution. Air pollution increases risk of lung cancer by 40% with highest pollution exposure. (*Am J Respir Crit Care Med.* 2006;173:667)

    iv. Occupational exposures (asbestos, arsenic, nickel, and chromium).

    v. Radiation exposure. (*Chest.* 2003;123:215)

i. Minimize Risk of Lung Cancer

    i. No evidence that vitamin E, tocopherol, retinoids, vitamin C, or beta-carotene in any dose reduces the risk of lung cancer. (*Ann Inter Med.* 2013;159:824)

    ii. Minimize indoor exposure to radon (can be measured in home), especially if smoker. Avoid occupational exposures (asbestos, arsenic, nickel, chromium, beryllium, and cadmium).

iii. Stopping tobacco use will lower the risk of lung and other cancers though at 15 y there is still a 2- to 3-fold increased risk of lung cancer.

iv. At least two-thirds of patients newly diagnosed with lung cancer will die of their disease. Early detection is critical. (*Chest.* 2017;151:193)

Renal Disorders

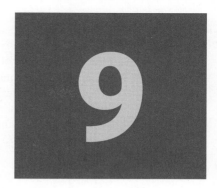

KIDNEY DISEASE, CHRONIC (CKD)

Population
–Adults.

Recommendations

▶ USPSTF 2012

–Insufficient evidence to recommend for or against routine screening.

Source
–USPSTF. *Chronic Kidney Disease (CKD): Screening.* 2012.

▶ ACP 2013, AAFP 2014

–Do not screen adults unless they have symptoms or risk factors.
–Adults taking an ACE inhibitor or ARB should not be tested for proteinuria, regardless of diabetes status.

Sources
–AAFP. *Clinical Recommendations: Chronic Kidney Disease.* 2014.
–*Ann Intern Med.* 2013;159(12):835.

▶ NICE 2014

–Monitor glomerular filtration rate (GFR) at least annually in people who are prescribed drugs known to be nephrotoxic.[a]
–Screen renal function in people at risk for CKD.[b]

Source
–NICE. *Early Identification and Management of Chronic Kidney Disease in Adults in Primary and Secondary Care.* London (UK): NICE; 2014.

---

[a]Examples: calcineurin inhibitors, lithium, or nonsteroidal anti-inflammatory drugs (NSAIDs).
[b]DM, HTN, CVD, structural renal disease, nephrolithiasis, benign prostatic hyperplasia (BPH), multisystem diseases with potential kidney involvement (eg, systemic lupus erythematosus [SLE]), FH of stage 5 CKD or hereditary kidney disease, or personal history of hematuria or proteinuria.

Comments

1. Diagnose CKD if either of the following present for >3 months:
   a. Markers of kidney damage such as albuminuria >30 mg/g, urinary sediment abnormalities, electrolyte abnormalities due to tubular disorders, histologic abnormalities, structural abnormalities by imaging, or kidney transplantation.
   b. GFR <60 mL/min/1.73 m².

Source

–Kidney Disease Improving Global Outcomes (KDIGO). *KDIGO 2012 Clinical Practice Guideline for the Evaluation and Management of Chronic Kidney Disease* 2013;3(1).

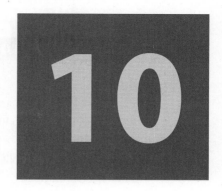

Special Population: Children and Adolescents

ALCOHOL ABUSE AND DEPENDENCE

Population
–Children and adolescents.

Recommendation

▶ **AAFP 2010, USPSTF 2018, ICSI 2010**
–Insufficient evidence to recommend for or against screening or counseling interventions to prevent or reduce alcohol misuse by adolescents.

Sources
–USPSTF. *Unhealthy Alcohol Use in Adolescents and Adults: Screening and Behavioral Counseling Interventions.* 2018.
–https://www.icsi.org/guidelines__more/catalog_guidelines_and_more/catalog_ guidelines/
–*Ann Fam Med.* 2010;8(6):484-492.

Comments
1. AUDIT and CAGE questionnaires have not been validated in children or adolescents.
2. Reinforce not drinking and driving or riding with any driver under the influence.
3. Reinforce to women the harmful effects of alcohol on fetuses.

ATTENTION-DEFICIT/HYPERACTIVITY DISORDER

Population

–Children age 4–18 y with academic or behavioral problems and inattention, hyperactivity, or impulsivity.

Recommendations

▶ AAFP 2016, AAP 2011, NICE 2018

–Do not screen routinely.

–Initiate an evaluation for ADHD for any child 4–18 y who presents with academic or behavioral problems and symptoms of inattention, hyperactivity, or impulsivity. Diagnosis requires that the child meets DSM-IV criteria[a] and direct supporting evidence from parents or caregivers and classroom teacher.

–Evaluation of a child with ADHD should include assessment for coexisting disorders and alternative causes of the behavior.

Sources

–AAFP. *Clinical Recommendation: ADHD in Children and Adolescents.* 2016.

[a]DSM-IV Criteria for ADHD:

I: Either A or B.

A: Six or more of the following symptoms of inattention have been present for at least 6 mo to a point that is disruptive and inappropriate for developmental level. Inattention: (1) Often does not give close attention to details or makes careless mistakes in schoolwork, work, or other activities. (2) Often has trouble keeping attention on tasks or play activities. (3) Often does not seem to listen when spoken to directly. (4) Often does not follow instructions and fails to finish schoolwork, chores, or duties in the workplace (not due to oppositional behavior or failure to understand instructions). (5) Often has trouble organizing activities. (6) Often avoids, dislikes, or does not want to do things that take a lot of mental effort for a long period of time (such as schoolwork or homework). (7) Often loses things needed for tasks and activities (eg, toys, school assignments, pencils, books, or tools). (8) Is often easily distracted. (9) Is often forgetful in daily activities.

B: Six or more of the following symptoms of hyperactivity-impulsivity have been present for at least 6 mo to an extent that is disruptive and inappropriate for developmental level. Hyperactivity: (1) Often fidgets with hands or feet or squirms in seat. (2) Often gets up from seat when remaining in seat is expected. (3) Often runs about or climbs when and where it is not appropriate (adolescents or adults may feel very restless). (4) Often has trouble playing or enjoying leisure activities quietly. (5) Is often "on the go" or often acts as if "driven by a motor." (6) Often talks excessively.

Impulsivity: (1) Often blurts out answers before questions have been finished. (2) Often has trouble waiting one's turn. (3) Often interrupts or intrudes on others (eg, butts into conversations or games).

II: Some symptoms that cause impairment were present before age 7 y.

III: Some impairment from the symptoms is present in two or more settings (eg, at school/work and at home).

IV: There must be clear evidence of significant impairment in social, school, or work functioning.

V: The symptoms do not happen only during the course of a pervasive developmental disorder, schizophrenia, or other psychotic disorder. The symptoms are not better accounted for by another mental disorder (eg, mood disorder, anxiety disorder, dissociative disorder, or a personality disorder).

–*Pediatrics.* 2011;128(5):1007.

–*Pediatrics.* 2000;105(5):1158.

–NICE. *Attention Deficit Hyperactivity Disorder: Diagnosis and Management.* 2018. nice.org.uk/guidance/ng87

Comments

1. Stimulant prescription rates continue to rise. (*Lancet.* 2016; 387(10024):1240-1250)
2. Current estimates are that 7.2% of children/adolescents meet criteria for ADHD. (*Pediatrics.* 2015;135(4):e994)
3. The U.S. Food and Drug Administration (FDA) approved a "black box" warning regarding the potential for cardiovascular side effects of ADHD stimulant drugs. (*N Engl J Med.* 2006;354:1445)

AUTISM SPECTRUM DISORDER

Population

–Children, age 12–36 mo.

Recommendations

▶ USPSTF 2016

–Insufficient evidence to screen routinely.

Source

–*JAMA.* 2016;315(7):691-696.

▶ AAP 2014

–Screen with autism-specific tool at 18 mo and 24 mo.

–M-CHAT is most commonly used (see page 711).

Sources

–*Pediatrics.* 2006;118(1):405.

–*Pediatrics.* 2014;135(5):e1520.

Comments

1. Listen and respond to concerns raised by caregivers; signs may be identifiable by 9 mo of age.
2. Prevalence is 1 in 68; 4.5:1 male:female ratio. (*MMWR Surveill Summ.* 2016;65(3):1–23)

CELIAC DISEASE

Population
–Children and adults.

Recommendations

▶ **USPSTF 2017, AAFP 2017**

–Insufficient evidence regarding screening of asymptomatic people.

Sources
–AAFP. *Clinical Recommendation: Screening for Celiac Disease.* 2017.
–*JAMA.* 2017;317(12):1252.

▶ **NICE 2015**

–Do not screen the asymptomatic general population.
–Serologic testing to rule out celiac disease should be performed for any of the following signs, symptoms, or associated conditions: persistent unexplained abdominal or gastrointestinal symptoms, faltering growth, prolonged fatigue, unexpected weight loss, severe or persistent mouth ulcers, unexplained iron, vitamin B12 or folate deficiency, type 1 diabetes, autoimmune thyroid disease, irritable bowel syndrome (in adults).
–Screen first-degree relatives of people with celiac disease.

Source
–NICE. *Coeliac Disease: Recognition, Assessment and Management.* 2015.

Comments
1. Patients must continue a gluten-containing diet during diagnostic testing.
2. IgA tissue transglutaminase (TTG) is the test of choice (>90% sensitivity/specificity), along with total IgA level.
3. IgA endomysial antibody test is indicated if the TTG test is equivocal.
4. Avoid antigliadin antibody testing.
5. Consider serologic testing for any of the following: Addison disease; amenorrhea; autoimmune hepatitis; autoimmune myocarditis; chronic immune thrombocytopenic purpura (ITP); dental enamel defects; depression; bipolar disorder; Down syndrome; Turner syndrome; epilepsy; lymphoma; metabolic bone disease; chronic constipation; poly-neuropathy; sarcoidosis; Sjögren syndrome; or unexplained alopecia.

CHOLESTEROL AND LIPID DISORDERS

Population
–Infants, children, adolescents, or young adults (age <20 y).

Recommendations

▶ **USPSTF 2016, NLA 2011**

–Insufficient evidence to recommend for or against routine universal lab screening.

–In familial hypercholesterolemia, screen at age 9–11 y with a fasting lipid panel or nonfasting non-HDL-C. If non-HDL-C ≥145 m/dL, perform fasting lipid panel.

–Genetic screening for familial hypercholesterolemia is generally not needed for diagnosis or clinical management.

–Cascade screening: testing lipid levels in all first-degree relatives of diagnosed familial hypercholesterolemia patients.

Sources
–*J Clin Lipidol.* 2011;5:S1-S8.
–*JAMA.* 2016;316:625-633.

▶ **AHA 2007**

–Screen selectively: obtain fasting lipid panel in patients age >2 y with a parent age <55 y with coronary artery disease, peripheral artery disease, cerebrovascular disease, or hyperlipidemia.

Source
–*Circulation.* 2007;115:1947-1967.

Comments

1. Childhood drug treatment of dyslipidemia lowers lipid levels but effect on childhood or adult outcomes is uncertain.
2. Lifestyle approach is recommended starting after age 2 y.

Recommendations

▶ **National Heart, Lung and Blood Institute Integrated Guidelines 2012**

–Selective screening age >2 y: positive family history (FH) of dyslipidemia, presence of dyslipidemia, or the presence of overweight, obesity, hypertension, diabetes, or a smoking history.

–Universal screening in adolescents regardless of FH between age 9 and 11 y and again between age 18 and 21 y.

Source
–*NHLBI. Expert Panel on Integrated Guidelines for Cardiovascular Health and Risk Reduction in Children and Adolescents.* 2012.

Comments

1. Fasting lipid profile is recommended. If within normal limits, repeat testing in 3–5 y is recommended.
2. Fasting lipid profile or nonfasting non-high-density lipoprotein (HDL) cholesterol level.

DEPRESSION

Population

–Children age 7–11 y.

Recommendation

▶ USPSTF 2016

–Insufficient evidence to recommend for or against routine screening.

Source

–*Ann Intern Med.* 2016;164(5):360-366.

Population

–Adolescents.

Recommendation

▶ USPSTF 2016

–Screen all adolescents age 12–18 y for major depressive disorder (MDD). Systems should be in place to ensure accurate diagnosis, appropriate psychotherapy, and adequate follow-up.

Sources

–*Ann Intern Med.* 2016;164(5):360-366.
–Wilkinson J, Bass C, et al. *Preventative Services for Children and Adolescents.* Bloomington: ICSI; 2013.

Comments

1. Screen in primary care clinics with the Patient Health Questionnaire for Adolescents (PHQ-A) (73% sensitivity; 94% specificity) or the Beck Depression Inventory-Primary Care (BDI-PC) (91% sensitivity; 91% specificity). See page 722.
2. Treatment options include pharmacotherapy (fluoxetine and escitalopram have FDA approval for this age group), psychotherapy, collaborative care, psychosocial support interventions, and CAM approaches.
3. SSRI may increase suicidality in some adolescents, emphasizing the need for close follow-up.

DIABETES

Population

–Children at start of puberty or age ≥10 y.

Recommendation

▶ ADA 2012

–Screen all children at risk for DM type 2.[a]

Source

–*Diabetes Care.* 2012; 35(suppl 1):S11-S63.

FAMILY VIOLENCE AND ABUSE

Population

–Children, women, and older adults.

Recommendation

▶ USPSTF 2018

–Insufficient evidence to recommend for or against routine screening of parents or guardians for the physical abuse or neglect of children.

Source

–USPSTF. *Interventions to Prevent Child Maltreatment.* 2018.

Comments

1. All providers should be aware of physical and behavioral signs and symptoms associated with abuse and neglect, including burns, bruises, and repeated suspect trauma.
2. CDC publishes a toolkit of assessment instruments: https://www.cdc.gov/violence prevention/pdf/ipv/ipvandsvscreening.pdf

[a]Risk factors for HIV: men who have had sex with men after 1975; multiple sexual partners; history of intravenous drug use; prostitution; history of sex with an HIV-infected person; history of sexually transmitted disease; history of blood transfusion between 1978 and 1985; or persons requesting an HIV test.

HUMAN IMMUNODEFICIENCY VIRUS (HIV)

Population
–Adolescents and adults.

Recommendations

▶ **AAFP 2013**

–Screen everyone age 18–65 y. Consider screening high-risk individuals[a] of other ages.

▶ **USPSTF 2019**

–Screen everyone age 15–65 y. Consider screening high-risk individuals of other ages.

▶ **CDC 2015**

–Screen everyone age 13–64 y. Consider screening high-risk individuals of other ages.

Sources

–AAFP. *Clinical Recommendations: HIV Infection, Adolescents and Adults.* 2013.

–CDC. *Sexually Transmitted Diseases Treatment Guidelines.* 2015.

–USPSTF. *HIV Infection: Screening.* 2019.

Comments

1. HIV testing should be voluntary and must have a verbal consent to test. Patients may "opt out" of testing.
2. Educate and counsel all high-risk patients regarding HIV testing, transmission, risk-reduction behaviors, and implications of infection.
3. If acute HIV is suspected, also use plasma RNA test.
4. False-positive results with electroimmunoassay (EIA): nonspecific reactions in persons with immunologic disturbances (eg, systemic lupus erythematosus or rheumatoid arthritis), multiple transfusions, recent influenza, or rabies vaccination.
5. Confirmatory testing is necessary using Western blot or indirect immunofluorescence assay.
6. Awareness of HIV positively reduces secondary HIV transmission risk and high-risk behavior and viral load if on highly active antiretroviral therapy (HAART). (CDC, 2006)

HYPERTENSION (HTN), CHILDREN AND ADOLESCENTS

Population
–Age 3–20 y.[a]

Recommendations
▶ Pediatrics 2017, NHLBI 2012, AAFP 2018
  –Measure BP only at preventative visits for children age ≥3 y. (Table 10-1)

Age	Boys		Girls	
	DBP	SBP	DBP	
1	98	52	98	54
2	100	55	101	58
3	101	58	102	60
4	102	60	103	62
5	103	63	104	64
6	105	66	105	67
7	106	68	106	68
8	107	69	107	69
9	107	70	108	71
10	108	72	109	72
11	110	74	111	74
12	113	75	114	75
13+	120	80	120	80

TABLE 10-1: REPRODUCED FROM TABLE 6 IN FLYNN ET AL. CLINICAL PRACTICE GUIDELINE FOR SCREENING AND MANAGEMENT OF BLOOD PRESSURE IN CHILDREN AND ADOLESCENTS. *PEDIATRICS.* 2017;140(3):E2017-1904

[a]In children age <3 y, conditions that warrant BP measurement include: prematurity, very low birth weight, or neonatal complications; congenital heart disease; recurrent urinary tract infections (UTIs), hematuria, or proteinuria; renal disease or urologic malformations; familial hypercholesterolemia of congenital renal disease; solid-organ transplant; malignancy or bone marrow transplant; drugs known to raise BP; systemic illnesses; and increased intracranial pressure.

–Measure BP at each encounter for children age ≥3 y who have obesity, renal disease, h/o aortic arch obstruction or coarctation, diabetes, or are taking medications known to raise blood pressure.

Sources

–*Pediatrics.* 2017;140(3):e2017-1904.

–NHLBI. *Expert Panel on Integrated Guidelines for Cardiovascular Health and Risk Reduction in Children and Adolescents.* 2012.

–NHLBI. *A Pocket Guide to Blood Pressure Management in Children.* 2012.

–AAFP. *High Blood Pressure in Children and Adolescents.* 2018.

Comments

1. Hypertension: average systolic blood pressure (SBP) or diastolic blood pressure (DBP) ≥95th percentile for gender, age, and height on 3 or more occasions. See pages 692–694.
2. Counsel children and adolescents who have been diagnosed with hypertension regarding lifestyle modifications including diet and physical activity.
3. Prescribe pharmacologic therapy to children and adolescents who fail lifestyle modifications.

ILLICIT DRUG USE

Population

–Adults, adolescents, and pregnant women.

Recommendation

▶ USPSTF 2014, ICSI 2014

–Insufficient evidence to recommend for or against routine screening for illicit drug use.

Sources

–*ICSI Preventive Services for Adults.* 20th ed. 2014.

–USPSTF. *Drug Use, Illicit: Screening.* 2014.

LEAD POISONING

Population
–Children age 1–5 y.

Recommendations

▶ AAFP 2006, USPSTF 2019, CDC 2000, AAP 2000
–Insufficient evidence to recommend for or against routine screening in asymptomatic children at increased risk.[a]
–Do not screen asymptomatic children at average risk.

Sources
–USPSTF. *Elevated Blood Lead Levels in Childhood and Pregnancy: Screening*. 2019.
–*Pediatrics*. 1998;101(6):1702.
–Advisory Committee on Childhood Lead Poisoning Prevention. Recommendations for blood lead screening of young children enrolled in Medicaid: targeting a group at high risk. *CDC MMWR*. 2000;49(RR14):1-13.
–AAFP. *Clinical Recommendations: Lead Poisoning*. 2006.

Comments

1. CDC recommends that children who receive Medicaid benefits should be screened unless high-quality, local data demonstrates the absence of lead exposure among this population.
2. Screen at ages 1 and 2 y, or by age 3 y if a high-risk child has never been screened.
3. As of 2012, the threshold for elevated blood lead level has been lowered to 5 µg/dL. (CDC. *Low Level Lead Exposure Harms Children: A Renewed Call for Primary Prevention*. 2012)
4. CDC personal risk questionnaire (http://www.cdc.gov/nceh/lead/publications/screening.htm):
   a. Does your child live in or regularly visit a house (or other facility, eg, daycare) that was built before 1950?
   b. Does your child live in or regularly visit a house built before 1978 with recent or ongoing renovations or remodeling (within the last 6 mo)?
   c. Does your child have a sibling or playmate who has or did have lead poisoning?

[a]Child suspected by parent, health care provider, or Health Department to be at risk for lead exposure; sibling or playmate with elevated blood lead level; recent immigrant, refugee, or foreign adoptee; child's parent or caregiver works with lead; household member uses traditional folk or ethnic remedies or cosmetics or who routinely eats food imported informally from abroad; residence near a source of high lead levels.

MOTOR VEHICLE SAFETY

Population
–Children and adolescents.

Recommendation
▶ ICSI 2013
  –Ask about
  - car seats,
  - booster seats,
  - seat belt use,
  - helmet use while riding motorcycles.

Source
–ICSI. *Preventive Services for Children and Adolescents*. 19th ed. 2013.

Comment
1. One study demonstrated a 21% reduction in mortality with the use of child restraint systems vs. seat belts in children age 2–6 y involved in motor vehicle collisions. (*Arch Pediatr Adolesc Med.* 2006;160:617-621)

OBESITY

Population
–Children age ≥6 y.

Recommendation
▶ USPSTF 2017
  –Screen children age 6 y and older for obesity.

Source
–*JAMA*. 2017;317(23):2417-2426.

Comments
1. Offer obese children intensive counseling and behavioral interventions to promote improvement in weight status.
2. Intensive interventions (>26 h) can improve weight status; less intensive interventions have not been proven but have little potential harm.

Population
–Children age ≥2 y.

Recommendation

▶ ICSI 2013

  –Record height, weight, and body mass index (BMI) annually starting at age 2 y.

  Source

  –ICSI. *Preventive Services for Children and Adolescents*. 19th ed. 2013.

Comments

  1. Children with a BMI ≥25 are 5 times more likely to be overweight as adults when compared with their normal-weight counterparts.
  2. Overweight children should be counseled about wholesome eating, 30–60 min of daily physical activity, and avoiding soft drinks.

SCOLIOSIS

Population

  –Adolescents.

Recommendation

▶ AAFP 2013, USPSTF 2017

  –Insufficient evidence to assess the balance of benefits and harms of screening for adolescent idiopathic scoliosis in children and adolescents age 10–18.

  Sources

  –AAFP. *Choosing Wisely: Scoliosis in Adolescents*. 2013.
  –USPSTF. *Screening for Adolescents Idiopathic Scoliosis*. 2017.

SPEECH AND LANGUAGE DELAY

Population

  –Preschool children.

Recommendation

▶ AAFP 2015, USPSTF 2015

  –Evidence is insufficient to recommend for or against routine use of brief, formal screening instruments in primary care to detect speech and language delay in children up to age 5 y.

  Sources

  –AAFP. *Clinical Recommendation: Speech and Language Delay*. 2015.
  –*Pediatrics*. 2015;136(2):e474-481.

Comments

1. Fair evidence suggests that interventions can improve the results of short-term assessments of speech and language skills; however, no studies have assessed long-term consequences.
2. In a study of 9000 toddlers in the Netherlands, 2-time screening for language delays reduced the number of children who required special education (2.7% vs. 3.7%) and reduced deficient language performance (8.8% vs. 9.7%) at age 8 y. (*Pediatrics.* 2007;120:1317)
3. Studies have not fully addressed the potential harms of screening or interventions for speech and language delays, such as labeling, parental anxiety, or unnecessary evaluation and intervention.
4. Insufficient evidence to recommend a specific test, but parent-administered tools are best (eg, Communicative Development Inventory, Infant-Toddler Checklist, Language Development Survey, Ages and Stages Questionnaire).

Population

–Children.

Recommendation

▶ AAP 2014

–Screen using validated test during well child checks at 9, 18, and 24/30 mo.

Sources

–*Pediatrics.* 2006;118(1):405.
–*Pediatrics.* 2015;136(2):e448.

SUICIDE RISK

Population

–Adolescents.

Recommendation

▶ AAP 2016

–Ask questions about suicidal thoughts in routine history taking throughout adolescence.

Source

–*Pediatrics.* 2016. Suicide and Suicide Attempts in Adolescents.

TOBACCO USE

Population
–Children and adolescents.

Recommendations

▶ USPSTF 2013

–Provide interventions, including education or brief counseling to prevent initiation of tobacco use in school-aged children and adolescents.

▶ ICSI 2013

–Screen for tobacco use beginning at age 10, and reassess at every opportunity.

Sources
–ICSI. *Preventive Services for Children and Adolescents.* 19th ed. 2013.
–USPSTF. *Tobacco Use Interventions: Children and Adolescents.* 2013.

Comment

1. Children and adolescents should avoid tobacco use. It is uncertain whether advice and counseling by health care professionals in this area is effective.

TUBERCULOSIS, LATENT

Population
–Persons at increased risk of developing tuberculosis (TB).

Recommendation

▶ USPSTF 2016, CDC 2010

–Screen by tuberculin skin test (TST) or interferon-gamma release assay (IGRA). Frequency of testing is based on likelihood of further exposure to TB and level of confidence in the accuracy of the results.

Sources
–*JAMA.* 2016;316(9):962-969.
–*CDC MWWR.* 2010;59(RR-5).

Comments

1. Risk factors include birth or residence in a country with increased TB prevalence and residence in a congregate setting (shelters, correctional facilities).
2. Typically, a TST is used to screen for latent TB.

3. IGRA is preferred if:
   a. Testing persons who have a low likelihood of returning to have their TST read.
   b. Testing persons who have received a bacille Calmette–Guérin (BCG) vaccination.

VISUAL IMPAIRMENT

Population
   –Children 3–5 y.

Recommendations
▶ USPSTF 2017
   –Screen vision for all children 3–5 y at least once to detect amblyopia.
   –Insufficient evidence for vision screening in children <3 y of age.

Sources
   –USPSTF. *Vision Screening in Children Aged 6 Months to 5 Years.* 2017.
   –*JAMA.* 2017;318(9):836-844.

Comment
   1. May screen with a visual acuity test, a stereoacuity test, a cover–uncover test, and the Hirschberg light reflex test.

Special Population: Newborns and Infants

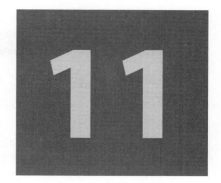

ANEMIA

Population
–Infants age 6–24 mo.

Recommendations

▶ USPSTF 2015, AAFP 2015

–Insufficient evidence to recommend for or against screening.
–Consider selective screening in high-risk children[a] with malnourishment, low birth weight, or symptoms of anemia.

▶ AAP 2010

–Universal screening of Hgb at 12 mo. If anemic, measure ferritin, C-reactive protein, and reticulocyte hemoglobin content.

Sources
–AAFP. *Clinical Recommendations: Iron Deficiency Anemia.* 2015.
–USPSTF. *Iron Deficiency in Young Children: Screening.* 2015.
–*Pediatrics.* 2010;126(5):1040-1050.

Comments

1. Reticulocyte hemoglobin content is a more sensitive and specific marker than is serum hemoglobin level for iron deficiency.
2. One-third of patients with iron deficiency will have a hemoglobin level >11 g/dL.
3. Use of transferring receptor 1 (TfR_1) assay as screening for iron deficiency is under investigation.

[a]Includes infants living in poverty, Blacks, Native Americans, Alaska natives, immigrants from developing countries, preterm and low-birth-weight infants, infants whose principal dietary intake is unfortified cow's milk or soy milk, bottle feeding beyond one year, having a mom who is currently pregnant, living in an urban area and having less than two servings per day of iron-rich foods (iron-fortified breakfast cereals or meats).

CRITICAL CONGENITAL HEART DISEASE

Population
–Newborns.

Recommendation
▶ AAP 2011

–All newborns should have pulse oximetry screening for CCHD at or greater than 24 h of life but prior to discharge home from the hospital.

Source
–AAP. *Endorsement of HHS Recommendation for Pulse Oximetry Screening for CCHD.* 2012.

Comment
1. Obtain oxygen saturations in the right hand and in one foot.

DEVELOPMENTAL DYSPLASIA OF THE HIP (DDH)

Population
–Infants.

Recommendations
▶ AAP 2017, AAFP 2017

–Examine newborn and continue periodic surveillance physical exam for DDH including length discrepancy, asymmetric thigh or buttock creases, performing Ortolani test, and observing for limited abduction.
–Selective ultrasonography for "high-risk" infants 6 wk to 6 mo of age: history of breech presentation, family history, parenteral concern, history of clinical hip instability on exam, or history of lower extremity swaddling.
–Radiography can be considered after 4 mo of age in high-risk infants without physical exam findings or any child with positive physical exam findings.
–Indication for orthopedic referral: unstable or dislocated hip in physical exam. Referral does not require any prior imaging.

Comment
1. There is evidence that screening leads to earlier identification; however, 60%–80% of the hips of newborns identified as abnormal or suspicious for DDH by physical examination, and >90% of those identified by ultrasound in the newborn period, resolve spontaneously, requiring no intervention.

Sources
  –*Pediatrics*. 2016;138(6):e20163107.
  –*Am Fam Physician*. 2017;96(3):196-197.

GROWTH ABNORMALITIES

Population
  –Children 0–59 mo.

Recommendation

▶ CDC 2010, AAP 2010

  –Use the 2006 World Health Organization (WHO) international growth charts for children age <24 mo.

Sources
  –CDC. Use of World Health Organization and CDC growth charts for children aged 0–59 mo in the United States. *MMWR* 2010;59 (No. RR-9):1-15.
  –AAP News. 2010;31(11).

Comments

1. The Centers for Disease Control and Prevention (CDC) and American Academy of Pediatricians (AAP) recommend the WHO as opposed to the CDC growth charts for children age <24 mo.
2. The CDC growth charts should still be used for children age 2–19 y.
3. This recommendation recognizes that breast-feeding is the recommended standard of infant feeding, and therefore the standard against which all other infants are compared.

HEARING IMPAIRMENT

Population
  –Newborns.

Recommendation

▶ AAP 1999, USPSTF 2008

  –Universal screening of all newborn infants for hearing loss.

Sources
  –*Pediatrics*. 1999;103(2).
  –*Pediatrics*. 2008;122(1).

Comments

1. Screening should be performed before 1 mo of age. Those infants who do not pass the initial screening should undergo audiologic and medical evaluation before 3 mo of age.
2. Screening involves either a 1-step or a 2-step process. The 2-step process includes otoacoustic emissions (OAEs) followed by auditory brainstem response (ABR) in those who fail the OAE test. The 1-step process uses either OAE or ABR testing.

HEMOGLOBINOPATHIES

Population

–Newborns.

Recommendation

▶ AAFP 2010, USPSTF 2007

–Screen all newborns for hemoglobinopathies (including sickle cell disease).

Sources

–http://www.guideline.gov/content.aspx?id=38619
–http://www.uspreventiveservicestaskforce.org/uspstf07/sicklecell/sicklers.htm

Comments

1. Screening for sickle cell disease is mandated in all 50 states and the District of Columbia.
2. Infants with sickle cell anemia should receive prophylactic Penicillin starting at 2 mo of age and pneumococcal vaccinations at recommended intervals.

NEWBORN SCREENING

Population

–Newborns.

Recommendation

▶ ICSI 2013

–Perform a metabolic screening test prior to hospital discharge for all newborns.

Source
- –ICSI. *Preventive Services for Children and Adolescents*. 19th ed. 2013.

Comment

1. The newborn screen should be performed after 24 h of age. Infants who receive their newborn screen before 24 h of age should have it repeated before 2 wk of age.

PHENYLKETONURIA (PKU)

Population
- –Newborns.

Recommendations

▶ Advisory Committee on Heritable Disorders in Newborns and Children 2015, USPSTF 2008

- –PKU screening is mandated in all 50 states.
- –Three main methods are used to screen for PKU in the United States: Guthrie Bacterial Inhibition Assay (BIA), automated fluorometric assay, tandem mass spectrometry.

Sources
- –Advisory Committee on Heritable Disorders in Newborns and Children. 2015.
- –USPSTF. *Phenylketonuria in Newborns: Screening*. 2008.

Comments

1. If infant is tested within 24 h of birth, testing should be repeated in 2 wk.
2. Optimal screening time for premature infants and infants with illnesses is within 7 d of birth, and in all cases before discharge from nursery.
3. If screening is positive, implement phenylalanine restrictions immediately after birth to prevent the neurodevelopmental effects of PKU.

THYROID DISEASE

Population
–Newborns.

Recommendation
▶ ICSI 2013, AAFP 2008, USPSTF 2008, AAP 2012, Discretionary Advisory Committee on Heritable Disorders in Newborns and Children 2015

–Screen for congenital hypothyroidism in newborns.

Sources
–ICSI. *Preventive Services for Children and Adolescents.* 19th ed. 2013.
–*Pediatrics.* 2006;119(6):2290.
–*Pediatrics.* 2012;129(4):e1103.
–AAFP. *Clinical Recommendations: Thyroid.* 2008.
–Advisory Committee on Heritable Disorders in Newborns and Children. 2015.
–USPSTF. *Congenital Hypothyroidism: Screening.* 2008.

Comments
1. Less than 1% of adults have subclinical hypothyroidism; outcomes data to support treatment are lacking.
2. Individuals with symptoms and signs potentially attributable to thyroid dysfunction and those with risk factors for its development may require TSH testing.
3. Higher risk individuals are those with an autoimmune disorder, pernicious anemia, history of neck radiation, first-degree relative with a thyroid disorder, and those with psychiatric disorders.

Special Population: Older Adults

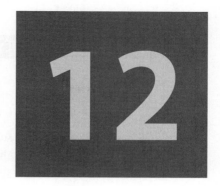

DEMENTIA

Population
–Adults.

Recommendations

▶ USPSTF 2014

–Insufficient evidence to recommend for or against routine screening for cognitive impairment or dementia.

▶ CTFPHC 2016

–Do not screen asymptomatic adults for cognitive impairment.

▶ AAN 2017

–Only assess for cognitive impairment when a patient or close contact voices concern about memory or impaired cognition. Use validated tools to assess cognitive impairment.

Sources
–*Neurology.* December 2017.
–*CMAJ.* 2016;188(1):37-46.
–*Ann Intern Med.* 2014;160(11):791-797.

Comments

1. False-positive rate for screening is high, and treatment interventions do not show consistent benefits.
2. Early recognition of cognitive impairment allows clinicians to anticipate problems that patients may have in understanding and adhering to recommended therapy and help patients and their caregivers anticipate and plan for future problems related to progressive cognitive decline.

FALLS IN THE ELDERLY

Population

–All older persons.

Recommendation

▶ NICE 2017, AAOS 2001, AGS 2010, British Geriatrics Society 2001, NFPCG/Public Health England 2017

–Ask at least yearly about falls.

Sources

–NICE. *Falls in Older People*. March 2015, updated January 2017.

–2010 AGS/BGS Clinical Practice Guideline: Prevention of Falls in Older Persons. http://www.americangeriatrics.org/files/documents/ health_care_pros/Falls.Summary.Guide.pdf

–*Public Health England/National Falls Prevention Coordination Group*. 2017. Falls and Fracture Consensus Statement, Supporting Commissioning for Prevention.

Population

–Community-dwelling older adults without known osteoporosis or vitamin D deficiency.

Recommendations

▶ USPSTF 2018

–Do not use vitamin D supplementation to prevent falls (Grade D).

–Encourage exercise interventions to prevent falls in older adults at increased risk for falls (Grade B).

–Selectively offer multifactorial interventions to prevent falls in older adults at increased risk for falls (Grade C).

Sources

–*JAMA*. 2018:319(15):1592-1599.

–*JAMA*. Published online April 17, 2018. doi:10.1001/jama.2017.21962.

Comments

1. Individuals are at increased risk if they report at least 2 falls in the previous year, or 1 fall with injury. Risk factors: Intrinsic: lower-extremity weakness, poor grip strength, balance disorders, functional and cognitive impairment, visual deficits. Extrinsic: polypharmacy ($\geq$4 prescription medications), environment (poor lighting, loose carpets, lack of bathroom safety equipment).

2. A fall prevention clinic appears to reduce the number of falls among the elderly. (*Am J Phys Med Rehabil*. 2006;85:882)

3. Effective exercise interventions include supervised individual and group classes and physical therapy.

4. Multifactorial interventions include initial assessment of modifiable fall risk factors (balance, vision, postural blood pressure, gait, medication, environment, cognition, psychological health) and interventions (nurses, clinicians, physical/occupational therapy, dietitian/nutritionist, CBT, education, medication management, urinary incontinence management, environmental modification, social/community resources, referral to specialist "ophthalmologist, neurologist, etc.").

5. All who report a single fall should be observed as they stand up from a chair without using their arms, walk several paces, and return (see Appendix II). Those demonstrating no difficulty or unsteadiness need no further assessment. Those who have difficulty or demonstrate unsteadiness, have ≥1 fall, or present for medical attention after a fall should have a fall evaluation.

6. Free "Tip Sheet" for patients from AGS (http://www.healthinaging. org/public_education/falls_tips.php).

7. Of US adults age ≥65 y, 15.9% fell in the preceding 3 mo; of these, 31.3% sustained an injury that resulted in a doctor visit or restricted activity for at least 1 d. (*MMWR Morb Mortal Wkly Rep.* 2008;57(9):225)

8. See also page 226 for Fall Prevention and Appendix II.

FAMILY VIOLENCE AND ABUSE

Population
–Women of reproductive age, older adults, and vulnerable adults.

Recommendations
▶ USPSTF 2018

–Insufficient evidence to recommend for or against routine screening of all older or vulnerable adults for abuse and neglect.

–Screen for intimate partner violence in women of reproductive age and provide or refer women who screen positive to ongoing support services.

Source
–*JAMA.* Screening for Intimate Partner Violence, Elder Abuse, and Abuse of Vulnerable Adults. 2018:320(16):1678-1787.

Comments

1. All providers should be aware of physical and behavioral signs and symptoms associated with abuse and neglect, including burns, bruises, and repeated suspect trauma.

2. CDC publishes a toolkit of assessment instruments: https://www.cdc. gov/violence prevention/pdf/ipv/ipvandsvscreening.pdf

OSTEOPOROSIS

Population
–Women age ≥65 y, and younger women at increased risk.

Recommendation

▶ **USPSTF 2018, ACPM 2009, ACOG 2012, NAMS 2010**

–Screen routinely using either dual-energy x-ray absorptiometry (DXA) of the hip and lumbar spine, or quantitative ultrasonography of the calcaneus.

Sources
–*JAMA*. Screening for Osteoporosis to Prevent Fractures. 2018:318(24):2521-2531.

–*Osteoporosis*. Washington (DC): ACOG; 2012. (ACOG practice bulletin; no. 129).

–*Menopause*. 2010;17(1):23.

–*Am J Prev Med*. 2009;36(4):366-375.

Comments

1. USPSTF specifically defines "increased risk" as having a fracture risk equivalent to that of a 65-y-old white woman.
2. The optimal screening interval is unclear, but should not be done more frequently than every 2 y.
3. ACOG: If FRAX score does not suggest treatment, DEXA should be repeated every 15 y if T-score ≥1.5, every 5 y if T-score is −1.5 to −1.99, and annually if T-score is −2.0 to −2.49.
4. Ten-year risk for osteoporotic fractures can be calculated for individuals by using the FRAX tool (http://www.shef.ac.uk/FRAX/).
5. Quantitative ultrasonography of the calcaneus predicts fractures of the femoral neck, hip, and spine as effectively as does DXA.
6. The criteria for treatment of osteoporosis rely on DXA measurements.

Population
–Older men.

Recommendations

▶ **USPSTF 2018**

–Insufficient evidence to recommend for or against routine osteoporosis screening.

▶ **NOF 2014, ACPM 2009, Endocrine Society 2012**

–Screen routinely over age 70 y via bone mineral density (BMD).

–Consider screening men age 50–69 with risk factors.

Sources
–*JAMA*. Screening for Osteoporosis to Prevent Fractures. 2018:318(24):2521-2531.
–*Am J Prev Med*. 2009;36(4).
–*Osteoporos Int*. 2014;25(10):2359-2381.
–*The Journal of Clinical Endocrinology & Metabolism*. Osteoporosis in Men: An Endocrine Society Clinical Practice Guideline. 2012;97(6):1802-1822.

Comment

1. Repeat every 3–5 y if "normal" baseline score; if high risk, then every 1–2 y.

VISUAL IMPAIRMENT, GLAUCOMA, OR CATARACT

Population

–Older adults.

Recommendation

▶ USPSTF 2016

–Insufficient evidence to recommend for or against visual acuity screening or glaucoma screening in older adults.

Source
–*JAMA*. Screening for Impaired Visual Acuity in Older Adults. 2016;315(9):908-914.

▶ ICSI 2014

–Objective vision testing (Snellen chart) recommended for adults age ≥65 y.

Source
–ICSI. *Preventive Services for Adults*. 20th ed. 2014.

▶ AAO 2015

–Individuals without risk factors 65 y and older should have an examination by an ophthalmologist every 1–2 y.

Source
–AAO Policy Statement. *Frequency of Ocular Examinations*. March 2015.

Comment

1. Adults with no signs or risk factors for eye disease should have a baseline comprehensive eye exam at age 40. Those with no signs or risk factors aged 40–54 should be examined by an ophthalmologist every 2–4 y, then every 1–3 y at age 55–64.

Special Population: Pregnant Women

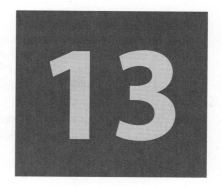

ANEMIA

Population
–Pregnant women.

Recommendation
▶ USPSTF 2015, AAFP 2014, ACOG 2008, CDC 1998
–Screen all women with hemoglobin or hematocrit at first prenatal visit.

Sources
–USPSTF. https://www.uspreventiveservicestaskforce.org/
–*Ann Intern Med.* 2015;163:529-536.
–ACOG. *Obstet Gynecol.* 2008;112(1):201.
–CDC. *MMWR Morb Mortal Wkly Rep.* 1998;47(RR-3):1.
–*Am Fam Physician.* 2014;89(3):199-208.

Comments
1. Insufficient evidence to recommend for or against routine screening for iron deficiency anemia (IDA) in pregnant women to prevent adverse maternal or birth outcomes. Insufficient evidence to recommend for or against use of iron supplements for non-anemic pregnant women. (USPSTF, 2015)
2. When acute stress or inflammatory disorders are not present, a serum ferritin level is the most accurate test for evaluating IDA. Among women of childbearing age, a cutoff of 30 ng/mL has sensitivity of 92%, specificity of 98%. (*Blood.* 1997;89:1052-1057)
3. Oral iron is first-line therapy for IDA in pregnancy. IV iron is preferred choice (after 13th wk) for those who have oral iron intolerance. Cobalamin and folate deficiency should be excluded. (*Blood.* 2017;129:940-949)

4. Decision to transfuse should be based on the hemoglobin, clinical context, and patient preferences. May be appropriate in severe anemia (<7 mg/dL according to WHO) in whom a 2-wk delay in Hb rise with oral iron may result in significant morbidity.

BACTERIAL VAGINOSIS

Population
–Pregnant women at high risk[a] for preterm delivery.

Recommendation
▶ USPSTF 2008

–Insufficient evidence to recommend for or against routine screening.

Population
–Low-risk pregnant women.

Recommendation
▶ USPSTF 2008

–Do not screen routinely.

Source
–USPSTF. *Bacterial Vaginosis in Pregnancy to Prevent Preterm Delivery: Screening.* 2008.

BACTERIURIA, ASYMPTOMATIC

Population
–Pregnant women.

Recommendations
▶ IDSA 2019, USPSTF 2008, AAFP 2006, ACOG/AAP 2012

–Screen for bacteriuria at first prenatal visit or at 12–16 wk gestation.
–Treat pregnant women who have asymptomatic bacteriuria with antimicrobial therapy for 4–7 d.

Sources
–USPSTF. *Asymptomatic Bacteriuria in Adults: Screening.* 2008.
–*Am Fam Physician.* 2006;74(6):985-990.
–*Clin Infect Dis.* 2019;68(10):e83-e110.

---

[a]Risk factors: African-American race or ethnicity, body mass index less than 20 kg/m², previous preterm delivery, vaginal bleeding, shortened cervix <2.5 cm, pelvic infection, bacterial vaginosis.

–American Academy of Pediatrics, American College of Obstetricians and Gynecologists. *Guidelines for Perinatal Care.* 7th ed. Elk Grove Village, Illinois and Washington, DC: AAP/ACOG, 2012:112-117.

Comment

1. Antibiotics for bacteriuria in pregnancy reduce the risk of pyelonephritis and low birth weight.

CHLAMYDIA AND GONORRHEA

Population

–Pregnant women.

Recommendations

▶ **CDC 2015, AAFP 2012, AAP/ACOG 2012**

–Screen all women at first prenatal visit.
–If infection detected, obtain test of cure 3–4 wk after treatment.
–If chlamydia detected during 1st trimester, repeat within 3–6 mo or re-test in 3rd trimester.

Sources

–CDC. *Sexually Transmitted Diseases Treatment Guidelines.* 2015.
–*Am Fam Physician.* 2012;86(12):1127-1132.
–AAP & ACOG. *Guidelines for Perinatal Care.* 7th ed. 2012.

DIABETES MELLITUS, GESTATIONAL (GDM)

Population

–Pregnant women after 24 wk of gestation.

Recommendation

▶ **USPSTF 2014**

–Recommends screening for gestational diabetes mellitus in asymptomatic pregnant women.

Source

–USPSTF. *Gestational Diabetes Mellitus: Screening.* 2014.

Recommendations

▶ **ACOG 2018**

–Perform 1-h glucose screening test with 50-g anhydrous glucose load between 24 and 28 gestational wk. Use a cutoff value of either 135 or 140 mg/dL.

–Perform early screening for undiagnosed diabetes, preferably at the initiation of prenatal care, in overweight and obese women with additional diabetic risk factors, including those with a prior history of GDM.

–Perform a 3-h glucose tolerance test if the 1-h glucose screening test is abnormal. Use either the Carpenter and Coustan criteria or the National Diabetes Data Group criteria.

–Target glucose values in women with GDM are <95 mg/dL fasting, <140 mg/dL 1-h postprandial, or <120 mg/dL 2-h postprandial.

–Screen women with GDM 6–12 wk postpartum for overt diabetes.

Source

–ACOG. *Gestational Diabetes Mellitus.* Washington (DC): American College of Obstetricians and Gynecologists (ACOG); 2018 (ACOG practice bulletin; no. 190).

Comments

1. Insufficient evidence to support screening for gestational diabetes prior to 24 gestational wk.
2. Insufficient evidence to define the optimal frequency of blood glucose testing in women with GDM. Based on the data available, consider glucose monitoring 4 times a day, once fasting and again after each meal.

DIABETES MELLITUS (DM), TYPE 2

Population

–Pregnant women.

Recommendations

▶ ADA 2018, ACOG 2018

–Screen for undiagnosed DM type 2 at first prenatal visit if risk factors for DM are present.[a]

–For all other women, screen at 24–28 wk with

- 75-g 2-h oral glucose tolerance test (OGTT) in the morning after an overnight fast of at least 8 h.
- 50-g 1-h OGTT followed by 100-g 3-h if 1 h is elevated (threshold: 130–140 mg/dL).

Sources

–*Diabetes Care* 2018;41(suppl 1).

–*Obstet Gynecol.* 2018;131(2):e49.

[a]Immigrants from Asia, Africa, South Pacific, Middle East (except Israel), Eastern Europe (except Hungary), the Caribbean, Malta, Spain, Guatemala, and Honduras.

Comments

1. Preexisting diabetes if:
   a. Fasting glucose ≥126 mg/dL.
   b. 2-h glucose ≥200 mg/dL after 75-g glucose load.
   c. Random glucose ≥200 mg/dL with classic hyperglycemic symptoms.
   d. Hemoglobin A1c ≥6.5%.
2. Criteria for GDM by 75-g 2-h OGTT if any of the following are abnormal:
   a. Fasting ≥92 mg/dL (5.1 mmol/L).
   b. 1 h ≥180 mg/dL (10.0 mmol/L).
   c. 2 h ≥153 mg/dL (8.5 mmol/L).
3. Criteria for GDM by 100-g 3-h OGTT
   a. Carpenter–Coustan:
      i. Fasting ≥95 mg/dL (5.3 mmol/L).
      ii. 1 h ≥180 mg/dL (10.0 mmol/L).
      iii. 2 h ≥155 mg/dL (8.6 mmol/L).
      iv. 3 h ≥140 mg/dL (7.8 mmol/L).
   b. National Diabetes Data Group
      i. Fasting ≥105 mg/dL (5.8 mmol/L).
      ii. 1 h ≥190 mg/dL (10.6 mmol/L).
      iii. 2 h ≥165 mg/dL (9.2 mmol/L).
      iv. 3 h ≥145 mg/dL (8.0 mmol/L).
4. A1c screening has lower sensitivity than OGTT and is not recommended as a sole screening tool.

FETAL ANEUPLOIDY

Population

–Pregnant women.

Recommendations

▶ ACOG 2016

–Offer screening to all women, ideally during first prenatal visit. The decision should be reached through informed patient choice, including discussion of sensitivity, positive screening and false-positive rates, and risks/benefits of diagnostic testing (amniocentesis and chorionic villous sampling).

–No one screening test is superior.

Source

–*Obstet Gynecol.* 2016;127(5):e123-e137.

Comment

1. Risk of chromosomal anomaly by maternal age at term:
    a. 20-y-old: 1 in 525.
    b. 30-y-old: 1 in 384.
    c. 35-y-old: 1 in 178.
    d. 40-y-old: 1 in 62.
    e. 45-y-old: 1 in 18.

GROUP B STREPTOCOCCAL (GBS) DISEASE

Population

–Pregnant women.

Recommendations

▶ CDC 2010, AAFP 2015

–Universal screening of all women at 35–37 gestational wk for GBS colonization with a vaginal–rectal swab.
–If screening is performed at 35 wk gestation, rescreening is not required for the remainder of the pregnancy.
–If screening is performed prior to 35 wk gestation, repeat screening 5 wk later or after 35 wk gestation.

Sources

–AAFP. *Clinical Recommendation: Group B Strep*. 2015.
–CDC. *Prevention of Perinatal Group B Streptococcal Disease: Revised Guidelines from CDC*. 2010.
–https://www.cdc.gov/groupbstrep/clinicians/qas-obstetric.html

Comments

1. Women who are colonized with GBS should receive intrapartum antibiotic prophylaxis to prevent neonatal GBS sepsis.
2. Even women planning a C-section benefit from GBS screening, in case of premature rupture of membranes.

HEPATITIS B VIRUS INFECTION

Population

–Pregnant women.

Recommendation

▶ USPSTF 2009, CDC 2015, ACOG 2015, AAP 2012, AAFP 2009

–Screen all women with HBsAg at their first prenatal visit.

Sources
- *Ann Intern Med.* 2009;150(12):874-876.
- ACOG/CDC. *Screening and Referral Algorithm for Hepatitis B Virus (HBV) Infection among Pregnant Women.* 2015.
- AAP/ACOG. *Guidelines for Perinatal Care.* 7th ed. 2012.
- AAFP. *Clinical Recommendation: Hepatitis.* 2009.
- CDC. *Sexually Transmitted Diseases Treatment Guidelines.* 2015.

Comments

1. Breast-feeding is not contraindicated in women with chronic HBV infection if the infant has received hepatitis B immunoglobulin (HBIG)-passive prophylaxis and vaccine-active prophylaxis.
2. All pregnant women who are HBsAg-positive should be reported to the local Public Health Department to ensure proper follow-up.
3. Immunoassays for HBsAg have sensitivity and specificity >98%. (*MMWR.* 1993;42:707)

HEPATITIS C VIRUS (HCV) INFECTION, CHRONIC

Population
- Pregnant women at increased risk.[a]

Recommendation

▶ ACOG 2012, CDC 2015
- Perform routine counseling and testing at the first prenatal visit.

Sources
- American College of Obstetricians and Gynecologists (ACOG). *Viral Hepatitis in Pregnancy.* Washington (DC): ACOG; 2007. (ACOG practice bulletin; no. 86)
- CDC. *Sexually Transmitted Diseases Treatment Guidelines.* 2015.

Comments

1. Route of delivery has not been shown to influence rate of vertical transmission of HCV infection. Reserve cesarean sections for obstetric indications only.
2. Breast-feeding is not contraindicated in women with chronic HCV infection.

---

[a]HCV risk factors: HIV infection; sexual partners of HCV-infected persons; persons seeking evaluation or care for STDs, including HIV; history of injection-drug use; persons who have ever been on hemodialysis; intranasal drug use; history of blood or blood component transfusion or organ transplant prior to 1992; hemophilia; multiple tattoos; children born to HCV-infected mothers; and health care providers who have sustained a needlestick injury.

3. HCV RNA testing should be performed for:
   a. Positive HCV antibody test result in a patient.
   b. When antiviral treatment is being considered.
   c. Unexplained liver disease in an immunocompromised patient
      with a negative HCV antibody test result.
   d. Suspicion of acute HCV infection.
4. HCV genotype should be determined in all HCV-infected persons
   prior to interferon treatment.
5. Seroconversion may take up to 3 mo.
6. Of persons with acute hepatitis C, 15%–25% resolve their
   infection; of the remaining, 10%–20% develop cirrhosis within
   20–30 y after infection, and 1%–5% develop hepatocellular
   carcinoma.
7. Patients testing positive for HCV antibody should receive a
   nucleic acid test to confirm active infection. A quantitative
   HCV RNA test and genotype test can provide useful prognostic information prior to initiating antiviral therapy. (*JAMA.*
   2007;297:724)

HERPES SIMPLEX VIRUS (HSV), GENITAL

Population
   –Pregnant women.

Recommendation

▶ CDC 2015, USPSTF 2016
   –Do not screen routinely for HSV with serologies.

Sources
   –*JAMA.* 2016;316(23):2525-2530.
   –CDC. *Sexually Transmitted Diseases Treatment Guidelines.* 2015.

Comments

1. In women with a history of genital herpes, routine serial cultures for
   HSV are not indicated in the absence of active lesions.
2. Women who develop primary HSV infection during pregnancy
   have the highest risk for transmitting HSV infection to their infants.

HUMAN IMMUNODEFICIENCY VIRUS (HIV)

Population
   –Pregnant women.

Recommendations

▶ **AAFP 2010, USPSTF 2013, ACOG 2015, CDC 2015**

–Screen all pregnant women for HIV as early as possible during each pregnancy, using an opt-out approach.

–Repeat HIV testing in 3rd trimester for women in areas with high HIV incidence or prevalence.

–Offer rapid HIV screening to women in labor who were not tested earlier in pregnancy or whose HIV is undocumented. If rapid HIV test is reactive, initiate antiretroviral prophylaxis immediately while waiting for supplemental test results.

Sources

–AAFP. *Clinical Recommendation: HIV Infection, Adolescents and Adults.* 2013.

–USPSTF. *HIV Infection: Screening.* 2013.

–CDC. *Sexually Transmitted Diseases Treatment Guidelines.* 2015.

–ACOG. Committee Opinion: Committee on Obstetric Practice and HIV Expert Work Group. *Obstet Gynecol.* 2015;125:1544-1547.

Comment

1. Rapid HIV antibody testing during labor identified 34 HIV-positive women among 4849 women with no prior HIV testing documented (prevalence: 7 in 1000). Eighty-four percent of women consented to testing. Sensitivity was 100%, specificity was 99.9%, positive predictive value was 90%. (*JAMA.* 2004;292:219)

INTIMATE PARTNER VIOLENCE

Population

–Pregnant women.

Recommendation

▶ **USPSTF 2018, ACOG 2012**

–Screen all pregnant women for intimate partner violence.

Sources

–*JAMA.* 2018;320(16):1678-1687.

–*Obstet Gynecol.* 2012;119(2):412-417.

Comments

1. Screening for intimate partner violence has the most robust evidence during pregnancy and the postpartum period.

2. Pregnant women may be at increased risk of intimate partner violence compared to their nonpregnant peers.

3. Validated interventions include home-visit interventions for psychosocial supports and brief counseling and referral to violence prevention organizations.

PREECLAMPSIA

Population
–Pregnant women.

Recommendation

▶ USPSTF 2017

–Screen with blood pressure measurements throughout pregnancy.

Source
–*JAMA.* 2017;317(16):1661-1667.

Comments

1. Screening for protein with urine dipstick has low accuracy.
2. Diagnose preeclampsia if blood pressure is $\geq$140/90 $\times$2, 4 h apart, after 20 wk gestation AND there is proteinuria ($\geq$300 mg/dL in 24 h or protein:creatinine ratio $\geq$0.3, or protein dipstick $\geq$1+), thrombocytopenia, renal insufficiency, impaired liver function, pulmonary edema, or cerebral/visual symptoms.

LEAD POISONING

Population
–Pregnant women.

Recommendations

▶ AAFP 2006, USPSTF 2006, CDC 2000, AAP 2000, ACOG 2012

–Insufficient evidence to recommend for or against routine screening for women at increased risk.[a]
–CDC and ACOG do not recommend blood lead testing of all pregnant women in the United States.
–For pregnant women with blood levels of 5 µg/dL or higher, sources of lead exposure should be identified and women should receive counseling.
  • Maternal or umbilical cord blood lead levels should be measured at delivery.

---

[a]Important risk factors for lead exposure in pregnant women include recent immigration, pica practices, occupational exposure, nutritional status, culturally specific practices such as the use of traditional remedies or imported cosmetics, and the use of traditional lead-glazed pottery for cooking and storing food.

Sources
- USPSTF. *Lead Levels in Childhood and Pregnancy: Screening.* 2006.
- *Pediatrics.* 1998;101(6):1702.
- Advisory Committee on Childhood Lead Poisoning Prevention. Recom-mendations for blood lead screening of young children enrolled in Medicaid: Targeting a group at high risk. *CDC MMWR.* 2000;49(RR14):1-13.
- AAFP. *Clinical Recommendations: Lead Poisoning.* 2006.
- *Obstet Gynecol.* 2012;120:416-420.

RH (D) INCOMPATIBILITY

Population
- Pregnant women.

Recommendations

▶ **AAFP 2010, USPSTF 2007, ACOG 2017**
- Order ABO type and Rh (D) antibody testing for all pregnant women at their first prenatal visit.
- Repeat Rh (D) antibody testing for all unsensitized Rh (D)-negative women at 24–28 wk gestation.

Sources
- http://www.guideline.gov/content.aspx?id=38619
- *Obstet Gynecol.* 2017;13:e57-70.
- http://www.uspreventiveservicestaskforce.org/3rduspstf/rh/rhrs.htm

Comment
1. Rh (D) antibody testing at 24–28 wk can be skipped if the biologic father is known to be Rh (D)-negative.

SYPHILIS

Population
- Pregnant women.

Recommendations

▶ **CDC 2015, AAFP 2018, USPSTF 2018, WHO 2017, AAP/ACOG 2017**
- Screen all pregnant women at the first prenatal visit.

–Screen again at 28 gestational wk if high risk[a] or previously untested.

Sources

–CDC. *Sexually Transmitted Diseases Treatment Guidelines*. 2015.

–USPSTF. *JAMA*. 2018;320(9):911-917.

–WHO. *Syphilis Screening and Treatment for Pregnant Woman*. 2017.

–https://www.aafp.org/patient-care/clinical-recommendations/all/syphilis.html.

–American Academy of Pediatrics; American College of Obstetricians and Gynecologists. *Guidelines for Perinatal Care*. 8th ed. Elk Grove Village, IL: American Academy of Pediatrics; American College of Obstetricians and Gynecologists; 2017.

Comments

1. A nontreponemal test (Venereal Disease Research Laboratory [VDRL] test or rapid plasma reagent [RPR] test) should be used for initial screening.
2. All reactive nontreponemal tests should be confirmed with a fluorescent treponemal antibody absorption (FTA-ABS) test.
3. If high risk, consider testing a third time at the time of delivery.
4. Syphilis is a reportable disease in every state.

THYROID DISEASE

Population

–Women who are pregnant or immediately postpartum.

Recommendations

▶ ATA 2017, AAFP 2014

–Insufficient evidence to recommend for or against routine screening of all women.

–Targeted screening of women at high risk.

–Obtain TSH levels at confirmation of pregnancy if:

- A history or current symptoms of thyroid dysfunction.
- Known thyroid antibody positivity or presence of a goiter.
- History of head or neck radiation or prior thyroid surgery.
- Age >30 y.
- Autoimmune disorders.
- History of pregnancy loss, preterm delivery, or infertility.
- Multiple prior pregnancies.

[a]High risk features include elevated community prevalence, concomitant HIV infection, and past incarceration or sex work.

- Family history of thyroid disease.
- BMI $\geq$40 kg/m^2.
- Use of amiodarone or lithium, or recent administration of iodinated radiologic contrast.
- Residing in an area of known moderate-to-severe iodine insufficiency.

Sources
  −*Thyroid*. 2017;27(3):315.
  −*Am Fam Physician*. 2014;89(4):273-278.

TOBACCO USE

Population
  −Adults.

Recommendation
▶ AAFP 2015, USPSTF 2015, ICSI 2014
  −Screen all adults for tobacco use and provide tobacco cessation interventions for those who use tobacco products.

Population
  −Pregnant women.

Recommendation
▶ AAFP 2015, USPSTF 2015, ICSI 2014
  −Screen all pregnant women for tobacco use and provide pregnancy-directed counseling and literature for those who smoke.

Sources
  −AAFP. *Clinical Preventive Service Recommendation: Tobacco Use*. 2015.
  −USPSTF. *Tobacco Smoking Cessation in Adults, Including Pregnant Women: Behavioral and Pharmacotherapy Interventions*. 2015.
  −ICSI. *Preventive Services for Adults*. 20th ed. 2014.

Comment
  1. The "5-A" framework is helpful for smoking cessation counseling:
     a. Ask about tobacco use.
     b. Advise to quit through clear, individualized messages.
     c. Assess willingness to quit.
     d. Assist in quitting.
     e. Arrange follow-up and support sessions.

Prevention

Cardiovascular Disorders

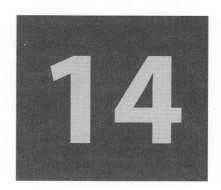

HYPERTENSION (HTN)

Population
–Persons at risk for developing HTN.[a]

Recommendations

▶ Hypertension Canada 2018, JNC 8, ACC/AHA 2014, 2017, ICSI 15th Ed 2014, ESC 2013

–Recommend weight loss, reduced sodium intake, moderate alcohol consumption, increased physical activity, potassium supplementation, and modification of eating patterns.

–Above the normal replacement levels, do not supplement K, Ca, and Mg for the prevention or treatment of HTN.

Sources
–Hypertension Canada 2018.
–*JAMA*. 2014;311(5):507-520.
–Kenning I, Kerandi H, Luehr D, et al. Institute for Clinical Systems Improvement. *Hypertension Diagnosis and Treatment*. 2014.
–*Eur Heart J*. 2013;34:2159-2219.

Population
–Patients age >65 y.

[a]Family history of HTN; African-American (black race) ancestry; overweight or obesity; sedentary lifestyle; excess intake of dietary sodium; insufficient intake of fruits, vegetables, and potassium; excess consumption of alcohol.

Comments

1. A 5 mm Hg reduction in systolic blood pressure in the population would result in a 14% overall reduction in mortality from stroke, a 9% reduction in mortality from CHD, and a 7% decrease in all-cause mortality.
2. Weight loss of as little as 10 lb (4.5 kg) reduces blood pressure and/or prevents HTN in a large proportion of overweight patients.

LIFESTYLE MODIFICATIONS FOR PREVENTION OF HYPERTENSION

- Maintain a healthy body weight for adults (BMI, 18.5–24.9 kg/m²; waist circumference <102 cm for men and <88 cm for women).
- Reduce dietary sodium intake to no more than 2000 mg sodium/d (approximately 5 g of sodium chloride). Per CHEP 2015: adequate intake 2000 mg daily (all >19-y-old) (80% in processed foods; 10% at the table or in cooking); 2000 mg sodium (Na) = 87 mmol sodium (Na) = 5 g of salt (NaCl) ~1 teaspoon of table salt.
- Engage in regular aerobic physical activity, such as brisk walking, jogging, cycling, or swimming (30–60 min per session, 4–7 d/wk or 90–150 min/wk), in addition to the routine activities of daily living. Higher intensities of exercise are not more effective. Weight training exercise does not adversely influence BP. Isometric exercise, eg, hand grip 4×2 min, 1 min rest between exercises, 3 sessions/wk shown to reduce BP.
- Limit alcohol consumption to no more than 2 drinks (eg, 24 oz [720 mL] of beer, 10 oz [300 mL] of wine, or 3 oz [90 mL] of 100-proof whiskey) per day in most men and to no more than one drink per day in women and lighter-weight persons (≤14/wk for men, ≤9/wk for women).
- Maintain adequate intake of dietary potassium (>90 mmol [3500 mg]/d). Above the normal replacement levels, do not supplement potassium, calcium, and magnesium for prevention or treatment of hypertension.
- Daily K dietary intake >80 mmol.
- Consume a diet that is rich in fruits and vegetables and in low-fat dairy products with a reduced content of saturated and total fat (Dietary Approaches to Stop Hypertension [DASH] eating plan).
- Offer advice in combination with pharmacotherapy (varenicline, bupropion, nicotine replacement therapy) to all smokers with a goal of smoking cessation.
- Consider stress management as an intervention in hypertensive patients in whom stress may be contributing to BP elevation.

Sources: CHEP 2015: http://guidelines.hypertension.ca
JACC. 2018;71(19):e127-e248

ATHEROSCLEROTIC CARDIOVASCULAR DISEASE (ASCVD), ASPIRIN THERAPY

Population
–Asymptomatic adults.

Recommendations

▶ **USPSTF 2016**

–Age 50–59 y: Initiate low dose aspirin (75–100 mg/d) if 10-y cardiovascular disease (CVD) risk is >10%, life expectancy is >10 y, and willing to take low-dose aspirin consistently for 10 y.

–Age 60–69 y: "Consider" aspirin if 10-y CVD risk is >10%, especially if at low risk for bleeding, have life expectancy >10 y, and are willing to take aspirin consistently for 10 y (fewer MIs are prevented and more GI bleeds are provoked compared to the 50–59 y age group).

–Age <50 y: evidence insufficient, benefit likely less because CVD risk is likely lower.

–Age >70 y: evidence insufficient, risk of bleeding increases significantly.

▶ **FDA 2016**

–Data do not support the general use of aspirin for primary prevention of a heart attack or stroke. Aspirin is associated with "serious risks," including increased risk of intracerebral and GI bleeding.

▶ **ACC/AHA 2019**

–Age 40–70 y: Low-dose aspirin (75–100 mg/d) might be considered for select adults who are at higher ASCVD risk[b] but not at increased bleeding risk.[c]

Sources

–USPSTF. *Aspirin Use to Prevent Cardiovascular Disease and Colorectal Cancer: Preventive Medication.* 2016.

–FDA. *Use of Aspirin for Primary Prevention of Heart Attack and Stroke.* 2016.

–*J Am Coll Cardiol.* 2019 [e-pub].

Comments

1. ACC/AHA "ABCS" of primary prevention presents risk reduction for ASCVD for mainstays of primary prevention: aspirin therapy in appropriate patients (RR 0.90), blood pressure control (RR 0.84

---

[b]A risk value is no longer given due to recent trials calling into question the value of aspirin for primary prevention. Recommend using all available risk factors when determining higher ASCVD risk.
[c]Examples of increased bleeding risk: history of previous GI or other sites bleeding, PUD, age >70 y, thrombocytopenia, coagulopathy, CKD, NSAID/steroid/anticoagulant use.

for CHD, 0.64 for stroke), cholesterol management (RR 0.75), and smoking cessation (RR 0.73). (*JACC.* 2017;69(12):1617-1636)

2. Risks of aspirin therapy: hemorrhagic stroke and GI bleeding (risk factors include age, male sex, GI ulcers, upper GI pain, concurrent NSAID/anticoagulant use, and uncontrolled hypertension).

3. Establish risk factors by the ACC/AHA pooled cohort equation (PCE) in all adults.

4. In a report showing a 50% reduction in the population's CHD mortality rate, 81% was attributable to primary prevention of CHD through tobacco cessation and lipid- and blood pressure–lowering activities. Only 19% of CHD mortality reduction occurred in patients with existing CHD (secondary prevention). (*BMJ.* 2005;331:614)

ATHEROSCLEROTIC CARDIOVASCULAR DISEASE (ASCVD), DIETARY THERAPY

Population
– All adults.

Recommendations

▶ USPSTF 2017

– Offer behavioral counseling to promote healthy diet and physical activity on an individualized basis, particularly to those interested and ready to make changes, even in the absence of obesity, abnormal blood glucose/diabetes, or dyslipidemia.

▶ AHA/ACC 2019, ESC 2016

– *Dietary guidelines:*
  • Balance calorie intake and physical activity to achieve or maintain a healthy body weight.
  • Consume diet rich in vegetables and fruits.
  • Choose whole grain, high-fiber foods.
  • Consume fish, especially oily fish, at least twice a week.
  • Limit intake of saturated fats to <7% energy, trans fats to <1% energy, and cholesterol to <300 mg/d by:
    ◦ Choosing lean meats and vegetable alternatives.
    ◦ Selecting fat-free (skim), 1% fat, and low-fat dairy products.
  • Minimize intake of beverages and foods with added sugars.
  • Choose and prepare foods with little or no salt.
  • If you consume alcohol, do so in moderation.
  • Follow these recommendations for food consumed/prepared inside *and* outside of the home.

–Recommended diets: DASH, USDA Food Pattern, or AHA Diet.

–Avoid use of and exposure to tobacco products.

▶ **CCS 2012**

–Recommend the Mediterranean, Portfolio, or DASH diets to improve lipid profiles or decrease CVD risk.

Comments

1. There is a strong correlation between healthy diet, physical activity, and incidence of CVD.
2. Behavioral counseling has shown to have a small benefit in the absence of metabolic disorders. There is better data to support behavioral interventions for patients with obesity (USPSTF, 2016) and adults with abnormal blood glucose (USPSTF, 2018).

Sources

–*J Am Coll Cardiol.* 2019 [e-pub].

–*Can J Cardiol.* 2013;29(2):151-167.

–*Eur Heart J.* 2016;37:2315-2381.

–*JAMA.* 2017:318:167-174.

–https://www.uspreventiveservicestaskforce.org/Page/Document/ RecommendationStatementFinal/obesity-in-adults-screening-and-management

–https://www.uspreventiveservicestaskforce.org/Page/Document/ RecommendationStatementFinal/screening-for-abnormal-blood-glucose-and-type-2-diabetes

ATHEROSCLEROTIC CARDIOVASCULAR DISEASE (ASCVD), STATIN THERAPY

Population

–Adults at risk for ASCVD.

Recommendations

▶ **USPSTF 2016**

–Use a low- to moderate-dose statin if age 40–75 y, and 1 or more CVD risk factors,[d] and have a calculated 10-year risk of CV event of 10% or greater.[e]

---

[d]Risk factors for CVD include dyslipidemia (LDL-C >130 mg/dL or HDL-C <40 mg/dL), diabetes, hypertension, or smoking.

[e]Use 2013 ACC/AHA PCE as a starting point for calculating risk assessment but be aware that the PCE has been shown to overestimate actual risk in multiple cohorts.

Source

–https://www.uspreventiveservicestaskforce.org/Page/Document/
UpdateSummaryFinal/statin-use-in-adults-preventive-medication1

ACC/AHA 2018

–Assess ASCVD risk:

- Adult age 40–75 with LDL-C $\geq$70 mg/dL: assess ASCVD risk using Risk Predictor Plus, http://tools.acc.org/ASCVD-Risk-Estimator-Plus/#!/calculate/estimate/
- No need for risk calculator if LDL-C $\geq$190 mg/dL or age 40–75 with diabetes, as these patients are already high-risk.

–Assess risk-enhancing factors and assess coronary calcium if risk is uncertain.[f]

–Recommend lifestyle management and drug therapy for high-risk groups.

–Statins are first-line therapy. Consider combination of statin and non-statin therapy in select patients.

–Use shared decision making when discussing use of statin. Discuss potential risk reduction, adverse effects, drug–drug interactions, out-of-pocket cost; encourage patient to verbalize what was heard; ask questions; express values and ability to adhere.

–Assess coronary artery calcium if risk is uncertain and additional information is needed.

Selected examples of candidates for coronary artery calcium measurement are:

1. Patients reluctant to start statin therapy, who want to understand risk/benefits.
2. Patients who may want to know the benefits of statin therapy after discontinuation due to side effects.
3. Older men age 55–80 or women age 60–80 with fewer risk factors, who question whether they would benefit from statin therapy.
4. Adults age 40–55 in borderline risk group (with ASCVD risk 5%–7.5%) with other factors that increase their risk.

[f]Risk enhancers: family hx premature ASCVD, persistent LDL-C $\geq$160 mg/dL, chronic kidney disease, metabolic syndrome, history of preeclampsia or premature menopause, inflammatory diseases esp. rheumatoid arthritis, psoriasis or HIV, ethnicity, eg, South Asian, persistent TG $\geq$175 mg/dL, and, in selected individuals if measured hs-CRP $\geq$2.0 mg/L, Lp(a) >50 mg/dL or >125 snmol/L, apoB $\geq$130 mg/dL, or Ankle Brachial Index (ABI) <0.9.

ASCVD GROUPS THAT BENEFIT FROM STATIN THERAPY

Risk Group	Statin Prescription
Very high-risk ASCVD[a]	High-intensity statin or maximal tolerated statin If LDL-C on statin is still ≥70 mg/dL, consider adding ezetimibe; if still ≥70, consider adding PCSK9-I
Clinical ASCVD not at very high-risk age ≤75 y	High-intensity statin or maximal tolerated statin; goal is to decrease LDL-C by ≥50%
Clinical ASCVD not at very high-risk age >75 y	If LDL-C on statin is still ≥70 mg/dL, consider adding ezetimibe
LDL-C ≥190 mg/dL	Continue high-intensity statin if tolerated or consider initiation of moderate- or high-intensity statin High-intensity statin
Diabetes (type 1 or 2) age 40–75 y	Moderate-intensity statin unless high-risk factors[b]
Diabetes age 40–75 with additional risk factors[b]	High-intensity statin
Age 0–19 y with familial hypercholesterolemia	Statin
	Consider statin
Age 20–39 y and family history, premature ASCVD and LDL-C ≥160 mg/dL	Risk discussion and consider moderate-intensity statin
Age 40–75 y and 10-y risk 5%–<7.5% with risk enhancers	Risk discussion, start moderate-intensity statin to reduce LDL-C by 30%–49%
Age 40–75 y and 10-y risk ≥7.5% to ≤20%	Risk discussion, start high-intensity statin to reduce LDL-C by ≥50%
Age 40–75 y and 10-y risk ≥20%	Clinical assessment and risk discussion
Age >75	

[a]Very high-risk ASCVD is history of multiple major ASCVD events or 1 major ASCVD event and multiple high-risk conditions. Major ASCVD events are ACS in past year, MI, ischemic stroke, symptomatic PAD. High-risk conditions are age ≥65 y, heterozygous familial hypercholesterolemia, prior CABG or PCI, diabetes, hypertension, CKD dGFR 15–59 mL/min/1.73 m^2, smoking, LDL-C ≥100 mg/dL despite statin and ezetimibe, CHF.
[b]Diabetes-specific risk enhancers are: duration of diabetes type 2 ≥10 y or type 1 ≥20 y, albuminuria ≥30 mcg/mg Cr, eGFR <60 mL/min/1.73 m^2, retinopathy, neuropathy, ABI <0.9.

STATIN INTENSITY DRUG LEVELS

High intensity (lowers LDL-C $\geq$50%)	Atorvastatin 40–80 mg Rosuvastatin 20–40 mg
Moderate intensity (lowers LDL-C 30%–49%)	Atorvastatin 10–20 mg Rosuvastatin 5–10 mg Simvastatin[a] 20–40 mg Pravastatin 40–80 mg Lovastatin 40 mg Fluvastatin XL 80 mg Fluvastatin 40 mg bid Pitavastatin 2–4 mg
Low intensity (lowers LDL-C <30%)	Simvastatin 10 mg Pravastatin 10–20 mg Lovastatin 20 mg Fluvastatin 20–40 mg Pitavastatin 1 mg

If unable to tolerate moderate- to high-intensity statin therapy, consider the use of low-intensity dosages to reduce ASCVD risk.

[a]Avoid Simvastatin 80 mg due to high risk of myopathy.

STATIN-ASSOCIATED SIDE EFFECTS

Side Effect	Frequency	Predisposing Factors	Evidence
Myalgias (no elevation CK)	1%–10%	Age, female, low BMI, Rx interactions, HIV, renal/liver/thyroid disease, Asian descent, alcohol, exertion, trauma	RCTs, observation
Myositis/Myopathy ($\uparrow$ CK)	Rare		RCTs, observation
Rhabdomyolysis ($\uparrow$ CK + renal injury)	Rare		RCTs, observation
Statin-associated autoimmune myopathy	Rare		Case reports
New-onset diabetes mellitus	More frequent if risk factors	BMI $\geq$30, FBG $\geq$100 mg/dL, metabolic syndrome, A1c $\geq$6%	RCTs, meta-analyses
Liver transaminases $\geq$3$\times$ ULN	Infrequent		RCTs, observation, case reports

Memory/Cognition	Rare: no increase in 3 RCTs		Case reports
Cancer, renal, cataracts, tendon rupture, hemorrhagic stroke, lung disease, low testosterone	Unfounded		

Source
  –*JACC.* 2019;73(24):e285-e350.

NON-STATIN CHOLESTEROL-LOWERING AGENTS

- In high-risk patients (clinical ASCVD, age <75 y; LDL-C ≥190 mg/dL; 40–75 y old with DM) who are intolerant to statins, may consider the use of non-statin cholesterol-lowering drugs.
- **Niacin**: Indicated for LDL-C elevation or fasting triglyceride ≥500 mg/dL; avoid with liver disease, persistent hyperglycemia, acute gout, or new-onset AF.
- **BAS**: Indicated for LDL-C elevation; avoid with triglycerides ≥300 mg/dL.
- **Ezetimibe**: Indicated for LDL-C elevation when combined with statin monitor transaminase levels.
- **Fibrates**: Indicated for fasting triglycerides ≥500 mg/dL; avoid the addition of Gemfibrozil to statin agent due to increased risk of muscle symptoms. Avoid fenofibrate if moderate/severe renal impairment. If needed, consider adding fenofibrate only to a low- or moderate-intensity statin.
- **Omega-3 fatty acids**: Indicated in severe fasting triglycerides ≥500 mg/dL.
- **PCSK9** (proprotein convertase subtilisin kexin 9). FDA-approved monoclonal antibodies including Alirocumab (Praluent®) and Evolocumab (Repatha®). Studies have shown decrease in LDL cholesterol most notably in patients with heterozygous familial hypercholesterolemia. FOURIER trial tested Evolocumab in combination with statin therapy against placebo plus statin therapy in patients with elevated cholesterol levels and existing cardiovascular disease. There was a modest additional reduction of LDL and composite cardiovascular events. (*NEJM* 2017;376:1713-1722)

COMPARISON OF ASCVD PREVENTION GUIDELINES

	ACC/AHA	CCS	ESC/EAS	USPSTF	VA-DoD
Risk estimator	PCE	Framingham	Score	PCE	PCE or Framingham
Treatment threshold (10-y risk)	≥7.5% age 40–75 LDL-C ≥190 mg/dL age ≥21	≥20% age 40–75 LDL-C ≥193 mg/dL	≥10% and LDL-C ≥70 mg/dL or 5%–10% and LDL-C ≥100 mg/dL age 40–65	≥10% and 1 risk factor age 40–75	≥12% for men >35 and women >45 or LDL-C ≥190 mg/dL
Treatment recommendations	Lifestyle ≥7.5% risk: M or H int. statin 5%–7.5% risk: M int. statin Select patients <5% risk or age <40 or >75 and LDL-C <190 mg/dL: consider M int. statin	Lifestyle Statin to reduce LDL-C ≥ 50% or <77 mg/dL	Lifestyle Maximally tolerated statin for target, goal of LDL-C ≤100 mg/dL reasonable for most	Lifestyle >10% risk: L to M int. statin 7.5%–10% risk: L to M int. statin for select patients	Lifestyle >12% risk: M int. statin 6%–12% risk: M int. statin for select patients
Treatment recommendations for patients with ASCVD (secondary prevention)	≤75 y: H int. statin >75 y: M int. statin	Target ≥50% reduction in LDL-C or LDL-C <77 mg/dL	Maximally tolerated statin for target Goal of LDL-C ≤70 mg/dL or ≥50% reduction reasonable	No recommendation	M int. statin Select patients with ACS, multiple uncontrolled risk factors, recurrent CV events: H int. statin

Note: H int, high intensity; M int, moderate intensity; L int, low intensity.
Source: Adapted from *JACC.* 2018;71:794-799.

Population
–Adults with diabetes.

Recommendations

▶ ADA 2019

–In all patients with hyperlipidemia and DM, recommend lifestyle modifications including:

- Diet: focusing on Mediterranean or DASH diet, the reduction of saturated fat, trans fat, and cholesterol intake; increase of n-3 fatty acids, viscous fiber, and plant stanols/sterols.
- Weight loss: if indicated.
- Physical activity.
- Smoking cessation.

–For patients of all ages with diabetes and ASCVD or 10-y risk >20%, use high-intensity statin. If LDL-C is still ≥70 mg/dL, consider adding ezetimibe (preferred) or PCSK9-I.

–For patients with diabetes and age <40 y + risk factors or >40 y without ASCVD, use moderate-intensity statin.

–Statin therapy is contraindicated in pregnancy.

–Although there is an increased risk of incident diabetes with statin use, the CV rate reduction with statins outweighed the risk of incident diabetes even for patient with a highest risk for diabetes.

–Use aspirin 25–162 mg/d in patients with diabetes and history of ASCVD. (Use clopidogrel 75 mg/d for patients with documented aspirin allergy.)

–Aspirin therapy may be considered for patients with diabetes and increased ASCVD risk, after discussion of benefits and increased risk of bleeding.

–In patients with diabetes and ASCVD, consider angiotensin-converting enzyme (ACE) inhibitor to reduce risk of CV events.

–In patients with diabetes and ASCVD, use SGLT2 I or GLP1 A as part of diabetes regimen to reduce risk.

Source
–*Diabetes Care.* 2019;42(suppl 1).

ATHEROSCLEROTIC CARDIOVASCULAR DISEASE (ASCVD), SPECIFIC RISK FACTORS

Population
  –Adults with HTN.

Recommendations

▶ **JNC 8, 2014**
  –See page 288 for JNC 8 treatment algorithms.

  Source
  –*JAMA.* 2014;311(5):507-520.

▶ **AHA/ACC 2017, Hypertension Canada 2018, ESC/ESH 2018**
  –Goal: blood pressure (BP) <140/90 mm Hg for population with stable CAD.
  –BP target <140/90 mm Hg is reasonable for the secondary prevention of CV events in patients with HTN and CAD.
  –BP target <130/80 mm Hg may be appropriate in some individuals with CAD, previous MI, stroke or transient ischemic attack (TIA), or CAD risk equivalents (carotid artery disease, PAD, abdominal aortic aneurysm), or 10-y CVD risk ≥10%.
  –In patients with an elevated DBP and CAD with evidence of myocardial ischemia, lower BP slowly, and use caution in inducing decreases in DBP <60 mm Hg in any patient with DM or who is >60 y. In older hypertensive patients with wide pulse pressures, lowering SBP may cause very low DBP values <60 mm Hg. This should alert clinicians to assess carefully any untoward signs or symptoms, especially those resulting from myocardial ischemia. Class IIa, level of evidence, C.
  –If ventricular dysfunction is present, lowering the goal to 120/80 mm Hg may be considered.

  Sources
  –*Canadian J Cardiol.* 2018;34(5):506-525.
  –Hypertension Canada 2018. http://www.hypertension.ca
  –*Eur Heart J.* 2018;39:3021-3104.
  –*JACC.* 2018;71(19):e127-e248.
  –*Circulation.* 2007;115:2761-2788.
  –*Circulation.* 2012;26:3097-3137.

Population
  –Diabetes mellitus.

Recommendations

▶ ADA 2019

–Diabetes and ASCVD or 10-y risk >15%, BP target is <130/80 if it can be safely attained.

–Diabetes and 10-y risk <15%, BP target is <140/90.

–Diabetes and BP >160/100, initiate 2 antihypertensive drugs.

–Diabetes and urinary albumin/Cr ratio >30 mg/gCr, first line are ACE inhibitors or angiotensin receptor blockers (ARBs) at maximum tolerated dose for BP treatment.

–Diabetes and pregnant, BP target is 120–160/80–105.

–Diabetes and BP >120/80, recommend lifestyle changes: weight loss, DASH diet pattern, reduce sodium and increase potassium intake, moderation of alcohol, increased physical activity.

Source

–*Diabetes Care.* 2019;42(suppl 1).

Comments

1. Avoid intensive glucose lowering in patients with a history of hypoglycemic spells, advanced microvascular or macrovascular complications, long-standing DM, or if extensive comorbid conditions are present.

2. Treat DM with BP readings of 130–139/80–89 mm Hg that persist after lifestyle and behavioral therapy with ACE inhibitor or ARB agents. Multiple agents are often needed. *Administer at least one agent at bedtime.*

3. No advantage of combining ACE inhibitor and ARB in HTN Rx (ONTARGET Trial). (*N Engl J Med.* 2008;358:1547-1559)

Population

–Adults who use tobacco.

Recommendations

▶ AHA 2019, USPSTF 2015

–Assess for tobacco use at every health care visit.

–All patients who use tobacco should be assisted and strongly advised to quit.

–Provide behavioral interventions and US FDA-approved pharmacotherapy to assist quitting.

–Recommended pharmacotherapy options for smoking cessation.

–Nicotine replacement: Patch (21, 14, 7 mg), Gum (2, 4 mg), Lozenge (2, 4 mg), Nasal spray (10 × 10 mg).

–Drug: Bupropion 150 mg SR, Varenicline (0.5, 1 mg).

Sources
-*JACC.* 2019;73(24):e285-e350.
-USPSTF. *Tobacco Smoking Cessation in Adults and Pregnant Women.* 2015.
-http://rxforchange.ucsf.edu

Recommendation

▶ ESC 2012

-Avoid passive smoking.

Source
-*Eur Heart J.* 2012;33:1635-1701.

Comment

1. New evidence on the health effects of passive smoking strengthens the recommendation on passive smoking. Smoking bans in public places, by law, lead to a decrease in incidence of myocardial infarction.

Population

-Women.

Recommendations

▶ AHA 2011, AHA 2019

-Standard CVD lifestyle recommendations.
-Limit alcohol consumption to ≤1 drink daily.
-Coronary artery calcium may further define risk in low-risk women (<7.5% 10 y).
-The benefit on perinatal outcomes of smoking cessation in pregnant women who smoke is substantial.

Sources
-*J Am Coll Cardiol.* 2011;57(12):1404-1423.
-*JACC.* 2019;73(24):e285-e350.

Comments

1. Estrogen plus progestin hormone therapy should not be used or continued.
2. Do not recommend antioxidants (vitamins E and C, and beta-carotene), folic acid, and B_{12} supplementation to prevent CHD.

STROKE

Population
–Adults.

Recommendations
▶ AHA/ASA 2014
–Treat known CV risk factors.[g]
–Obtain family history, identify high risk.
–Recommend physical activity, eg, 40 min/d, 3–4 d/wk of moderate-vigorous activity.
–Diet as in CVD prevention.
–Target BP <140/90.
–Statin therapy per AHA guidelines.

▶ FDA 2014
–FDA does not support the general use of aspirin for primary prevention of strokes or heart attacks, given risk of cerebral and gastrointestinal bleeding.

Sources
–FDA Consumer Updates 2014. https://www.fda.gov/Drugs/ResourcesForYou/Consumers/ucm390574.htm
–*Stroke*. 2011;42:517-584.
–*Stroke*. 2014;45:3754-3832.

STROKE, ATRIAL FIBRILLATION

Population
–Adults with atrial fibrillation.

Recommendations
▶ AAFP 2017
–Choose rate control, not rhythm control, for most patients.
–Prefer lenient rate control (<110), not strict rate control (<80).
–Discuss risk of stroke and bleeding with patients considering anticoagulation.

---

[g]Major modifiable risk factors: hypertension, cigarette smoke exposure, diabetes, atrial fibrillation, dyslipidemia, carotid artery stenosis, sickle cell disease, postmenopausal hormone therapy, poor diet, physical inactivity, obesity.

–Prescribe chronic anticoagulation unless low stroke risk ($CHADS_2$ <2) or specific contraindications. Options include warfarin, apixaban, dabigatran, edoxaban, or rivaroxaban.

–Do not give dual treatment with anticoagulant and antiplatelet therapy.

Source

–*Am Fam Physician*. 2017;96(5):332-333.

▶ AHA/ACC 2014, 2015

–Prioritize rate control; consider rhythm control if this is the first event, and if it occurs in a young patient with minimal heart disease or if symptomatic.

–Rate control goal is <110 beats/min in patients with stable ventricular function (ejection fraction [EF] >40%).

–Antithrombotic therapy is required. Anticoagulation or antiplatelet therapy is determined by ACC/AHA or CHA_2DS_2VASc (nonvalvular atrial fibrillation) guidelines.

–For patients with AF who have mechanical valves, use warfarin with an international normalized ratio (INR) target of 2–3 or 2.5–3.5, depending on the type and location of prosthesis.

–For patients with nonvalvular AF with a history of stroke, TIA or $CHA_2DS_2VASc \geq 2$, use oral anticoagulation: warfarin (INR: 2–3) or direct oral anticoagulants (DOACs) (novel oral anticoagulation agents)—see treatment.

–In patients treated with warfarin, perform INR weekly until INR is stable and at least monthly when INR is in range and stable.

–Evaluate renal function prior to initiation of direct thrombin or factor Xa inhibitors and reevaluate when clinically indicated and at least annually.

–Initially identify low-risk AF patients who do not require antithrombotic therapy (CHA_2DS_2VASc score, 0 for men, 1 for women). Offer oral anticoagulant (OAC) to patients with at least 1 risk factor (except when the only risk is being a woman). Address patient's individual risk of bleeding (BP control, discontinuing unnecessary medications such as ASA or nonsteroidal anti-inflammatory drugs).

–In nonvalvular AF with $CHA_2DS_2VASc = 0$, consider no antithrombotic therapy or treatment with ASA or an OAC.

–Following coronary revascularization (PCI or surgical) in patients with $CHA_2DS_2VASc \geq 2$, consider using Clopidogrel with OAC but without ASA.

Sources

–*Circulation*. 2014;130(23):e199-e267.

–*JAMA*. 2015;313(19):1950-1962.

Comments

1. Strokes and nonfatal strokes are reduced in diabetic patients by lower BP targets (<130/80 mm Hg). In the absence of harm, this benefit appears to justify the lower BP goal.
2. Average stroke rate in patients with risk factors is approximately 5% per year.
3. Adjusted-dose warfarin and antiplatelet agents reduce absolute risk of stroke.
4. Women have a higher prevalence of stroke than men.
5. Women have unique risk factors for stroke, such as pregnancy, hormone therapy, and higher prevalence of hypertension in older ages.

▶ **ESC 2012, 2016**

–ESC recommends the CHA_2DS_2VASc score as more predictive for stroke risk, especially with a low $CHADS_2$ score. DOACs offer better efficacy, safety, and convenience compared with OAC with VKAs.
–In high-risk patients unsuitable for anticoagulation, dual antiplatelet therapy (ASA plus clopidogrel) is reasonable.

Sources

–*Eur Heart J.* 2016;37:2893-2962.
–*Eur Heart J.* 2012;33:2719-2747.

Comments

1. Absolute CVA risk reduction with dual antiplatelet Rx is 0.8% per year balanced by increased bleeding risk 0.7% ACTIVE Trial.
2. In high-risk patients with history of TIA/minor ischemic stroke, dual antiplatelet therapy (ASA + Plavix), started in the first 24 h, is superior to ASA alone in preventing stroke in the first 90 d, without having increased risk of hemorrhage.

Recommendations

▶ **HRS 2014, 2015**

–Given the impact of AF on stroke and the association of AF with cognitive dysfunction, brain imaging may improve the care of AF patients by helping to stratify stroke risk in AF patients. Presence of subclinical brain infarcts is robustly associated with the subsequent risk of stroke. Short-term risk of stroke after TIA was 3-fold higher in patients with a brain infarct on MRI compared to those without.
–Compared to warfarin, DOACs offer relative efficacy, safety, and convenience. Warfarin efficacy and safety depend on the quality of anticoagulation control, as reflected by the average time in therapeutic range (TTR). Due to the difficulty of achieving therapeutic INRs

quickly after starting warfarin, an increased risk of stroke has been observed in the 30 d after initiation of warfarin.

–In patients with nonvalvular atrial fibrillation, a high SAMe-TT2R2 score (reflecting poor anticoagulation control with poor time in therapeutic range) was associated with more bleeding, adverse cardiovascular events, and mortality during follow-up.

Sources
–*Heart Rhythm.* 2015;12(1):e5-e25.
–*Am J Med.* 2014;127(11):1083-1088.

Recommendations
▶ CCS 2012

–Stratify all patients using $CHADS_2$ and HASBLED risk scores. Calculate $CHADS_2$-VaSc score if $CHADS_2 = 0$. Recommend OAC therapy to all patients with $CHADS_2 = 2$ and most of the patients with $CHADS_2 = 1$.
–When OAC therapy is recommended, prefer dabigatran and rivaroxaban over warfarin. Rate control goal is <100 beats/min. In stable CAD, give ASA (75–325 mg) for $CHADS_2 = 0$, OAC for most $CHADS_2 = 1$. In high-risk patients with ACS, consider ASA + clopidogrel + OAC (with adequate assessment of risk of stroke, recurrent CAD events, and hemorrhage).

Source
–*Can J Cardiol.* 2012;28:125-136.

STROKE, SPECIFIC RISK FACTORS

Population
–HTN.

Recommendations
▶ JNC 8

–Treat to goal SBP <140 mm Hg.
–If age ≥60 y, treat to <150/90 mm Hg.
–If comorbid diabetes or chronic kidney disease, treat to <140/90 mm Hg.

▶ ACC/AHA 2017

–Treat to goal <130/80 mm Hg.
–If ASCVD risk <10%, treat to goal <140/90.

Comment
1. See page 288 for JNC-8 treatment algorithms.

Sources
- *JACC*. 2018;71(19):e127-e248.
- *JAMA*. 2014;311(5):507-520.
- *Stroke*. 2011;42:517-584.

Population
- DM.

Recommendations

▶ AHA/ASA 2011

- Sixfold increase in stroke.
- Short-term glycemic control does not lower macro vascular events.
- HgA1c goal is <6.5%.
- Goal is <130/80 mm Hg.
- Statin therapy.
- Consider ACE inhibitor or ARB therapy for further stroke risk reduction.

Source
- *Stroke*. 2011;42:517-584.

Population
- Asymptomatic carotid artery stenosis (CAS).

Recommendations

▶ USPSTF 2014, AHA/ASA 2014

- No indication for general screening for CAS with ultrasonography.
- Screen for other stroke risk factors and treat aggressively.
- ASA and statin unless contraindicated.
- Prophylactic carotid endarterectomy (CEA) for patients with high-grade (>70%) CAS by ultrasonography when performed by surgeons with low (<3%) morbidity/mortality rates may be useful in selected cases depending on life expectancy, age, sex, and comorbidities.
- However, recent studies have demonstrated that "best" medical therapy results in a stroke rate <1%.
- The number needed to treat (NNT) in published trials to prevent 1 stroke in 1 y in this asymptomatic group varies from 84 up to 2000. (*J Am Coll Cardiol*. 2011;57(8):e16-e94)

Sources
- USPSTF. *Carotid Artery Stenosis*. https://www. uspreventiveservicestaskforce.org/Page/Document/ RecommendationStatementFinal/carotid-artery-stenosis-screening
- *Neurology*. 2011;77:751-758.
- *Neurology*. 2011;77:744-750.

–*Stroke*. 2011;42:517-584.
–*Stroke*. 2014;45:3754-3832.

Population

–Symptomatic CAS.

Recommendations

▶ ASA/ACCF/AHA/AANN/AANS/ACR/CNS 2011

–Optimal timing for CEA is within 2 wk of posttransient ischemic attack.
–CEA plus medical therapy is effective within 6 mo of symptom onset with >70% CAS.
–Intense medical therapy alone is indicated if the occlusion is <50%.
–Intensive medical therapy plus CEA may be considered with obstruction 50%–69%.
–Limit surgery to male patients with a low perioperative stroke/death rate (<6%) and should have a life expectancy of at least 5 y.

Sources

–*J Am Coll Cardiol*. 2011;57(8):1002-1038.
–*Neurology*. 2005;65(6):794-801.
–*Arch Intern Med*. 2011;171(20):1794-1795.
–*Stroke*. 2011;42:227-276, 517-584.

Comments

1. Treat asymptomatic CAS aggressively.
2. Individualize surgical intervention, guided by comparing comorbid medical conditions and life expectancy to the surgical morbidity and mortality.
3. Atherosclerotic intracranial stenosis: Use ASA in preference to warfarin.
4. Warfarin—significantly higher rates of adverse events with no benefit over ASA. (*N Engl J Med*. 2005;352(13):1305-1316)
5. Qualitative findings (embolic signals and plaque ulceration) may identify patients who would benefit from asymptomatic CEA.

Population

–Cryptogenic CVA.
–Hyperlipidemia.

Recommendations

▶ ASA/ACCF/AHA/AANN/AANS/ACR/CNS 2011

–Carotid artery stenting is associated with increased nonfatal stroke frequency but this is offset by decreased risk of MI post-CEA.
–Cryptogenic CVA with patent foramen ovale (PFO) should receive ASA 81 mg/d.

Sources
- –*J Am Coll Cardiol.* 2011;57(8):1002-1044.
- –*J Am Coll Cardiol.* 2009;53(21):2014-2018.
- –*N Engl J Med.* 2012;366:991-999.
- –*N Engl J Med.* 2013;368:1083-1091.

Comments

1. Consider referral to tertiary center for enrollment in randomized trial to determine optimal Rx.
2. Closure I trial demonstrated no benefit at 2 y of PFO closure device over medical therapy.
3. In 2013, the PC Trial also failed to demonstrate significant benefit in reducing recurrent embolic events in patients undergoing PFO closure compared to medical therapy, at 4 y follow-up.

Population

–Sickle cell disease.

Recommendations

▶ ASA/ACCF/AHA/AANN/AANS/ACR/CNS 2011

- –Transfusion therapy (target reduction of hemoglobin S from a baseline of >90% to <30%) is effective for reducing stroke risk in those children at elevated stroke risk (*Class I; level of evidence, B*).
- –Begin screening with transcranial Doppler (TCD) at age 2 y.
- –Use transfusion therapy for patients at high-stroke risk per TCD (high cerebral blood flow velocity >200 cm/s).
- –Frequency of screening not determined.

Sources
- –*J Am Coll Cardiol.* 2011;57(8):1002-1044.
- –*ASH Education Book.* 2013;2013(1):439-446.

Population

–Primary prevention in women.

Recommendations

▶ ACC/ASA 2014

- –Higher lifetime risk, third leading cause of death in women, 53.5% of new recurrent strokes occur in women.
- –Sex-specific risk factors: pregnancy, preeclampsia, gestational diabetes, oral contraceptive use, postmenopausal hormone use, changes in hormonal status.
- –Risk factors with a stronger prevalence in women: migraine with aura, atrial fibrillation, diabetes, hypertension, depression, psychosocial stress.

Source
   –*Circulation.* 2011;123:1243-1262.

Population
   –Oral contraceptives/menopause, postmenopausal hormone therapy.

Recommendations

▶ ACC/ASA 2014
   –Stroke risk with low-dose OC users is about 1.4–2 times that of non-OC users.
   –Measure BP prior to initiation of hormonal contraception therapy.
   –Routine screening for prothrombotic mutations prior to initiation of hormonal contraception is not useful.
   –Among OC users, aggressive therapy of stroke risk factors may be reasonable.
   –Hormone therapy (conjugated equine estrogen with or without medroxyprogesterone) should not be used for primary or secondary prevention of stroke in postmenopausal women.
   –Selective estrogen receptor modulators, such as raloxifene, tamoxifen, or tibolone, should not be used for primary prevention of stroke.

Source
   –*Stroke.* 2014;45:1545-1588.

$SAM_E TT_2 R_2$ SCORE	
Sex (female)	1
Age >60	1
Medical history (>2 comorbidities: HTN, DM, CAD/MI, PAD, CHF, history of stroke, pulmonary disease, hepatic or renal disease)	1
Treatment (rhythm control strategy) (interacting medications, eg, beta-blocker, verapamil, amiodarone)	1
Tobacco use (within 2 y)	2
Race (non-white)	2
Maximum points	8
Interpretation	Score >2 = DOAC
	Score 0–2 = VKA with TTR
	>65%–70%

Source: Fauchier L, Angoulvant D, Lip GY. The SAM_E-$TT_2 R_2$ score and quality of anticoagulation in atrial fibrillation: a simple aid to decision-making on who is suitable (or not) for vitamin K antagonists. doi: http://dx.doi.org/10.1093/europace/euv088.

VENOUS THROMBOEMBOLISM (VTE) PROPHYLAXIS IN NONSURGICAL PATIENTS

Population
–Hospitalized medical patients.

Recommendations

▶ ASH 2018

–In acutely ill patients (hospitalized, not in ICU/CCU), determine risk for VTE using Padua Prediction Score or IMPROVE score (Table I).

–Consider determining risk of bleeding using IMPROVE bleeding score or risk factors (Table II, Table III).

–If acutely ill, use UFH, LMWH, or fondaparinux. Prefer LMWH or fondaparinux over UFH.

–If critically ill (in ICU/CCU), use UFH or LMWH, prefer LMWH.

–If acutely or critically ill, prefer pharmacologic over mechanical prophylaxis. If not using pharmacological prophylaxis, prefer mechanical over none.

–Do not use both pharmacological and mechanical prophylaxis together.

–For mechanical prophylaxis, use pneumatic compression or graduated compression stockings.

–Do not use DOACs for prophylaxis unless on DOAC for some other reason.

–If acutely ill, do not use extended duration outpatient prophylaxis. Give only while inpatient.

–High VTE risk, high bleeding risk: use mechanical prophylaxis.

–High VTE risk, unable to use pharmacologic or mechanical: use aspirin.

–Do not use VTE prophylaxis in chronically ill (including nursing home), outpatients with minor risk factors, or low-risk long-distance travelers (>4 h).

–For high-risk long-distance travelers: use graduated compression stockings or LMWH.

Sources

–*Blood Adv.* 2018;2:3198-3225.

–American Society of Hematology 2018. *Guidelines for Management of Venous Thromboembolism: Prophylaxis for Hospitalized and Nonhosptialized Medical Patients.*

–*JAMA.* 2012;307:306.

TABLE I: RISK FACTORS FOR VTE IN HOSPITALIZED MEDICAL PATIENTS—PADUA PREDICTIVE SCALE	
Risk Factor	**Points**
Active cancer[a]	3
Previous VTE	3
Reduced mobility[b]	3
Underlying thrombophilic disorder[c]	3
Recent (<1 mo) trauma or surgery	2
Age (>70 y)	1
Congestive heart failure (CHF) or respiratory failure	1
Acute MI or stroke	1
Acute infection or inflammatory disorder	1
Obesity (BMI >30)	1
Thrombophilic drugs (hormones, tamoxifen, erythroid stimulating agents, lenalidomide, bevacizumab)	1
High risk: >4 points—11% risk of VTE without prophylaxis	
Low risk: <3 points—0.3% risk of VTE without prophylaxis	
IMPROVE VTE RISK SCALE	
Risk Factor	**Points**
Previous VTE	3
Known thrombophilia	2
Lower limb paralysis	2
Active cancer	2
Immobilization ≥7 d	1
ICU/CCU stay	1
Age >60 y	1
Score	Risk of VTE
0–1	0.5%
2–3	1.5%
≥4	5.7%

[a]Local or distant metastases and/or chemotherapy or radiation in prior 6 mo.
[b]Bedrest with bathroom privileges for at least 3 d.
[c]Antithrombin, protein C/S, factor V leiden, prothrombin or antiphospholipid defects.

TABLE II: RISK FACTORS FOR BLEEDING (*CHEST.* 2011;139:69-79)

Risk Factor[a,b]	N = % of Patients	Overall Risk
Active gastroduodenal ulcer	2.2	4.15
GI bleed <3 mo previous	2.2	3.64
Platelet count <50 K	1.7	3.37
Age ≥85 y (vs. 40 y)	10	2.96
Hepatic failure (INR[c] >1.5)	2	2.18
Renal failure (GFR[d] <30 mL/min)	11	2.14
ICU admission	8.5	2.10
Current cancer	10.7	1.78
Male sex	49.4	1.48

[a]Although not studied in medical patients, antiplatelet therapy would be expected to increase risk of bleeding.
[b]Go to www.outcomes-umassmed.org/IMPROVE/risk_score/vte/index.html to calculate the risk of bleeding for individual patients.
[c]International normalized ratio.
[d]Glomerular filtration rate.

TABLE III: IMPROVE BLEEDING RISK SCALE

Risk Factor	Points
Renal failure (GFR 30–59)	1
Male vs. female	1
Age 40–80 y	1.5
Current cancer	2
Rheumatic disease	2
Central venous catheter	2
ICU/CCU stay	2.5
Renal failure (GFR <30)	2.5
Hepatic failure (INR >1.5)	2.5
Age >85 y	3.5
Platelets <50k	4
Bleeding in last 3 mo	4
Active gastroduodenal ulcer	4.5
Score	Bleeding Risk (major/any)
<7	0.4%/1.5%
≥7	4.1%/7.9%

Recommendations

▶ ACCP 2016, ACP 2011

–Do not use pharmacologic prophylaxis or mechanical prophylaxis in low-risk patients.

–Give anticoagulant therapy to high-risk patients.

- Thromboprophylaxis with low-molecular-weight heparin (LMWH)—equivalent of enoxaparin 40 mg SQ daily; fondaparinux 2.5 mg SQ daily. Only use low-dose unfractionated heparin (UFH) 5000 units bid or tid in patients with significant renal disease. UFH has a 10-fold increased risk of heparin-induced thrombocytopenia (HIT). Women are 2.5 times likely to develop HIT compared to men.
- If patient is bleeding or at high risk of bleeding (see Table II), give mechanical prophylaxis with graduated compression stockings (GCS) or intermittent pneumatic compression (IPC).
- When bleeding risk decreases, substitute pharmacologic thromboprophylaxis for mechanical prophylaxis.
- Continue thromboprophylaxis for duration of hospital stay.
- Do not offer extended prophylaxis after discharge for medical patients, but consider it if patient has underlying thrombotic risk (see Table IV).

Sources

–*Ann Intern Med.* 2011;155:625-632.

–*Chest.* 2016;149:315-352.

–http://www.uwhealth.org/files/uwheath/docs/anticoagulation/VTE

TABLE IV: HEREDITARY THROMBOPHILIC DISORDERS		
Disorder	% of US Population	Increase in Lifetime of Risk of Clot
Resistance to activated protein C (factor V Leiden mutation)	5–6	3×
Prothrombin gene mutation	2–3	2.5×
Elevated factor 8 (>175% activity)	6–8	2–3×
Elevated homocysteine	10–15	1.5–2×
Protein C deficiency	0.37	10×
Protein S deficiency	0.5	10×
Antithrombin deficiency	0.1	25×
Homozygous factor V Leiden	0.3	60×

Comments

1. **Clinical perspective**

   a. Routine ultrasound screening for DVT is not recommended in any group.

   b. 150–200,000 deaths from VTE in the United States per year. Hospitalized patients have a VTE risk which is 130-fold greater than that of community residents. (*Mayo Clin Proc.* 2001;76:1102)

   c. Neither heparin nor warfarin is recommended prophylactically for patients with central venous catheters.

   d. In higher risk long-distance travelers, frequent ambulation, calf muscle exercises, aisle seat, and below-the-knee graduated compression stockings (GCS) are recommended over aspirin or anticoagulants.

   e. Treat hospitalized inpatients with solid tumors without additional risk factors for VTE (history of DVT, thrombophilic drugs, immobilization) with prophylactic dose LMWH.

   f. Be cautious in patients with Ccr <20–30 mL/min—UFH or dalteparin (half dose) preferred.

   g. Consider adjusted LMWH dose in patients <50 kg or >110 kg in weight. Monitor with heparin anti 10a activity testing.

   h. Inferior vena cava (IVC) filter indicated in patients with diagnosed DVT with or without pulmonary embolism (PE) who cannot be anticoagulated because of bleeding. There are no other situations where a filter has been proven to be beneficial.

   i. Do not use IVC filter prophylactically.

   j. Although several studies have shown survival benefit for VTE prophylaxis in surgical patients, this has not been proven in medical patients. (*N Engl J Med.* 2011;365:2463) (*N Engl J Med.* 2007;356:1438)

   k. In patients with cancer and VTE, use LMWH. The new OACs are being tested and will probably have a role in cancer-related VTE in the near future. Warfarin is inferior to LMWH. (*Lancet Oncol.* 2008;9:577) (*Thromb Res.* 2012;130:853)

   l. In patients with mechanical heart valves, use warfarin for anticoagulation. The direct oral anticoagulants (DOACs) are inferior. (*N Engl J Med.* 2013;369:1206)

VENOUS THROMBOEMBOLISM (VTE) IN SURGICAL PATIENTS

Population
–Adults preparing for surgery.

Recommendations

▶ ACCP 2016

–Stratify surgical risk

- Low risk—<40 y, minor surgery[h], no risk factors[i], Caprini score <2 (see Table V).
- Intermediate risk—minor surgery plus risk factors, age 40–60 y, major surgery with no risk factors, Caprini score 3–4.
- High risk—major surgery plus risk factors, high-risk medical patient, major trauma, spinal cord injury, craniotomy, total hip or knee arthroplasty (THA, TKA), thoracic, abdominal, pelvic cancer surgery.

–Employ preventive measures

- Early ambulation—consider mechanical prophylaxis and intermittent pneumatic compression, graduated compression stocking (IPC or GCS).
- UFH 5000 U SQ q 8–12 h should ONLY be used in patients with renal disease with a Ccr <20–30 mL/min.
- LMWH equivalent to enoxaparin 40 mg SQ 2 h before surgery then daily or 30 mg q12h SQ starting 8–12 h postop.
- Fondaparinux 2.5 mg SQ daily starting 8–12 h postop.
- LMWH—equivalent to enoxaparin 40 mg SQ 2 h preoperative then daily or 30 mg SQ q12h starting 8–12 h postop and also use mechanical prophylaxis with IPC or GCS.
- Extend prophylaxis for as long as 28–35 d in high-risk patients. In THA, TKA ortho patients, acceptable VTE prophylaxis also includes rivaroxaban 10 mg/d, dabigatran 225 mg/d, adjusted dose warfarin, and aspirin, although LMWH is preferred. DOACs are likely to play a larger role in the future as trials continue to show superiority over warfarin. (*Ann Int Med.* 2013;159:275) (*Thromb Haemot.* 2011;105:444)
- If high risk of bleeding, use IPC alone. (*Ann Intern Med.* 2012;156:710, 720) (*JAMA.* 2012;307:294)

---

[h]Eye, ear, laparoscopy, cystoscopy, and arthroscopic operations.
[i]Prior VTE, cancer, stroke, obesity, congestive heart failure pregnancy, thrombophilic medications (tamoxifen, raloxifene, lenalidomide, thalidomide, erythroid-stimulating agents).

TABLE V: CAPRINI RISK STRATIFICATION MODEL			
1 Point	**2 Points**	**3 Points**	**5 Points**
• Age 41–60 y • Minor surgery • BMI >251 g/m² • Swollen legs • Varicose veins • Pregnancy or postpartum • History of recurrent spontaneous abortion • Sepsis (<1 mo) • Lung disease • History of acute MI • Congestive heart failure (CHF) (<1 mo) • History of inflammatory bowel disease • Medical patient at bed rest	• Age 61–74 y • Arthroscopic surgery • Major open surgery >45 min • Laparoscopic surgery • Malignancy • Confined to bed • Immobilizing cast • Central venous catheter	• Age >75 y • History VTE • Family history of VTE • Factor V Leiden • Prothrombin gene mutation • Lupus anticoagulant • Elevated homocysteine • Other congenital or acquired thrombophilia	• Stroke (<1 mo) • Elective arthroplasty; hip, pelvis, or leg fracture • Acute spinal cord injury (<1 mo)
		Caprini score <3: low risk Caprini score 3–4: intermediate risk Caprini score >5: high risk	

- Do not use UFH for prophylaxis if Ccr is >20 cc/min. There is a 10-fold increased risk of HIT compared to LMWH.

Sources
  –*Chest.* 2016;149:315.
  –http://www.fda.gov/Drugs/ResourcesForYou/Consumers/ucm390574.htm

Comments
1. **Clinical points**
   a. 75%–90% of surgical bleeding is structural. VTE prophylaxis adds minimally to risk of bleeding.
   b. With creatinine clearance <20 to 30 cc/min UFH with partial thromboplastin time (PTT) monitoring is preferred (decrease dose if PTT prolonged). In all other situations LMWH or DOACs are preferred to reduce the risk HIT.

    c. Patients with liver disease and prolonged INR are still at risk for clot. Individualize risk-to-benefit ratio of VTE prophylaxis.

    d. Epidural anesthesia—to place catheter wait 18 h after daily prophylactic dose of LMWH, and 24 h after prophylactic dose of fondaparinux. For patients on BID therapeutic LMWH anticoagulation or once daily LMWH, wait more than 24 h before placing epidural catheter. Patients on DOACs should hold their anticoagulation for 3–5 days. After placing or removing an epidural catheter hold on starting anticoagulation for 6–8 h.

    e. Do not place prophylactic IVC filter for high-risk surgery.

    f. For cranial and spinal surgery patients at low risk for VTE use mechanical prophylaxis—high-risk patients should have pharmacologic prophylaxis added to mechanical prophylaxis once hemostasis is established and bleeding risk decreased.

    g. Patients at high risk of bleeding[j] with major surgery should have mechanical prophylaxis (IPC, GCS)—initiate anticoagulant prophylaxis if risk is lowered.

    h. Surgical patients receive indicated prophylaxis 60% of the time compared to 40% in medical patients.

[j]SELECTED FACTORS IN THE RISING RISK OF MAJOR BLEEDING COMPLICATIONS:

General Risk Factors:

Active bleeding, previous major bleed, known untreated bleeding disorder, renal or liver failure, thrombocytopenia, acute stroke, uncontrolled high BP, concomitant use of anticoagulants, or antiplatelet therapy.

Procedure-Specific Risk Factors:

Major abdominal surgery—extensive cancer surgery, pancreatic-duodenectomy, hepatic resection, cardiac surgery, thoracic surgery (pneumonectomy or extended resection). Procedures where bleeding complications have especially severe consequences: craniotomy, spinal surgery, spinal trauma.

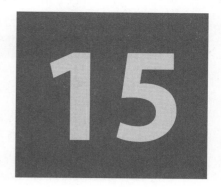

Disorders of the Skin, Breast, and Musculoskeletal System

BACK PAIN, LOW

Population
–Adults.

Recommendation

▶ AAFP 2004, USPSTF 2004

–Insufficient evidence for or against the use of interventions to prevent low-back pain in adults in primary care settings.

Sources
–AAFP. *Clinical Recommendations: Low Back Pain.* 2004.
–USPSTF. *Low Back Pain.* 2004.

Comments
1. Topic is now inactive at USPSTF.
2. Insufficient evidence to support back strengthening exercises, mechanical supports, or increased physical activity to prevent low-back pain.
3. Meta-analyses in *Lancet* 2018;391:2368-2383, *Am J Epidemiol.* 2018;187(5):1093-1101, and *JAMA Intern Med.* 2016;176(2):199-208:
   a. Conclude that exercise alone or exercise in combination with education are effective for preventing low-back pain.
   b. Evidence that education alone, back belts, and shoe insoles are not effective.
   c. Exercises that were studied and shown to be effective are a combination of strengthening with either stretching or aerobic exercise, 2–3 times/wk.

BREAST CANCER

Population
–Adult women.

Recommendations

▶ NCCN 2019

–If a woman is at high risk secondary to a strong family history or very early onset of breast or ovarian cancer, offer genetic counseling.

–Healthy lifestyle:

- Breast cancer risks associated with combined estrogen/ progesterone therapy ≥3–5 y duration of use.
- Limit alcohol consumption.
- Exercise: at least 150 min/wk of moderate intensity, or at least 75 min/wk of vigorous aerobic physical activity.
- Weight control.
- Breast-feeding.

–Risk-reducing agents:

- Discussion of relative and absolute risk reducing with tamoxifen, raloxifene, or aromatase inhibitors.
- Contraindications to tamoxifen or raloxifene: history of deep vein thrombosis, pulmonary embolus, thrombotic stroke, transient ischemic attack, or known inherited clotting trait.
- Contraindications to tamoxifen, raloxifene, and aromatase inhibitors: current pregnancy or pregnancy potential without effective nonhormonal method of contraception. Common and serious adverse effects of tamoxifen, raloxifene, or aromatase inhibitors with emphasis on age-dependent risks.

–Risk-reducing surgery:

- Risk-reducing mastectomy should generally be considered only in women with a genetic mutation conferring a high risk for breast cancer, compelling family history, or possibly with prior thoracic RT at <30 y of age. While this approach has been previously considered for LCIS, the currently preferred approach is risk-reducing therapy. The value of risk-reducing mastectomy in women with deleterious mutations in other genes associated with a 2-fold or greater risk for breast cancer (based on large epidemiologic studies) in the absence of a compelling family history of breast cancer is unknown.

▶ Minimize Known Risk Factor Exposure

–Hormone Replacement Therapy

- Approximately 26% increased incidence of invasive breast cancer with combination hormone replacement therapy (HRT) (estrogen and progesterone-Prempro).
- Estrogen alone with mixed evidence—unlikely to increase risk of breast cancer significantly (decreases risk in African-Americans).

–Ionizing Radiation to Chest and Mediastinum

- Increased risk begins approximately 10 y after exposure. Risk depends on dose and age at exposure (woman with radiation from age 15 to 30 y at highest risk). These patients often have received mediastinal radiation for Hodgkin Lymphoma.

–Obesity

- In Women's Health Initiative (WHI), relative risk (RR) = 2.85 for breast CA for women >82.2 kg compared with women <58.7 kg only in postmenopausal women.

–Alcohol

- RR for intake of 4 alcoholic drinks/day is 1.32.
- RR increases approximately 7% for each drink per day.
- Family history—risk is doubled if a single first-degree relative develops breast cancer. Fivefold increased risk if 2 first-degree relatives are diagnosed with breast cancer. (*Breast CA Res Treat.* 2012;133:1097)

–Factors of Unproven or Disproven Association

- Abortions.
- Environmental factors.
- Diet and vitamins.
- Underarm deodorant/antiperspirants—no evidence to support increased risk of breast CA. (*J Natl Cancer Inst.* 2002;94:1578)

▶ Therapeutic Approaches to Reduce Breast Cancer Risk

–Tamoxifen (Postmenopausal and High-Risk Premenopausal Women)

- Treatment with tamoxifen for 5 y reduced breast CA risk by 40%–50%. (*Ann Intern Med.* 2013;159:698-718)
- Meta-analysis shows RR = 2.4 (95% confidence interval [CI], 1.5–4.0) for endometrial CA and 1.9 (95% CI, 1.4–2.6) for venous thromboembolic events.

–Raloxifene (Postmenopausal Women)

- Similar effect as tamoxifen in reduction of invasive breast CA, but does not reduce the incidence of noninvasive tumors—studied only in postmenopausal women.

- Similar risks as tamoxifen for venous thrombosis, but no risk of endometrial CA or cataracts. (*Lancet.* 2013;381:1827)

–**Aromatase Inhibitors**
- Anastrozole reduces the incidence of new primary breast CAs by 50% compared with tamoxifen; similar results have been reported with letrozole and exemestane treatment (*Lancet.* 2014;383:1041). Aromatase inhibitor use as a prevention of breast cancer will reduce the risk of developing breast cancer by 3%–5%.
- Harmful effects of aromatase inhibitors include decreased bone mineral density and increased risk of fracture, hot flashes, increased falls, decreased cognitive function, fibromyalgia, and carpal tunnel syndrome. There are no life-threatening side effects.

–**Prophylactic Bilateral Mastectomy (High-Risk Women)**
- Reduces risk of breast cancer as much as 90%.
- Approximately 6% of high-risk women undergoing bilateral mastectomies were dissatisfied with their decision after 10 y. Regrets about mastectomy were less common among women who opted not to have breast reconstruction.

–**Prophylactic Salpingo-oophorectomy among *BRCA*-Positive Women**
- Breast CA incidence decreased as much as 50%.
- Nearly all women experience some sleep disturbances, mood changes, hot flashes, and bone demineralization, but the severity of these symptoms varies greatly.
- Perform salpingo-oophorectomy in BRCA 1 patients at 35 y of age and >40 y of age in BRCA 2 patients.
- In patients who have uterus removed as well, it is safe to give estrogen replacement. (*Eur J Cancer.* 2016;52:138)

–**Exercise**
- Exercising >120 min/wk results in average risk reduction of developing breast cancer by 30%–40%. There is also a 30% reduction in breast cancer recurrence in patients who have had breast CA. (*Eur J Cancer.* 2016;52:138)
- The effect may be greatest for premenopausal women of normal or low body weight.

–**Breast-Feeding**
- The RR of breast CA is decreased 4.3% for every 12 mo of breast-feeding, in addition to 7% for each birth.

–**Pregnancy before Age 20 y**
- Approximately 50% decrease in breast CA compared with nulliparous women or those who give birth after age 35 y.

–**Dense Breasts**

- Women have increased risk of breast CA proportionate to breast density. Relative risk 1.79 for 50% density and 4.64 for women with >75% breast density. (*Cancer Epidemiol Biomarkers Prev.* 2006;15:1159) (*Br J Cancer.* 2011;104:871)
- No known interventional method to reduce breast density.
- Adding ultrasound to mammography will improve sensitivity and specificity and is more accurate than tomosynthesis without radiation exposure. (*J Clin Oncol.* 2016;34:1840, 1882)

▶ **USPSTF 2013**

Population

–Women age ≥35 y.

Recommendations

–Shared informed decision making.

–Tamoxifen or Raloxifene for women at increased risk and at low risk for adverse medication effects.

–If patient has a family history of breast cancer or personal history of breast biopsy, consider using risk assessment tool for assessing risk, eg, www.cancer.gov/bcrisktool.

–If 5-y risk of breast cancer is 3% or greater, benefits more likely to outweigh risk.

–Daily doses: Tamoxifen 20 mg, Raloxifene 60 mg, either for 5 y.

–Tamoxifen approved for women ≥35 y, increased risk for VTE, especially older or personal/family hx VTE.

–Increased risk for endometrial cancer, perform baseline exam and regular follow-up.

–Raloxifene approved for use in postmenopausal women.

–Not recommended in combination with other hormonal therapy/hormonal contraception or in pregnancy, risk of pregnancy, breast-feeding.

GOUT

Population

–Adults with history of gout.

Recommendations

▶ **American College of Rheumatology 2012, ACP 2017**

–Recommend a urate-lowering diet and lifestyle measures for patients with gout to prevent exacerbations.

–Do not initiate urate-lowering therapy in most patients after a first gout attack or with infrequent attacks.

–Discuss benefits, harms, costs, and preferences before initiating urate-lowering therapy.

–Urate-lowering medications[c] are indicated for gout with Stage 2–5 CKD or recurrent gout attacks and hyperuricemia (uric acid >6 mg/dL).

–Anti-inflammatory prophylaxis[d] indicated for 6 mo after an attack and for 3 mo after uric acid level falls <6 mg/dL.

Sources

–*Arthritis Care Res.* 2012;64(1):1431-1446.

–*Ann Intern Med.* 2017;166:58-68.

–*BMJ.* 2018;362:k2893.

Comments

1. ACP states that evidence is insufficient to determine efficacy of dietary therapies.
2. Limit consumption of high-fructose corn syrup–sweetened soft drinks and energy drinks.
3. Increase low-fat dairy products and vegetable intake.
4. Manage weight, increase exercise, and reduce alcohol consumption.

ORAL CANCER

Population

–Adults.

Recommendations

▶ National Cancer Institute 2018

–Minimize Risk Factor Exposure. Risk factors include:

- Tobacco (in any form, including smokeless).
- Alcohol and dietary factors—double the risk for people who drink 3–4 drinks/d vs. nondrinkers. (*Cancer Causes Control.* 2011;22:1217)
- Betel-quid chewing. (*Cancer.* 2014;135:1433)
- Oral HPV infection—found in 6.9% of general population and found in 70%–75% of patients with oropharyngeal squamous cell cancer. (*N Engl J Med.* 2007;356:1944)
- Lip cancer—avoid chronic sun exposure and smokeless tobacco.

---

[c]Colchicine 0.6 mg daily-bid; naproxen 250 mg bid is second-line; low-dose prednisone is third-line.
[d]Allopurinol, febuxostat, probenecid; goal uric acid level <6 mg/dL.

Source

–https://www.cancer.gov/types/head-and-neck/hp/oral-prevention-pdq

Comments

1. Oropharyngeal squamous cell CAs (tonsil and base of tongue) are related to HPV infection (types 16 and 18) in 75% of patients. This correlates with sexual practices, number of partners, and may be prevented by HPV vaccine. HPV (+), nonsmokers have improved cure rate by 35%–45%. (*N Engl J Med.* 2010;363:24, 82)
2. There is inadequate evidence to suggest change in diet will reduce risk of oral cancer.

OSTEOPOROSIS

Population

–Adults and children.

Recommendations

▶ Osteoporosis International 2014, ACOG 2014

–Counsel on the risk of osteoporosis and fractures.

–Diet with adequate calcium and vitamin D (respectively):

- Age 9–18y: 1300 mg/d and 600 U/d.
- Age 19–50 y: 1000 mg/d and 600 U/d.
- Age 51–70 y: 1200 mg/d and 600 U/d (1000 mg/d for men 50–70 y).
- Age ≥71 y: 1200 mg/d and 800–1000 U/d with dietary supplements if needed.

–Regular weight-bearing and muscle-strengthening exercise.

–Assess risk factors for falls and offer modifications (eg, home safety, balance training, vitamin D deficiency, CNS depressant medications, antihypertensive medication monitoring, vision correction).

–Target a serum vitamin D level of 20 ng/mL.

–Tobacco cessation.

–Avoid excess alcohol intake.

–In patients with low bone mass (T-score on screening DXA scan of ≤2.5), consider pharmacologic therapy—see Chapter 29, section: Osteoporosis.

Sources

–*Osteoporos Int.* 2014: doi:10.1007/s00198-014-2794-2

–*Obstet & Gyn.* 120(3):718-734.

–*Am Fam Phys.* 2015;92(4):261-268.

Population

–Adults and children being treated with glucocorticoids (GC).

Recommendations

▶ ACR 2017

–Assess clinical fracture risk within 6 mo of starting GC treatment.

–Include history of dose and duration of steroids, falls, fractures, frailty.

–High risk of fracture: malnutrition, weight loss/low body weight, hypogonadism, hyperparathyroidism, thyroid disease, family hx hip fracture, alcohol use, smoking.

–For adults ≥40 y, use FRAX to assess risk (https://www.shef.ac.uk/FRAX/tool.jsp).

–For adults <40 y with hx osteoporotic (OP) fracture or high risk, perform bone mineral density testing.

–For adults taking >7.5 mg/d prednisone, FRAX risk increases by 15% for major OP fracture and 20% for hip fracture.

–High fracture risk: hx OP fracture, T-score ≤−2.5 (postmenopausal or male ≥50 y), FRAX 10-y risk OP fracture ≥20% or hip fracture ≥3%.

–Moderate fracture risk: FRAX 10-y risk OP fracture 10%–19% or hip fracture 1%–3% (or if <40 y Z-score <−3 or ≥10% bone loss over 1 y and continued GC ≥7.5 mg/d for ≥6 mo).

–Low fracture risk: lower FRAX risk.

–Adults taking prednisone ≥2.5 mg/d for ≥3 mo: calcium (1000–1200 mg/d), vitamin D (600–800 U/d), healthy diet, normal weight, no smoking, exercise, alcohol ≤1–2 drinks/d.

–Adults at low risk of fracture: Ca, VitD, lifestyle as above.

–Adults at moderate or high risk of fracture: add oral bisphosphonate.

–If GC treatment continued, reassess risk every 12 mo.

–Continue bisphosphonate treatment for 5 y if continues to be at moderate-to-high risk or continues to take GC.

–Treat with another class of OP medication (teriparatide or denosumab) or IV bisphosphonate if malabsorption of oral form, if fracture after 18 mo of oral bisphosphonate, ≥10% bone loss after 1 y, or continue to be moderate-to-high risk after 5 y.

Source

–*Arthritis Rheumatol.* 2017:69(8):1521-1537.

PRESSURE ULCERS

Population
–Adults or children with impaired mobility.

Recommendations
▶ NICE 2014, ACP 2015
–Assess risk for in both outpatient and inpatient settings (eg, the Braden Scale in adults and Braden Q Scale in children).
–Educate patient, family, and caregivers regarding the causes and risk factors of pressure ulcers.
–Use compression stockings cautiously in patients with lower-extremity arterial disease. Avoid thigh-high stockings when compression stockings are used.
–Move patients with caution
  • Avoid dragging patient when moving.
  • Lubricate or powder bed pans prior to placing under patient.
–Minimize pressure on skin, especially areas with bony prominences.
  • Turn patient side-to-side every 2 h.
  • Pad areas over bony prominences.
  • Pad skin-to-skin contact.
  • Use heel protectors or place pillows under calves.
  • Consider a bariatric bed for patients weighing over 300 lb.
  • Consider high-specification foam (not air) mattress for high-risk patients admitted to secondary care or who are undergoing surgery.
–Manage moisture.
  • Moisture barrier protectant on skin.
  • Frequent diaper changes.
  • Scheduled toileting.
  • Treat candidiasis if present.
  • Consider a rectal tube for stool incontinence with diarrhea.
–Maintain adequate nutrition and hydration.
–Keep the head of the bed at or <30° elevation.

Sources
–National Clinical Guideline Centre. *Pressure Ulcers: Prevention and Management of Pressure Ulcers.* London (UK): National Institute for Health and Care Excellence; 2014.
–*Ann Intern Med.* 2015;162(5):359-369.

Comments
1. Outpatient risk assessment for pressure ulcers:
   a. Is the patient bed or wheel chair bound?

      b. Does the patient require assistance for transfers?

      c. Is the patient incontinent of urine or stool?

      d. Any history of pressure ulcers?

      e. Does the patient have a clinical condition placing the patient at risk for pressure ulcers?

         i. DM.

         ii. Peripheral vascular disease.

         iii. Stroke.

         iv. Polytrauma.

         v. Musculoskeletal disorders (fractures or contractures).

         vi. Spinal cord injury.

         vii. Guillain–Barré syndrome.

         viii. Multiple sclerosis.

         ix. CA.

         x. Chronic obstructive pulmonary disease.

         xi. Coronary heart failure.

         xii. Dementia.

         xiii. Preterm neonate.

         xiv. Cerebral palsy.

      f. Does the patient appear malnourished?

      g. Is equipment in use that could contribute to ulcer development (eg, oxygen tubing, prosthetic devices, urinary catheter)?

SKIN CANCER

Population

    –All people.

Recommendations

▶ USPSTF 2018

    –Counsel to minimize UV exposure for people age 6 mo to 24 y with fair skin types.

    –Offer selective counseling to adults over 24 y with fair skin types.

    –Insufficient evidence to recommend skin self-exam.

▶ National Cancer Institute 2019

    –Avoid sunburns and tanning booths,[c] especially severe blistering sunburns at a younger age.

---

[c]Twenty-eight million Americans per year use indoor tanning salons—increased risk of squamous cell and basal cell cancers greater than melanoma. Source: http://www.cancer.gov/cancertopics/pdq/prevention

Sources

–*JAMA.* 2018;319(11):1134-1142.

–http://www.cancer.gov/types/skin/hp/skin-prevention-pdq

Comments

1. Use sunscreen (SPF ≥15) and protective clothing, spend limited time in the sun, avoid indoor tanning and blistering sunburn in adolescents and young adults.
2. Phenotypic risk factors (fair skin) include ivory or pale skin color, light eye color, red or blond hair, freckles, or easily sunburned skin.
3. Nicotinamide (Vitamin B_3) shows promise in preventing skin cancers but further studies are required. (*J Invest Dermatol.* 2012;132:1498)
4. Chemopreventive agents (beta carotene, isoretinoin, selenium, and celecoxib) have not shown prevention of new skin cancers in randomized clinical trials. (*Arch Dermatol.* 2000;136:179)

Endocrine and Metabolic Disorders

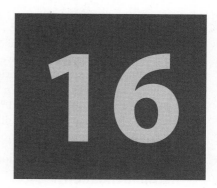

DIABETES MELLITUS (DM), TYPE 2

Population
–Persons with pre-diabetes or impaired glucose tolerance (IGT).[a]

Recommendations

▶ ADA 2019

–Structured behavioral weight loss therapy with a reduced calorie meal plan such as the Mediterranean or low-calorie, low-fat eating plan. Quality of the food is important; avoid refined and processed foods.

–Intensive lifestyle modification with a goal of sustained 7% weight loss.

–Moderate physical activity such as brisk walking at least 150 min/wk.

–Consider metformin for patients at highest risk for developing diabetes (eg, BMI 35 kg/m^2 or greater, those age 60 y or younger, and women with prior gestational diabetes mellitus [GDM]).

–Based on patient preference, technology-assisted diabetes prevention interventions (eg, SBGM) may be effective in preventing type 2 diabetes and should be considered.

–At least annual monitoring for the development of type 2 diabetes.

–Screening for and treatment of modifiable risk factors for cardiovascular disease.

Source
–*Diabetes Care.* 2018;41(suppl 1):S1-S159.

Comments
1. Recommendations for disease prevention:
   a. Annual influenza vaccine.

[a]IGT, or pre-diabetes, if fasting glucose 100–125 mg/dL, 2-h glucose after 75-g anhydrous glucose load 140–199 mg/dL, or HgbA1c 5.7%–6.4%.

b. Pneumococcal polysaccharide vaccine if 2 y or older with one-time revaccination when over 64 y.
c. Hepatitis B vaccine series if unvaccinated and 19–59 y of age.
d. Aspirin 81 mg daily for primary prevention if 10-y risk of significant CAD is at least 10% (by Framingham Risk Score); includes most men over 50 y and most women over 60 y.

Population

–Persons with abnormal blood glucose or BMI >25.

Recommendation

▶ USPSTF 2015

–Intensive behavioral intervention to promote healthy diet and physical activity.

Source

–*Ann Intern Med.* 2015;163(11):861-868.

Population

–Children of ethnicities with higher prevalence of diabetes, such as American Indian, Alaskan Native, Mexican-American, and African-American.

Recommendations

▶ AAP 2009

–Counsel children with BMI >85th percentile on weight control, physical activity, and nutrition.
–Do not use medications to prevent diabetes.
–Nutritional interventions require familiarity with family and community culture and rely on the entire family making changes.

Source

–*Pediatrics.* 2003;112(4):e328-e347.

HORMONE REPLACEMENT THERAPY TO PREVENT CHRONIC CONDITIONS

Population

–Postmenopausal women.

Recommendation

▶ USPSTF 2017

–Do not use combined estrogen and progestin to prevent chronic conditions, including osteoporosis, coronary artery disease, breast cancer, and cognitive impairment.

Source
- *JAMA.* 2017;318(22):2224-2233.

Population
- Postmenopausal women who have had a hysterectomy.

Recommendation

▶ USPSTF 2017
- Do not use estrogen to prevent chronic conditions, including osteoporosis, coronary artery disease, breast cancer, and cognitive impairment.

Source
- *JAMA.* 2017;318(22):2224-2233.

Comment
1. This recommendation does not apply to women under the age of 50 y who have undergone a surgical menopause and require estrogen for hot flashes and vasomotor symptoms.

OBESITY

Population
- Adolescents and adults.

Recommendations

▶ ICSI 2013, CDC 2011
- Recommends a team approach for weight management in all persons of normal weight (BMI 18.5–24.9) or overweight (BMI 25–29.9), including:
  - Nutrition.
  - Physical activity. 150 minutes of moderate-intensity aerobic exercise/wk.
  - Lifestyle changes. Avoid inactivity.
  - Screen for depression.
  - Screen for eating disorders.
  - Review medication list and assess if any medications can interfere with weight loss.
- Recommends regular follow-up to reinforce principles of weight management.

Source
- Fitch A, Everling L, Fox C, et al. *Prevention and Management of Obesity for Adults.* Bloomington (MN): ICSI; 2013.

Comments

1. Recommend 30–60 min of moderate physical activity on most days of the week.
2. Nutrition education focused on decreased caloric intake, encouraging healthy food choices, and managing restaurant and social eating situations. Eat 5–6 servings of fruits and vegetables daily.
3. Weekly weight checks.
4. Encourage nonfood rewards for positive reinforcement.
5. Stress management techniques.
6. 5%–10% weight loss can produce a clinically significant reduction in heart disease risk.

Population

–Children.

Recommendations

▶ Endocrine Society 2017, AAP 2015, CDC 2011

–Educate children and parents about healthy diets and the importance of regular physical activity. 60 minutes or more/d of aerobic activity of a moderate or vigorous intensity.
–Encourage school systems to promote healthy eating habits and provide health education courses.
–Foster healthy sleep patterns. Children should sleep 9 h or more/night.
–Balance screen time with opportunities for physical activity.
–Avoid using food as a reward or withholding food as punishment.
–Breast-feed infants 6 months or longer.

Sources

–*J Clin Endocrinol Metab.* 2017;102(3):709-757.
–Stanford Health Care.

Comments

1. Avoid the consumption of calorie-dense, nutrient-poor foods (eg, juices, soft drinks, "fast food" items, and calorie-dense snacks). Consume whole fruits rather than juices.
2. Control calorie intake by portion control.
3. Reduce saturated dietary fat intake for children age >2 y.
4. Increase dietary fiber, fruits, and vegetables to 5 servings daily.
5. Eat regular, scheduled meals and avoid snacking.
6. Limit television, video games, and computer time to 2 h daily.

Gastrointestinal Disorders

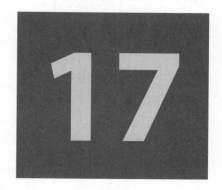

COLORECTAL CANCER

Population
–Adults.

Recommendations

▶ AAFP 2018

–**Modifiable Risk Factors**

Diet:

- Advise patients to increase consumption of fruits, non-starchy vegetables, and whole grains to reduce risk of colorectal cancer (CRC) (*Gastroenterology.* 2015;148(6):1244-1260)
- Cholesterol: 2-fold increased risk of CRC with increased intake.
- Fat: 25% increased risk of serrated polyps with increased fat intake.
- Dairy: 15% reduced risk of CRC with >8 oz of cow's milk daily.
- Fiber: No reduced risk of CRC or adenomatous polyps with increased fiber intake.
- Red meat: 22% increased risk of CRC with increased red meat and processed meat intake.

Lifestyle:

- Alcohol: 8% increased risk of CRC and 24% increased risk of serrated polyps. Reducing alcohol intake does not clearly lower risk for CRC or polyps.
- Cigarettes: 114% increased risk of high-risk adenomatous polyps and CRC in current smokers.
- Obesity: Bariatric surgery associated with 27% reduced risk of CRC in obese individuals. Increased BMI is associated with increased mortality from CRC.

- Occupational physical activity: 25% decreased risk of colon cancer and 12% decreased risk of rectal cancer.
- Recreational physical activity: 20% decreased risk of colon cancer and 13% decreased risk of rectal cancer.

Medications:

- Statins: Weak evidence that statin use ≥ 5 y is associated with decreased risk of advanced adenomatous polyps.
- Calcium: 26% reduced risk of adenomatous polyps; 22% reduced risk of CRC in individuals taking 1400 mg daily calcium compared to 600 mg.

–**Polyp Removal**

- Based on fair evidence, removal of adenomatous polyps reduces the risk of CRC, especially polyps >1 cm. (*Ann Intern Med.* 2011;154:22) (*Gastrointest Endosc.* 2014;80:471)
- Based on fair evidence, complications of polyp removal include perforation of the colon and bleeding estimated at 7–9 events per 1000 procedures.

–**Interventions without Benefit**

- Vitamin D.
- Folic acid.
- Antioxidants.

▶ USPSTF 2016

–Aspirin: Associated with 40% decreased CRC incidence after 5–10 y of use.

- Initiate low-dose aspirin for primary prevention of cardiovascular disease and CRC in persons aged 50–59 y with a 10-y cardiovascular event risk of $\geq 10\%$, no increased risk for bleeding, life expectancy of ≥ 10 y, and who are willing to take low-dose aspirin daily for 10 y. (USPSTF. *Aspirin Use to Prevent Cardiovascular Disease and Colorectal Cancer.* 2016.)
- Individualize decision to initiate low-dose aspirin for persons 60–69 y of age with similar risk profile, as there is increased risk for bleeding and decreased CRC prevention benefit.
- Do not initiate aspirin in persons <50 or ≥ 70 y of age.

Sources

–USPSTF. *Aspirin Use to Prevent Cardiovascular Disease and Colorectal Cancer.* 2016.
–*Am Fam Physician.* 2018;97(10):658-665.

ESOPHAGEAL CANCER

▶ AAFP 2017

–**Adenocarcinoma Risk Factors**
- Age 50–60 y.
- Male sex (8-fold risk).
- White race (5-fold risk).
- Gastroesophageal reflux disease (5- to 7-fold risk, depending on symptom frequency).
- Obesity (2.4-fold risk with BMI ≥30), particularly central adiposity.
- Smoking (2-fold risk).
- Barrett's esophagus (BE) (premalignant).

–**Squamous Cell Carcinoma Risk Factors**
- Age 60–70 y.
- Achalasia (10-fold risk).
- Smoking (9-fold risk).
- Alcohol use (3- to 5-fold risk with ≥3 drinks per day).
- Black Race (3-fold risk).
- High-starch diet without fruits or vegetables.

Source
–*Am Fam Physician.* 2017;95(1):22-28.

Comments
1. Minimize exposure to risk factors.
2. Longstanding GERD associated with BE and increased risk of esophageal CA. (*PLOS.* 2014;9:e103508)
3. Radiofrequency ablation of BE with moderate or severe dysplasia may reduce risk of progression to malignancy. (*N Engl J Med.* 2009;360:2277-2288)
4. Uncertain if elimination of GERD by surgical or medical therapy will reduce the risk of esophageal adenocarcinoma although a few trials show benefit. (*Gastroenterology.* 2010;138:1297)
5. No trials in the United States have shown any benefit from the use of chemoprevention with vitamins and/or minerals to prevent esophageal cancer. (*Am J Gastroenterol.* 2014;109:1215) (*Gut.* 2016;65:548)

GASTRIC CANCER

-**Modifiable Risk Factors**
- *H. pylori*: Classified as Group 1 (definite) carcinogen by World Health Organization (WHO), *H. pylori* triggers a series of inflammatory reactions leading to chronic gastritis, stomach atrophy, and early steps in the carcinogenesis sequence.
  - Screen for *H. pylori* in patients with peptic ulcer disease or gastric MALT lymphoma. (*Am J Gastroenterol.* 2007;102:1808-1825)
  - A study over 15 y showed a 40% reduction in risk of gastric cancer with *H. pylori* eradication. (*Ann Intern Med.* 2009;151:121) (*J Natl Cancer Inst.* 2012;104:488)
- Diet: Increased risk with smoked foods (N-nitroso compounds), high salt diet. Decreased risk with fruit and non-starch vegetable intake.
- Cigarette use: 60% increased risk in current male smokers and 20% increased risk in female smokers, compared to non-smokers.
- Obesity: Increased risk with BMI $\geq$30.
- Physical activity: 21% decreased risk.
- Male sex: 2-fold to 5-fold risk compared to women, though postmenopausal women have increased risk approaching that of men.
- First-degree relative with gastric cancer: 2.6-fold to 3.5-fold risk.

-**Clinical Consideration**
- Patients with hereditary susceptibility (HNPCC, e-cadherin mutation, Li–Fraumeni syndrome), pernicious anemia, atrophic gastritis, partial gastrectomy, or gastric polyps should be followed carefully for early cancer symptoms and for upper endoscopy at intervals according to risk.

Sources
-*Am Fam Physician.* 2017;95(1):22-28.
-*Gastrointest Endosc.* 2016;84(1):18-28.

HEPATOCELLULAR CANCER

▶ AASLD 2018, NCI 2019

–**Modifiable Risk Factors**

Cirrhosis and associated risk factors:

- Chronic Hepatitis B (HBV) infection.
- Hepatitis C (HCV) infection.
- Extensive alcohol use.
- Non-alcoholic steatohepatitis (NASH).
- Hereditary hemochromatosis.
- Primary biliary cholangitis.
- Wilson's disease.
- Aflatoxin B1 (fungal toxin that contaminates corn, grains and nuts that are not stored properly).

–**Prevention**

- Vaccinate against Hepatitis B.
- Treat Hepatitis C infection.
- Achieve alcohol cessation.
- Treat underlying risk factors as applicable.

Sources

–AASLD. *Hepatology.* 2018;68(2):723-750.
–NCI. *Adult Primary Liver Cancer Treatment (PDQ).* 2019.

Genitourinary Disorders

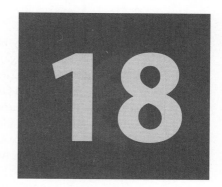

CERVICAL CANCER

▶ Minimize Risk Factor Exposure

–**Human Papillomavirus (HPV) Infection**[a]
  • Abstinence from sexual activity; condom and/or spermicide use (RR, 0.4).
  • HPV vaccination per CDC schedule.

–**Cigarette Smoke (Active or Passive)**
  • Increased risk of high-grade cervical intraepithelial neoplasia (CIN) or invasive cancer 2- to 3-fold among HPV-infected women.

–**High Parity**
  • HPV-infected women with 7 or more full-term pregnancies have a 4-fold increased risk of squamous cell CA of the cervix compared with nulliparous women.

–**Long-Term Use of Oral Contraceptives (>5 y)**
  • Increases risk by 3-fold.
  • Longer use related to even higher risk.

▶ Therapeutic Approaches

–**HPV-16/HPV-18 Vaccination**[b]
  • Reduces incidence and persistent infections with efficacy of 91.6% (95% CI, 64.5–98.0) and 100% (95% CI, 45–100), respectively; duration of efficacy is not yet known; impact on long-term cervical CA rates also unknown but likely to be significant. Two doses

---

[a]Methods to minimize risk of HPV infection include abstinence from sexual activity and the use of barrier contraceptives and/or spermicidal gel during sexual intercourse.
[b]On June 8, 2006, the US Food and Drug Administration (FDA) announced approval of Gardasil, the first vaccine developed to prevent cervical CA, precancerous genital lesions, and genital warts caused by HPV types 6, 11, 16, and 18. The vaccine is approved for use in females age 9–26 y (http://www.fda.gov). A bivalent vaccine, Cervarix, is also FDA approved with activity against HPV subtypes 16 and 18 (*N Engl J Med*. 2006;354:1109-1112).

of vaccine if 9- to 14-y-old, 3 doses if 15- to 26-y-old. (*Lancet.* 2009;374:1975) (*N Engl J Med.* 2015;372:711, 775)

- Also will likely decrease risk of other HPV-driven malignancies (oropharynx and anal CA).

–**Screening with PAP Smears**

- Estimates from population studies suggest that screening may decrease CA incidence and mortality by <80%. Adding screening for HPV after age 30 y increases sensitivity and reduces frequency of screening to every 5 y if both are negative.
- HPV screening only, without a PAP smear, is being studied in developing countries.

ENDOMETRIAL CANCER

▶ Minimize Risk Factor Exposure

–**Unopposed estrogen is a significant risk factor for the development of uterine cancer**

- Unopposed estrogen use in postmenopausal women for 5 or more years more than doubled the risk of endometrial CA compared to women who did not use estrogen. Other significant events include stroke (39% relative increase) and pulmonary embolus (34% relative increase). (*Lancet.* 2005;365:1543) (*JAMA.* 2004;291:1701)
- Obesity—risk increases 1.59-fold for each 5 kg/m^2 change in body mass.
- Lack of exercise—regular exercise (2 h/wk) with 38%–48% decrease in risk.
- Tamoxifen—used for >2 y has a 2.3- to 7.5-fold increased risk of endometrial CA (usually stage I—95% cure rate with surgery).
- Nulliparous women have a 35% increased risk of endometrial CA.
- Endometrial hyperplasia and atypia—50% go on to develop uterine cancer. Most often occurs in women over 50-y-old. (*Gynecol.* 1995;5:233)

▶ Therapeutic Approaches

–**Oral Contraception (Estrogen and Progesterone Containing)**

- Use of oral contraceptives for 4 y reduces the risk of endometrial CA by 56%; 8 y, by 67%; and 12 y, by 72%, but will increase risk of breast cancer by 26%.

–**Increasing Parity and Lactation**

- 35% reduction vs. nulliparous women-increasing length of breast-feeding with decreasing risk.

–**Weight Loss**

- Insufficient evidence to conclude weight loss is associated with a decreased incidence of endometrial cancer.

OVARIAN CANCER

▶ Minimize Risk Factor Exposure

–**Risk Factors**

- Postmenopausal use of unopposed estrogen replacement will lead to a 3.2-fold increased risk of ovarian cancer after >20 y of use.
- Talc exposure and use of fertility drugs have inadequate data to show increased risk of ovarian cancer—remains controversial.
- If a woman is newly diagnosed with ovarian cancer, she should be tested for *BRCA 1* or *2* at any age—if positive, family members should be tested for that specific gene mutation and undergo genetic counseling.

–**Obesity and Height of Ovarian Cancer**

- Elevated BMI including during adolescence associated with increased mortality from ovarian cancer. (*J Natl Cancer Inst.* 2003;95:1244)
- Taller women with higher risk of ovarian cancer. RR of ovarian cancer per 5 cm increase in height is 1.07.

▶ Therapeutic Approaches

–**Risk Reduction**

–**Oral Contraceptives**

- 5%–10% reduction in ovarian cancer per year of use, up to 80% maximum risk reduction.
- Increased risk of deep venous thrombosis (DVT) with oral contraceptive pill (OCP). The risk amounts to about 3 events per 10,000 women per year; increased breast CA risk among long-term OCP users of about 1 extra case per 100,000 women per year.
- Tubal ligation decreases the risk of ovarian cancer (30% reduction).
- Breast-feeding associated with an 8% decrease in ovarian cancer with every 5 mo of breast-feeding.

–**Prophylactic Salpingo-oophorectomy**—in high-risk women (eg, *BRCA 1* or *2* gene mutation).

- Ninety percent reduction in ovarian cancer risk and 50% reduction in breast cancer with bilateral salpingo-oophorectomy.
- If prophylactic salpingo-oophorectomy is done prior to menopause, approximately 50% of women experience vasomotor symptoms; there is a 4.5-fold increased risk of heart disease especially in women <40-y-old following oophorectomy.

PROSTATE CANCER

▶ Minimize Risk Factor Exposure

–Family history of prostate CA in men age <60 y defines risk. One first-degree relative with prostate CA increases the risk 3-fold, 2 first-degree relatives increase the risk 5-fold. The incidence of prostate CA in African-Americans is increased by 2-fold, occurs at a younger age, and is more virulent with increased death rate compared to Caucasian men.

–High dietary fat intake does not increase risk for prostate CA but is associated with more aggressive cancers and shorter survivals.

▶ Therapeutic and Preventive Approaches

–**Finasteride**
  • Decreased 7-y prostate CA incidence from 25% (placebo) to 18% (finasteride), but no change in mortality.
  • Trial participants report reduced ejaculate volume (47%–60%); increased erectile dysfunction (62%–67%); increased loss of libido (60%–65%); increased gynecomastia (3%–4.5%).

–**Dutasteride**
  • Absolute risk reduction of 22.8%.
  • No difference in prostate CA-specific or overall mortality. Concern raised by mild increase in more aggressive cancers in patients on dutasteride (Gleason score of 7–10). (*N Engl J Med*. 2013;369:603) (*N Engl J Med*. 2010;302:1192)

–**Vitamins and Minerals**
  • Vitamin E/alfa-tocopherol—inadequate data—one study showed a 17% increase in prostate CA with vitamin E alone. (*JAMA*. 2011;306:1549)
  • Selenium—no study shows benefit in reducing risk of prostate CA.
  • Lycopene—largest trials to date show no benefit. (*Am J Epidemiol*. 2010;172:566)

Infectious Diseases

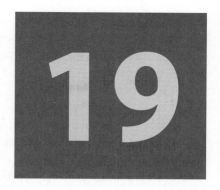

CATHETER-RELATED BLOODSTREAM INFECTIONS

Population
–Adults and children requiring intravascular catheters.

Recommendations

▶ IDSA 2009, CDC 2011

- Educate staff regarding proper procedures for insertion and maintenance of intravascular catheters.
- Do not place a central venous catheter if peripheral venous access is a safe and effective option.
- Use an upper extremity site for catheter insertion instead of a lower extremity in adults.
- Use a midline catheter or peripherally inserted central catheter (PICC) when the duration of IV therapy is likely to exceed 6 d.
- Avoid the femoral vein for central venous access in adult patients.
- Place nontunneled CVC in the subclavian vein, rather than the internal jugular vein or femoral vein, to minimize infection risk.
- Use a CVC with the minimum number of ports or lumens essential for management.
- Use ultrasound guidance to place CVCs to minimize mechanical complications.
- Promptly remove a CVC that is no longer essential.
- Replace catheters which were placed emergently within 48 h.
- Wash hands before and after catheter insertion, replacement, accessing, or dressing an intravascular catheter.
- Use maximal sterile barrier precautions including a cap, mask, sterile gown, sterile gloves, and a sterile full-body drape for the insertion of CVCs.

–Avoid antibiotic ointments on insertion sites.

–Use chlorhexidine-impregnated dressings to protect the insertion site of short-term, nontunneled CVCs only in patients aged 18 y or older.

Sources
  –*Clin Infect Dis.* 2011;52(9):e162-e193.
  –CDC Intravascular Catheter-related Infection: https://www.cdc.gov/infectioncontrol/guidelines/BSI/index.html

▼ COLITIS, *CLOSTRIDIUM DIFFICILE*

Population
  –Adults and children with no prior history of CDI.

Recommendations
▶ ACG 2013, CID 2018

  –Develop antibiotic stewardship programs to minimize the frequency and duration of high-risk antibiotic therapy.
  –Place patients with suspected CDI preemptively on contact precautions pending the *C. difficile* test results.
  –Maintain contact precautions for at least 48 h after diarrhea has resolved.
  –Treat patients with CDAD in a private room.
  –Perform hand hygiene before and after contact of a patient with CDI and after removing gloves with either soap or water.
  –Use gloves and gowns on entry to the room of a patient with known or suspected CDI (*C. difficile* infection) and remove gowns and glovers before leaving the patient's room.
  –Prevent transmission by using single-use disposable equipment. Thoroughly clean and disinfect reusable medical equipment, preferentially with a sporicidal disinfectant. Dedicated nondisposable equipment should be kept in the patient's room.
  –Disinfect environmental surfaces using an Environmental Protective Agency (EPA)–registered disinfectant with *C. difficile* sporicidal label claim or minimum chlorine concentration of 5000 ppm.
  –Although there is an epidemiological association between proton pump inhibitor (PPI) use and CDI, there is insufficient evidence for discontinuation of PPIs as a measure for preventing CDI.
  –Although there is moderate evidence that probiotics containing *Lactobacillus rhamnosus* GG and *Saccharomyces boulardii* decrease the incidence of antibiotic-associated diarrhea, there is insufficient data at this time to recommend administration of probiotics for primary prevention of *C. difficile* infection. Still, short-term use of probiotics appears to be safe and effective when used along with antibiotics in patients who are not immunocompromised or severely ill.

Sources

–*Am J Gastroenterol.* 2013;108(4):478.

–*Clin Infect Dis.* 2018;66(7):e1-e48.

–Goldenberg JZ, et al. Probiotics for the prevention of Clostridium difficile-associated diarrhea in adults and children. *Cochrane Database Syst Rev.* 2017;12:CD006095.

ENDOCARDITIS PREVENTION

Population

–Adults and children with underlying cardiac conditions associated with the highest risk of adverse outcomes from infective endocarditis (IE) undergoing specific procedures.

Recommendations

▶ AHA 2007, AHA/ACC 2014, AHA/ACC 2017, AAPD 2014

–Maintenance of optimal oral health and hygiene is more important in reducing the risk of IE than prophylactic antibiotics for dental procedures.

–There is insufficient evidence to support the use of topical antiseptics for IE prevention.

–Prevent rheumatic fever by promptly recognizing and treating streptococcal pharyngitis.

–The effectiveness of antibiotic prophylaxis in preventing IE in patients undergoing dental procedures is unknown.

–Antibiotic prophylaxis is no longer recommended for mitral valve prolapse (MVP), rheumatic heart disease (RHD), and most cases of congenital heart disease,[a] despite an increased lifetime risk of acquisition of IE when these conditions are present.

–IE prophylaxis[b] is indicated only for patients with underlying cardiac conditions that have the highest risk of morbidity and mortality from

---

[a]Exceptions: (1) Unrepaired cyanotic congenital heart disease, including palliative shunts and conduits; (2) completely repaired congenital heart defect with prosthetic material or device, whether placed by surgery or by catheter intervention, during first 6 mo after the procedure; (3) repaired CHD with residual defects (eg, shunts or valvular regurgitation) at the site of or adjacent to the site of a prosthetic patch or prosthetic device.

[b]Standard prophylaxis regimen: amoxicillin (adults 2 g; children 50 mg/kg orally 1 h before procedure). If unable to take oral medications, give ampicillin (adults 2.0 g IM or IV; children 50 mg/kg IM or IV within 30 min of procedure). If penicillin-allergic, give clindamycin (adults 600 mg; children 20 mg/kg orally 1 h before procedure) or azithromycin or clarithromycin (adults 500 mg; children 15 mg/kg orally 1 h before procedure). If penicillin-allergic and unable to take oral medications, give clindamycin (adults 600 mg; children 20 mg/kg IV within 30 min before procedure. If allergy to penicillin is not anaphylaxis, angioedema, or urticaria, options for nonoral treatment also include cefazolin (1 g IM or IV for adults, 50 mg/kg IM or IV for children); and for penicillin-allergic, oral therapy includes cephalexin 2 g PO for adults or 50 mg/kg PO for children (IM, intramuscular; IV, intravenous; PO, by mouth, orally).

IE who will undergo selected dental, respiratory, GI, GU, skin, and soft tissue procedures. These include patients with prosthetic valves,[c] previous history of IE, certain cardiac transplant recipients,[d] and selected patients with CHD and residual defects.

–Consider antibiotic prophylaxis for dental procedures that involve the gingival tissues or periapical region of a tooth and for those procedures that perforate the oral mucosa only for patients with underlying cardiac conditions associated with the highest risk of adverse outcomes from IE.

–Consider antibiotic prophylaxis for invasive respiratory tract procedures that involve incision or biopsy of the respiratory mucosa only for patients with underlying cardiac conditions associated with the highest risk of adverse outcomes from IE.

–Antibiotic prophylaxis solely to prevent IE is not recommended for GU or GI tract procedures, unless there is ongoing enterococcal infection in patients with underlying cardiac conditions associated with the highest risk of adverse outcomes from IE. Treat patients with an enterococcal urinary tract infection (UTI) or whose urine is colonized with *Enterococcus* with an antibiotic to eradicate enterococci from the urine prior to an elective cystoscopy or other urinary tract manipulation. If the urinary tract procedure is not elective, treat concurrently with antibiotics which are active against enterococci.

–Consider antibiotic prophylaxis for surgical procedures involving infected skin, skin structure, or musculoskeletal tissue using an agent that is active against staphylococci and beta-hemolytic streptococci, only in patients with underlying cardiac conditions associated with the highest risk of adverse outcomes from IE.

–Advise against body piercing in patients with underlying cardiac conditions associated with the highest risk of adverse outcomes from IE.

–A careful preoperative dental evaluation is recommended before cardiac valve surgery or replacement or repair of CHD.

–Perioperative prophylactic antibiotics with staphylococcal coverage are recommended for patients undergoing surgery for placement of prosthetic intravascular or intracardiac materials (eg, prosthetic valves).

–Long-term antistreptococcal prophylaxis is indicated for secondary prevention of rheumatic fever in patients with rheumatic heart disease, specifically mitral stenosis.

---

[c]Prosthetic cardiac valves, including transcatheter-implanted prostheses and homografts, or prosthetic material used for cardiac valve repair (annuloplasty rings, chords).
[d]Only those who develop cardiac valvulopathy.

–IE prophylaxis should be continued indefinitely in postcardiac transplant patients with a structurally abnormal valve.

–Antibiotic prophylaxis is not recommended for the following procedures and events: routine anesthetic injections through noninfected tissue, taking dental radiographs, placement of removable prosthodontic or orthodontic appliances, adjustment of orthodontic appliances, placement of orthodontic brackets, shedding of deciduous teeth, bleeding from trauma to the lips or oral mucosa, bronchoscopy without incision of the respiratory tract mucosa, diagnostic esophagogastroduodenoscopy or colonoscopy, vaginal delivery, Cesarean delivery, hysterectomy, tattooing, coronary artery bypass graft surgery.

Sources

–*Circulation.* 2007;116:1736-1754.

–Nishimura RA, et al. *J Am Coll Cardiol.* 2014;63(22):e57.

–Nishimura RA, et al. *J Am Coll Cardiol.* 2017;70(2):252-289.

–American Academy of Pediatric Dentistry. 2014;40(6):386-391.

Comment

1. IE is much more likely to result from frequent exposure to random bacteremia associated with daily activities (eg, chewing food, tooth brushing, flossing, use of toothpicks, use of water irrigation devices) and dental disease than from bacteremia caused by a dental, GI, or GU procedure. Antibiotic prophylaxis may reduce the incidence and duration of bacteremia but does not eliminate bacteremia. Only an extremely small number of cases of IE might be prevented by antibiotic prophylaxis even if it were 100% effective.

HUMAN IMMUNODEFICIENCY VIRUS (HIV), OPPORTUNISTIC INFECTIONS

Population

–Primary prevention in HIV-infected adults and adolescents.

Recommendation

▶ CDC 2009, WHO 2018, NIH 2018

–See the following table (from the clinical practice guidelines at *CDC MMWR.* 2009;58(RR04);1-198).

Sources

–*CDC MMWR.* 2009;58(RR04):1-198.

-NIH. *Guidelines for the Prevention and Treatment of Opportunistic Infections in HIV-Infected Adults and Adolescents.* March 2018. https://aidsinfo.nih.gov/contentfiles/lvguidelines/adultoitablesonly.pdf

Population

-Primary prophylaxis in HIV-infected children.

Recommendation

▶ CDC 2014, WHO 2018, NIH 2013

-See table below (from the clinical practice guidelines at *CDC MMWR.* 2009;58(RR04):1-198).

-Antiretroviral therapy to avoid advanced immune deficiency constitutes primary prophylaxis against candidiasis, coccidioidomycosis, cryptococcosis, cryptosporidiosis, cystoisosporiasis, and giardiasis in children.

Sources

-Centers for Disease Control and Prevention. Revised Surveillance Case Definition for HIV Infection—United States, 2014. *MMWR Recomm Rep.* 2014;63(RR-03):1-10.

-NIH. *Guidelines for the Prevention and Treatment of Opportunistic Infections in HIV-Exposed and HIV-Infected Children.* November 2013.

PROPHYLAXIS TO PREVENT FIRST EPISODE OF OPPORTUNISTIC DISEASE AMONG HIV-INFECTED ADULTS			
Pathogen	**Indication**	**First Choice**	**Alternative**
Pneumocystis carinii pneumonia (PCP)	CD4+ count <200 cells/µL or oropharyngeal candidiasis CD4+ <14% or history of AIDS-defining illness CD4+ count ≥200 but <250 cells/µL if monitoring CD4+ count every 3 mo is not possible and ART initiation delayed Note: Additional PCP prophylaxis is not needed if already receiving pyrimethamine/sulfadiazine for treatment/suppression of toxoplasmosis	Trimethoprim-sulfamethoxazole (TMP-SMX), 1 DS PO daily or 1 SS daily	• TMP-SMX 1 DS PO TI, *or* • Dapsone 100 mg PO daily or 50 mg PO bid, *or* • Dapsone 50 mg PO daily + pyrimethamine 50 mg PO weekly + leucovorin 25 mg PO weekly, *or* • [Dapsone 200 mg + pyrimethamine 75 mg + leucovorin 25 mg] PO weekly, *or* • Aerosolized pentamidine 300 mg via Respirgard II nebulized every month, *or* • Atovaquone 1500 mg PO daily, *or* • [Atovaquone 1500 mg + pyrimethamine 25 mg + leucovorin 10 mg] PO daily

PROPHYLAXIS TO PREVENT FIRST EPISODE OF OPPORTUNISTIC DISEASE AMONG HIV-INFECTED ADULTS (Continued)

Pathogen	Indication	First Choice	Alternative
Toxoplasma gondii encephalitis	*Toxoplasma* IgG-positive patients with CD4+ count <100 cells/μL Seronegative patients receiving PCP prophylaxis not active against toxoplasmosis should have toxoplasma serology retested if CD4+ count declines to <100 cells/ μL; prophylaxis should be initiated if seroconversion occurred Note: Patients receiving primary prophylaxis for *Toxoplasma gondii* are also covered for PCP prophylaxis	TMP-SMX 1 DS PO daily	• TMP-SMX 1 DS PO TIW, or • TMP-SMX 1 SS PO daily, or • Dapsone 50 mg PO daily + pyrimethamine 50 mg PO weekly + leucovorin 25 mg PO weekly, or • [Dapsone 200 mg + pyrimethamine 75 mg + leucovorin 25 mg] PO weekly, or • Atovaquone 1500 mg PO daily, or • [Atovaquone 1500 mg + pyrimethamine 25 mg + leucovorin 10 mg] PO daily Note: (1) Screen for G6PD prior to administration with dapsone or primaquine. (2) Screen for latent TB prior to initiating treatment with pyrimethamine

Mycobacterium tuberculosis infection (TB) (treatment of latent TB infection [LTBI])	(+) Screening test for LTBI, no evidence of active TB, and no prior treatment for active or latent TB (−) Diagnostic test for LTBI and no evidence of active TB, but close contact with a person with infectious pulmonary TB A history of untreated or inadequately treated healed TB (ie, old fibrotic lesions) regardless of diagnostic tests for LTBI and no evidence of active TB (AII)	Isoniazid (INH) 300 mg PO daily or 900 mg PO biw by DOT + pyridoxine 25–50 mg PO daily × 9 mo For persons exposed to drug-resistant TB, selection of drugs after consultation with public health authorities	• Rifampin (RIF) 600 mg PO daily × 4 mo, or • Rifabutin (adjust dose based on concomitant ART) × 4 mo, or • [Rifapentine PO (750 mg if 32.1–49.9 kg or 900 mg if ≥50 kg) + INH 900 mg PO + pyridoxine 50 mg PO] once weekly × 12 wk (only administer rifapentine if receiving raltegravir or efavirenz-based ART regimen)
Disseminated *Mycobacterium avium* complex (MAC) disease	CD4+ count <50 cells/µL in those who are not on fully suppressive ART—after ruling out active MAC infection Not recommended for those who immediately initiate ART	Azithromycin 1200 mg PO once weekly; or clarithromycin 500 mg PO bid; or azithromycin 600 mg PO twice weekly	• Rifabutin 300 mg PO daily (dosage adjustment based on drug–drug interactions with ART); rule out active TB before starting RFB
Streptococcus pneumoniae infection	Patients who have not received any pneumococcal vaccine Patients with previous PPSV23 vaccine	PCV13 0.5 mL IM × 1, followed by 1. If CD4 ≥200 cells/µL: PPSV23 0.5 mL IM 8 wk after PCV13 2. If CD4 <200 cells/µL: PPV23 at least 8 wk after receiving PCV13 or after CD4 rises ≥200 cells/µL (BIII)	PPSV23 0.5 mL IM × 1 (BII)

PROPHYLAXIS TO PREVENT FIRST EPISODE OF OPPORTUNISTIC DISEASE AMONG HIV-INFECTED ADULTS *(Continued)*

Pathogen	Indication	First Choice	Alternative
		If previously vaccinated with PPSV23, administer PCV13 × 1 at least 1 y after last PPSV23 If age 19–64 y and ≥5 y since first PPSV23 or age ≥65 y and ≥5 y since previous PPSV23, revaccinate with PPSV23 0.5 mL IM or SQ × 1	
Influenza A and B virus infection	All HIV-infected patients	Inactivated influenza vaccine 0.5 mL IM annually Do not use live-attenuated influenza vaccine	
Syphilis	For patients with exposure to a partner diagnosed with syphilis <90 d prior or for partners diagnosed >90 d prior with unknown serologic tests or uncertain follow-up	Benzathine penicillin G 2.4 million units IM × 1	For penicillin allergy: Doxycycline 100 mg PO BID × 14 d, or Ceftriaxone 1 g IM/IV daily × 8–10 d, or Azithromycin 2 g PO × 1 (BII) (not recommended for MSM or pregnant women)
Histoplasma capsulatum infection	CD4+ count < 150 cells/μL and at high risk because of occupational exposure or live in a community with a hyperendemic rate of histoplasmosis (>10 cases/100 patient-y)	Itraconazole 200 mg PO daily	

Coccidioidomycosis	New positive IgM or IgG serologic test in a patient from a disease-endemic area, and CD4+ count <250 cells/µL	Fluconazole 400 mg PO daily	
Varicella-zoster virus (VZV) infection	*Preexposure prevention:* Patient with CD4+ count >200 cells/µL who have not been vaccinated, have no history of varicella or herpes zoster, or who are seronegative for VZV. Note: Routine VZV serologic testing in HIV-infected adults/adolescents is not recommended. *Postexposure prevention:* Close contact in susceptible persons (not vaccinated, no history of chickenpox or shingles, or VZV seronegative) with a person who has active varicella or herpes zoster	*Preexposure prevention:* Primary varicella vaccination (Varivax), 2 doses (0.5 mL SQ) administered 3 mo apart. If vaccination results in disease because of vaccine virus, treat with acyclovir. *Postexposure prevention:* Varicella-zoster immune globulin (VZIG) 125 IU/10 kg (maximum of 625 IU) IM, administered as soon as possible within 10 d after exposure. Note: VZIG can be obtained only under a treatment IND (1-800-843-7477, FFF Enterprises). No need to redose if patient receives monthly IVIG >400 mg/kg with last dose within previous 3 wk	*Preexposure prevention:* VZV-susceptible household contacts of susceptible HIV-infected persons should be vaccinated to prevent potential transmission of VZV to their HIV-infected contacts. *Alternative postexposure prevention* (not studied in the HIV population): • Preemptive acyclovir 800 mg PO 5 ×/d for 5–7 d • Valacyclovir 1 g PO TID × 5–7 d • Varicella vaccines should be delayed >72 h after administration of antivirals • These two alternatives have not been studied in the HIV population
Human papillomavirus (HPV) infection	Patients age 13–26 y	HPV recombinant vaccine 9 valent (types 6, 11, 16, 18, 31, 33, 45, 52, 58) 0.5 mL IM at 0, 1–2, and 6 mo	Consider additional vaccination with recombinant 9-valent vaccine for patients who completed vaccination with recombinant bivalent or quadrivalent series (unclear who benefits or how cost-effective this is)

PROPHYLAXIS TO PREVENT FIRST EPISODE OF OPPORTUNISTIC DISEASE AMONG HIV-INFECTED ADULTS *(Continued)*			
Pathogen	**Indication**	**First Choice**	**Alternative**
Hepatitis A virus (HAV) infection	HAV-susceptible patients with chronic liver disease, or who are injection-drug users, or men who have sex with men	Hepatitis A vaccine 1 mL IM × 2 doses—at 0 and 6–12 mo Reassess IgG antibody response 1 mo after vaccination; revaccinate nonresponders when CD4 count >200 cells/µL	If susceptible to both HAV and HBV, combined vaccine (Twinrix) 1 mL IM as a 3-dose series (0, 1, and 6 mo) or 4-dose series (day 0, day 7, day 21–30, and 12 mo)
Hepatitis B virus (HBV) infection	No evidence of prior exposure to HBV (anti-HBs <10 IU/mL) should be vaccinated with HBV vaccine, including patients with CD4+ count <200 cells/µL Vaccinate early before CD4 falls <350 cells/µL Patients with CD4 <200 cells/µL may not respond to vaccination; consider delayed revaccination Vaccine nonresponders (anti-HBs <10 1–2 mo after vaccine series)	HBV vaccine IM (Engerix-B 20 µg/mL or Recombivax HB 10 µg/mL) at 0, 1, and 6 mo or 0, 1, 2, and 6 mo or Vaccine conjugated to CpG (Heplisav-B) IM at 0 and 1 mo (2-dose series can only be used if both doses are Heplisav-B) *or* Combined HAV and HBV vaccine (Twinrix) 1 mL IM as a 3-dose (0, 1, and 6 mo) or 4-dose series (days 0, 7, 21–30, and 12 mo) If anti-HBs ≤10 IU/mL after 1–2 mo from receipt of the vaccine, revaccinate with additional 4-dose series; consider delayed revaccination until sustained increase in CD4 count on ART *Patients with isolated anti-HBc:* Vaccinate × 1 standard dose of HBV. If anti-HBs <100 IU in × 1–2 mo, vaccinate with full series and retest anti-HBs	Some experts recommend doses of double dose of either HBV vaccine

	Vaccine nonresponders: Defined as anti-HBs <10 IU/mL 1 mo after a vaccination series For patients with low CD4+ count at the time of first vaccination series, certain specialists might delay revaccination until after a sustained increase in CD4+ count with ART (CIII)	Revaccinate with a second vaccine series (BIII)	Consider double doses of either HBV vaccine (BI)
Malaria	Travel to disease-endemic area	Recommendations are the same for HIV-infected and noninfected patients. One of the following three drugs is usually recommended, depending on location: atovaquone/proguanil, doxycycline, or mefloquine. Refer to the following website for the most recent recommendations based on region and drug susceptibility: http://www.cdc.gov/malaria/	
Penicilliosis (talaromycosis)	Patients with CD4 <100 cells/μL who have extended exposure to rural areas of Thailand, Vietnam, or Southern China (BI)	Itraconazole 200 mg PO daily	Fluconazole 400 mg PO once weekly

BID, twice daily; BIW, two times weekly; DS, double strength; IM, intramuscular; PO, by mouth; SS, single strength; SQ, subcutaneous; TIW, three times weekly.

PROPHYLAXIS TO PREVENT FIRST EPISODE OF OPPORTUNISTIC INFECTIONS AMONG HIV-EXPOSED AND HIV-INFECTED INFANTS AND CHILDREN, UNITED STATES

Pathogen	Indication	Preventive Regimen	
		First Choice	Alternative
		STRONGLY RECOMMENDED AS STANDARD OF CARE	
Pneumocystis pneumoniae	• HIV-infected or HIV-indeterminate infants age 1–12 mo • HIV-infected children age 1–5 y with CD4 count of <500 cells/mm³ or CD4 percentage of <15% • HIV-infected children age 6–12 y with CD4 count of <200 cells/mm³ or CD4 percentage of <15%	• TMP-SMX [2.5–5 mg/kg]/[12.5–25 mg/kg] body weight/dose (max: 320/1600 mg) PO BID TIW on consecutive or alternative days (AI) • Acceptable alternative dosage schedules: 2 d/wk on consecutive or alternative days; single dose orally daily (TDD TMP 5–10 mg/kg body weight)	• Dapsone: children age ≥1 mo, 2 mg/kg body weight (max 100 mg) orally daily; or 4 mg/kg body weight (max 200 mg) orally once weekly • Atovaquone: children age 1–3 mo and >24 mo to 12 y: 30 mg/kg body weight orally daily; children age 4–24 mo: 45 mg/kg body weight orally daily; children aged ≥ 13 y: 1500 mg (10 cc oral yellow suspension) per dose by mouth once daily • Aerosolized pentamidine: children age ≥5 y, 300 mg every month by Respirgard II (Marquest, Englewood, CO) nebulizer

Malaria	Travel to area in which malaria is endemic	• Recommendations are the same for HIV-infected and HIV-uninfected children. Refer to http://www.cdc.gov/malaria/ for the most recent recommendations based on region and drug susceptibility	• Chloroquine base 5 mg/kg base orally up to 300 mg weekly for sensitive regions only (7.5 mg/kg chloroquine phosphate)
		• Chloroquine phosphate 7.5 mg/kg = chloroquine base 5 mg/kg (up to 300 mg) once weekly. Start 1–2 wk before leaving, take weekly while away, and then take once weekly for 4 wk after returning home	
		• Doxycycline 2.2 mg/kg body weight (max 100 mg) by mouth once daily for children aged ≥8 y. Must be taken 1–2 d before travel, daily while away, and then up to 4 wk after returning	
		• Mefloquine 5 mg/kg body weight orally 1 time weekly (max 250 mg)	
		• Atovaquone/proguanil (Malarone) 1 time daily. Start 1–2 d before travel, for duration of stay, and then for 1 wk after returning home	
		• 11–20 kg = 1 pediatric tablet (62.5 mg/25 mg)	
		• 21–30 kg = 2 pediatric tablets (125 mg/50 mg)	
		• 31–40 kg = 3 pediatric tablets (187.5 mg/75 mg)	
		• >40 kg = 1 adult tablet (250 mg/100 mg)	
		• *For areas with mainly P. vivax:* primaquine phosphate 0.6 mg/kg body weight base once daily by mouth, up to a max of 30 mg base/d. Starting 1 d before leaving, taken daily, and for 3–7 d after return (G6PD screening must be performed prior to primaquine use)	

PROPHYLAXIS TO PREVENT FIRST EPISODE OF OPPORTUNISTIC INFECTIONS AMONG HIV-EXPOSED AND HIV-INFECTED INFANTS AND CHILDREN, UNITED STATES (Continued)

Pathogen	Indication	Preventive Regimen	
		First Choice	Alternative
		STRONGLY RECOMMENDED AS STANDARD OF CARE	
Mycobacterium tuberculosis (postexposure prophylaxis)	• Tuberculin skin test (TST) reaction >5 mm or IGRA without prior TB treatment, regardless of current TST result • Close contact with any person who has contagious TB • TB disease must be excluded before start of treatment	*If source case is drug-susceptible,* isoniazid 10–15 mg/kg body weight (max 300 mg daily) PO daily for 9 mo *Adjunctive treatment:* Pyridoxine 1–2 mg/kg body weight once daily (maximum 25–50 mg/d) with INH; pyridoxine supplementation is recommended for exclusively breast-fed infants and for children and adolescents on meat- and milk-deficient diets; children with nutritional deficiencies, including all symptomatic HIV-infected children; and pregnant adolescents and women *If source case is drug resistant (MDR),* choice of drugs requires consultation with ID expert and public health authorities and depends on susceptibility of isolate from source patient	• INH 20–30 mg/kg body weight (max 900 mg/d) orally BIW for 9 mo via DOT • Isoniazid 10–15 mg/kg body weight (max 300 mg daily) PO daily + rifampin 10–20 mg/kg body weight (max 600 mg/d) orally daily for 3–4 mo • Rifampin 10–20 mg/kg body weight (max 600 mg) orally daily for 4–6 mo (drug–drug interactions with cART should be considered for all rifamycin-containing alternatives; infectious disease specialist consultation recommended)
Mycobacterium avium complex	For children age >6 y with CD4 count of <50 cells/mm³; age 2–5 y with CD4 count of <75 cells/mm³; age 1–2 y with CD4 count of <500 cells/mm³; age <1 y with CD4 count of <750 cells/mm³	• Clarithromycin 7.5 mg/kg body weight (max 500 mg) PO BID, or azithromycin 20 mg/kg body weight (max 1200 mg) PO once weekly	• Azithromycin 5 mg/kg body weight (max 250 mg) PO daily; children age >6 y, rifabutin 300 mg orally daily

Varicella-zoster virus	*Preexposure prophylaxis:* VZV vaccine *Postexposure prophylaxis:* Substantial exposure to chickenpox or shingles with no history of varicella or zoster or seronegative status for VZV by a sensitive, specific antibody assay or lack of evidence for age-appropriate vaccination. Some experts limit this to apply only to patients with severe immunocompromise or high viral load	• VZIG 125 IU/10 kg (max 625 IU) IM, administered within 96 h after exposure (potentially beneficial up to 10 d) • If VZIG is not available or >96 h have passed since exposure, administer IVIG 400 mg/kg × 1. When VZIG or IVIG is not available, some experts recommend prophylaxis with acyclovir 20 mg/kg body weight (max 800 mg) per dose PO QID for 5–7 d, to be started 7–10 d after exposure. If VZIG is intravenous immune globulin (IVIG), IVIG should be administered within 96 h after exposure (CIII)
Vaccine-preventable pathogens	Standard recommendations for HIV-exposed and HIV-infected children	Routine vaccinations

PROPHYLAXIS TO PREVENT FIRST EPISODE OF OPPORTUNISTIC INFECTIONS AMONG HIV-EXPOSED AND HIV-INFECTED INFANTS AND CHILDREN, UNITED STATES (Continued)

Pathogen	Indication	Preventive Regimen	
		First Choice	**Alternative**
		STRONGLY RECOMMENDED AS STANDARD OF CARE	
Toxoplasma gondii	IgG to Toxoplasma and severe immunosuppression: • HIV-infected children age <6y with CD4 <15%; • HIV-infected children age ≥6 y with CD4 <100 cells/mm³	• TMP-SMX, 150/750 mg/m² body surface area PO daily	• Dapsone (children age >1 mo) 2 mg/kg body weight or 15 mg/m² body surface area (max 25 mg) orally daily + pyrimethamine 1 mg/kg body weight (max 25 mg) orally daily + leucovorin 5 mg orally every 3 d • Atovaquone: children age 1–3 mo and >24 mo, 30 mg/kg body weight orally daily; children age 4–24 mo, 45 mg/kg body weight orally daily with or without pyrimethamine 1 mg/kg body weight or 15 mg/m² body surface area (max 25 mg) orally daily; plus leucovorin 5 mg orally every 3 d • Acceptable alternative dosage schedules for TMP-SMX: TMP-SMX 150/750 mg PO TIW on consecutive days; TMP-SMX 75/375 mg PO BID; TMP-SMX 75/375 mg PO BID TIW on alternate days
Invasive bacterial infections (S. pneumoniae)	Hypogammaglobulinemia (IgG <400 mg/dL)	• IVIG (400 mg/kg body weight) every 2–4 wk • Pneumococcal, meningococcal, and Hib vaccines	• TMP-SMX 75/375 mg/m² BSA/dose PO BID

Cytomegalovirus (CMV)	+ CMV Ab and severe immunosuppression (CD4 <50 cells/mm^3 in children ≥6 y or %CD4 <5% in children <6 y)	• Valganciclovir 900 mg PO daily with food for older children who can receive adult dosing • For children aged 4 mo to 16 y, valganciclovir PO soln 50 mg/mL (dose in mg = 7 × BSA × CrCl) PO daily with food (max dose 900 mg/d)
Influenza	*Preexposure prophylaxis:* Severely immunosuppressed children while influenza circulating in community *Postexposure prophylaxis:* only if chemoprophylaxis can be started within 48 h of exposure • Children >3 mo with severe immunosuppression regardless of influenza vaccination status	Oseltamivir • 3 mo to 1 y: 3 mg/kg BW/dose once daily • ≥1 to 12 y: weight-based dosing (<15 kg: 30 mg PO daily; >15 to 23 kg: 45 mg PO daily; >23 to 40 kg: 60 mg PO daily) • >13 y or > 40 kg: 75 mg PO daily Zanamivir (≥5 y): 10 mg (2 inhalations) once daily Note: dose adjustments required for premature infants and renal insufficiency (CrCl <30) Duration • If influenza vaccine provided after contact, chemoprophylaxis should continue for 2 wk after vaccine • If household contact is the exposure, chemoprophylaxis duration should be 7 d • If chemoprophylaxis is given in the setting of an institutional outbreak, duration either 14 or 7 d after onset of symptoms in the last person infected, whichever is longer

PROPHYLAXIS TO PREVENT FIRST EPISODE OF OPPORTUNISTIC INFECTIONS AMONG HIV-EXPOSED AND HIV-INFECTED INFANTS AND CHILDREN, UNITED STATES (Continued)

Pathogen	Indication	Preventive Regimen	
		First Choice	**Alternative**
		STRONGLY RECOMMENDED AS STANDARD OF CARE	
	• Children >3 mo with moderate to no immunosuppression if (a) influenza vaccination is contraindicated or unavailable; (b) low vaccine effectiveness		
HPV	Children aged 9–26 y old	Quadrivalent HPV vaccine (0, 1–2, 6 mo)	
Hepatitis B	• All patients negative for HBV infection	• Hepatitis B vaccine	HBV Ig following exposure
	• Infants born to mothers with HBV infection	• *For infants born to HBV-positive mothers:* HBV Ig + HBV vaccine	

CMV, cytomegalovirus; FDA, Food and Drug Administration; HIV, human immunodeficiency virus; IgG, immunoglobulin G; IM, intramuscularly; IVIG, intravenous immune globulin; PCP, *P. pneumoniae*; TB, tuberculosis; TMP-SMX, trimethoprim-sulfamethoxazole; TST, tuberculin skin test; VZV, varicella-zoster virus.

IMMUNIZATIONS

Population

–Adults, adolescents, and children.

Recommendation

▶ **CDC 2019**

–Immunize according to the Centers for Disease Control and Prevention (CDC) recommendations, unless contraindicated (see Appendix IX).

Sources

–CDC. *Adult Immunization Schedule.* 2019.
–CDC. *Child and Adolescent Immunization Schedule.* 2019.

INFLUENZA, CHEMOPROPHYLAXIS

Population

–Children ≥3 mo and adults.

Recommendations

▶ **AAP 2016**

The following situations warrant chemoprophylaxis:

–Children at high risk for complications who cannot receive vaccine, or within 2 wk of receiving vaccine.

–Family members or health care providers who are unimmunized and likely to have ongoing exposure to high-risk or unimmunized children younger than 24 mo of age.

–Supplement vaccination in high-risk immunocompromised children.

▶ **IDSA 2018, CDC 2011, AAP 2016**

–Consider preexposure antiviral chemoprophylaxis for adults and children aged ≥3 mo at highest risk of influenza complications as soon as influenza activity is detected in the community, in the absence of an outbreak.

  • Continue chemoprophylaxis for the duration of the influenza season when influenza vaccination is contraindicated, unavailable, or expected to have low effectiveness.

    ◦ Anaphylactic hypersensitivity to prior influenza vaccine

    ◦ Acute febrile illness

    ◦ History of Guillain–Barré syndrome within 6 wk of a previous influenza vaccination

    ◦ Persons who are severely immunocompromised

- Recipients of hematopoietic stem cell transplant in the first 6–12 mo posttransplant
- Lung transplant recipients
- Short-term chemoprophylaxis is indicated for unvaccinated adults and children aged ≥3 mo during periods of influenza activity.
  - Promptly administer inactivated influenza vaccine in conjunction with chemoprophylaxis in patients in whom influenza vaccination is expected to be effective.
  - Consider chemoprophylaxis for health care personnel and others who are in close contact with persons at high risk of developing influenza complications (but who cannot take antiviral chemoprophylaxis) when influenza vaccination is contraindicated or unavailable.

–Start postexposure antiviral chemoprophylaxis no later than 48 hours for asymptomatic adults and children aged ≥3 mo who are

- At high risk of developing complications from influenza (eg, severely immunocompromised persons) and for whom influenza vaccination is contraindicated, unavailable, or expected to have low effectiveness, after household exposure to influenza.
- Unvaccinated household contacts of a person at very high risk of complications from influenza (eg, severely immunocompromised persons).
- Exposed residents of an extended-care facility or hospitalized patients during an institutional outbreak, regardless of influenza vaccination history.
- Unvaccinated staff in whom prophylaxis is indicated based on their underlying conditions or those of their household members (duration: throughout outbreak).
- Staff who received inactivated influenza vaccine during an institutional outbreak (duration: 14 d post-vaccination).

Sources
–Uyeki T, et al. *Clinical Practice Guidelines by the Infectious Diseases Society of America: 2018 Update on Diagnosis, Treatment, Chemoprophylaxis, and Institutional Outbreak Management of Seasonal Influenza.* CID 2018.
–CDC. https://www.cdc.gov/flu/professionals/antivirals/summary-clinicians.htm

Comments
1. Influenza vaccination is the best way to prevent influenza.
2. Antiviral chemoprophylaxis is not a substitute for influenza vaccination.
3. Agents for chemoprophylaxis of influenza A (H1N1) and B: inhaled zanamivir or oral oseltamivir.

4. Children at high risk of complications include those with chronic diseases such as asthma, diabetes, cardiac disease, immune suppression, and neurodevelopmental disorders.

INFLUENZA, VACCINATION

Population
–All persons age $\geq$6 mo.

Recommendations
▶ CDC 2018, AAP 2018

–All persons age >6 mo should receive the seasonal influenza vaccine annually.

–All children age 6 mo to 8 y should receive 2 doses of the vaccine (>4 wk apart) during their first season of vaccination.

–The live attenuated influenza vaccine (Flumist quadrivalent) should not be used due to low efficacy.

–Offer vaccines before onset of influenza activity (by end of October, if possible) and continue vaccinations as long as influenza virus circulates and vaccine is available.

–High-dose vaccine is more effective for adults $\geq$65 y old.

–Influenza vaccine is contraindicated only if history of severe allergic reaction is found. Egg allergy is not a contraindication, though persons with history of severe reaction should be monitored after receiving the vaccine.

–Do not vaccinate persons who have experienced GBS within 6 wk of a previous influenza vaccine if not at higher risk for influenza complications. Consider influenza chemoprophylaxis as an alternative. Benefits of influenza vaccination might outweigh risks for certain persons with a history of GBS who are also at higher risk for severe complications from influenza.

–Do not vaccinate with live-attenuated influenza vaccine (LAIV) in children (1) younger than 2 y; (2) with a moderate-to-severe febrile illness; (3) with an amount of nasal congestion that would notably impede vaccine delivery; (4) aged 2 through 4 y with a history of recurrent wheezing or a wheezing episode in the previous 12 mo; (5) with asthma; (6) who have received other live-virus vaccines within the previous 4 wk; (7) who have an immunodeficiency or who are receiving immunosuppressive therapies; (8) who are receiving aspirin or other salicylates; (9) with any condition that can compromise respiratory function or the handling of secretions or can increase the risk for aspiration, such as neurodevelopmental disorders, spinal cord injuries, seizure disorders, or neuromuscular abnormalities; (10) children taking an influenza antiviral medication (oseltamivir, zanamivir, or peramivir) until 48 h after stopping the influenza antiviral therapy; (11) with chronic underlying medical conditions that may predispose them to complications after wild-type influenza infection.

Sources

–*Pediatrics.* 2018;142(4):e2018-2367.

–Grohskopft L, et al. Prevention and Control of Seasonal Influenza with Vaccines: Recommendations of the Advisory Committee on Immunization Practices—United States, 2018–19 Influenza Season. *CDC MMWR.* 2018;67(3):1-20.

Comment

1. Highest-risk groups for influenza complications are:
   a. Pregnant women.
   b. Children age 6 mo to 5 y.
   c. Adults age ≥50 y.
   d. Persons with chronic medical conditions or who are immunocompromised.[e]
   e. Pregnant females or women who will be pregnant during the influenza season or breast-feeding.
   f. Residents of extended-care facilities.
   g. Morbidly obese (BMI >40) persons.
   h. Health care personnel.
   i. Household contacts of persons with high-risk medical conditions or caregivers of children age <5 y or adults age >50 y.
   j. Children and adolescents receiving long-term aspirin therapy.
   k. American Indians or Alaska Natives.
   l. People with a history of influenza-associated encephalopathy.

---

[e]Chronic heart, lung, renal, liver, hematologic, cancer, metabolic, neuromuscular or neurodevelopmental, or seizure disorders, severe cognitive dysfunction, diabetes, HIV infection, or immunosuppression.

Renal Disorders

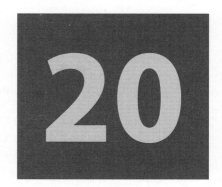

20

Population

–Adults and children.

Recommendations

▶ NICE 2013, VA/DoD 2014, KDIGO 2012

–Acute kidney injury (AKI) is defined as the increase in the SCr by equal to or greater than 0.3 mg/dL over 48 h, or increase in SCr to equal to or greater than 1.5 times baseline within the past 7 d, or urine volume <0.5 mL/kg/h for 6 h.

–Recommendations for acute management:

• In the absence of hemorrhagic shock, use of isotonic crystalloids rather than colloids for intravascular volume expansion.

• Do not use diuretics to prevent or treat AKI except in the management of volume overload.

• Do not use low-dose dopamine in either the prevention or treatment of AKI.

• Use vasopressors in addition to fluids for management of vasomotor shock with or at risk for AKI.

–Recommend volume expansion to at-risk adults who will receive intravenous iodinated contrast.

• CKD with eGFR <40 mL/min.

• CHF.

• Renal transplant.

• 75 y or over.

–Consult a pharmacist to assist with drug dosing in adults or children at risk for AKI.

Sources

–NICE. *Acute Kidney Injury: Prevention, Detection and Management of Acute Kidney Injury up to the Point of Renal Replacement Therapy.* London (UK): National Institute for Health and Care Excellence (NICE); 2013.

–VA/DoD. *Clinical Practice Guideline for the Management of Chronic Kidney Disease in Primary Care.* Washington (DC): Department of Veterans Affairs, Department of Defense; 2014.

–Kidney Disease Improving Global Outcomes (KDIGO). *KDIGO Clinical Practice Guideline for Acute Kidney Injury: Kidney International Supplements*; March 2012;2(1).

Comment

1. Inconsistent evidence for *N*-acetylcysteine use to prevent contrast-induced nephropathy.

Special Population: Children and Adolescents

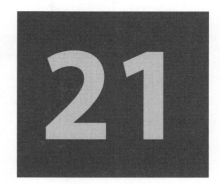

ASTHMA

Population
–Children.

Recommendations

▶ Global Initiative for Asthma (GINA) 2017
–Advise pregnant women and parents of young children not to smoke.
–Encourage vaginal delivery.
–Minimize use of acetaminophen and broad-spectrum antibiotics during first year of life.
–Avoid maternal obesity and excessive prepartum weight gain.

Source
–Global Initiative for Asthma. 2017.

Comments

1. Environmental exposures such as automobile exhaust and dust mites are associated with higher rates of asthma, while others (household pets and farm animals) may be protective. Avoiding tobacco smoke and air pollution is protective, but allergen avoidance measures have not been shown to be effective primary prevention.
2. Public health interventions to reduce childhood obesity, increase fruit and vegetable intake, improve maternal-fetal health, and reduce socioeconomic inequality would address major risk factors. (*Lancet.* 2015;386:1075-1085)
3. Maternal intake of allergenic food likely decreases the risk of allergy and asthma in offspring.
4. Breast-feeding is generally advisable, but not for the specific purpose of preventing allergies and asthma.

ATHEROSCLEROTIC CARDIOVASCULAR DISEASE

Population
–Children and adolescents.

Recommendations

▶NIH/NHLBI 2012

–Screen all children for cholesterol once between age 9 and 11 y and once between age 17 and 21 y.
–Use nonfasting total cholesterol and HDL cholesterol as the screening tests.
–Clinicians may recommend low-fat or nonfat dairy at age 1 y for high-risk patients.
–If lifestyle changes are not effective, consider a lipid-lowering agent at age 10 y.

Lifestyle Therapies

–If LDL elevated, refer to a registered dietitian for family medical nutrition therapy:
  • 25%–30% of calories from fat,[a] ≤7% from saturated fat, approximately 10% from monounsaturated fat; <200 mg/d of cholesterol; avoid trans fats as much as possible.
–Plant sterol esters and/or plant stanol esters[b] up to 2 g/d as replacement for usual fat sources can be used after age 2 y in children with familial hypercholesterolemia.
–Plant stanol esters as part of a regular diet are marketed directly to the public. Short-term studies show no harmful effects in healthy children.
–The water-soluble fiber psyllium can be added to a low-fat, low-saturated-fat diet as cereal enriched with psyllium at a dose of 6 g/d for children 2–12 y, and 12 g/d for those ≥12 y.
–If TG elevated, refer to a registered dietitian for family medical nutrition therapy:
  • 25%–30% of calories from fat, ≤7% from saturated fat, ~10% from monounsaturated fat; <200 mg/d of cholesterol; avoid trans fats as much as possible.

[a] The 2010 USDA Dietary Guidelines for Americans supports the IOM recommendations for 30%–40% of calories from fat for ages 1–3 y, 25%–35% of calories from fat for ages 4–18 y, and 20%–35% of calories from fat for adults (https://health.gov/dietaryguidelines/dga2010/dietaryguidelines2010.pdf).
[b] Can be found added to some foods, such as some margarines.

–Decrease sugar intake by replacing simple with complex carbohydrates and eliminating sugar sweetened beverages.

–Increase dietary fish to increase omega-3 fatty acids.[c]

–As in all children, recommend physical activity. Age 5–10, 1 h/d of moderate-to-vigorous physical activity and <2 h/d of sedentary screen time are recommended. Age 11–21, 1 h/d of moderate-to-vigorous activity with vigorous intensity 3 d/wk, with <2 h of screen time with quality programming daily.

Pharmacologic Therapies

–Birth–10 y: Only use medications for children with severe primary hyperlipidemia (homozygous familial hypercholesterolemia, primary hypertriglyceridemia with TG ≥500 mg/dL) or a high-risk condition or evident cardiovascular disease; all under the care of a lipid specialist.

–≥10–21 y: Perform detailed FH and risk factor (RF) assessment before initiation of drug therapy. Consider drug therapy based on the average of at least 2 fasting lipid panels obtained between 2 wk and 3 mo apart.

–LDL-C:

- If average LDL-C ≥250 mg/dL, consult a lipid specialist.
- If average LDL-C ≥130–250 mg/dL, or non-HDL ≥145 mg/dL, refer to a dietitian for medical nutrition therapy with Cardiovascular Health Integrated Lifestyle Diet (CHILD 1) and CHILD 2-LDL diet × 6 mo repeat fasting lipid panel (FLP).
- If repeat FLP shows LDL-C <130 mg/dL, continue CHILD 2-LDL diet, reevaluate in 12 mo.
- If repeat FLP shows LDL-C ≥190 mg/dL, consider initiation of statin therapy.
- If repeat FLP shows LDL-C ≥130–189 mg/dL, FH (–), no other RF or RC, continue CHILD 2-LDL diet, reevaluate q 6 mo.
- If repeat FLP shows LDL-C = 160–189 mg/dL + FH positive or ≥1 high-level RF/RC or ≥2 moderate-level RFs/RCs, consider statin therapy.
- If repeat FLP shows LDL-C ≥130–159 mg/dL + ≥2 high-level RFs/RCs or 1 high-level + 2 moderate-level RFs/RCs, consider statin therapy.

[c]The Food and Drug Administration (FDA) and the Environmental Protection Agency are advising women of childbearing age who may become pregnant, pregnant women, nursing mothers, and young children to avoid some types of fish and shellfish and eat fish and shellfish that are low in mercury. For more information, call the FDA's food information line toll free at 1-888-SAFEFOOD or visit http://www.fda.gov/downloads/Food/FoodborneIllnessContaminants/UCM312787.pdf-page=21

–Children on statin therapy should be counseled and carefully monitored.

–TG:

- If average TG ≥500 mg/dL, consult a lipid specialist.
- If average TG ≥100 mg/dL in a child <10 y, ≥130 mg/dL in a child age 10–19 y, TG <500 mg/dL, refer to a dietitian for medical nutrition therapy with CHILD 1 diet and CHILD 2-TG diet × 6 mo.
- If repeat FLP shows TG <100 mg/dL, continue CHILD 2-TG diet, monitor 6–12 mo.
- If repeat FLP shows TG >100 mg/dL, reconsult dietitian for intensified CHILD 2 TG diet counseling.
- If repeat FLP shows TG ≥200–499 mg/dL, non-HDL ≥145 mg/dL, consider fish oil ± consult a lipid specialist.

Source

–Expert Panel on Integrated Guidelines for Cardiovascular Health and Risk Reduction in Children and Adolescents. *Pediatrics.* 2011;128(5):S213-S258. https://www.nhlbi.nih.gov/files/docs/peds_guidelines_sum.pdf

CONCUSSION

Population

–Children and young adults.

Recommendations

▶ AAN 2013

–School-based professionals should be educated by licensed health care professionals to understand the risks of a concussion.

–Licensed health care professionals should educate athletes about concussion risks.

–Athletes with a concussion should be prohibited from returning to play or practice in contact sports until a licensed health care provider has cleared them to return.

–Licensed health care providers should recommend retirement for any athlete with repeated concussions who has chronic, persistent neurologic or cognitive deficits.

Source

–*Neurology.* 2013;80(24):2250.

DENTAL CARIES

Population
  –Infants and children up to age 5 y.

Recommendations

▶ **USPSTF 2014, AAP 2014, AAFP 2014, Bright Futures Oral Health Guide**
  –Clean infant gums with clean, soft, damp cloth once daily.
  –Apply fluoride varnish to the primary teeth of all infants and children starting at the age of primary teeth eruption.
  –Supplement with oral fluoride starting at age 6 mo where water supply is fluoride deficient ($\leq$0.6 mg/L).

  Sources
  –AAFP. *Clinical Recommendation.* 2014.
  –*Pediatrics.* 2014;133(5):s1-s10.

Comments
  1. Fluoride mouthwash used regularly by children under 16 reduces risk of dental caries by >25%. (*Cochrane Database Syst Rev.* 2016;7:CD002284)
  2. The CDC's My Water's Fluoride resource provides county-level information on content of fluoride in the water system. https://nccd.cdc.gov/DOH_MWF/
  3. Brush infant teeth with a smear of fluoridated toothpaste at eruption of first tooth twice per day up to age 3. Children aged 3–6 years should brush with a pea-sized amount of fluoridated toothpaste twice daily; parents should be brushing child's teeth once daily until age 7.
  4. Caries risk assessment tool can be found at: https://www.aapd.org/globalassets/media/policies_guidelines/bp_cariesriskassessment.pdf

TABLE I: RECOMMENDED FLUORIDE SUPPLEMENTATION BY AGE AND FLUORIDE LEVEL IN COMMUNITY WATER SUPPLY		
Age	**Fluoride Level in Drinking Water <0.3 ppm**	**Fluoride Level in Drinking Water 0.3–0.6 ppm**
6 mo–3 y	0.25 mg/d	None
3–6 y	0.5 mg/d	0.25 mg/d
6–16 y	1.0 mg/d	0.5 mg/d

Adapted from Table 1 in CDC MMWR. 2001;50(RR14):1-42. https://www.cdc.gov/mmwr/preview/mmwrhtml/rr5014a1.htm

TABLE II: CLINICAL RECOMMENDATIONS FOR USE OF PROFESSIONALLY APPLIED OR PRESCRIPTION-STRENGTH, HOME-USE TOPICAL FLUORIDE AGENTS FOR CARIES PREVENTION IN PATIENTS AT ELEVATED RISK OF DEVELOPING CARIES

Age Group or Dentition Affected	Professionally Applied Topical Fluoride Agent	Prescription-Strength, Home-Use Topical Fluoride Agent
Younger than 6 y	2.26% fluoride varnish at least every 3 to 6 mo (**In Favor**)	
6–18 y	2.26% fluoride varnish at least every 3 to 6 mo (**In Favor**) or 1.23% fluoride (acidulated phosphate fluoride [APF]) gel for 4 min at least every 3 to 6 mo (**In Favor**)	0.09% fluoride mouthrinse at least weekly (**In Favor**) or 0.5% fluoride gel or paste twice daily (**Expert Opinion For**)
Older than 18 y	2.26% fluoride varnish at least every 3 to 6 mo (**Expert Opinion For**) or 1.23% fluoride (APF) gel for at least 4 min every 3 to 6 mo (**Expert Opinion For**)	0.09% fluoride mouthrinse at least weekly (**Expert Opinion For**) or 0.5% fluoride gel or paste twice daily (**Expert Opinion For**)
Adult Root Caries	2.26% fluoride varnish at least every 3 to 6 mo (**Expert Opinion For**) or 1.23% fluoride (APF) gel for 4 min at least every 3 to 6 mo (**Expert Opinion For**)	0.09% fluoride mouthrinse daily (**Expert Opinion For**) or 0.5% fluoride gel or paste twice daily (**Expert Opinion For**)

Additional Information:
· **Patients at low risk of developing caries may not need additional topical fluorides other than over-the-counter fluoridated toothpaste and fluoridated water.**

Source: Weyant RJ, et al. *Topical Fluoride for Caries Prevention.* Chicago, IL: American Dental Association; 2013. http://www.guideline.gov/content.aspx?id=47553

DIABETES MELLITUS (DM), TYPE 2

Population
–Children at start of puberty or age ≥10 y.

Recommendation
▶ ADA 2012
–Screen all children at risk for DM type 2.[d]

Source
–*Diabetes Care.* 2012;35(suppl 1):S11-S63.

Comments
1. Preexisting diabetes if:
   a. Fasting glucose ≥126 mg/dL.
   b. 2-h glucose ≥200 mg/dL after 75-g glucose load.
   c. Random glucose ≥200 mg/dL with classic hyperglycemic symptoms.
   d. Hemoglobin A1c ≥6.5%.
2. Criteria for GDM by 75-g 2-h OGTT if any of the following are abnormal:
   a. Fasting ≥92 mg/dL (5.1 mmol/L).
   b. 1 h ≥180 mg/dL (10.0 mmol/L).
   c. 2 h ≥153 mg/dL (8.5 mmol/L).

DOMESTIC VIOLENCE

Population
–Adolescents and adult women.

Recommendation
▶ WHO 2010
–Institute school-based programs that emphasize preventing dating violence.

Source
–World Health Organization. *Preventing Intimate Partner and Sexual Violence against Women.* 2010.

[d]Test asymptomatic children if BMI >85% for age/gender, weight for height >85th percentile, or weight >120% of ideal for height plus any two of the following: FH of DM in first- or second-degree relative; high-risk ethnic group (eg, Native American, African-American, Latino, Asian-American, or Pacific Islander); Acanthosis nigricans; HTN; dyslipidemia, polycystic ovary syndrome; small-for-gestational-age birth weight; maternal history of DM or GDM during the child's gestation.

Comment

1. Interventions with possible but not proven efficacy include:
   a. School-based programs that teach children to recognize and avoid sexually abusive situations.
   b. Empowerment and relationship skills training for women.
   c. Programs that change social and cultural gender norms.

IMMUNIZATIONS, INFANTS AND CHILDREN

Population

–Infants and children age 0–18 y.

Recommendation

▶ CDC 2018

–Immunize infants and children according to the CDC recommendations unless contraindicated (see Appendix IX).

Sources

–CDC. Child and Adolescent Schedule.
–CDC. Catch-Up Immunization Schedule.

INFLUENZA, CHEMOPROPHYLAXIS

Population

–Children and adults.

Recommendations

▶ AAP 2016

The following situations warrant chemoprophylaxis:

–Children at high risk for complications who cannot receive vaccine, or within 2 wk of receiving vaccine.

–Family members or health care providers who are unimmunized and likely to have ongoing exposure to high-risk or unimmunized children younger than 24 mo of age.

–Unimmunized staff and children in an institutional setting during an outbreak.

–Postexposure prophylaxis for close contacts of infected person who are at high risk of complications if less than 48 h since exposure.

▶ IDSA 2009, CDC 2011, AAP 2016

–Consider antiviral chemoprophylaxis for adults and children age >1 y at high risk of influenza complications (see the Influenza, Vaccination section) when any of the following conditions are present:

- Influenza vaccination is contraindicated (anaphylactic hypersensitivity to eggs, acute febrile illness, history of Guillain–Barré syndrome within 6 wk of a previous influenza vaccination).
- Unvaccinated adults or children when influenza activity has been detected in the community. Vaccinate simultaneously.
- Unvaccinated adults and children in close contact with people diagnosed with influenza.
- Residents of extended-care facilities with an influenza outbreak.

Sources

–CID. 2009;48:1003-1032.

–CDC. https://www.cdc.gov/flu/professionals/antivirals/summary-clinicians.htm

Comments

1. Influenza vaccination is the best way to prevent influenza.
2. Antiviral chemoprophylaxis is not a substitute for influenza vaccination.
3. Agents for chemoprophylaxis of influenza A (H1N1) and B: zanamivir or oseltamivir.
4. Children at high risk of complications include those with chronic diseases such as asthma, diabetes, cardiac disease, immune suppression, and neurodevelopmental disorders.
5. If child <3 mo, use of oseltamivir for chemoprophylaxis is not recommended unless situation is judged critical due to limited data in this age group.

INFLUENZA, VACCINATION

Population

–All persons age >6 mo.

Recommendations

▶ CDC 2016, AAP 2016

–All persons age >6 mo should receive the seasonal influenza vaccine annually.

–All children age 6 mo to 8 y should receive 2 doses of the vaccine (>4 wk apart) during their first season of vaccination.

–The live attenuated influenza vaccine (Flumist quadrivalent) should not be used due to low efficacy.

Sources
–*Pediatrics*. 2016;138(4):e20162527.
–CDC. https://www.cdc.gov/vaccines/hcp/acip-recs/vacc-specific/flu.html

Comment

1. Highest-risk groups for influenza complications are:
   a. Pregnant women.
   b. Children age 6 mo to 5 y.
   c. Adults age >50 y.
   d. Persons with chronic medical conditions.[e]
   e. Residents of extended-care facilities.
   f. Morbidly obese (BMI >40) persons.
   g. Health care personnel.
   h. Household contacts of persons with high-risk medical conditions or caregivers of children age <5 y or adults age >50 y.
   i. Children and adolescents receiving long-term aspirin therapy.
   j. American Indians or Alaska Natives.

MOTOR VEHICLE INJURY

Population
–Infants, children, and adolescents.

Recommendations
▶ ICSI 2013
–Ask the family about the use of car seats, booster seats, and seat belts.
–Ask children and adolescents about helmet use in recreational activities.

Source
–ICSI. *Preventive Services for Children and Adolescents*. 19th ed. 2013.

Comments

1. Head injury rates are reduced by approximately 75% in motorcyclists who wear helmets compared with those who do not.
2. Properly used child restraint systems can reduce mortality up to 21% compared with seat belt usage in children age 2–6 y.

[e]Chronic heart, lung, renal, liver, hematologic, cancer, neuromuscular, or seizure disorders, severe cognitive dysfunction, diabetes, HIV infection, or immunosuppression.

3. All infants and toddlers should ride in a rear-facing car safety seat until they are age 2 or until they have met the max height or weight allowed by car seat manufacturer.

OBESITY

Population
–Children age ≥ 6 y.

Recommendation
▶ AAFP 2010, USPSTF 2017
–Screen children age 6 y and older for obesity.

Source
–USPSTF. *Obesity in Children and Adolescents: Screening.* 2017.

Comment
1. Obese children should be offered intensive counseling and behavioral interventions to promote improvement in weight status.

Population
–Children age ≥ 2 y.

Recommendation
▶ ICSI 2013
–Record height, weight, and body mass index (BMI) annually starting at age 2 y.

Source
–ICSI. *Preventive Services for Children and Adolescents.* 19th ed. 2013.

Comments
1. Children with a BMI ≥ 25 are 5 times more likely to be overweight as adults when compared with their normal-weight counterparts.
2. Overweight children should be counseled about wholesome eating, 30–60 min of daily physical activity, and avoiding soft drinks.

Population
–Adolescents.

Recommendations
▶ ICSI 2013
–Employ a team approach to manage weight in all persons of normal weight (BMI 18.5–24.9) or overweight (BMI 25–29.9) including:
- Nutrition.
- Physical activity.

- Lifestyle changes.
- Screen for depression.
- Screen for eating disorders.
- Review medication list and assess if any medications can interfere with weight loss.

–Follow up regularly to reinforce principles of weight management.

Source

–Fitch A, Everling L, Fox C, et al. *Prevention and Management of Obesity for Children and Adolescents.* Bloomington (MN): ICSI; 2013.

Comments

1. Recommend 30–60 min of moderate physical activity on most days of the week.
2. Nutrition education focused on decreased caloric intake, encouraging healthy food choices, and managing restaurant and social eating situations.
3. Limit screen time to less than 2 h per day.
4. Encourage nonfood rewards for positive reinforcement.
5. Stress management techniques.
6. 5%–10% weight loss can produce a clinically significant reduction in heart disease risk.

Population

–Children.

Recommendations

▶ Endocrine Society 2017

–Educate children and parents about healthy diets and the importance of regular physical activity.
–Encourage school systems to promote healthy eating habits and provide health education courses.
–Foster healthy sleep patterns.
–Balance screen time with opportunities for physical activity.
–Clinicians should help educate families and communities about healthy dietary and activity habits.

Source

–*J Clin Endocrinol Metab.* 2017;102(3):709-757.

Comments

1. Avoid the consumption of calorie-dense, nutrient-poor foods (eg, juices, soft drinks, "fast food" items, and calorie-dense snacks). Consume whole fruits rather than juices.

2. Control calorie intake by portion control.
3. Reduce saturated dietary fat intake for children age >2 y.
4. Increase dietary fiber, fruits, and vegetables.
5. Eat regular, scheduled meals and avoid snacking.
6. Limit television, video games, and computer time to 2 h daily.

OTITIS MEDIA

Population
–Children 6 mo to 12 y.

Recommendations
▶ AAP 2013

–Do not use prophylactic antibiotics to reduce the frequency of episodes of AOM in children with recurrent AOM.
–Exclusive breast-feeding for at least the first 6 mo of life.
–Vaccinate all children to prevent bacterial AOM with pneumococcal and influenza vaccines.
–Avoid tobacco exposure.

Source
–*Pediatrics.* 2013;131(3):e964-e999.

SEXUALLY TRANSMITTED INFECTIONS (STIs)

Population
–Sexually active adolescents and high-risk adults.

Recommendation
▶ USPSTF 2014

–Employ high-intensity behavioral counseling to prevent STIs for all sexually active adolescents and for adults at increased risk for STIs. Include basic information about STIs, condom use, communication about safe sex, problem solving, and goal setting.

Source
–USPSTF. *Sexually Transmitted Infections.* 2014.

TOBACCO USE

Population
–School-aged children and adolescents.

Recommendation
▶ AAFP/USPSTF 2013
–Provide interventions including education or brief counseling to prevent the initiation of tobacco use.

Source
–USPSTF. *Tobacco Use in Children and Adolescents: Primary Care Interventions.* 2013.

Comment
1. The efficacy of counseling to prevent tobacco use in children and adolescents is uncertain.

Special Population: Newborns and Infants

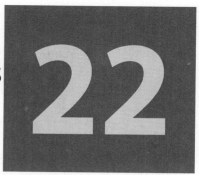

IMMUNIZATIONS, INFANTS AND CHILDREN

Population
–Infants and children age 0–18 y.

Recommendations

▶ **Advisory Committee on Immunization Practices (ACIP) 2017**
–Immunize infants and children based on the 2018 immunization schedule.
–Centers for Disease Control (CDC), the American Academy of Pediatrics (AAP), the American Academy of Family Physicians (AAFP), and the American College of Obstetricians and Gynecologists (ACOG) have approved the schedule.

Source
–*MMWR Morb Mortal Wkly Rep.* 2018;67:156-157.

SUDDEN INFANT DEATH SYNDROME (SIDS)

Population
–Newborns and infants.

Recommendations

▶ **AAP 2016**
–Place their infants to sleep on their backs.
–Use a firm sleep surface without soft objects or loose bedding.
–Breastfeed.
–For the first 6–12 m, infants should sleep in parents' room (but not in parents' bed).
–Avoid smoke exposure, alcohol and illicit drug use, overheating.

Source

–*Pediatrics.* 2016;138(5):e20162938.

Comments

1. Stomach and side sleeping have been identified as major risk factors for SIDS.
2. Pacifiers may be protective.

GONORRHEA, OPHTHALMIA NEONATORUM

Population

–Newborns.

Recommendation

▶ USPSTF 2019

–Give all newborns prophylactic ocular topical medication against gonococcal ophthalmia neonatorum.

Source

–USPSTF. *Gonorrhea Prophylactic Medication: Newborns.* 2019.

Comments

1. Erythromycin 0.5% ointment is only agent available in the United States for this application.
2. Canadian Paediatric Society now recommends against universal prophylaxis, given incomplete efficacy of erythromycin, rarity of the condition, and disruption in maternal-infant bonding. Instead, they recommend screening mothers for gonorrhea and chlamydia infection and, if infected with gonorrhea at the time of delivery, treating the infant with ceftriaxone. (*Paediatr Child Health.* 2015;20:93-96)

Special Population: Older Adults

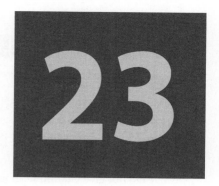

DRIVING RISK

Population
–Adults with dementia.

Recommendation
▶ AAN 2019

–Assess patients with dementia for the following characteristics that place them at increased risk for unsafe driving (Clinical Dementia Rating Scale):

- Caregiver's assessment that the patient's driving ability is marginal or unsafe.
- History of traffic citations and motor vehicle collisions.
- Self-reported situational avoidance.
- Reduced driving mileage (<60 miles/wk).
- Self-reported situational avoidance.
- Mini-Mental Status Exam score ≤24.
- Aggression or impulsivity.
- Alcohol, medications, sleep disorders, visual impairment, motor impairment.

Sources
–*Neurology.* 2010;74(16):1316.
–https://www.aan.com/Guidelines/home/GuidelineDetail/396

FALLS IN THE ELDERLY

Population
–Older adults.

Recommendations

▶ **USPSTF 2018, Cochrane Database of Systematic Reviews 2012**

–Do not give vitamin D supplementation to community-dwelling older adults without vitamin D deficiency or osteoporosis for fall prevention.
–Recommend vitamin D supplementation to elderly patients in care facilities. This reduces the rate of falls by 37%.
–Recommend home-hazard modification (eg, adding nonslip tape to rugs and steps, provision of grab bars, etc) for all homes of persons age >65 y.
–Recommend exercise or physical therapy interventions targeting gait and balance training.
–Selectively offer a multifactorial assessment and management approach in community-dwelling older adults at increased risk for falls.

Sources
–USPSTF. *Falls Prevention in Older Adults: Counseling and Preventive Medication.* 2018.
–Cochrane Collaborative. *Interventions for Preventing Falls in Older People in Care Facilities and Hospitals.* 2012.
–Public Health England. *Falls and Fracture Consensus Statement: Supporting Commissioning for Prevention.* 2012.

Comments
1. 30%–40% of all community-dwelling persons age >65 y fall at least once a year.
2. Falls are the leading cause of fatal and nonfatal injuries among persons age >65 y.
3. A review and modification of chronic medications, including psychotropic medications, is important although not proven to reduce falls. Please see appendix for Beers List of potentially problematic medications.
4. Public Health England (2017): Older adults should aim for at least 150 min of moderate activity or 75 min of vigorous activity per week. Strength/balance training is recommended at least 2 d/wk. Extended sedentary periods should be minimized.

OSTEOPOROTIC HIP FRACTURES

Population

–Noninstitutionalized postmenopausal women.

Recommendation

▶ USPSTF 2018

–Screen for osteoporosis with bone measurement testing to prevent osteoporotic fractures in older women.

Source

–*JAMA*. 2018;319(24):2521-2531.

Recommendation

▶ USPSTF 2018

–Do not supplement daily with ≤400 IU vitamin D and ≤1000 mg calcium for primary prevention of fractures. Insufficient evidence for higher doses.

Source

–*JAMA*. 2018;319(15):1592-1599.

Comments

1. Insufficient evidence for vitamin D and calcium supplementation for anyone for the primary prevention of fractures.
2. These recommendations do not apply to individuals with history of osteoporotic fractures, increased risk for fall, diagnosis of osteoporosis, or vitamin D deficiency.

Population

–Postmenopausal women.

Recommendation

▶ USPSTF 2017

–Recommends against the routine use of combined estrogen and progestin for the prevention of chronic conditions including osteoporotic fractures.

Population

–Postmenopausal women who have had a hysterectomy.

Recommendation

▶ USPSTF 2017

–Do not use estrogen routinely to prevent chronic conditions in postmenopausal women who have had a hysterectomy.

Source
–*JAMA*. 2017;318(22):2224-2233.

Comment

1. The results of studies including the WHI and the Heart and Estrogen/Progestin Replacement Study reveal that HRT probably reduces osteoporotic hip and vertebral fractures and may decrease the risk of colon CA; however, HRT may lead to an increased risk of breast CA, stroke, cholecystitis, dementia, and venous thromboembolism. HRT does not decrease the risk of coronary artery disease (CAD).

Special Population: Pregnant Women

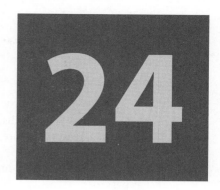

CESAREAN SECTION

Population
  –Pregnant women with history of prior cesarean delivery.

Recommendations

▶ AAFP 2014, ACOG 2017
  –Attempting a vaginal birth after cesarean (VBAC) is safe and appropriate for most women.
  –Encourage and facilitate planning for VBAC. If necessary, refer to a facility that offers trial of labor after cesarean (TOLAC).

Sources
  –AAFP. *Clinical Recommendation: Vaginal Birth After Cesarean.* 2014.
  –*Obstet Gynecol.* 2017;130(5):1167-1169.

Comments

1. Provide counseling, encouragement, and facilitation for a planned vaginal birth after cesarean (PVBAC) so that women can make informed decisions. If PVBAC is not locally available, offer women who desire it referral to a facility or clinician who offers the service.
2. Obtain informed consent for PVBAC, including risk to patient, fetus, future fertility, and the capabilities of local delivery setting.
3. Develop facility guidelines to promote access to PVBAC and improve quality of care for women who elect TOLAC.
4. Assess the likelihood of PVBAC as well as individual risks to determine who is an appropriate candidate for TOLAC.
5. A calculator for probability for successful VBAC is available here: https://mfmunetwork.bsc.gwu.edu/PublicBSC/MFMU/VGBirthCalc/vagbirth.html

Population

–Women in labor.

Recommendations

▶ ACOG 2012

–Induce labor only for medical indications. If induction is performed for nonmedical reasons, ensure that gestational age is >39 wk and cervix is favorable.

–Do not diagnose failed induction or arrest of labor until sufficient time[a] has passed.

–Consider intermittent auscultation rather than continuous fetal monitoring if heart rate is normal.

Source

–*Obstet Gynecol.* 2012;120(5):1181.

▶ WHO 2018

–Implement prenatal education programs including childbirth training, nurse-led relaxation, couple-based support, and psychoeducation.

–Consider mandatory second opinion for cesarean section decisions.

–Give timely feedback to health care professionals regarding cesarean section decision making.

Source

–World Health Organization. *WHO Recommendations Non-Clinical Interventions to Reduce Unnecessary Cesarean Sections.* 2018.

Comments

1. If fetal heart rate variability is moderate, other factors have little association with fetal neurologic outcomes.

2. Doctors who are salaried have lower cesarean rates than those paid fee-for-service.

3. As part of informed consent for the first cesarean, discuss effect on future pregnancies including risks of uterine rupture and abnormal implantation of placenta.

---

[a]Failed induction: inability to generate contractions every 3 min and cervical change after 24 h of oxytocin administration and rupture of membranes, if feasible. Arrest of labor, first stage: 6 cm dilation, membrane rupture, and 4 h of adequate contractions or 6 h of inadequate contractions without cervical change. Arrest of labor, second stage: no descent or rotation for 4 h (nulliparous woman with epidural), 3 h (nulliparous woman without epidural or multiparous woman with epidural), or 2 h (multiparous woman without epidural).

GROUP B STREPTOCOCCAL (GBS) INFECTION

Population
–Pregnant women.

Recommendations

▶ ACOG 2019, AAP 2019

–Obtain vaginal-rectal swab specimen for GBS culture at 36 0/7–37 6/7 wk gestation.

–Intrapartum antibiotic prophylaxis (IAP) to prevent early-onset invasive GBS disease in newborns is indicated for high-risk pregnancies, including those with positive GBS culture, GBS bacteriuria during pregnancy, or history of previous GBS-infected newborn.

–If a woman presents in labor with unknown GBS colonization status this pregnancy, but has a history of GBS in a prior pregnancy, can offer IAP.

–Do not give IAP if a cesarean delivery is performed with intact membranes and before the onset of labor.

Sources
–https://www.acog.org/GBS
–https://pediatrics.aappublications.org/content/144/2/e20191881

Comments

1. Penicillin G is the agent of choice for IAP.
2. Ampicillin is an acceptable alternative to penicillin G.
3. Use cefazolin if the patient has a penicillin allergy that does not cause anaphylaxis, angioedema, urticaria, or respiratory distress.
4. Use clindamycin[b] or vancomycin if the patient has a penicillin allergy that causes anaphylaxis, angioedema, urticaria, or respiratory distress.

NEURAL TUBE DEFECTS

Population
–Women of childbearing age.

Recommendation

▶ USPSTF 2016, AAFP 2016, ACOG 2017

–Women should take a daily supplement containing 400–800 µg of folic acid if planning or capable of pregnancy.

---

[b]Use clindamycin if isolate is sensitive to both clindamycin and erythromycin. If not, use vancomycin.

Sources

–*Obstet Gynecol.* 2017;130:e279-e290. [lww.com]

–https://journals.lww.com/greenjournal/Fulltext/2017/12000/Practice_ simplein_No__187___Neural_Tube_Defects.41.aspx

–*JAMA.* 2017;317(2):183-189. [uspstf] https://www.uspreventiveservices taskforce.org/Page/Document/RecommendationStatementFinal/folic-acid-for-the-prevention-of-neural-tube-defects-preventive-medication

–AAFP. *Clinical Recommendation.* [aafp.org] https://www.aafp.org/ patient-care/clinical-recommendations/all/neural-tube-defects.html

POSTPARTUM DEPRESSION

Population

–Pregnant women.

Recommendations

▶ USPSTF 2019

–Refer those at increased risk of perinatal depression to counseling interventions.

–No accurate screening tool to identify those at risk. Consider providing counseling to women with 1 or more of the following risk factors: history of depression, current depressive symptoms, certain socioeconomic risk factors such as low income or adolescent or single parenthood, recent intimate partner violence, or mental health–related factors.

Source

–https://jamanetwork.com/journals/jama/fullarticle/2724195

POSTPARTUM HEMORRHAGE

Population

–Pregnant women.

Recommendations

▶ ACOG 2017

–Give uterotonic medications to all women during the third stage of labor.

• Oxytocin 10 IU, IV, or IM is first choice.

• Methylergometrine or oral/rectal misoprostol is an alternative.

–Perform uterine massage.

–Use controlled cord traction to remove the placenta.

Source
–*Obstet Gynecol.* 2017;183(130):e168-e186.

Comment

1. ACOG defines maternal hemorrhage as cumulative blood loss of ≥1000 mL or blood loss accompanied by signs or symptoms of hypovolemia within 24 h after birth.

PREECLAMPSIA

Population

–Pregnant women at increased risk of preeclampsia.

Recommendation

▶ USPSTF 2014

–Use aspirin 81 mg/d after 12th wk of gestation if ≥1 major risk factor for preeclampsia.

Source
–*Ann Intern Med.* 2014;161:819-826.

Comment

1. Major risk factors: personal history of preeclampsia, multifetal gestation, chronic hypertension, DM, renal disease, autoimmune disease.

PRETERM BIRTH

Population

–Pregnant women.

Recommendations

▶ ACOG 2012

–Do not use maintenance tocolytics to prevent preterm birth.
–Do not give antibiotics for the purpose of prolonging gestation or improving neonatal outcome in preterm labor with intact membranes.
–In women with prior spontaneous preterm delivery, start progesterone therapy between 16 and 24 wk gestation.
–Consider cerclage placement to improve preterm birth outcomes in women with prior spontaneous preterm delivery <34 wk, current singleton pregnancy, short cervical length (<25 mm) before 24 wk gestation.

Source
–*Obstet Gynecol.* 2012;120(4):964-973.

Comments

1. No evidence to support the use of prolonged tocolytics for women with preterm labor.
2. No evidence to support strict bed rest for the prevention of preterm birth.
3. The positive predictive value of a positive fetal fibronectin test or a short cervix for preterm birth is poor in isolation.

Rh ALLOIMMUNIZATION

Population
–Pregnant women.

Recommendations

▶ ACOG 2018

–Screen ABO blood group and Rh-D type at first prenatal visit of each pregnancy.
–Repeat antibody screen before giving anti-D immune globulin (28 wk gestation, postpartum, and pregnancy events).

Source
–*Obstet Gynecol.* 2018;131:e8.

SURGICAL SITE INFECTIONS (SSI)

Population
–Women undergoing abdominal procedures.

Recommendations

▶ Cochrane Database of Systematic Reviews 2014, ACOG 2018

–Treat remote infections prior to elective operations.
–Do not shave incision site unless hair interferes with operation. If necessary, remove hair immediately before operation with clippers.
–Control serum blood glucose levels and avoid perioperative hyperglycemia.
–Patients should shower or bathe (full body) on at least the night before abdominal surgery.
–Prepare the surgical site preoperatively with an alcohol-based agent unless contraindicated.

–Use a vaginal preparation with povidone-iodine solution immediately prior to hysterectomy or vaginal surgery.
–Give prophylactic IV antibiotics preoperatively within 60 min of skin incision as opposed to administration after cord clamping.

Sources
–*Obstet Gynecol.* 2018;131:e172-e189.
–http://www.cochrane.org/CD007892/PREG_vaginal-cleansing-before-cesarean-delivery-to-reduce-post-cesarean-infections

Comments

1. A vaginal prep prior to cesarean section reduces the incidence of postpartum endometritis. This benefit was especially true for women in active labor or with rupture membranes.
2. The incidence of maternal infectious morbidity is decreased (RR 0.54) when prophylactic antibiotics are administered preoperatively as opposed to after cord clamping.

THROMBOEMBOLISM IN PREGNANCY

Population
–Pregnant women.

Recommendations

▶ ACOG 2018
–Consider thromboprophylaxis for patients at increased risk of thromboembolism.
–There is not sufficient evidence for routine prophylaxis in pregnancy.
–No risk assessment tool has been sufficiently validated, but risk factors include: personal history of thrombosis, thrombophilia, cesarean delivery, obesity, hypertension, autoimmune disease, heart disease, sickle cell disease, multiple gestations, preeclampsia.

TOBACCO USE

Population
–Pregnant women.

Recommendation

▶ AAFP 2015, USPSTF 2015, ICSI 2014
–Screen all pregnant women for tobacco use and provide pregnancy-directed counseling and literature for those who smoke.

Sources
   –AAFP. *Clinical Preventive Service Recommendation: Tobacco Use.* 2015.
   –USPSTF. *Tobacco Smoking Cessation in Adults, Including Pregnant Women: Behavioral and Pharmacotherapy Interventions.* 2015.
   –ICSI. *Preventive Services for Adults.* 20th ed. 2014.

Comment

1. The "5-A" framework is helpful for smoking cessation counseling:
   a. Ask about tobacco use.
   b. Advise to quit through clear, individualized messages.
   c. Assess willingness to quit.
   d. Assist in quitting.
   e. Arrange follow-up and support sessions.

Population

   –School-aged children and adolescents.

Recommendation

▶ AAFP/USPSTF 2013

   –Recommend that primary care clinicians provide interventions including education or brief counseling to prevent the initiation of tobacco use.

Comment

1. The efficacy of counseling to prevent tobacco use in children and adolescents is uncertain.

Source
   –USPSTF. *Tobacco Use in Children and Adolescents: Primary Care Interventions.* 2013.

Management

Behavioral Health Disorders

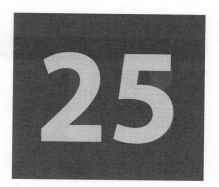

ADULT PSYCHIATRIC PATIENTS IN THE EMERGENCY DEPARTMENT

Populations
- Adult patients presenting to ED with psychiatric symptoms.
- Adults with abnormal liver chemistries.

Recommendations
- No role for routine laboratory testing. Medical history, examination, and previous psychiatric diagnoses should guide testing.
- No role for routine neuroimaging studies in the absence of focal neurological deficits.
- Risk assessment tools should not be used in isolation to identify low-risk adults who are safe for ED discharge if they present with suicidal ideations.

Source
- Nazarian DJ, Broder JS, Thiessen ME, Wilson MP, Zun LS, Brown MD; American College of Emergency Physicians. Clinical policy: critical issues in the diagnosis and management of the adult psychiatric patient in the emergency department. *Ann Emerg Med.* 2017;69(4):480-498.

ALCOHOL USE DISORDERS

Population
–Adults.

Recommendations

▶ USPSTF 2018, APA 2018

–For patients identified with an Alcohol Use Disorder, provide a brief intervention and schedule follow-up via SBIRT (Screening Brief Intervention, and Referral to Treatment) model.
–Refer all patients with life-threatening withdrawal such as seizure or delirium tremens to a hospital for admission.
–Refer more stable outpatients to a behavioral therapy such as the IOP (Intensive Outpatient Program), an RTC (residential treatment center), or a Sober Living facility.
–Recommend prophylactic thiamine for all harmful alcohol use or alcohol dependence.
–Refer suitable patients with decompensated cirrhosis for consideration of liver transplantation once they have been sober from alcohol for ≥3 mo.
–Recommend pancreatic enzyme supplementation for chronic alcoholic pancreatitis with steatorrhea and malnutrition.

Sources
–*JAMA.* 2018;320(18):1899-1909.
–*Am J Psychiatr.* 2018;175(1):86-90.

Comments

1. Assess all patients for a coexisting psychiatric disorder (dual diagnosis).
2. Addiction-focused psychosocial intervention is helpful for patients with alcohol dependence.
3. Consider adjunctive pharmacotherapy under close supervision for alcohol dependence:
   a. Naltrexone and Acamprosate have the best evidence (COMBINE Trial https://www.ncbi.nlm.nih.gov/pubmed/16670409).
   b. Consider gabapentin or topiramate if patient has not responded to above (https://psychiatryonline.org/doi/pdf/10.1176/appi.books.9781615371969)

ANXIETY

Population
–Adults.

Recommendations
▶ NICE 2011, amended 2018
–Recommends cognitive behavioral therapy for generalized anxiety disorder (GAD).
–Consider sertraline first if drug treatment is needed.
–If sertraline is ineffective, recommend a different selective serotonin reuptake inhibitor (SSRI) or selective noradrenergic reuptake inhibitor (SNRI).
–Avoid long-term benzodiazepine use or antipsychotic therapy for GAD.

Source
–nice.org.uk/guidance/cg113

ATTENTION-DEFICIT HYPERACTIVITY DISORDER (ADHD)

Population
–Children age 4–18 y.

Recommendations
▶ AAP 2011
–Initiate an evaluation for ADHD in any child who presents with academic or behavioral problems and symptoms of inattention, hyperactivity, or impulsivity.
–Consider children with ADHD as children with special health care needs.
–For children age 4–5 y, parent- or teacher-administered behavior therapy is the treatment of choice.
–Methylphenidate is reserved for severe refractory cases.
–For children age 6–18 y, first-line treatment is with FDA-approved medications for ADHD ± behavior therapy.

Source
–http://pediatrics.aappublications.org/content/early/2011/10/14/peds.2011-2654.full.pdf

Population
–Children, young adults, and adults.

Recommendations

▶ NICE 2018

- Health care and education professionals require training to better address the needs of people with ADHD.
- Recommends against universal screening for ADHD in nursery, primary, and secondary schools.
- A diagnosis of ADHD should only be made by a specialist psychiatrist, pediatrician, or other appropriately qualified health care professional with training and expertise in the diagnosis of ADHD.
- Health care professionals should stress the value of a balanced diet, good nutrition, and regular exercise for children, young people, and adults with ADHD.
- Drug treatment is not recommended for preschool children with ADHD.
- Drug treatment is not indicated as the first-line treatment for all school-age children and young people with ADHD. It should be reserved for those with severe symptoms and impairment or for those with moderate levels of impairment who have refused nondrug interventions.
- Where drug treatment is considered appropriate, methylphenidate, atomoxetine, and dexamfetamine are recommended, within their licensed indications, as options for the management of ADHD in children and adolescents.
- For adults with ADHD, drug treatment should be the first-line treatment.
  - Following a decision to start drug treatment in adults with ADHD, lisdexamfetamine or methylphenidate should normally be tried first.
  - Atomoxetine or dexamfetamine should be considered in adults unresponsive or intolerant to an adequate trial of methylphenidate.
- For all patients, obtain a second opinion or refer to a tertiary service if ADHD symptoms are not controlled on one or more stimulants and one nonstimulant.
- Do not offer any of the following medications for ADHD without advice from a tertiary ADHD service:
  - Guanfacine for adults.
  - Clonidine for children with ADHD and sleep disturbances, rages, or tics.
  - Atypical antipsychotics in addition to stimulants for people with ADHD or coexisting pervasive aggression, rages, or irritability.

Source
-https://www.nice.org.uk/guidance/ng87/chapter/
Recommendations#medication

Comments

1. Essential to assess any child with ADHD for concomitant emotional, behavioral, developmental, or physical conditions (eg, mood disorders, tic disorders, seizures, sleep disorders, learning disabilities, or disruptive behavioral disorders).
2. For children 6–18 y, evidence is best to support stimulant medications and less strong to support atomoxetine, ER guanfacine, and ER clonidine for ADHD.

AUTISM SPECTRUM DISORDERS

Population

-Children and young adults.

Recommendations

▶ NICE 2011, updated 2017

-Consider autism for regression in language or social skills in children <3 y.
-Clinical signs of possible autism have to be seen in the context of a child's overall development, and account for cultural variations.
-An autism evaluation by a specialist is indicated for any of the following signs of possible autism:
  - Language delay.
  - Regression in speech.
  - Echolalia.
  - Unusual vocalizations or intonations.
  - Reduced social smiling.
  - Rejection of cuddles by family.
  - Reduced response to name being called.
  - Intolerance of others entering into their personal space.
  - Reduced social interest in people or social play.
  - Reduced eye contact.
  - Reduced imagination.
  - Repetitive movements like body rocking.
  - Desire for unchanged routines.
  - Immature social and emotional development.

Source
  –https://www.nice.org.uk/guidance/cg128

American College of Medical Genetics and Genomics 2013

  –Every child with an ASD should have a medical home.
  –A genetic consultation should be offered to all patients with an ASD and their families.
  –Initial evaluation to identify known syndromes or associated conditions.
   • Three-generation family history with pedigree analysis.
   • Examination with special attention to dysmorphic features.
   • If specific syndromic diagnosis is suspected, proceed with targeted testing.
   • If appropriate clinical indicators are present, perform metabolic and/or mitochondrial testing (alternatively, consider a referral to a metabolic specialist).
   • Chromosomal microarray: oligonucleotide array-comparative genomic hybridization or single-nucleotide polymorphism array.
   • Deoxyribonucleic acid (DNA) testing for fragile X (to be performed routinely for male patients only).
  –*Methyl-CPG-binding protein 2* (*MECP2*) sequencing to be performed for all females with autism spectrum disorders (ASDs).
  –*MECP2* duplication testing in males, if phenotype is suggestive.
  –*Phosphatase and tensin homolog* (*PTEN*) testing only if the head circumference is >2.5 standard deviation (SD) above the mean.

Source
  –https://www.nature.com/articles/gim201332

DEPRESSION

Population
  –Children and adolescents.

Recommendations
▶ USPSTF 2016
  –Adequate evidence showed that SSRIs, psychotherapy, and combined therapy will decrease symptoms of major depressive disorder in adolescents age 12–18 y.
  –Insufficient evidence to support screening and treatment of depression in children age 7–11 y.

Source

−USPSTF. *Depression in Children and Adolescents: Screening.* 2016.

Comment

1. Good evidence showed that SSRIs may increase absolute risk of suicidality in adolescents by 1%–2%. Therefore, SSRIs should be used only if close clinical monitoring is possible.

EATING DISORDERS

Population

−Adults and children with eating disorders.

Recommendations

▶ **APA, accessed 2018**

−Psychiatric management begins with the establishment of a therapeutic alliance.

−Recommend a multidisciplinary approach with a psychiatrist, dietician, social worker, and physician.

−Components of the initial evaluation include:

- A thorough history and physical examination.
- Assessment of the social history.
- An evaluation of the height and weight history.
- Any family history of eating disorders or mental health disorders.
- Assess attitude of eating, exercising, and appearance.
- Assess for suicidality.
- Assess for substance abuse.
- Recommend nutritional rehab for seriously underweight patients.
  ○ Recommend nasogastric tube feeding over parenteral nutrition for patients not meeting caloric requirements with oral feeds alone.
- Psychosocial rehab for patients with both anorexia nervosa and bulimia nervosa.
- Prozac is preferred agent to prevent relapse during maintenance phase of bulimia nervosa.
- Labs
  ○ CBC.
  ○ Chemistry panel.
  ○ TSH.
- Additional testing
  ○ Bone mineral densitometry if amenorrhea for more than 6 mo.
  ○ Dental evaluation for history of purging.

Source

–http://psychiatryonline.org/pb/assets/raw/sitewide/practice_guidelines/
guidelines/eatingdisorders.pdf

OPIOID USE DISORDER

Population

–Adults.

Recommendations

▶ ASAM 2015

–Obtain medical history to assess for concomitant medical conditions
including infectious diseases (TB, HIV, hepatitis), acute trauma, and
pregnancy. Assess mental health status, possible psychiatric disorders,
past and current substance use, and social and environmental factors.

–Include CBC, liver function tests, hepatitis C, HIV, and urine drug
testing in initial lab evaluation. Consider testing for STIs and TB. Offer
hepatitis B vaccination if appropriate.

–Consider use of clinical scales that measure withdrawal symptoms, like
the Clinical Opioid Withdrawal Scale (COWS).

–Choose medications to manage opioid withdrawal, including
methadone, buprenorphine, and naltrexone, rather than abrupt
cessation. Consider non-narcotic medications like clonidine,
benzodiazepines, loperamide, acetaminophen or NSAIDs, and
ondansetron to target specific opioid withdrawal symptoms.

–Provide psychosocial treatment for patients on opioid agonist
treatment.

Source

–https://www.asam.org/docs/default-source/practice-support/
guidelines-and-consensus-docs/asam-national-practice-guideline-
supplement.pdf

Population

–Nonpregnant adults electing buprenorphine therapy for opiate use
disorder.

Recommendations

▶ US Dept Health and Human Services 2004, ASAM 2015

–Physicians prescribing outpatient medication-assisted opioid therapy
with buprenorphine must complete training compliant with the Drug
Addiction Treatment Act of 2000.

–Consider patients to be candidates for buprenorphine therapy if they want treatment, have no contraindications, can be expected to be compliant, provide informed consent, and are willing to follow safety precautions.

–Consider alternatives to office-based buprenorphine if patients use high doses of benzodiazepines, alcohol, or other CNS depressants; have significant untreated psychiatric disease; have frequently relapsed despite maintenance therapy previously; have previously had poor response to buprenorphine; have significant medical illness.

–Use buprenorphine/naloxone combination for maintenance in most patients rather than buprenorphine monotherapy.

–For buprenorphine induction, wait until patient has early withdrawal symptoms (typically 12–24 h after short-acting opioids) before giving first dose to avoid precipitated withdrawal. Give initial dose of 4/1–8/2 mg buprenorphine/naloxone in an observed setting (ASAM: initial dose 2/0.5–4/1 mg; home induction may be considered). If 4 mg is given initially, give another 4 mg dose after 2 h if withdrawal symptoms persist, with a maximum dose of 8 mg in the first day. If symptoms are not sufficiently controlled with 8 mg, use adjunctive nonopioid medications.

–If transitioning from methadone to buprenorphine, taper methadone to 30 mg or less per day at least 1 wk prior to induction, and wait at least 24 h after last dose of methadone, and start 2 mg of buprenorphine monotherapy to minimize the chance of precipitated withdrawal.

–On day 2 of induction, if symptoms are controlled, administer the total dose from day 1 as the initial dose. If withdrawal symptoms are persistent, give the day 1 dose plus an additional 4/1 mg. If symptoms persist after 2 h, give an additional 4/1 mg dose for daily maximum of 16/4 mg. This process may continue on subsequent days, increasing by a maximum of 8 mg/d up to a maximum total daily dose of 24/6 mg/d (FDA approval limit).

–Once a dose is achieved that eliminates withdrawal symptoms, titrate dose weekly to a minimum effective dose that eliminates cravings and opioid use (by urine toxicology). Most patients will stabilize between 16/4 and 24/6 mg.

–The maintenance phase may be indefinite. Relapse remains a risk of therapy. Attend to psychiatric comorbidities, psychosocial support, legal and financial issues to maximize opportunity for abstinence. Consider tapering after 12 mo if patient and physician agree that tapering is likely to succeed. Taper slowly (ie, several months).

–Monitor for diversion by testing for buprenorphine and metabolites, counting pills, accessing the Prescription Drug Monitoring Program and arranging frequent visits (weekly at onset of therapy).

Sources

–McNicholas L. *Clinical Guidelines for the Use of Buprenorphine in the Treatment of Opioid Addiction.* U.S. Department of Health and Human Services, Rockville, MD. 2004.

–https://www.samhsa.gov/medication-assisted-treatment/training-materials-resources/buprenorphine-waiver

–American Society of Addiction Medicine. *The ASAM National Practice Guideline for the Use of Medications in the Treatment of Addiction Involving Opioid Use.* 2015. https://www.asam.org/docs/default-source/practice-support/guidelines-and-consensus-docs/asam-national-practice-guideline-supplement.pdf

PREGNANCY, SUBSTANCE ABUSE

Population

–Pregnant or postpartum patients using alcohol or illicit drugs.

Recommendations

▶ WHO 2014, ASAM 2017

–Health care providers should ask all pregnant women about their use of alcohol and other illicit drugs at prenatal visits.

–Health care providers should offer a brief intervention and individualized care to all pregnant women using alcohol or drugs.

–Health care providers should refer pregnant women with alcohol or cocaine or methamphetamine abuse to a detoxification center.

- Women with opioid addiction should continue a structured opioid maintenance program with either methadone or buprenorphine.
- Women with a benzodiazepine addiction should gradually wean the dose.

–Mothers with a substance abuse history should be encouraged to breast-feed unless the risks outweigh the benefits.

–Carefully monitor and treat infants of substance abusing mothers.

Sources

–ASAM. https://www.asam.org/advocacy/find-a-policy-statement/view-policy-statement/public-policy-statements/2017/01/19/substance-use-misuse-and-use-disorders-during-and-following-pregnancy-with-an-emphasis-on-opioids

–http://www.who.int/substance_abuse/activities/pregnancy_substance_use/en/

POSTTRAUMATIC STRESS DISORDER (PTSD)

Population
–Adults.

Recommendations

▶ VA 2017, NICE 2018

–For suspected PTSD, determine DSM criteria, acute risk of harm to self or others, functional status, medical history, treatment history, and relevant family history.

–Establish a risk management and safety plan as part of initial treatment planning if there is a risk of harm to self or others.

–Do not offer psychologically focused debriefing for the prevention or treatment of PTSD.

–Treat PTSD initially with individual, manualized trauma-focused psychotherapy.

–When trauma-focused psychotherapy is unavailable or not preferred, use pharmacotherapy or other psychotherapy. Recommended medications include sertraline, paroxetine, fluoxetine, or venlafaxine.

Sources
–https://www.healthquality.va.gov/guidelines/MH/ptsd/
–nice.org.uk/guidance/ng116

TOBACCO ABUSE, SMOKING CESSATION

Population
–Adults, including pregnant women who smoke tobacco.

Recommendations

▶ USPSTF 2015, AAFP 2015, ACOG 2017

–Current evidence is insufficient to recommend electronic nicotine delivery systems for tobacco cessation in adults, including pregnant women.

–Current evidence is insufficient to assess the benefits and harms of pharmacotherapy interventions for tobacco cessation in pregnant women.

Sources
–USPSTF. *Tobacco Smoking Cessation in Adults, Including Pregnant Women: Behavioral and Pharmacotherapy Interventions.* 2015.
–*Am Fam Physician.* 2016;93(10).

–ACOG. https://www.acog.org/Clinical-Guidance-and-Publications/Committee-Opinions/Committee-on-Obstetric-Practice/Smoking-Cessation-During-Pregnancy

TOBACCO CESSATION TREATMENT ALGORITHM

Five A's

1. Ask about tobacco use.
2. Advise to quit through clear, personalized messages.
3. Assess willingness to quit.
4. Assist to quit,[a] including referral to Quit Lines (eg, 1-800-NO-BUTTS).
5. Arrange follow-up and support.

[a]Physicians can assist patients to quit by devising a quit plan, providing problem-solving counseling, providing intratreatment social support, helping patients obtain social support from their environment/friends, and recommending pharmacotherapy for appropriate patients. Use caution in recommending pharmacotherapy in patients with medical contraindications, those smoking <10 cigarettes per day, pregnant/breast-feeding women, and adolescent smokers. As of March 2005, Medicare covers costs for smoking cessation counseling for those who (1) have a smoking-related illness; (2) have an illness complicated by smoking; or (3) take a medication that is made less effective by smoking (http://www.cms.hhs.gov).

Source: Fiore MC, Jaén CR, Baker TB, et al. *Treating Tobacco Use and Dependence: Quick Reference Guide for Clinicians*. Rockville, MD: U.S. Department of Health and Human Services. Public Health Service; 2008 (http://www.ahrq.gov/legacy/clinic/tobacco/tobaqrg.pdf).

MOTIVATING TOBACCO USERS TO QUIT

Five R's

1. Relevance: personal
2. Risks: acute, long term, environmental
3. Rewards: have patient identify (eg, save money, better food taste)
4. Road blocks: help problem-solve
5. Repetition: at every office visit

TOBACCO CESSATION TREATMENT OPTIONS[a]

First-Line Pharmacotherapies (approved for use for smoking cessation by the FDA)

Pharmacotherapy	Precautions/ Contraindications	Side Effects	Dosage	Duration	Availability
Bupropion SR	History of seizure History of eating disorder	Insomnia Dry mouth	150 mg every morning for 3 d, then 150 mg bid (Begin treatment 1–2 wk prequit)	7–12 wk maintenance up to 6 mo	Zyban (prescription only)
Nicotine gum	—	Mouth soreness Dyspepsia	1–24 cigarettes/d: 2-mg gum (up to 24 pieces/d) 25+ cigarettes/d: 4-mg gum (up to 24 pieces/d)	Up to 12 wk	Nicorette, Nicorette Mint (OTC only)
Nicotine inhaler	—	Local irritation of mouth and throat	6–16 cartridges/d	Up to 6 mo	Nicotrol Inhaler (prescription only)
Nicotine nasal spray	—	Nasal irritation	8–40 doses/d	3–6 mo	Nicotrol NS (prescription only)
Nicotine patch	—	Local skin reaction Insomnia	21 mg/24 h 14 mg/24 h 7 mg/24 h 15 mg/16 h	4 wk Then 2 wk Then 2 wk 8 wk	NicoDerm CQ (OTC only), generic patches (prescription and OTC) Nicotrol (OTC only)

	Precautions/Contraindications	Side Effects	Dosage	Duration	Availability
Varenicline	Renal impairment	Nausea, Abnormal dreams	0.5 mg qd for 3 d, then 0.5 mg bid for 4 d, then 1.0 mg PO bid	12 wk or 24 wk	Chantix (prescription only)
Second-Line Pharmacotherapies (not approved for use for smoking cessation by the FDA)					
Clonidine	Rebound hypertension	Dry mouth, Drowsiness, Dizziness, Sedation	0.15–0.75 mg/d	3–10 wk	Oral clonidine—generic, Catapres (prescription only), transdermal Catapres (prescription only)
Nortriptyline	Risk of arrhythmias	Sedation, Dry mouth	75–100 mg/d	12 wk	Nortriptyline HCL—generic (prescription only)

bid, twice daily; FDA, Food and Drug Administration; OTC, over-the-counter; PO, by mouth; qd, every day.

[a]The information contained within this table is not comprehensive. Please see package inserts for additional information.

Source: U.S. Public Health Service.

Cardiovascular Disorders

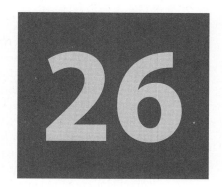

ABDOMINAL AORTIC ANEURYSM (AAA)

Population
–Adults.

Recommendations

▶ ACCF/AHA 2005/2011

Pharmacologic Therapy

–Monitor and control BP and fasting serum lipids as recommended for patients with atherosclerotic disease (Class I, LOE C).

–Smoking cessation: Provide counseling and medications to all patients with AAA or family history of AAA.

–Monitor patients with infrarenal or juxtarenal AAA 4.0–5.4 cm in diameter with ultrasound or CT scan every 6–12 mo to detect expansion (Class I, LOE A).

–Monitor patients with AAA <4.0 cm in diameter with ultrasound every 2–3 y (Class IIa, LOE B).

–In patients undergoing surgical repair of AAA, administer beta-adrenergic blocking agents perioperatively, in the absence of contraindications, to reduce the risk of adverse cardiac events and mortality (Class I, LOE A).

Surgical Therapy

–Repair infrarenal or juxtarenal AAA ≥5.5 cm in diameter to eliminate risk of rupture (Class I, LOE B).

–Consider repair of suprarenal or type IV thoracoabdominal aortic aneurysm >5.5–6.0 cm diameter (Class IIa, LOE B).

–Do not repair asymptomatic infrarenal or juxtarenal AAA if <5.0 cm in diameter in men or <4.5 cm in diameter in women (Class III, LOE A).

–Obtain immediate surgical evaluation for patients with clinical triad of abdominal and/or back pain, a pulsatile abdominal mass, and hypotension (Class I, LOE B).

–Repair symptomatic AAA regardless of diameter (Class I, LOE C).

–In patients who are good surgical candidates, recommend open repair or EVAR[a] of infrarenal and/or common iliac aneurysms.

–After EVAR of infrarenal aortic and/or iliac aneurysms, perform periodic long-term surveillance imaging to monitor for vascular leak, document shrinkage/stability of the excluded aneurysm sac, confirm graft position, and determine the need for further intervention (Class I, LOE A).

–Consider open aneurysm repair for patients who are good surgical candidates but who cannot comply with the periodic long-term surveillance required after endovascular repair (Class IIa, LOE C).

–Endovascular repair of infrarenal aortic aneurysm in patients who are at high surgical or anesthetic risk (presence of coexisting severe cardiac, pulmonary, and/or renal disease) is of uncertain effectiveness (Class IIb, LOE B).

▶ ESC 2014

Pharmacologic Therapy

–Recommend smoking cessation slow the growth of the AAA.

–In patients with HTN and AAA, give beta-blockers as first-line treatment.

–Consider ACEI and statins in patients with AAA to reduce cardiovascular risk.

–Consider aspirin therapy. Enlargement of AAA is usually associated with the development of an intraluminal mural thrombus. Overall data on the benefits of ASA in reducing AAA growth are contradictory; however, given the strong association between AAA and other atherosclerotic diseases, the use of ASA may be advisable.

–Surveillance without intervention is indicated and safe in patients with AAA with a maximum diameter <5.5 cm and slow growth <1 cm/y.

–In patients with small AAA, monitor with imaging at the following frequencies:

- Every 4 y for AAA 2.5–2.9 cm diameter.
- Every 3 y for AAA 3.0–3.9 cm diameter.
- Every 2 y for AAA 4.0–4.4 cm diameter.
- Every year for AAA >4.5 cm diameter.

Surgical Therapy

–Repair an AAA in the following circumstances:

- AAA >5.5 cm in diameter.
- Aneurysm growth >1 cm/y.

–If a large aneurysm is anatomically suitable for EVAR, recommend either open or EVAR in patients with acceptable surgical risk.

–If a large aneurysm is anatomically unsuitable for EVAR, open aortic repair is recommended.

[a]EVAR, endovascular aortic repair.

–In patients with asymptomatic AAA who are unfit for open repair, consider EVAR along with optimal medical treatment.

–In patients with suspected rupture of AAA, obtain immediate abdominal ultrasound or CT.

–Repair ruptured AAA emergently.

–In patients with symptomatic but nonruptured AAA, repair urgently. If anatomically suitable for EVAR, recommend either open or EVAR.

Comments

Risk Factors for Developing AAA

1. Age >60 y. About 1 person in 1000 develops an abdominal aortic aneurysm between the ages of 60 and 65. Abdominal aortic aneurysms occur in 2%–13% of men and 6% of women >65 y.
2. Smoking. The risk is directly related to number of years smoking and decreases in the years following smoking cessation.
3. Men develop AAA 4–5 times more often than women.
4. Ethnicity. AAA is more common in the white population.
5. History of CHD, PAD, HTN, and hypercholesterolemia.
6. Family history of AAA. Accentuates the risks associated with age and gender. The risk of developing an aneurysm among brothers of a person with a known aneurysm who are >60 y of age is as high as 18%.

Risk Factors for AAA Expansion

1. Age >70 y, cardiac or renal transplant, previous stroke, severe cardiac disease, tobacco use.

Risk Factors for AAA Rupture

1. Aneurysms expand at an average rate of 0.3–0.4 cm/y.
2. The annual risk of rupture based upon aneurysm size is estimated as follows:
   a. <4.0 cm diameter = <0.5%.
   b. Between 4.0 and 4.9 cm diameter = 0.5%–5%.
   c. Between 5.0 and 5.9 cm diameter = 3%–15%.
   d. Between 6.0 and 6.9 cm diameter = 10%–20%.
   e. Between 7.0 and 7.9 cm diameter = 20%–40%.
   f. ≥8.0 cm diameter = 30%–50%.
3. Aneurysms that expand rapidly (>0.5 cm over 6 mo) are at high risk of rupture.
4. Growth tends to be more rapid in smokers and less rapid in patients with peripheral artery disease or diabetes mellitus.
5. The risk of rupture of large aneurysms (≥5.0 cm) is significantly greater in women (18%) than in men (12%).
6. Other risk factors for rupture: cardiac or renal transplant, decreased forced expiratory volume in 1 s, higher mean BP, larger initial AAA diameter, current tobacco use. Duration of smoking is more significant than quantity smoked.

Sources
- −Adapted from http://www.uptodate.com/contents/abdominal-aortic-aneurysm-beyond-the-basics.
- −Hirsch AT, Haskal ZJ, Hertzer NR, et al. ACC/AHA guidelines for the management of patients with peripheral arterial disease (lower extremity, renal, mesenteric, and abdominal aortic). *J Vasc Inter Radiol.* 2006;17:1383-1398.
- −Rooke TW, Hirsch AT, Misra S, et al. 2011 ACCF/AHA focused update of the guideline for the management of patients with peripheral artery disease (updating the 2005 guideline). *JACC.* 2011;58(19):2020-2045.
- −Erbel R, Aboyans V, Boileau C, et al. 2014 ESC guidelines on the diagnosis and treatment of aortic diseases. Document covering acute and chronic aortic diseases of the thoracic and abdominal aorta of the adult. The Task Force for the diagnosis and treatment of aortic disease of the European Society of Cardiology (ESC). *Eur Heart J.* 2014;35:2873-2926. doi:10.1093/eurheartj/ehu281.

ANAPHYLAXIS

Population
- −Children and adults.

Recommendations
▶ NICE 2011, EACCI 2014
- −Obtain blood samples for mast cell tryptase testing at onset and after 1–2 h.
- −Administer epinephrine (1:1000) 0.01 mg/kg (maximum 0.5 mg) SC; repeat as necessary IM every 15 min.
- −If circulatory instability, place patient supine with lower extremities raised and given intravenous saline 20 mL/kg bolus.
- −Give inhaled beta-2 agonists and glucocorticoids for wheezing or signs of bronchoconstriction.
- −Consider H1- and H2-blockers for cutaneous signs of anaphylaxis.
- −Observe all people ≥16 y suspected of having an anaphylactic reaction for at least 6–12 h before discharge.
- −Admit All children younger than age 16 y suspected of having an anaphylactic reaction for observation.
- −Refer all patients treated for an anaphylactic reaction to an allergy specialist.
- −Prescribe an epinephrine injector (eg, EpiPen).

Sources
- −http://www.nice.org.uk/nicemedia/live/13626/57474/57474.pdf
- −http://www.guideline.gov/content.aspx?id=48690

Comment

1. Anaphylaxis is a severe, life-threatening, generalized hypersensitivity reaction. It is characterized by the rapid development of:
   a. Airway edema.
   b. Bronchospasm.
   c. Circulatory dysfunction.

ATRIAL FIBRILLATION

Population

–All adults.

Recommendations

▶ 2019 AHA/ACC/HRS, 2016 ESC

Management of Stroke Risk

–Decide whether to anticoagulate after discussion of risks of stroke and bleeding, regardless of whether AF is paroxysmal or persistent. Estimate stroke risk with CHA_2DS_2-VASc score.

–Give oral anticoagulants to patients with AF and an elevated CHA2DS2-VASc score (≥2 in men, ≥3 in women). Options include: warfarin, dabigatran, rivaroxaban, apixaban, edoxaban. For patients who meet this criteria but have CKD (CrCl<15 mL/min), consider warfarin (INR 2–3) or apixaban.

–Use NOACs instead of warfarin in NOAC-eligible patients with AF (except with moderate-to-severe mitral stenosis or mechanical heart valve).

–Use warfarin in patients with AF who have mechanical heart valves.

–If PCI is required in a patient anticoagulated for AF, consider using clopidogrel acutely without aspirin in addition to anticoagulation rather than antithrombotic therapy.

–Consider percutaneous LAA occlusion in patients with AF at increased risk of stroke who have contraindications to long-term anticoagulation.

Management of Rate

–Acutely, if hemodynamically stable, slow the rate to <110 bpm with IV beta-blocker or calcium channel blocker.[b] These are preferred to digoxin for their rapid onset of action and effectiveness at high sympathetic tone.

–In critically ill patients and those with severely impaired LV systolic function in whom excess heart rate is leading to hemodynamic instability, consider intravenous amiodarone.

[b]Dosing: metoprolol 2.5–10 mg IV bolus repeated prn; esmolol 0.5 mg/kg IV bolus over 1 min then 0.05–0.25 mg/kg/min; diltiazem 15–25 mg IV bolus repeated prn; verapamil 2.5–10 mg IV bolus repeated prn; digoxin 0.5 mg IV bolus, then 0.75–1.5 mg divided over 24 h; amiodarone 300 mg IV over 30–60 min, preferably via central line.

–Acutely, if hemodynamically stable, slow the rate to <110 bmp with IV beta blocker or calcium channel blocker. These are preferred to digoxin for their rapid onset of action and effectiveness at high sympathetic tone (See Table 1).

–Long term, use beta-blocker or nondihydropyridine calcium channel blocker to control rate in both persistent and paroxysmal AF. If unsuccessful or contraindicated, use amiodarone (ACC/AHA) or digoxin (ESC).

–If symptomatic, titrate medication to a resting heart rate <80.

–If asymptomatic and LVEF is preserved, titrate medication to a resting heart rate <110.

–If rate and/or rhythm control strategies fail, consider AV nodal ablation and pacemaker placement.

Management of Rhythm

–Choose rhythm control over rate control only if symptoms persist after efforts to control rate. Various studies (AFFIRM, RACE, PIAF, STAF, etc.) have failed to show quality of life difference for rhythm control vs. rate control. Rhythm control is more likely to be effective in symptomatic patients who are younger with minimal heart disease, few comorbid conditions, and recent onset of AF.

–For patients with AF or atrial flutter of 48 h duration or longer, or when the duration of AF is unknown, anticoagulate with warfarin (INR 2.0–3.0), a factor Xa inhibitor, or direct thrombin inhibitor for at least 3 wk before and at least 4 wk after cardioversion, regardless of the CHA2DS2-VASc score or the method (electrical or pharmacological).

–For patients with AF or atrial flutter of more than 48 h duration or unknown duration that required immediate cardioversion because of hemodynamic instability, start anticoagulation as soon as possible and continue for at least 4 wk after cardioversion unless contraindicated

–For patients with AF or atrial flutter of more than 48 h duration or unknown duration who have not been anticoagulated for the preceding 3 wk, consider transesophageal echocardiography before cardioversion and proceed with cardioversion if no left atrial thrombus is identified.

–If duration of AF is <48 h with a CHA2DS2-VASc score of 2 or greater in men and 3 or greater in women, give heparin, a factor Xa inhibitor, or a direct thrombin inhibitor as soon as possible before cardioversion, followed by long-term anticoagulation therapy.

–Options for pharmacologic cardioversion include flecainide, dofetilide, propafenone, ibutilide, and amiodarone. Choose amiodarone if LVH, HF, or CAD.

–Long-term antiarrhythmic options include dronedarone, flecainide, propafenone, and sotalol. Avoid amiodarone unless heart failure because of side effect profile.

TABLE I: RATE CONTROL THERAPY IN ATRIAL FIBRILLATION

Therapy	Acute Intravenous Rate Control	Long-term Oral Rate Control	Side Effect Profile	Comments
Beta-blockers[a]				
Bisoprolol	Not available	1.25–20 mg once daily or split.	Most common reported adverse symptoms are lethargy, headache, peripheral oedema, upper respiratory tract symptoms, gastrointestinal upset and dizziness. Adverse effects include bradycardia, atrioventricular block, and hypotension.	Bronchospasm is rate – in cases of asthma, recommended beta-1 selective agents (avoid carvedilol). Contra-indicated in acute cardiac failure and a history of severe bronchospasm.
Carvedilol	Not available	3.125–50 mg twice daily.		
Metoprolol	2.5–10 mg intravenous bolus (repeated as required).	100–200 mg total daily dose (according to preparation).		
Nobivolol	Not available	2.5–10 mg once daily or split.		
Esmolol	0.5 mg/kg intravenous bolus over 1 min; than 0.05–0.25 mg/kg/min.			
Calcium-channel blockers				
Diltiazem	15–25 mg intravenous bolus (repeated as required).	60 mg 3 times daily up to 360 mg total daily dose (120–360 mg once daily modified release).	Most common reported adverse symptoms are dizziness, mobilize, lethargy, headache, hot flushes, gastrointestinal upset, and oedema. Adverse effects include bradycardia, atrioventricular block, and hypotension (prolonged hypotension possible with verapamil).	Use with caution in combination with beta-blockers. Reduce dose with hepatic impairment and start with smaller dose in renal impairment. Contra-indicated in LV failure with pulmonary congestion or LVEF <40%.
Verapamil	2.5–10 mg intravenous bolus (repeated as required).	40–120 mg 3 times daily (120–190 mg once daily modified release).		

TABLE I: RATE CONTROL THERAPY IN ATRIAL FIBRILLATION (Continued)

Therapy	Acute Intravenous Rate Control	Long-term Oral Rate Control	Side Effect Profile	Comments
Cardiac glycosides				
Digoxin	0.5 mg intravenous bolus (0.75–1.5 mg over 24 hours in divided doses).	0.0625–0.25 mg daily dose.	Most common reported adverse symptoms are gastrointestinal upset, dizziness, blurred vision, headache, and rash. In toxic states (serum level >2 ng/mL), digoxin is proarrhythmic and can aggravate heart failure, particularly with co-existent hypokalaemia.	High plasma levels associated with increased risk of death. Check real function before starting and adapt dose in patients with CKD. Contra-indicated in patients with accessory pathways, ventricular tachycardia and hypertrophic cardiomyopathy with outflow tract obstruction.
Digitoxin	0.4–0.6 mg intravenous bolus.	0.05–0.3 mg daily dose.		
Specific indications				
Amiodarone	300 mg intravenously diluted in 250 ml. 5% dextrose over 30–60 min (preferably via central venous cannula).[b]	200 mg daily.	Hypotension, bradycardia, nausea, QT prolongation, pulmonary toxicity, skin discolouration, thyroid dysfunction, corneal deposits, and cutaneous reaction with extravasation.	Suggested as adjunctive therapy in patients where heart rate control cannot be achieved using combination therapy.

AF, atrial fibrillation; CKD, chronic kidney disease; i.v., intravenous; LV, left ventricular; LVEF, left ventricular ejection fractions.

[a]A number of other beta-blockers are also available, but are not recommended an specific rate control therapy in AF. These include atenolol (25–100 mg once daily with a short biological half-life), propranolol [non-selective, 1 mg over 1 min and repeat up to 3 mg at 2-min intervals (acure) or 10–10 mg three times daily (long term)], or labetalol [non-selective, 1–2 mg/min (acute)].

[b]If ongoing requirement for $$, follow with 900 mg i.v. over 2.1 h diluted in 500–1000 mL via a control venous $$.

European Heart Journal (2016) 37, 2893-2962.

–Consider catheter ablation of AF as initial rhythm-control strategy,[c] or after failure of an antiarrhythmic medication. Do not offer ablation to patients who cannot be anticoagulated for at least 8 wk after ablation.[d]

–Consider AF catheter ablation in selected patients with symptomatic AF and HF with reduced left ventricular (LV) ejection fraction (HFrEF) to potentially lower mortality rate and reduce hospitalization for HF.

▶ Heart Rhythm Society 2014

–Do not use Class Ic antiarrhythmic drugs (Vaughan–Williams) as a first-line agent for the maintenance of sinus rhythm in patients with ischemic heart disease who have experienced prior MI.

Population

–Adults without valvular heart disease.

Recommendations

Management of Stroke Risk

▶ 2016 ESC, 2018 ACCP

–If nonvalvular AF and CHA_2DS_2-VASc ≥ 2, anticoagulate with warfarin titrated to INR of 2.0–3.0, dabigatran, rivaroxaban, or apixaban. If unable to maintain a therapeutic INR with warfarin, switch to a direct thrombin inhibitor or factor Xa inhibitor. If anticoagulation must be interrupted for a procedure, consider risks of stroke and bleeding before deciding whether to bridge. If CKD, safety, and efficacy of oral anticoagulants other than warfarin is not well established, but they may be considered as alternatives (except rivaroxaban and dabigatran, which do not have effect). Consider left atrial appendage occlusion if anticoagulation is contraindicated.

–If nonvalvular AF and CHA_2DS_2-VASc 1 or more in men and 2 or more in women, recommend oral anticoagulation.

[c]ESC guidelines observe that if ablation is done in expert centers, ablation reduces recurrence rate much more than antiarrhythmics for paroxysmal AF. The long-term benefit is less certain for persistent AF.

[d]Data suggest that stopping anticoagulation with warfarin prior to the ablation (even if patients are bridged with low-molecular-weight heparin) is associated with an increased risk of complications compared with an uninterrupted anticoagulation approach. In COMPARE study, patients with CHADS2 score of >1 undergoing catheter ablation for nonvalvular AF, bridged with low-molecular-weight heparin, had a >10-fold increased risk of ischemic stroke or transient ischemic attack in the 48 h after ablation compared with those on uninterrupted warfarin. Patients with atrial fibrillation frequently stop oral anticoagulation therapy following radiofrequency catheter ablation despite an increased risk for stroke, transient ischemic attack, or systemic embolism in the first 3 mo after the procedure, according to the results of a new analysis. If the patient is at a lower risk for stroke, the type of patient that might not need to be anticoagulated to begin with, then the medication can be stopped after 3 mo. Everybody else should remain on oral anticoagulation for at least 12 mo after the ablation. At that point, physicians can reassess a patient's risk factors to determine whether the oral anticoagulation should continue.

Source: O'Riordan M. Stopping anticoagulation after ablation increases stroke risk in first 3 mo. May 21, 2015. (http://www.medscape.com/viewarticle/845106?src=confwrap&uac=91737BX)

For patients undergoing catheter ablation for nonvalvular atrial fibrillation, continuing with uninterrupted rivaroxaban appears to be as safe as uninterrupted oral anticoagulant therapy with warfarin. Source: O'Riordan M. Uninterrupted rivaroxaban feasible for patients undergoing AF ablation. VENTURE-AF Study. (http://www.medscape.com/viewarticle/845168?src=confwrap&uac=91737BX)

–If nonvalvular AF and CHA$_2$DS$_2$-VASc 0, antithrombotic therapy is not necessary. ESC recommends against aspirin, while AHA/ACC recommends it to be considered.

▶ 2019 ACC/AHA/HRS, 2018 ESC

–If anticoagulation is indicated, choose non-vitamin K antagonists preferably over warfarin (unless patient has mechanical heart valves or moderate or severe mitral stenosis).

–When switching from vitamin K antagonist to non-vitamin K antagonist, start the NOAC as soon as the INR is <2.0. If INR 2.0–2.5, start NOAC the following day. If INR ≥2.5, recheck INR in 1–3 days.

–When switching from non-vitamin K antagonist to warfarin, administer both concomitantly until the INR is in the therapeutic range.

–If mild-to-moderate CKD, use NOACs with dose adjustments according to drug label.

–If severe CKD or ESRD (GFR <30 mL/min), consider avoiding NOACs as they have not been studied for safety and efficacy in this population with AF.

–If chronic liver disease with coagulopathy, avoid NOACs.

–Observe drug–drug interactions. Diltiazem mildly elevates the plasma levels of apixaban but not dabigatran or rivaroxaban. Verapamil mildly elevates the plasma levels of dabigatran and edoxaban but not rivaroxaban. HIV protease inhibitors and most antifungal medications markedly increase activities of all NOACs.

–Reversal of anticoagulation in life-threatening bleeding:
  • Direct thrombin inhibitor (dabigatran): use idarucizumab.
  • Factor Xa inhibitors (apixaban, edoxaban, or rivaroxaban): use andexanet alpha.
  • If the above are not available, consider prothrombin complex concentrate (PCC) and replacement of platelets where appropriate.

Population
–Adults with mechanical valve or severe mitral stenosis.

Recommendations
Management of Stroke Risk
▶ 2014 AHA/ACC/HRS, 2016 ESC, 2018 ACCP

–If mechanical valve present, anticoagulate with warfarin titrated to INR goal of 2.0–3.0 or 2.5–3.5 (depending on location and type of replacement valve) and bridge with heparin or low-molecular-weight heparin for procedures that require warfarin to be held. Do not use direct thrombin inhibitors or factor Xa inhibitors.

▶ 2019 ACC/AHA/HRS, 2018 ESC

–Do not use non-vitamin K antagonist oral anticoagulants if moderate-to-severe mitral stenosis or mechanical prosthetic valve. They may be used in mild-to-moderate valvular disease. They are also likely acceptable in aortic stenosis (including severe) and >3 mo after mitral valve repair or bioprosthetic valve placement.

Population

–Adults with heart failure with reduced ejection fraction.

Recommendations

Management of Rate

▶ 2016 ESC

–Acutely, avoid calcium channel blockers in patients with left ventricular ejection fraction <40%.

–Only beta-blockers and digoxin are suitable in HFrEF because of the negative inotropic potential of verapamil and diltiazem.

Management of Rhythm

▶ 2014 AHA/ACC/HRS, 2016 ESC

–Choose rhythm control over rate control only if symptoms persist after efforts to control rate. Various studies (AFFIRM, RACE, PIAF, STAF, etc.) have failed to show quality-of-life difference for rhythm control vs. rate control. Rhythm control is more likely to be effective in symptomatic patients who are younger with minimal heart disease, few comorbid conditions, and recent onset of AF.

–Long-term, choose amiodarone rather than other antiarrhythmics only in patients with heart failure because of side effect profile.

–Catheter ablation may be a useful method to restore LV function in AF patients with HFrEF but further data still needed.

Population

–Adults with atrial fibrillation and heart failure with preserved ejection fraction.

Recommendations

–It may be difficult to separate symptoms that are due to HF from those due to AF.

–Focus on the control of fluid balance and concomitant conditions such as hypertension and myocardial ischemia.

Population

–Patients with atrial fibrillation and acute TIA or ischemic stroke.

Recommendations

–When to start OAC:
  • TIA: 1 d after acute event.
  • Mild stroke (NIHSS <8): 3 d after acute event.
  • Moderate stroke (NIHSS 8–15): evaluate hemorrhagic transformation by CT or MRI at day 6, then start OAC 6 d after acute event.
  • Severe stroke (NIHSS >16): evaluate hemorrhagic transformation.

Sources

  –*JACC.* 2014;64(21):2246-2280. http://www.onlinejacc.org/content/64/21/2246

  –*Eur Heart J.* 2016;37:2893-2962.

  –*Eur Heart J.* 2018;39(16):1330-1393. https://academic.oup.com/
  eurheartj/article/39/16/1330/4942493

  –*Chest.* 2018;154(4):1121-1201.

  –http://www.choosingwisely.org/societies/heart-rhythm-society/

  –2016 ESC guidelines for the management of atrial fibrillation developed
  in collaboration with EACTS.

  –2019 AHA/ACC/HRS Focused Update of the 2014 AHA/ACC/HRS.
  Guideline for the Management of Patients with Atrial Fibrillation.

Comments

1. Atrial fibrillation guidelines apply to patients with atrial flutter as well.
2. Risk factors for AF include age >60, CKD, COPD, valvular heart
   disease, OSA, tobacco use, MI, HF, hyperthyroidism, obesity, HTN,
   and heavy alcohol use.
3. ACC/AHA definitions of atrial fibrillation:
   a. Paroxysmal: Terminates within 7 d of onset.
   b. Persistent: Sustained continuously >7 d.
   c. Long-standing persistent: Sustained continuously >12 mo.
   d. Permanent: Declared once patient and physician decide to stop
      trying to restore sinus rhythm.
   e. Nonvalvular: Mitral stenosis, prosthetic valve, or mitral valve repair
      absent.
4. Expected ventricular heart rate (HR) in untreated AF is between 110
   and 210 beats/min.
   a. If HR <110 beats/min, atrioventricular (AV) node disease present.
   b. If HR >220 beats/min, preexcitation syndrome (WPW) present.
5. Initial choice of AV nodal slowing agent to be determined by:
   a. Ventricular rate/blood pressure (BP).
   b. Presence of heart failure (HF) or asthma.
   c. Associated cardiovascular (CV) symptoms (chest pain/shortness
      of breath [SOB]).
6. Holter monitor best measures the adequacy of the chronic HR
   control. In acute medical conditions when the patient has noncardiac
   illness (ie, pneumonia), the resting HR may be allowed to increase
   to simulate physiologic demands (mimic HR if sinus rhythm was
   present). (ESC recommends HR target <110 beats/min; CCS
   recommends <100 beats/min; ACCF/AHA/HRS recommends HR
   target <110 beats/min only if EF >40%.)
7. Choosing Wisely: American Society of Echocardiography (2013)
   recommends against transesophageal echocardiography to detect
   cardiac sources of embolization if a source has been identified and
   patient management will not change. (http://www.choosingwisely.org/
   sourcessocieties/american-society-of-echocardiography/)

DOAC COMPARISON CHART

	Warfarin	Dabigatran	Rivaroxaban	Apixaban	Edoxaban
Molecular target	Vitamin-dependent clotting factor	Thrombin	Factor Xa	Factor Xa	Factor Xa
Dosing in AF	Once daily	Twice daily	Once daily	Twice daily	Once daily
Time to peak plasma concentration (min)	240	85–150	30–180	30–120	30–60
Time to peak effect (h)	96–120	2	2–3	1–2	1–2
Half-life (h)	40	14–17	5–9 (increased to 11–13 in elderly)	8–15	9–11
Renal clearance	<1%	80%	33%	25%	35%
Hepatic excretion		20%	66%	75% (hepatic-biliary-intestinal)	65%
Food and drug interactions	Foods rich in vitamin K, substrates of CYP2C9, CYP3A4, and CYP1A2	Strong P-gp inhibitors and inducers	Strong CYP3A4 inducers, strong inhibitors of both CYP3A4 and P-gp	Strong inhibitors and inducers of CYP3A4 and P-gp	Strong P-gp inhibitors
Creatinine clearance below which drug is contraindicated	n/a	<30 mL/min	<15 mL/min	<15 mL/min	<30 mL/min (Japan)

Sources: Lip et al. J Intern Med. 2015; Shields AM, Lip GY. Which drug should we use for stroke prevention in atrial fibrillation? *Curr Opin Cardiol.* 2014;29(4):293-300.

ANTITHROMBOTIC STRATEGIES FOLLOWING CORONARY ARTERY STENTING IN PATIENTS WITH AF AT MODERATE-TO-HIGH THROMBOEMBOLIC RISK (IN WHOM ORAL ANTICOAGULATION THERAPY IS REQUIRED)

Hemorrhagic Risk	Clinical Setting	Stent Implanted	Anticoagulation Regimen
Low or intermediate (eg, HASBLED score 0–2)	Elective	Bare metal	1 mo: triple therapy of VKA (INR 2.0–2.5) + aspirin ≤100 mg/d + clopidogrel 75 mg/d Up to 12th mo: combination of VKA (INR 2.0–2.5) + clopidogrel 75 mg/d (or aspirin 100 mg/d) Lifelong: VKA (INR 2.0–3.0) alone
	Elective	Drug eluting	3 (-olimus[a] group) to 6 (paclitaxel) mo: triple therapy of VKA (INR 2.0–2.5) + aspirin ≤100 mg/d + clopidogrel 75 mg/d Up to 12th mo: combination of VKA (INR 2.0–2.5) + clopidogrel 75 mg/d (or aspirin 100 mg/d) Lifelong: VKA (INR 2.0–3.0) alone
	ACS	Bare metal/ drug eluting	6 mo: triple therapy of VKA (INR 2.0–2.5) + aspirin ≤100 mg/d + clopidogrel 75 mg/d Up to 12th mo: combination of VKA (INR 2.0–2.5) + clopidogrel 75 mg/d (or aspirin 100 mg/d) Lifelong: VKA (INR 2.0–3.0) alone
High (eg, HAS-BLED score ≥3)	Elective	Bare metal[b]	2–4 wk: triple therapy of VKA (INR 2.0–2.5) + aspirin ≤100 mg/d + clopidogrel 75 mg/d Lifelong: VKA (INR 2.0–3.0) alone
	ACS	Bare metal[b]	4 wk: triple therapy of VKA (INR 2.0–2.5) + aspirin ≤100 mg/d + clopidogrel 75 mg/d Up to 12th mo: combination of VKA (INR 2.0–2.5) + clopidogrel 75 mg/d[c] (or aspirin 100 mg/d) Lifelong: VKA (INR 2.0–3.0) alone

[a]Sirolimus, everolimus, and tacrolimus.

[b]Drug-eluting stents should be avoided as far as possible, but, if used, consideration of more prolonged (3–6 mo) triple antithrombotic therapy is necessary.

[c]Combination of VKA (INR 2.0–3.0) + aspirin ≤100 mg/d (with PPI, if indicated) may be considered as an alternative.

Source: Adapted from Lip GY, Huber K, Andreotti F, et al. European Society of Cardiology Working Group on Thrombosis. Management of antithrombotic therapy in atrial fibrillation patients presenting with acute coronary syndrome and/or undergoing percutaneous coronary intervention/stent. *Thromb Haemost.* 2010;103:13-28.

HAS-BLED BLEEDING RISK SCORE FOR WARFARIN THERAPY

Letter	Clinical Characteristics	Points Awarded
H	Hypertension (systolic blood pressure [SBP] >160 mm Hg)	1
A	Abnormal renal function (presence of chronic dialysis or renal transplantation or serum creatinine ≥2.6 mg/dL and abnormal liver function; chronic hepatic disease or biochemical evidence of significant hepatic derangement; bilirubin >2× upper limit of normal, in association with glutamic-oxaloacetic transaminase [GOT]/glutamic-pyruvic transaminase [GPT] >3× upper limit normal) 1 point each	1 or 2
S	Stroke	1
B	Bleeding (previous bleeding history and/or predisposition to bleeding, eg, bleeding diathesis, anemia)	1
L	Labile INRs (unstable/high INRs or poor time in therapeutic range, eg, <60%)	1
E	Elderly (age >65 y)	1
D	Drugs or alcohol (concomitant use of drugs such as antiplatelet agents, nonsteroidal anti-inflammatory drugs, or alcohol abuse) 1 point each	1 or 2
		Maximum 9 points

Interpretation

The risk of (spontaneous) major bleeding (intracranial, hospitalization, hemoglobin decrease 2 g/L, and/or transfusion) within 1 y in patients with atrial fibrillation enrolled in the Euro Heart Survey expressed as bleeds per 100 patient-years:

Score 0:1.13   Score 1:1.02
Score 2:1.88   Score 3:3.74
Score 4:8.70   Score 5:12.50
Score 6–9: insufficient data to quantify risk

Sources: 2010 Guidelines for the management of atrial fibrillation. *Eur Heart J.* 2010;31:2369-2429; Table 10; Pisters R, Lane DA, Nieuwlaat R, de Vos CB, Crijns HJ, Lip GY. A novel user-friendly score (HAS-BLED) to assess 1-y risk of major bleeding in atrial fibrillation patients: the Euro Heart Survey. *Chest.* 2010;138:1093-1100; Table 5.

THROMBOEMBOLIC RISK SCORES IN NONVALVULAR ATRIAL FIBRILLATION

	CHADS$_2$	Points	CHA$_2$DS$_2$-VASc	Points
C	Congestive heart failure	1	Congestive heart failure (or left ventricular systolic dysfunction [LVEF] ≤40%)	1
H	Hypertension (blood pressure [BP] consistently >140/90 mm Hg or treated hypertension [HTN] on medication)	1	Hypertension (BP consistently >140/90 mm Hg or treated HTN on medication)	1
A	Age ≥75 y	1	Age ≥75 y	2
D	Diabetes mellitus	1	Diabetes mellitus	1
S2	Prior stroke or transient ischemic attack (TIA)	2	Prior stroke or TIA or thromboembolism	2
V			Vascular disease (eg, coronary artery disease, peripheral artery disease, myocardial infarction [MI], aortic plaque)	1
A			Age 65–74 y	1
Sc			Sex category (ie, female gender)	1
Max.		6		9

STROKE RISK STRATIFICATION WITH THE CHADS$_2$ AND CHA$_2$DS$_2$-VASC SCORES

CHADS$_2$ score acronym^a	Adjusted Stroke Rate (% per year)
0	1.9
1	2.8
2	4.0
3	5.9
4	8.5
5	12.5
6	18.2

STROKE RISK STRATIFICATION WITH THE CHADS$_2$ AND CHA$_2$DS$_2$-VASC SCORES (Continued)

CHADS$_2$-VAS$_c$ score acronym[b]	Adjusted Stroke Rate (% per year)
0	0
1	1.3
2	2.2
3	3.2
4	4.0
5	6.7
6	9.8
7	9.6
8	6.7
9	15.20

[a]C, CHF; H, hypertension; A, age >75 y; D, diabetes mellitus; S, history of stroke or TIA.
[b]C, CHF; H, hypertension; A, age 65–74 y; D, diabetes mellitus; S, history of stroke or TIA; V, vascular disease; A, age 75 y or older; S, female sex.

RISK FACTORS FOR STROKE AND THROMBOEMBOLISM IN NONVALVULAR AF

"Major" Risk Factors	"Clinically Relevant Nonmajor" Risk Factors
Previous Stroke TIA Systemic embolism Age ≥75 y	Heart failure or moderate-to-severe left ventricular (LV) systolic dysfunction (LVEF ≤40%) Hypertension Diabetes mellitus Female sex Age 65–74 y Vascular disease

Sources: 2010 Guidelines for the management of atrial fibrillation. Eur Heart J. 2010;31:2369-2429; Tables 8(a) and (b). Gage BF, Waterman AD, Shannon W, Boechler M, Rich MW, Radford MJ. Validation of clinical classification schemes for predicting stroke. Results from the National Registry of Atrial Fibrillation. JAMA. 2001;285:2864-2870.

BRADYCARDIA

Population
–Adults.

Recommendations

▶ ACC/AHA/HRS 2018

–Consider evaluating for and treating sleep apnea if nocturnal bradycardia.

–Consider evaluating for structural heart disease.

–Evaluate for systemic conditions that may contribute such as medications (many antihypertensives, antiarrhythmics and psychoactive medications), rheumatologic conditions and inflammatory disorders, physical conditioning, carotid sinus hypersensitivity, syncope disorders, sleep, and sleep apnea.

–Give atropine for sinus node disease causing bradycardia with symptoms or hemodynamic instability.

–If bradycardia is caused by medication, use a reversal agent (10% calcium chloride or gluconate for calcium channel blocker overdose, glucagon or high-dose insulin for beta-blocker overdose, and digoxin antibody fragment for digoxin overdose).

–Use transcutaneous pacing for patients who remain hemodynamically unstable after medical therapy.

–Refer for pacemaker regardless of symptoms for second-degree Mobitz type II, high-grade atrioventricular (AV) block or third-degree AV block without reversible etiology.

–Refer for pacemaker if symptomatic from bradycardia with other etiologies that are not reversible.

–There is no minimum duration of pause that indicates the need for pacemaker, but rather the correlation between the pause and symptoms.

Source
–*JACC*. 2018;74(4):e51-e156.

CAROTID ARTERY DISEASE

CAROTID ARTERY STENOSIS

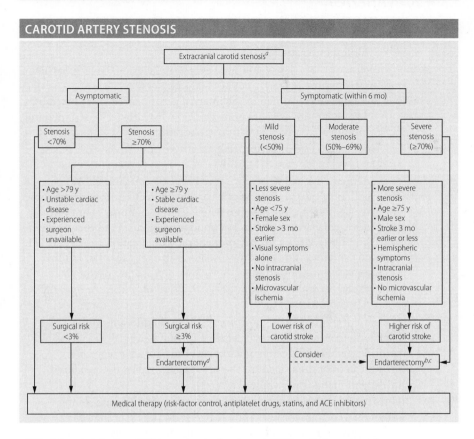

[a]Critical stenosis defined as >70% by noninvasive imaging or >50% by catheter angiography.

[b]Carotid endarterectomy (CEA) in symptomatic patients with average or low surgical risk should generally be reserved for patients with >5 y expectancy, and perioperative stroke/death rate <6%. When CEA is indicated, it should be performed within 2 wk after an ischemic central nervous system (CNS) event.

[c]Carotid artery stenting (CAS) with an embolic protection device is an alternative to CEA in symptomatic patients with average or low surgical risk when >70% obstruction is present, and the periprocedural stroke and mortality rate is <6%. CAS may be chosen over CEA if the neck anatomy is surgically unfavorable or if comorbid conditions make CEA a very high risk.

[d]The annual rate of stroke in asymptomatic patients treated with optimal medical therapy for carotid artery stenosis has decreased to <1%. Therefore, the benefit of CEA or CAS remains controversial in asymptomatic patients. (*Stroke*. 2010;41:975-979)

Sources: AHA/ASA 2005 Guidelines. *Circulation*. 2006;113:e872. *Stroke*. 2006;37:577. ASA/ACCF/AHA/AANN/AANS/ACR/ASNR/CNS/SAIP/SCAI/SIR/SNIS/SVM/SVS 2011 Guidelines. *J Am Coll Cardiol*. 2011;57:e16-e94. ACCF/SCAI/SVMB/SIR/ASITN 2007 Consensus. *J Am Coll Cardiol*. 2007;49(1):126-168.

Recommendations

▶ 2014 AHA/ASA

–Use CAS (carotid artery stenting) as an alternative to CEA (carotid endarterectomy) if all of the following:

- Symptomatic patient.
- Average or low risk of complications associated with endovascular intervention.
- Diameter of the lumen of the internal carotid artery is reduced by >70% by noninvasive imaging or >50% by catheter-based imaging or noninvasive imaging with corroboration.
- Anticipated rate of periprocedural stroke or death is <6% (Class IIa; Level of Evidence (LOE) B).

–Consider patient's age when choosing between CAS and CEA. For older patients (≥70 y), CEA may be associated with improved outcome compared with CAS, particularly when arterial anatomy is unfavorable for endovascular intervention. For younger patients, CAS is equivalent to CEA in terms of risk for periprocedural complication (ie, stroke, MI, or death) and long-term risk for ipsilateral stroke (Class IIa; LOE B).

–Do not perform routine, long-term follow-up imaging of the extracranial carotid circulation with carotid duplex ultrasonography (Class III; LOE B).

–For patients with recurrent or progressive ischemic symptoms ipsilateral to a stenosis or occlusion of a distal (surgically inaccessible) carotid artery, or occlusion of a midcervical carotid artery after institution of optimal medical therapy, EC/IC bypass is considered investigational only (Class IIB; LOE C).

–For patients with a stroke or TIA attributable to moderate stenosis (50%–69%) of a major intracranial artery, do not offer angioplasty or stenting given the low rate of stroke on medical management and the inherent periprocedural risk of endovascular treatment.

–For patients who have experienced an acute ischemic stroke or TIA with no other apparent cause, consider prolonged rhythm monitoring (approx. 30 d) for AF within 6 mo of the index event.

–In patients with ischemic stroke or TIA in the setting of acute anterior STEMI without demonstrable left ventricular mural thrombus formation but with anterior apical akinesis or dyskinesis identified by echo or other imaging modality, consider treatment with VKA therapy (target INR 2.5, range 2.0–3.0) for 3 mo.

–In patients with ischemic stroke or TIA in sinus rhythm who have left atrial or left ventricular thrombus demonstrated by echo or another imaging modality, anticoagulate with a VKA for >3 mo.

–For patients with ischemic stroke or TIA and a PFO who are not undergoing anticoagulation therapy, give antiplatelet therapy.

Women only:

–For women with recent TIA or IS and ipsilateral moderate (50%–69%) carotid stenosis, consider CEA depending on patient-specific factors such as age and comorbidities, if the perioperative morbidity and mortality risk is estimated to be <6%.

–For women with recent TIA or IS within the past 6 mo and ipsilateral severe (70%–99%) carotid artery stenosis, recommend CEA if the perioperative morbidity and mortality risk is estimated to be <6%.

–In women who are to undergo CEA, give aspirin unless contraindicated. Aspirin was used in every major trial that demonstrated efficacy of CEA.

–If a high-risk female patient (ie, 10-y predicted CVD risk ≥10%) has an indication for aspirin but is intolerant to it, use clopidogrel.

–When CEA is indicated for women with TIA or stroke, perform surgery within 2 wk rather than delaying surgery if there are no contraindications to early revascularization.

–Give aspirin therapy to women >65 y of age (81 mg daily or 100 mg every other day) if blood pressure is controlled and benefit for ischemic and myocardial infarction prevention is likely to outweigh risk of gastrointestinal bleeding and hemorrhagic stroke (Class IIa; LOE B). It may also be reasonable for women <65 y of age for ischemic stroke prevention.

Sources

–Guidelines for the prevention of stroke in patients with stroke and transient ischemic attack: a guideline for healthcare professionals from the American Heart Association/American Stroke Association. *Stroke.* 2014;45.

–Bushnell C, McCullough LD, Awad IA, et al. Guidelines for the prevention of stroke in women: a statement for healthcare professionals from the American Heart Association/American Stroke Association. *Stroke.* 2014;45. doi: 10.1161/01.str.0000442009.06663.48.

CORONARY ARTERY DISEASE (CAD)

Population
–Patients with stable coronary disease experiencing angina.

Recommendations
▶ 2012,2014 ACCF/AHA/ACP/AATS/PCNA/SCAI/STS

–Classify patients presenting with angina pectoris as stable or unstable.
–Acute coronary syndrome (ACS) includes high-risk unstable angina, non-ST-segment elevation myocardial infarction (NSTEMI) or ST-segment elevation myocardial infarction (STEMI).
–Obtain resting ECG with all symptoms of chest pain (typical or atypical in nature).
–Choose exercise treadmill test if the baseline ECG is normal, the patient can exercise, and the pretest likelihood of coronary disease is intermediate (10%–90%).
–If unable to perform an exercise treadmill and the pretest likelihood is >10%, choose either a nuclear myocardial perfusion imaging study (MPI) or exercise echocardiogram.
–Repeat exercise and imaging studies when there is a change in clinical status or if needed for exercise prescription.
–Consider coronary computed tomography angiogram (CTA) in patients with an intermediate pretest probability of CAD (FRS) in whom symptoms persist despite prior normal testing, with equivocal stress tests, or in patients who cannot be studied otherwise. Coronary CTA is not indicated if known moderate or severe coronary calcification or in the presence of prior stents.
–An echocardiogram is recommended to assess resting LV function and valve disease in patients with suspected CAD, pathological Q waves, presence of heart failure, or ventricular arrhythmias.
–Treat patients who have stable coronary disease with:
  • Lifestyle guidance (diet, weight loss, smoking cessation, and exercise education).
  • Blood pressure control per JNC guidelines.
  • Associated risk factor assessment: Presence of chronic kidney disease and psychosocial factors such as depression, anxiety, and poor social support have been added to the classic risk factors.
  • Appropriate medications: (ASA 75–162 mg daily, moderate-dose statin, BP control, blood glucose control, beta-blocker therapy, and sublingual NTG).

–Consider coronary angiography in patients who survive sudden cardiac death, who have high-risk noninvasive test results (large areas of silent ischemia are often associated with malignant ventricular arrhythmias) and in whom anginal symptoms cannot be controlled with optimal medical therapy.[e]

–Coronary bypass grafting surgery (CABG) is preferred to angioplasty in diabetic patients with multivessel disease (FREEDOM trial 2012).[f]

Population

–Patients with stable coronary disease experiencing unstable angina or non-ST elevation MI (NSTEMI).

Recommendations

▶ 2014 ACC/AHA, 2015 ESC

–Include in initial evaluation an ECG, cardiac troponin I or T levels (obtained at symptom onset and 3–6 h later, with levels beyond 6 h if EKG or clinical presentation suggest a high probability of ACS), and assess prognosis with risk scores such as TIMI[g] or GRACE.[h]

–Give sublingual nitroglycerin q5min x3 for ongoing ischemic pain. Use IV nitroglycerin for persistent ischemia, heart failure, or hypertension.

–Give dual antiplatelet therapy in likely or definite NSTE-ACS. Aspirin (162–325 mg, non-enteric-coated) and clopidogrel (300–600 mg loading dose, then maintenance) or ticagrelor (180 mg loading dose, then maintenance). After stabilization, consider dual antiplatelet therapy (clopidogrel or ticagrelor in addition to aspirin) "up to" 12 mo if not stented, "at least" 12 mo if stented.

---

[e]Coronary angiography is useful in patients with presumed SIHD who have unacceptable ischemic symptoms despite GDMT (guideline determined medical therapy) and who are amenable to, and candidates for, coronary revascularization. Coronary angiography is reasonable to define the extent and severity of coronary artery disease (CAD) in patients with suspected SIHD whose clinical characteristics and results of noninvasive testing (exclusive of stress testing) indicate a high likelihood of severe IHD and who are amenable to, and candidates for, coronary revascularization. Coronary angiography is reasonable in patients with suspected symptomatic SIHD who cannot undergo diagnostic stress testing, or have indeterminate or nondiagnostic stress tests, when there is a high likelihood that the findings will result in important changes to therapy. Coronary angiography might be considered in patients with stress test results of acceptable quality that do not suggest the presence of CAD when clinical suspicion of CAD remains high and there is a high likelihood that the findings will result in important changes to therapy.
[f]A Heart Team approach to revascularization is recommended in patients with diabetes mellitus and complex multivessel CAD. CABG is generally recommended in preference to PCI to improve survival in patients with diabetes mellitus and multivessel CAD for which revascularization is likely to improve survival (3-vessel CAD or complex 2-vessel CAD involving the proximal LAD), particularly if a LIMA graft can be anastomosed to the LAD artery, provided the patient is a good candidate for surgery.
[g]TIMI Risk Score predicts 30-d and 1-y mortality in ACS (mortality rises at TIMI = 3–4). 1 point each for age $\geq$65, $\geq$3 risk factors for CAD, known CAD, ST changes on EKG ($\geq$0.5 mm), active angina ($\geq$2 episodes in past 24 h), aspirin in past 7 d, elevated cardiac marker.
[h]GRACE risk model predicts in-hospital and postdischarge mortality or MI. Downloadable tool: http://www.outcomes-umassmed.org/grace/

–Anticoagulate, in addition to dual antiplatelet therapy. Use unfractionated heparin, enoxaparin, or fondaparinux. The strongest evidence supports enoxaparin.

–Give oral beta-blockers in the first 24 h, unless signs of heart failure, low output state, risk factors for cardiogenic shock, or other contraindications to beta-blockade. If contraindicated or if ischemia persists despite beta-blockers and nitrates, give nondihydropyridine calcium channel blocker.

–If patients already on beta-blockers with normal LVEF or stable reduced LVEF, continue home dose of long-acting metoprolol succinate, carvedilol, or bisoprolol.

–Block the renin-angiotensin-aldosterone system with an ACE inhibitor. Continue after stabilization if LVEF <40%, HTN, DM, or stable CKD.

–Start or continue high-intensity statin, unless contraindicated, and continue indefinitely.

–Give supplemental oxygen if SaO_2 <= 90% or respiratory distress.

–Give IV morphine for analgesia if anti-ischemic medications have been maximized. Do not give NSAIDs.

–After stabilization, continue aspirin (81–325 mg/d) indefinitely.

Sources
–*Eur Heart J.* 2016;37(3):267-315. https://academic.oup.com/eurheartj/article/37/3/267/2466099;

–*J Am Coll Cardiol.* 2014;64(24):e139-e228. http://content.onlinejacc.org/article.aspx?articleid=1910086;

–*Am Coll Cardiol.* 2016;68(10):1082-1115. http://content.onlinejacc.org/article.aspx?articleid=2507082

Population
–Patients with stable coronary disease experiencing ST Elevation MI (STEMI).

Recommendations
▶ 2013 ACC/AHA, 2012 ESC, NICE 2013

–Draw serum markers routinely, but do not wait for results to initiate reperfusion therapy.

–Elect PCI rather than fibrinolysis for all patients with STEMI if an experienced team is available within 120 min of first medical contact.

–Give aspirin (162–325 mg) and a loading dose of an ADP-receptor inhibitor (clopidogrel 600 mg, prasugrel 60 mg, or ticagrelor 180 mg) as early as possible.

–Anticoagulate with unfractionated heparin (UFH), enoxaparin, or bivalirudin. A glycoprotein IIb/IIIa inhibitor (abciximab, eptifibatide, tirofiban) may be added to UFH.

–If hypertensive or with ongoing ischemia, give beta-blocker at presentation.

–In PCI for STEMI, use either a bare metal or drug-eluting stent. Use a bare metal stent in patients with high bleeding risk, inability to comply with 1 y of dual antiplatelet therapy, or upcoming invasive procedure.

–After PCI, give dual antiplatelet therapy for 1 y.

–If PCI is not available, treat instead with fibrinolytics. Give a loading dose of clopidogrel (300 mg; 75 mg if >75 y of age) with aspirin. Anticoagulate with heparin, enoxaparin, or fondaparinux until hospital discharge (minimum 48 h, up to 8 d) or until revascularization is performed. Give fibrinolytic therapy within 30 min of hospital arrival. It is most useful if ischemic symptoms started within the past 12 h and is a reasonable choice between 12 and 24 h if there is evidence of ongoing ischemia or a large area of myocardium at risk. Transfer to a PCI-capable facility if fibrinolysis fails.

–Give patients who have undergone PCI for STEMI dual antiplatelet therapy for 1 y. Continue aspirin indefinitely. Initiate beta-blockers within 24 h of admission, high-intensity statin, and if LVEF <40% an ace inhibitor or angiotensin receptor blocker.

Sources

–*J Am Coll Cardiol.* 2013;61(4). https://www.guideline.gov/summaries/summary/39429?

–*Eur Heart J.* 2012;33(20):2569-619. https://www.guideline.gov/summaries/summary/39353?

–National Institute for Health and Care Excellence (NICE); 2013:28. https://www.guideline.gov/summaries/summary/47019?

–*Am Coll Cardiol.* 2016;68(10):1082-1115. http://content.onlinejacc.org/article.aspx?articleid=2507082

Population

–Patients with elevated cardiac troponin level.

Recommendations

▶ 2012 ACC

–Elevated troponin levels are an imperfect diagnostic test and are dependent upon the probability of underlying CAD.

–Establish high pretest probability and global risk scores (TIMI, GRACE, PERSUIT) to determine the significance of elevated troponin levels.

–Clinical factors that establish a high pretest probability include a history of typical angina, typical ECG changes consistent with ischemia (ST-segment changes), history of established coronary risk factors, or the history of known CAD.

–Elevated troponin levels in patients with high pretest probability of CAD (typical chest pain and ECG changes of ischemia) have a predictive accuracy of ≥95% to establish acute coronary syndrome.

–Elevated troponin levels in patients with low pretest probability of CAD (atypical chest pain and nonspecific ECG changes) have a predictive accuracy of only 50% to establish ACS.

–Use global risk scores to further establish the role of early conservative vs. early invasive therapy in patients with elevated troponin levels and a high pretest probability.

–Cardiac causes for elevated troponin levels include ACS, coronary spasm or embolism, cocaine or methamphetamine use, stress cardiomyopathy, congestive heart failure, myocarditis or pericarditis, trauma, infiltrative diseases, postprocedure (ablation, electric shock, coronary bypass surgery, and postcoronary angioplasty).

–Noncardiac causes for elevated troponin levels include pulmonary embolus, renal failure, stroke, sepsis, drug toxicity (anthracycline), and hypoxia.

Source

–Newby LK, Jesse RL, Babb JD, et al. ACCF 2012 expert consensus document of practical clinical considerations in the interpretation of troponin elevations: a report of the American College of Cardiology Foundation task force on Clinical Expert Consensus Documents. *J Am Coll Cardiol.* 2012;60:2427-2463.

Population

–Patients with stable coronary disease experiencing sexual dysfunction.

Recommendations

▶ 2013 AHA/Princeton Consensus Panel

–Erectile dysfunction (ED) is associated with CAD and often precedes the diagnosis of CAD.

–ED is associated with an increased risk for CV events and all-cause mortality.

–Angina pectoris during sexual activity represents <5% of all angina attacks.

–Patients with CAD with angina pectoris should undergo full medical evaluation prior to partaking in sexual activity.

–Patients should be able to perform 3–5 metabolic equivalents (METs) on a treadmill or climb 2 flights of stairs or walk briskly without angina before engaging in sexual activity.

-After uncomplicated MI if no symptoms on mild-to-moderate activity exist >1 wk, patient may resume sexual activity.

-After angioplasty, sexual activity is reasonable within 1 wk if the radial groin site is healed.

-After coronary bypass, sexual activity is reasonable after 6–8 wk, being limited by the sternal healing or pain.

-If residual coronary lesions persist post revascularization, perform exercise stress testing to evaluate for significant ischemia.

-Sexual activity is contraindicated in patients with angina at low effort, refractory angina, or unstable angina.

-Nitrate therapy is contraindicated with phosphodiesterase 5 (PDE5) inhibitor therapy. Following sildenafil (Viagra) or vardenafil (Levitra) at least 24 h must elapse before nitrates can be started; ≥48 h if tadalafil (Cialis) is used.

-Beta-blockers, calcium channel blockers, and Ranolazine are not contraindicated; however, they may exacerbate erectile dysfunction.

Sources

-Schwartz BG, Kloner RA. Clinical cardiology: physician update: erectile dysfunction and cardiovascular disease. *Circulation.* 2011;123:98-101.

-Nehra A, Jackson G, Martin Miner, et al. The Princeton III consensus recommendations for the management of erectile dysfunction and cardiovascular disease. *Mayo Clin Proc.* 2012;87:766-778.

-Kloner RA, Henderson L. Sexual function in patients with chronic angina pectoris. *Am J Cardiol.* 2013;111:1671-1676.

Population

-Patients with coronary artery disease and atrial fibrillation.

Recommendations

▶ 2014 ACC/AHA/ESC

-The prudent use of triple anticoagulation therapy with aspirin, clopidogrel, and warfarin in AF patients at high risk of thromboembolism and recent coronary stent placement remains a matter of clinical judgment, balancing the risk of thrombotic vs. bleeding events.

-Choose bare-metal stents if triple anticoagulation therapy is required.

-Reserve drug-eluting stents for high-risk clinical or anatomic situations (diabetic patients or if the coronary lesions are unusually long, totally occlusive, or in small blood vessels) if triple anticoagulation therapy is required.

-Dual antiplatelet therapy with clopidogrel (75 mg/d) and ASA (81 mg/d) is the most effective therapy to prevent coronary stent thrombosis.

–Warfarin anticoagulation is the most effective therapy to prevent thromboembolism in high-risk AF patients as defined by the CHA2DS2-VASC risk score ($\geq$2).

–In nonvalvular AF consider NOACs. Following coronary revascularization, in high-risk patients with AF consider clopidogrel 75 mg daily concurrently with OAC but without ASA.

–Triple anticoagulation therapy is the most effective therapy to prevent both coronary stent thrombosis and the occurrence of embolic strokes in high-risk patients. However, the addition of warfarin to DAPT increases the bleeding risk by 3.7-fold. Therefore, awaiting a definitive clinical trial (WOEST trial), perform a risk stratification of patients to evaluate the thromboembolic potential of AF vs. the bleeding potential. The HAS-BLED (see table on page 267) bleeding risk score is the best measure of bleeding risk. A high risk of bleeding is defined by a score >3.

–If dual antiplatelet or triple anticoagulation therapy, maintain prophylactic GI therapy with an H2-blocker (except cimetidine) or PPI agent. If considering omeprazole (Prilosec), review the risk-to-benefit ratio because of its possible interference with clopidogrel function.

–In patients with a high risk of bleeding, triple anticoagulation therapy should be reserved for AF patients with a high thromboembolic risk. If the bleeding risk is high but the AF thromboembolic risk is low, choose dual antiplatelet therapy.

Sources

–*Circulation* 2014;130(23).

–*Eur Heart J.* 2010;31:2369-2429.

–*BMJ.* 2008;337:a840.

–*Chest.* 2011;139:981-987.

–*J Am Coll Cardiol.* 2008;51:172-208; 2009;54:95-109; 2010;56:2051-2066; 2011;57:1920-1959.

CORONARY ARTERY DISEASE: STENT THERAPY USE OF TRIPLE ANTICOAGULATION TREATMENT

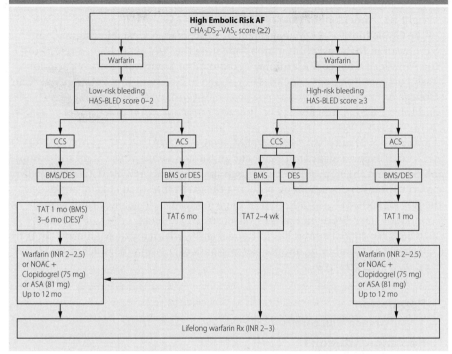

ACS, acute coronary syndrome; AF, atrial fibrillation; ASA, aspirin; BMS, bare-metal stent; CCS, patient with chronic coronary syndrome (stable coronary artery disease); DES, drug eluting stent; INR, international normalized ratio; Rx, therapy [warfarin (INR 2–2.5) + aspirin (81 mg daily) + clopidogrel (75 mg daily)]; TAT, triple anticoagulation therapy.

[a]DES stents if sirolimus, everolimus, or tacrolimus require 3-mo dual platelet therapy (ASA plus clopidogrel). If DES stent is paclitaxel, 6-mo dual therapy is required.

Sources

– European Heart Rhythm Association; European Association for Cardio-Thoracic Surgery, Camm AJ, Kirchhof P, Lip GY, et al. Guidelines for the management of atrial fibrillation: the Task Force for the Management of Atrial Fibrillation of the European Society of Cardiology (ESC). *Eur Heart J.* 2010;31:2369-2429.
– Lip GY. Managing the anticoagulated patient with atrial fibrillation at high risk of stroke who needs coronary intervention. *BMJ.* 2008;337:a840.
– Rubboli A, Kovacic JC, Mehran R, Lip GY. Coronary stent implantation in patients committed to long-term oral anticoagulation: successfully navigating the treatment options. *Chest.* 2011;139:981-987.
– King SB III, Smith SC Jr, Hirshfeld JW Jr, et al. 2007 focused update of the ACC/AHA/SCAI 2005 guideline update for percutaneous coronary intervention: a report of the American College of Cardiology/American Heart Association Task Force on Practice guidelines. *J Am Coll Cardiol.* 2008;51:172-208. 2014 AHA/

ACC/HRS Guideline for the Management of Patients With Atrial Fibrillation.
- CT January, LS Wann, JS Alpert, et al. *Circulation.* 2014. http://circ.ahajournals. org/content/early/2014/04/10/CIR.0000000000000041.
- Wright RS, Anderson JL, Adams CD, et al. 2011 ACCF/AHA focused update of the Guidelines for the Management of Patients with Unstable Angina/Non-ST-Elevation Myocardial Infarction (updating the 2007 guideline): a report of the American College of Cardiology Foundation/American Heart Association Task Force on Practice Guidelines developed in collaboration with the American College of Emergency Physicians, Society for Cardiovascular Angiography and Interventions, and Society of Thoracic Surgeons. *J Am Coll Cardiol.* 2011;57:1920-1959.
- Abraham NS, Hlatky MA, Antman EM, et al. ACCF/ACG/AHA. ACCF/ACG/AHA 2010 expert consensus document on the concomitant use of proton pump inhibitors and thienopyridines: a focused update of the ACCF/ACG/AHA 2008 expert consensus document on reducing the gastrointestinal risks of antiplatelet therapy and NSAID use. A Report of the American College of Cardiology Foundation Task Force on Expert Consensus Documents. *J Am Coll Cardiol.* 2010;56:2051-2066. Holmes DR Jr, Kereiakes DJ, Kleiman NS, Moliterno DJ, Patti G, Grines CL. Combining antiplatelet and anticoagulation therapies. *J Am Coll Cardiol.* 2009;54:95-109.

Population
–Women with coronary artery disease.

Recommendations
▶ 2011 AHA

–CVD is the leading cause of mortality in women.

–AHA recommends the risk assessment of CVD in women should begin at age 20 y, identifying women at higher risk.

–There are racial/ethnic differences in risk factors, with black and Hispanic women having a higher prevalence of hypertension and diabetes. The highest CVD morbidity and mortality occurs in black women.

–Autoimmune diseases (systemic lupus erythematosus, rheumatoid arthritis) and preeclampsia are significant risk factors for CVD in women.

–Psychological stress (anxiety, depression) and socioeconomic disadvantages are associated with a higher CVD risk in women.

–Microvascular disease with endothelial dysfunction, also known as female pattern disease, is the etiology of ischemia in more women than men.

–Women are more likely to have atypical cardiovascular symptoms such as sudden or extreme fatigue, dyspnea, sleep disturbances, anxiety, nausea, vomiting, and indigestion.

–ACC/AHA guidelines recommend a routine exercise stress test as the initial evaluation in symptomatic women who have a good exercise capacity and a normal baseline ECG. Exercise stress perfusion study (myocardial perfusion scintigraphy [MPS]) or exercise echo should be reserved for symptomatic women with higher pretest likelihood for CAD or indeterminate routine testing.

–Women often receive less medical therapy and lifestyle counseling than men.

–After PCI procedure, women experience higher rate of complications and mortality than men.

–Management of stable CAD should be the same as in men which include ASA, beta-blocker, statin, ACE inhibitor (ejection fraction [EF] <40%), and nitrate/calcium channel blocker (CCB) for angina management.

–In microvascular disease, beta-blockers have shown to be superior to CCB for angina management. Statins, ACE inhibitors, ranolazine, and exercise can improve angina scores and endothelial dysfunction in female pattern disease.

Sources

–Moasca L, Benjamin EJ, Berra K, et al. Effectiveness-based guidelines for the prevention of cardiovascular disease in women—2011 update: a guideline from the American Heart Association. *Circulation.* 2011;123:1243-1262.

–Gulati M, Shaw LJ, Bairey Merz CN. Myocardial ischemia in women: lessons from the NHLBI wise study. *Clin Cardiol.* 2012;35:141-148.

HEART FAILURE

HEART FAILURE STAGING

Stage A: Patients with hypertension, atherosclerotic disease, diabetes mellitus, metabolic syndrome, or those using cardiotoxins or having a family history of cardiomyopathy.

Stage B: Patients with previous MI, LV remodeling including LVH and low EF, or asymptomatic valvular disease.

Stage C: Patients with known structural heart disease; shortness of breath and fatigue, reduced exercise tolerance.

Stage D: Patients who have marked symptoms at rest despite maximal medical therapy (eg, those who are recurrently hospitalized or cannot be safely discharged from the hospital without specialized interventions).

Source: Adapted from the American College of Cardiology, American Heart Association, Inc. *Circulation.* 2017. doi:10 .1161/CIR.0000000000000509.

Population

–Adults with heart failure.

Recommendations

▶ 2013, 2017 ACC/AHA, 2018 NICE

Assessment

–Classify heart failure as reduced or preserved ejection fraction:
  - Heart failure with reduced ejection fraction (HFrEF), referred to as systolic heart failure, when LVEF $\leq$40%.
  - Heart failure with preserved ejection fraction (HFpEF), referred to as diastolic dysfunction, when LVEF >40%.

–Diagnosing heart failure:
  - Measure N-terminal pro-B-type natriuretic peptide.
  - If BNP >2000 ng/L, obtain transthoracic echo within 6 wk (of note, other causes of high BNP include age over 70 y, LVH, tachycardia, RV overload, hypoxemia, pulmonary embolism, renal dysfunction, COPD, DM, and cirrhosis).
  - If BNP <400 in an untreated person, heart failure is less likely (of note, obesity, African or African-Carribbean family origin, or treatment with diuretics can reduce levels of BNP).

–Obtain CXR, blood tests (renal function, thyroid function, liver function, lipid profile, A1c, complete blood count), urine analysis, and peak flow or spirometry. Identify prior cardiac or noncardiac disease that may lead to HF. For patients at risk of developing HF (Stage A/B), natriuretic peptide biomarker–based screening (BNP or NT-pro-BNP) and optimizing GDMT can help prevent the development of left ventricular dysfunction (systolic or diastolic) or new-onset HF.

–Obtain history to include diet or medicine nonadherence; current or past use of alcohol, illicit drugs, and chemotherapy; or recent viral illness.

–If idiopathic dilated cardiomyopathy, obtain a three-generational family history to exclude familial disease.

–Consider risk score evaluation to help predict outcomes, chronic heart failure—Seattle Heart Failure Model. (http://depts.washington.edu/shfm/)

–Identify the patient's present activity level and desired post-treatment level.

–Assess the patient's volume status, orthostatic BP changes, height and weight, and body mass index.

–Control hypertension and lipid disorders in accordance with contemporary guideline to lower the risk of HF. Control or avoid other risk factors.

–In initial blood work, measure N-terminal pro-brain natriuretic peptide (NT-proBNP) or BNP levels to support clinical judgment for diagnosis, especially if diagnosis is uncertain. Also include CBC, chemistry panel, lipid profile, troponin I level, and TSH level.

–Obtain 12-lead ECG.

–Obtain 2D echocardiogram to determine the systolic function, diastolic function, valvular function, and pulmonary artery pressure.

–In patients with angina or significant ischemia, perform coronary arteriography unless the patient is not eligible for surgery.

Management

–If volume overloaded, initiate diuretic therapy and salt restriction. Diuretics do not improve long-term survival, but improve symptoms and short-term survival. Once euvolemic and symptoms have resolved, carefully wean dosage as an outpatient to lowest dose possible to prevent electrolyte disorders and activation of the renin-angiotensin system.

–Give ACE inhibitor or ARB or ARNI (ARB plus a neprilysin inhibitor, such as valsartan/sacubitril) early in the initial course if ejection fraction reduced to decrease afterload. Titrate dosage every 2 wk to target dose in clinical studies as BP allows. Measure renal function and electrolytes 1–2 wk after each change.

–In patients with chronic symptomatic HFrEF NYHA Class II or III who tolerate an ACE inhibitor or ARB, replace with an ARNI to further reduce morbidity and mortality.

–Add beta-blockers (specifically carvedilol, sustained release metoprolol succinate, or bisoprolol) to reduce morbidity and mortality. These beta-blockers improve survival the most in systolic heart failure. Start with low dose, and titrate dosage gradually to heart rate 65–70 beats/min.

–Start aldosterone antagonist in patients with moderate or severe symptoms (NYHA Class II–IV) and reduced ejection fraction. Creatinine should be <2.5 mg/dL in men and <2 mg/dL in women, and the potassium should be <5 mEq/L.

–Consider ivabradine to reduce HF hospitalization in select patients: symptomatic stable chronic HFrEF (EF <35%) at least 4 wk removed from exacerbation on optimal medical therapy including optimal dosing of ACE inhibitor and beta-blocker at maximal tolerated dose in sinus rhythm with resting HR >70.

–Use the combination of hydralazine and nitrates to improve outcomes in African-Americans with moderate-to-severe HF with decreased ejection fraction, in addition to optimal therapy. If ACE inhibitor or ARB agent is contraindicated, hydralazine and nitrates may be used as alternative therapy.

–Consider digoxin if severe or worsening HFrEF despite optimal first-line therapies.

–Statins are not beneficial as adjunctive therapy when prescribed solely for the diagnosis of HF. In all patients with a recent or remote hx of CAD, CVA, PAD, or hyperlipidemia, use statins according to guidelines.

–Discontinue anti-inflammatory agents, diltiazem, and verapamil.

–Nutritional supplements are not useful therapy for patients with current or prior symptoms of systolic dysfunction (HFrEF).

–Avoid calcium channel blockers in the routine treatment for patients with HFrEF.

–Recommend exercise training, which is beneficial in HF patients with decreased ejection fraction (systolic dysfunction) or preserved ejection fraction (diastolic dysfunction) once therapy is optimized.

–Refer for intracardiac cardiac defibrillator to obtain secondary survival benefit in patients who survive cardiac arrest, ventricular fibrillation, or hemodynamically significant ventricular tachycardia.

–Refer for intracardiac cardiac defibrillator to obtain primary survival benefit in patients with ischemic or nonischemic cardiomyopathy with EF ≤35% with New York Heart Association (NYHA) class II or III. The patient should be stable on GDMT (guideline-determined medical therapy) optimal chronic medical HF therapy and at least 40 d post-MI and have a life-expectancy of at least 1 y.

–Consider biventricular heart pacemaker (CRT) in refractory HF with ejection fraction equal to or less than 35% with NYHA class II and III or ambulatory class IV on GDMT. The rhythm should be sinus, with a QRS ≥150 ms, ± LBBB.

–Do not administer long-term anticoagulation therapy in patients with chronic systolic function while in sinus rhythm in the absence of AF, a prior thromboembolic event, or cardioembolic source.

–Maintain blood pressure less than 130/80 mm Hg.

–In HF patients with preserved systolic function (diastolic dysfunction), randomized data on therapy are lacking. The goal is to control blood volume (diuretic), keep systolic blood pressure <130 mm Hg (beta-blocker, ACE inhibitor, ARB agent, or diuretic), slow heart rate (beta-blocker), and treat coronary artery ischemia. Whether beta-blockers, ACE inhibitors, ARB agents, or aldosterone antagonists improve survival independently is yet to be proven.

–Give all patients comprehensive written discharge instruction. Emphasize diet, weight monitoring, medicine, and salt adherence. Discuss activity along with education of symptoms of worsening HF.

–During an HF hospitalization, consider obtaining a predischarge natriuretic peptide level (BNP or NT-pro-BNP) to establish a postdischarge prognosis.

–Arrange postdischarge appointment with physician and health care team with attention to information on discharge medications.

Comments

1. Lifetime risk of developing HF for Americans $\geq$40-y-old is 20%.
2. Overall mortality is 50% in 5 y; varies with HF stage:
   a. Stage B: 5-y mortality 4%.
   b. Stage C: 5-y mortality 25%.
   c. Stage D: 5-y mortality 80%.

Sources

–ACCF/AHA 2017 Guidelines. *Circulation*. 2017. doi: 10.1161/ CIR.0000000000000509.

–*N Engl J Med*. 2012.

–WARCET Trial; American Academy of Family Physicians; American Academy of Hospice and Palliative Medicine; American Nurses Association; American Society of Health-System Pharmacists; Heart Rhythm Society; Society of Hospital Medicine, Bonow RO, Ganiats TG, Beam CT, et al. ACCF/AHA/AMA-PCPI 2011 performance measures for adults with heart failure: a report of the American College of Cardiology Foundation/American Heart Association Task Force on Performance Measures and the American Medical Association-Physician Consortium for Performance Improvement. *J Am Coll Cardiol*. 2012;59(20):1812-1832.

–Yancy CW, Jessup M, Bozkurt B, et al. 2013. ACCF/AHA guideline for the management of heart failure: a report of the American College of Cardiology Foundation/American Heart Association Task Force on practice guidelines. *Circulation*. 2013;128:e240-e327.

HYPERLIPIDEMIA

The risk assessment and management of ASCVD risk factors, including hyperlipidemia, is detailed in Chapter 14: Cardiovascular Disorders.

HYPERTENSION

HYPERTENSION TREATMENT—JNC 8 2014

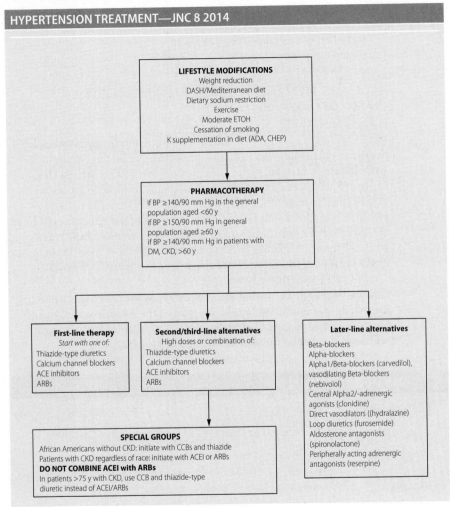

LIFESTYLE MODIFICATIONS
Weight reduction
DASH/Mediterranean diet
Dietary sodium restriction
Exercise
Moderate ETOH
Cessation of smoking
K supplementation in diet (ADA, CHEP)

PHARMACOTHERAPY
if BP ≥140/90 mm Hg in the general
population aged <60 y
if BP ≥150/90 mm Hg in general
population aged ≥60 y
if BP ≥140/90 mm Hg in patients with
DM, CKD, >60 y

First-line therapy
Start with one of:
Thiazide-type diuretics
Calcium channel blockers
ACE inhibitors
ARBs

Second/third-line alternatives
High doses or combination of:
Thiazide-type diuretics
Calcium channel blockers
ACE inhibitors
ARBs

Later-line alternatives
Beta-blockers
Alpha-blockers
Alpha1/Beta-blockers (carvedilol),
vasodilating Beta-blockers
(nebivolol)
Central Alpha2/-adrenergic
agonists (clonidine)
Direct vasodilators ((hydralazine)
Loop diuretics (furosemide)
Aldosterone antagonists
(spironolactone)
Peripherally acting adrenergic
antagonists (reserpine)

SPECIAL GROUPS
African Americans without CKD: initiate with CCBs and thiazide
Patients with CKD regardless of race: initiate with ACEI or ARBs
DO NOT COMBINE ACEI with ARBs
In patients >75 y with CKD, use CCB and thiazide-type
diuretic instead of ACEI/ARBs

Source: James PA, Oparil S, Carter BL. 2014 evidence-based guideline for the management of high blood pressure in adults. Report from the panel members appointed to the Eighth Joint National Committee (JNC8). *JAMA.* 2014;311(5):507-520. doi:10.1001/jama.2013.284427.

Population

–All adults.

Recommendations

▶ **2017 ACC/AHA**

–Initiate therapy

- BP 120–129/<80: lifestyle changes, follow-up 3–6 mo.
- BP 130–139/80–89, 10-y ASCVD risk ≥10%: lifestyle changes and medications, follow-up 1 mo.
- BP 130–139/80–89, 10-y ASCVD risk <10%: lifestyle changes and medications, follow-up 3–6 mo.
- BP ≥140/90: lifestyle changes and medications, follow-up 1 mo.

–Goal therapy

- <130/80 for CVD or 10-y ASCVD risk ≥10%; consider <130/18 for all.

–Choice of antihypertensive therapy

- Choose from thiazide diuretics, calcium channel blockers ACE inhibitors, and angiotensin receptor blockers for first drug therapy. Begin therapy with two drugs initially if desired BP reduction is more than 20/10 mm Hg.
- If stable ischemic heart disease, prioritize medications indicated by CAD/CHF as first drugs.
- If ischemic heart disease and angina, add nondihydropyridine calcium channel blockers to beta-blockers.
- If CKD, target BP <130/80 and favor ACE inhibitor or ARB if proteinuria.

▶ **2014 JNC8**

–Initiate therapy

- BP ≥140/90 mm Hg in the general population age <60-y-old.
- BP ≥150/90 mm Hg in general population age ≥60-y-old.

–Goal therapy

- BP <140/90 mm Hg in patients <60-y-old.
- BP <150/90 mm Hg in patients ≥60-y-old.
- BP <140/90 mm Hg in patients with DM, CKD who are <60-y-old.

–Choice of antihypertensive therapy

- In the general non-black population, including those with DM, initial treatment should include a thiazide-type diuretic, CCB, ACEI, or ARB. In the general black population, including those with DM, initial treatment should include a thiazide-type diuretic or CCB. In all population age ≥18-y-old with CKD (+/−DM), treatment should include an ACEI/ARB to improve kidney outcomes.

- Patients with CKD regardless of race: initiate with ACEI or ARBs.
- In patients >75-y-old with CKD, use CCB and thiazide-type diuretic instead of ACEI/ARBs.
- If BP cannot be reached within 1 mo, increase the dose of the initial drug or add a second and then third drug from the recommended classes.
- Do not use an ACEI and ARB together!
- beta-blockers, alpha-blockers, central alpha-2-adrenergic agonists (eg, clonidine), direct vasodilators (eg, hydralazine), aldosterone receptor antagonists (eg, spironolactone), peripherally acting adrenergic antagonists (eg, reserpine), and loop diuretics (eg, furosemide) are not recommended as a first-line therapy.

▶ 2018 ESC/ESH

– Initiate therapy
  - BP 130–139/85–89: lifestyle modification (salt restriction <5 g/d, alcohol intake <14 drinks/wk for men and <8 drinks/wk for women, increasing fruits/vegetables/fish/nuts/olive oil in diet, controlling BMI, regular physical activity, and smoking cessation.
  - BP 140–159/90–99: lifestyle modification; medications if high cardiovascular risk, hypertension-mediated organ damage, or persistent elevation after 3–6 mo lifestyle changes.
  - BP 160+/100+: lifestyle modification and drug therapy.
– Goal therapy
  - Target <140/90 in all patients.
  - If tolerating 140/90, target SBP 120–129 if <65 y and 130–139 if ≥65 y.
– Choice of antihypertensive therapy
  - Start with combination pill including ACE inhibitor (ACEi) or angiotensin receptor blocker (ARB) plus a calcium channel blocker (CCB) or diuretic. Consider using a single agent in older/frailer patients or those with mild elevations.
  - If not controlled with initial therapy, switch to a three-drug combination pill including ACEi/ARB + CCB + diuretic.
  - If not controlled on three drugs, add spironolactone, diuretic, alpha-blocker or beta-blockers and consider further investigation for resistant hypertension.
  - If CAD, initial combination should be ACEi/ARB or diuretic plus beta-blocker or CCB.
  - If CKD, consider adding loop diuretic.
  - If HFrEF, avoid CCB.

▶ 2014 ASH

–Goal therapy

- BP <150/90 mm Hg in patients ≥80-y-old.
- BP <140/90 mm Hg in patients 60- to 79-y-old.
- BP <140/90 mm Hg or <130/80 mm Hg (if tolerated), in patients <50-y-old.
- In patients with CKD or diabetes:
  ○ BP <140/90 mm Hg (without proteinuria).
  ○ BP <130/80 mm Hg (with proteinuria) or if they are at "high risk of cardiovascular disease"—no consensus.

–Antihypertensive therapy

- Start lifestyle changes.
- In stage I (140–159/90–99) in patients without CV risks, some months of regularly monitored lifestyle management without drugs can be considered.
- In black patients initiate with CCB or thiazide. If unable to control BP, add ACEI/ARB. If needed, add spironolactone, centrally acting agents, and beta-blockers.
- In non-black patients <60-y-old initiate with ACEI/ARB. If uncontrolled, add CCB or thiazide. If needed, add spironolactone, centrally acting agents, and beta-blockers. In non-black patients ≥60-y-old initiate with CCB or thiazide. If needed, add spironolactone, centrally acting agents, and beta-blockers.

▶ 2015 CHEP

–The diagnosis of HTN should be based on out-of-office measurements (home or ambulatory). Electronic (oscillometric) measurement methods are preferred to manual measurements. HBPM and ABPM identify white-coat hypertension (as well as diagnose masked hypertension). (10% may have marked hypertension.)

–Risk factors cluster; therefore, the management of HTN is combining global cardiovascular risk management and vascular protection including advice and treatment for smoking cessation.

–Structured exercise prescription as lifestyle modification.

–Resistance or weight training does not adversely affect BP in normotensive or mildly hypertensive individuals.

–Stress management should be considered as an intervention in hypertensive patients in whom stress may be contributing to BP elevation.

Initiate therapy

–BP ≥160/100 mm Hg in patients without macrovascular target organ damage or other CV risk factors.

–BP ≥140/90 mm Hg in patients with macrovascular target organ damage or high cardiovascular risk.

–BP >130/80 mm Hg in patients with diabetes.

–SBP >160 mm Hg in elderly (≥60 y).

Goal therapy

–BP <140/90 mm Hg in the general population, including those with CKD.

–BP <130/80 mm Hg in patients with DM.

–SBP <150 mm Hg in the elderly (≥60 y).

–SBP <140 mm Hg in the elderly with cerebrovascular disease (history of CVA/TIA).

–Caution in elderly patients who are frail and in patients with CAD and have low DBP <60 mm Hg.

Choice of antihypertensive therapy

–Combination of both lifestyle modifications and antihypertensive medicines is generally necessary to achieve target blood pressures. Adopting health behaviors is integral to the management of hypertension.

–Optimum management of the hypertensive patient requires assessment and communication of overall cardiovascular risk.

–Initial therapy should be monotherapy with a thiazide diuretic, a beta-blocker, an ACEI in non-black patients, a long-acting CCB or an ARB in patients <60 y.

–First-line combinations: thiazide diuretic or CCB with an ACEI, ARB, or beta-blocker. Do not combine ACEI and ARB. Caution in combination of nondihydropyridine and a beta-blocker.

–In patients with diabetes, the combination is preferred: ACEI with dihydropyridine rather than ACEI with HCTZ.

–Single-pill combination therapies improve achieving optimal BP control.

–ISH: initial monotherapy with a thiazide diuretic, a long-acting dihydropyridine CCB, or an ARB. Combination of 2 or more first-line agents or other classes like alpha-blockers, ACEI, centrally acting agents, or nondihydropyridine CCBs.

–Beta-blockers are not recommended as first-line therapy for uncomplicated hypertension/uncomplicated ISH in patients ≥60 y. ACEIs are not recommended as first-line therapy for uncomplicated hypertension in black patients. Alpha-blockers are not recommended as first-line agents for uncomplicated hypertension/uncomplicated ISH.

–The patient with hypertension attributable to atherosclerotic renal artery stenosis should be primarily medically managed, because renal angioplasty and stenting offer no benefits over optimal medical therapy alone. Renal artery angioplasty and stenting for atherosclerotic hemodynamically significant renal artery stenosis could be considered for patients with uncontrolled HTN resistant to maximally tolerated pharmacotherapy, progressive renal function loss, and acute PE.

–Global cardiovascular risk should be assessed in all hypertensive patients. Informing patients of their global risk improves the effectiveness of risk factor modification.

–Statin therapy is recommended in high-risk hypertensive patients based on having established atherosclerotic disease or at least 3 of the following: male, $\geq$55 y, smoking, type 2 diabetes, total-C/HDL-C ratio $\geq$6, premature family history of CV disease, previous stroke or TIA, LVH, ECG abnormalities, microalbuminuria or proteinuria, and peripheral vascular disease.

–Low-dose ASA should be started in hypertensive patients $\geq$50 y for vascular protection. Caution should be exercised if BP is not controlled.

–Advice in combination with pharmacotherapy (eg, varenicline, bupropion, nicotine replacement therapy) should be offered to all smokers with a goal of smoking cessation. ABPM, ambulatory BP measurement; HBPM, home BP measurement.

Sources

–Whelton et al. *JACC.* 2018:71(19);e127-e248.

–James PA, Oparil S, Carter BL. 2014 Evidence-based guideline for the management of high blood pressure in adults. Report from the panel members appointed to the Eighth Joint National Committee (JNC8). *JAMA.* 2014;311(5):507-520. doi:10.1001/jama.2013.284427.

–*Eur Heart J.* 2018;39:3021–3104. doi:10.1093/eurheartj/ehy339.

–Clinical practice guidelines for the management of hypertension in the community: a statement by the American Society of Hypertension and the International Society of Hypertension. *J Clin Hypertens.* 2014. doi: 10.1111/jch.12237.

–https://www.hypertension.ca/en/chep. The 2015 Canadian Hypertension Education Program recommendations. *Can J Cardiol.* 2015;31(5):549-568. https://www.onlinecjc.ca/article/S0828-282X(15)00130-0/fulltext

Population
–Adults with CAD.

Recommendations
▶ 2017 ACC/AHA/ASH

–Patients with HTN and chronic stable angina:
- Goal therapy: <140/90 mm Hg for secondary prevention of CV events on patients with HTN and CAD.
- For adults with 10-y ASCVD event risk of 10% or higher or with patients with CAD, previous MI, stroke or TIA, or CAD equivalents (CAD, PAD, AAA), BP goal is <130/80 mm Hg. Medication choices should include:
  ◦ Beta-blocker in patients with a history of prior MI.
  ◦ ACEI/ARB if prior MI, LV systolic dysfunction, DM, or CKD.
  ◦ A thiazide or thiazide-like diuretic.
- If beta-blocker is contraindicated or produce intolerable side effects, a nondihydropyridine CCB may be substituted but if there is no LV dysfunction.
- If either angina or HTN remains uncontrolled, a long-acting dihydropyridine CCB can be added to the basic regimen of beta-blocker, ACEI/ARB, and thiazide/thiazide-like diuretic. Combination of beta-blocker and either of the nondihydropyridine CCB should be used with caution in patients with symptomatic CAD and HTN because of the increased risk of significant bradyarrhythmias and HF.
- There are no special contraindications in HTN patients for the use of antiplatelet or anticoagulant drugs, except that in patients with uncontrolled severe HTN who are taking antiplatelet or anticoagulant drugs, the BP should be lowered without delay to reduce the risk of hemorrhagic stroke.

–Patients with HTN and ACS:
- BP target <140/90 mm Hg in patients with HTN and ACS that are hemodynamically stable. BP target <130/80 mm Hg at the time of hospital discharge is reasonable. BP should be lowered slowly and caution is advised to avoid decreases in DBP to <60 mm Hg because this may reduce coronary artery perfusion and worsen ischemia.
- If no contraindication to beta-blockers, the initial therapy of HTN should include a short-acting beta-1-selective beta-blocker without intrinsic sympathomimetic activity (metoprolol tartrate or bisoprolol). Beta-blocker therapy should typically be initiated orally within 24 h of presentation. For patients with severe HTN or ongoing ischemia, an intravenous beta-blocker (esmolol) can be

considered. For hemodynamically unstable patients or when decompensated HF exists, the initiation of beta-blocker therapy should be delayed until stabilization has been achieved.

- Nitrates should be considered to lower BP or relieve ongoing ischemia or pulmonary congestion. Nitrates should be avoided in patients with suspected RV infarction and in those with hemodynamic instability. Sublingual or IV nitroglycerin therapy is preferred for initial treatment and can be transitioned later to a longer-acting form if needed.

- If contraindication/intolerance/side effects to beta-blocker and no presence of LV dysfunction or HF, okay to substitute with nondihydropyridine CCB (verapamil, diltiazem). If the angina or HTN is not controlled on beta-blocker alone, a longer-acting dihydropyridine CCB may be added after optimal use of ACEI. ACEI/ARB should be added if anterior MI, persistent HTN, LV dysfunction, HF, or DM. For lower-risk ACS patients with preserved LV function and no DM, ACEI can be considered a first-line agent for BP control.

- Aldosterone antagonists are indicated for patients who are already receiving a beta-blocker and ACEI after MI and have LV dysfunction and either HF or DM. Serum K levels must be monitored. These agents should be avoided in patients with elevated serum creatinine levels ($\geq$2.5 mg/dL in men, $\geq$2.0 mg/dL in women) or elevated K levels ($\geq$5.0 mEq/L).

- Loop diuretics are preferred over thiazide/thiazide-type diuretics for patients with ACS who have HF (NYHA III or IV) or for patients with CKD and estimated glomerular filtration rate <39 mL/min. If HTN remains uncontrolled despite a beta-blocker, an ACEI, and an aldosterone antagonist, a thiazide/thiazide-type diuretic may be added in selected patients for BP control.

- In adults with hypertension (SBP >130 mm Hg or DBP >80 mm Hg) and a high risk of CVD, a strong body of evidence supports treatment with more intensive intervention. SPRINT Trial: targeted an SBP <120 mm Hg, this reduced CVD by 25%, HF was also decreased.

–Patients with HTN and HF of ischemic origin:

- BP target is <130/80 mm Hg, but consideration can be given to lowering the BP even further, to <130/80 mm Hg. In patients with an elevated DBP who have CAD and HF with evidence of myocardial ischemia, the BP should be lowered slowly. In older hypertensive individuals with wide pulse pressures, lowering SBP may cause very low DBP values (<60 mm Hg). This should alert the clinician to assess carefully any untoward signs or symptoms, especially those caused by myocardial ischemia and worsening HF. Octogenarians should be checked for orthostatic changes with standing, and an SBP <130 mm Hg and a DBP <65 mm Hg should be avoided.

- Treatment should include management of risk factors (dyslipidemia, obesity, DM, smoking, dietary sodium, and closely monitored exercise program).

- The patient should be treated with ACEI/ARB, beta-blocker (carvedilol, metoprolol succinate, bisoprolol, or nebivolol), and aldosterone receptor antagonists. These drugs have shown to improve outcomes for patients with HF and reduced EF.

- Thiazide/thiazide-type diuretic should be used for BP control and to reverse volume overload and associated symptoms. In patients with severe HF (NYHA III or IV), or those with severe renal impairment (eGFR <30 mL/min), loop diuretics should be used for volume control, but they are less effective than thiazide/thiazide-type diuretics in lowering BP. Diuretics should be used together with an ACE/ARB and a beta-blocker.

- Do not use nondihydropyridine CCBs in the treatment of HTN in adults with HFrEF.

- Studies have shown equivalence of benefit of ACEI and ARB (candesartan or valsartan) in HF with reduced EF. Either class of agents is effective in lowering BP.

- The aldosterone receptor antagonists spironolactone and eplerenone have been shown to be beneficial in HF and should be included in the regimen if there is HF (NYHA III or IV) with reduced EF <40%. One or the other may be substituted for a thiazide diuretic in patients requiring a K-sparing agent. If an aldosterone receptor antagonist is administered with an ACEI/ARB in the presence of renal insufficiency, serum K level should be monitored frequently. Should not be used if creatinine level ≥2.5 mg/dL in men or ≥2.0 mg/dL in women, or if serum K level ≥5 mEq/L. Spironolactone or eplerenone may be used with a thiazide/thiazide-type diuretic in resistant HTN.

- Hydralazine plus isosorbide dinitrate should be added to the regimen of diuretic, ACE inhibitor, or ARB, and beta-blocker in African-American patients with NYHA class III or IV HF with reduced ejection fraction. Others may benefit similarly, but this has not yet been tested.

- In patients who have hypertension and HF with preserved ejection fraction, the recommendations are to control systolic and diastolic hypertension, ventricular rate in the presence of atrial fibrillation, and pulmonary congestion and peripheral edema.

- Use of beta-adrenergic blocking agents, ACEI/ARBs, or CCB in patients with HF with preserved ejection fraction and hypertension may be effective to minimize symptoms of HF.
- In IHD, the principles of therapy for acute hypertension with pulmonary edema are similar to those for STEMI and NSTEMI, as described above. If the patient is hemodynamically unstable, the initiation of these therapies should be delayed until stabilization of HF has been achieved.
- Drugs to avoid in patients with hypertension and HF with reduced ejection fraction are nondihydropyridine CCBs (such as verapamil and diltiazem), clonidine, moxonidine, and hydralazine without a nitrate. Alpha-adrenergic blockers such as doxazosin should be used only if other drugs for the management of hypertension and HF are inadequate to achieve BP control at maximum tolerated doses. Nonsteroidal anti-inflammatory drugs should also be used with caution in this group, given their effects on BP, volume status, and renal function.

Sources

–Rosendorff C, Lackland DT, Allison M, et al. Treatment of hypertension in patients with coronary artery disease: a scientific statement from the American Heart Association, American College of Cardiology, and American Society of Hypertension. *JACC*. 2015;65(18):1998-2038.

–*Circulation*. 2017. doi: 10.1161/CIR.0000000000000509.

Population

–Adults with diabetes.

Recommendations

▶ 2017 ADA

–Goal therapy
- BP <140/80 mm Hg in patients with diabetes and HTN.
- BP <130/80 mm Hg in young patients and those at "high risk of cardiovascular disease."
- BP 110–129/65–79 in pregnant patients with diabetes and chronic HTN (lower than this may be associated with impaired fetal growth).

–Antihypertensive therapy
- Start lifestyle changes.
- Initiate with ACEI or ARB.
- Administer one or more antihypertensive medications at bedtime. Closely monitor eGFR, serum K levels if any ACEI/ARB/ diuretic is used.
- Safe in pregnancy: methyldopa, labetalol, diltiazem, clonidine, and prazosin.

Source
  –Standards of medical care in diabetes. *Diabetes Care*. 2017;40(suppl 1):S1–S142. (www.care.diabetesjournals.org).

Population
  –Adults.

Recommendation

IMPACT OF HEALTH BEHAVIOR MANAGEMENT ON BLOOD PRESSURE

Intervention	Systolic BP (mm Hg)	Diastolic BP (mm Hg)
Diet and weight control	−6.0	−4.8
Reduced salt/sodium intake <2000 mg sodium (Na)[a]	−5.4	−2.8
Reduced alcohol intake (<2 drinks/d)	−3.4	−3.4
DASH diet	−11.4	−5.5
Physical activity (30–40 min 5–7× wk)	−3.1	−1.8
Relaxation therapies	−5.5	−3.5

[a]2000 mg sodium (Na) = 87 mmol sodium (Na) = 5 g of salt (NaCl) ~1 teaspoon of table salt.

Source: Adapted from Canadian Hypertension Education Program (CHEP) Recommendations. 2015. (www.hypertension.ca/en/chep).

LIFESTYLE MODIFICATIONS FOR TREATMENT OF HYPERTENSION

Modification	Recommendation[a]	Approximate SBP Reduction (Range)
Weight reduction	Maintain normal body weight (BMI 18.5–24.9 kg/m^2)	5–20 mm Hg per 10-kg weight loss
Adopt DASH eating plan	Consume diet rich in fruits, vegetables, and low-fat dairy products with a reduced content of saturated and total fat	8–14 mm Hg
Dietary sodium reduction	Reduce dietary sodium intake to less than 100 mmol/d (2.4 g sodium or 6 g sodium chloride)	2–8 mm Hg

LIFESTYLE MODIFICATIONS FOR TREATMENT OF HYPERTENSION (Continued)

Physical activity	Engage in regular aerobic physical activity such as brisk walking (at least 30 min/d, most days of the week)	4–9 mm Hg
Moderation of alcohol consumption	Limit consumption to no more than 2 drinks (1 oz or 30 mL ethanol; eg, 24 oz beer, 10 oz wine, or 3 oz 80-proof whiskey) per day in most men and to no more than 1 drink per day in women and lighter-weight persons	2–4 mm Hg

DASH, dietary approaches to stop hypertension.

[a]The effects of implementing these modifications are dose- and time-dependent and could be greater for some individuals. DASH diet found to be effective in lowering SBP in adolescents.

Sources: Couch SC, Saelens BE, Levin L, Dart K, Falciglia G, Daniels SR. The efficacy of a clinic-based behavioral nutrition intervention emphasizing a DASH-type diet for adolescents with elevated blood pressure. *J Pediatr.* 2008;152:494-501.

Aronow WS, Fleg JL, Pepine CJ, et al. ACCF/AHA 2011 expert consensus document on hypertension in the elderly: a report of the American College of Cardiology Foundation Task Force on Clinical Expert Consensus documents developed in collaboration with the American Academy of Neurology, American Geriatrics Society, American Society for Preventive Cardiology, American Society of Hypertension, American Society of Nephrology, Association of Black Cardiologists, and European Society of Hypertension. *J Am Coll Cardiol.* 2011:57:2037-2110.

RECOMMENDED MEDICATIONS FOR COMPELLING INDICATIONS

Compelling Indication	Diuretic	BB	ACEI	ARB	CCB	AldoANT
Heart failure	X	X	X	X		X
Post-MI		X	X			X
High coronary disease risk	X	X	X		X	
Diabetes	X	X	X	X	X	
Chronic kidney disease[a]			X	X		
Recurrent stroke prevention	X		X			

ACEI, ACE inhibitor; AldoANT, aldosterone antagonist; ARB, angiotensin receptor blocker; BB, beta-blocker; CCB, calcium channel blocker.

[a]ALLHAT: Patients with hypertension and reduced GFR: no difference in renal outcomes (development of end-stage renal disease [ESRD] and/or decrement in GFR of ≥50% from baseline) comparing amlodipine, lisinopril, and chlorthalidone. (*Arch Intern Med.* 2005;165:936-946) Data do not support preference for CCB, alpha-blockers, or ACEI compared with thiazide diuretics in patients with metabolic syndrome. (*Arch Intern Med.* 2008;168:207-217; *J Am Coll Cardiol.* 2011;57:2037-2110; 2012 CHEP Recommendations, http://www. hypertension.ca).

Population
–Adults with comorbidities.

Recommendations
▶ 2014 CHEP

–HTN and documented CAD:
- ACEI is recommended for patients with HTN and documented CAD.
- For patients with stable angina, beta-blockers are preferred as initial therapy.
- Combination of ACEI with ARB is not recommended in HTN patients with CAD but absence of LV systolic dysfunction.
- In high-risk patients, combination of ACEI and a dihydropyridine CCB is preferable to an ACEI and a thiazide/thiazide-like diuretic in selected patients.
- Myocardial ischemia may be exacerbated when DBP ≤60 mm Hg—caution in lowering DBP too much (grade D).

–HTN and recent STEMI/NSTEMI:
- Initial therapy should include beta-blocker and an ACEI or ARB. CCB may be used if beta-blockers are contraindicated. Should not use nondihydropyridine CCBs with heart failure.

–HTN with heart failure:
- When LVEF <40%, ACEI/ARBs and beta-blockers are recommended as initial therapy.
- Aldosterone antagonists may be added for patients with a recent CV hospitalization, acute MI, elevated BNP/NT-proBNP levels, or symptomatic cardiomyopathy NYHA class II–IV. Diuretics can be used if needed: thiazide/thiazide-like diuretic for BP control, loop diuretics for volume control.
- If ACEI/ARB contraindicated or not tolerated, a combination of hydralazine and isosorbide dinitrate is recommended.
- For HTN patients whose BP is not controlled, ARB may be added to an ACEI and other antihypertensive drug treatment (grade A). (Watch for hypotension, hyperkalemia, and worsening renal function.)

–HTN with stroke/TIA Acute stroke (72 h) after acute stroke:
- For patients eligible for thrombolytic therapy very high BP >185/110 mm Hg should be treated concurrently in patient receiving thrombolytic therapy for acute ischemic stroke to reduce the risk of intracranial hemorrhage.
- For patients not eligible for thrombolytic therapy, extreme SBP elevation >220 or DBP>120 mm Hg may be treated to reduce BP by 15% and not more than 25% over the first 24 h.

- Strong consideration should be given to the initiation of antihypertensive therapy after the acute phase of a stroke or TIA.

–HTN with LVH:
- Initial therapy with ACEI/ARB, long-acting CCB, or thiazide/thiazide-like diuretics. Hydralazine and minoxidil should not be used.

–HTN with nondiabetic CKD:
- Goal BP <140/90 mm Hg.
- If proteinuric CKD, initiate with ACEI or ARB.
- ACEI in combination with ARB is not recommended for patients with nonproteinuric CKD.

–HTN with diabetes:
- Goal BP 130/80 mm Hg.
- Initiate with ACEI, dihydropyridine CCBS, thiazide/thiazide-like diuretic, or ARB.
- If additional CVD, CKD, microalbuminuria, or CV risk factors, initiate with an ACEI or ARB.
- Combination preferred: ACEI with dihydropyridine rather than ACEI with HCTZ.

Source
–http://www.hypertension.ca/en/chep.

REFRACTORY HYPERTENSION

Definition: Failure to reach BP goal (<140/90 mm Hg, or 130/80 mm Hg in patients with diabetes, heart disease, or chronic kidney disease) using three different antihypertensive drug classes.

Incidence: 20%–30% of HTN patients.

Common causes:

1. Nonadherence to drugs/diet.
2. Suboptimal therapy/BP measurement (fluid retention, inadequate dosage).
3. Diet/drug interactions (caffeine, cocaine, alcohol, nicotine, NSAIDs, steroids, BCP, erythropoietin, natural licorice, herbs).
4. Common secondary causes:
   a. Obstructive sleep apnea.
   b. Diabetes.
   c. Chronic kidney disease.
   d. Renal artery stenosis.
   e. Obesity.
   f. Endocrine disorders (primary hyperaldosteronism, hyperthyroidism, hyperparathyroidism, Cushing syndrome), pheochromocytoma.

Therapy:
- Exclude nonadherence and incorrect BP measurement.
- Review drug and diet history.
- Screen for secondary causes: History of sleep disorders/daytime sleepiness/tachycardias/BPs in both arms; routine labs: sodium, potassium, creatinine, CBC, ECG, urinalysis, blood glucose, cholesterol; additional evaluation: aldosterone: renin ratio, renal ultrasound with Doppler flow study, serum or urine catecholamine levels, morning cortisol level.
- Lifestyle therapy: Weight loss (10-kg weight loss results in a 5–20 mm Hg decrease in SBP); diet consult for low sodium (2.3 g daily), high fiber, and high potassium (DASH diet results in an 8–14 mm Hg decrease in SBP); exercise aerobic training results in a 4–9 mm Hg decrease in SBP; and restriction of excess alcohol (1 oz in men and 0.5 oz in women) results in a 2–4 mm Hg decrease in SBP.
- Pharmacologic therapy: Consider volume overload.
- Switch from HCTZ to chlorthalidone (especially if GFR <40 mL/min).
- Switch to loop diuretic if GFR <30 mL/min (eg, furosemide 40 mg bid).
- Use CCB (amlodipine or nifedipine) + ACE inhibitor or ARB: Consider catecholamine excess.
- Switch to vasodilating beta-blocker (carvedilol, labetalol, nebivolol): Consider aldosterone excess (even with normal serum K+ level).
- Spironolactone or eplerenone.
- Finally, consider hydralazine or minoxidil.
- If already on beta-blocker, clonidine adds little BP benefit.
- Nonpharmacologic therapy: Still under investigation.
- Carotid baroreceptor stimulation (*Hypertension*. 2010;55:1-8): May lower BP 33/22 mm Hg.
- Renal artery nerve denervation (SYMPLICITY HTN-3) did not show a significant reduction of SBP in patients with resistant hypertension, 6 mo after the procedure.

ACE, angiotensin-converting enzyme; ARB, angiotensin receptor blocker; BCP, birth control pill; bid, twice a day; BP, blood pressure; CBC, complete blood count; CCB, calcium channel blocker; DASH diet, Dietary Approaches to Stop Hypertension diet; ECG, electrocardiogram; GFR, glomerular filtration rate; HCTZ, hydrochlorothiazide; HTN, hypertension; NSAIDs, nonsteroidal anti-inflammatory drugs; SBP, systolic blood pressure.

Sources:
- Bhatt DL, Kandzari DE, O'Neill WW, et al. A controlled trial of renal denervation for resistant hypertension. *N Engl J Med*. 2014;370:1393-1401.
- Calhoun DA, Jones D, Textor S, et al; American Heart Association Professional Education Committee. Resistant hypertension: diagnosis, evaluation, and treatment: a scientific statement from the American Heart Association Professional Education Committee of the Council for High Blood Pressure Research. *Circulation*. 2008;117:e510-e526.

– JNC VII. *Arch Intern Med.* 2003;289:2560-2572.
– European 2007 Guidelines. 2007;28:1462-1536. American College of Cardiology/American Heart Association/European Society of Cardiology.

Population
–Children and adolescents with hypertension.

Recommendations

| | BP, mm Hg | | | |
| | Boys | | Girls | |
Age, y	Systolic	DBP	Systolic	DBP
1	98	52	98	54
2	100	55	101	58
3	101	58	102	60
4	102	60	103	62
5	103	63	104	64
6	105	66	105	67
7	106	68	106	68
8	107	69	107	69
9	107	70	108	71
10	108	72	109	72
11	110	74	111	74
12	113	75	114	75
≥13	120	80	120	80

TABLE II: SCREENING BP VALUES REQUIRING FURTHER EVALUATION

–The current definition of HTN in children and adolescents is based on the normative distribution per above; "normal BP" was initially defined as SBP and DBP values <90th percentile (on the basis of age, sex, and height percentiles).
–For adolescents, "prehypertension" was defined as BP >120/80 mm Hg to <95th percentile or >90th and <95th percentile.
–Indications for antihypertensive therapy in children and adolescents:
  • Symptomatic hypertension.
  • Secondary hypertension.
  • Hypertensive target organ damage.
  • Diabetes (types 1 and 2).

- Persistent hypertension despite nonpharmacologic measures (weight management counseling if overweight; physical activity; diet management).

Sources
  –*Pediatrics.* 2011;128(5):S213-S258.
  –Kavey RE, Allada V, Daniels SR, et al; American Heart Association Expert Panel on Population and Prevention Science; American Heart Association Council on Cardiovascular Disease in the Young; American Heart Association Council on Epidemiology and Prevention, et al. Cardiovascular risk reduction in high-risk pediatric patients: a scientific statement from the American Heart Association Expert Panel on Population and Prevention Science; the Councils on Cardiovascular Disease in the Young, Epidemiology and Prevention, Nutrition, Physical Activity and Metabolism, High Blood Pressure Research, Cardiovascular Nursing, and the Kidney in Heart Disease; and the Interdisciplinary Working Group on Quality of Care and Outcomes Research: endorsed by the American Academy of Pediatrics. *Circulation.* 2006;114:2710-2738.

Population
  –Special populations with hypertension.

Recommendations
  ▶ 2018 ESC/ESH
  –White-coat HTN is defined as elevated BP in doctor's office with normal home BPs. It is more common with increasing age, in women, and in nonsmokers.
   - White-coat hypertension at low risk (unassociated with additional risk factors) should receive lifestyle intervention and close follow-up.
   - White-coat hypertension at higher risk (associated with additional risk factors, metabolic disorders, or organ damage) should receive lifestyle intervention and drug therapy.
  –Masked HTN is defined as normal BP in the doctor's office with elevated BPs at home.
   - Masked hypertension at low risk (with or without additional risk factors) should receive lifestyle intervention and drug therapy due to the higher CV risk.
  –Elderly HTN occurs in patients ≥65-y-old.
   - In all elderly hypertensive patients SBP >160 mm Hg should be reduced to SBP between 140 and 150 mm Hg based upon good evidence.
   - In fit elderly hypertensive patients <80-y-old, SBP >160 mm Hg may be reduced to <140 mm Hg if therapy is well tolerated.

- Diuretics and calcium antagonist may be preferred in isolated systolic hypertension, although all medications have been used with success.
- Very elderly HTN occurs in patients ≥80-y-old.
  - In fit very elderly patients >80-y-old, SBP should be reduced to 140–150 mm Hg.
  - In frail very elderly patients >80-y-old, SBP goal needs to be individualized.
- Hypertensive therapy during pregnancy.
  - Drug therapy should be started with persistent BP ≥150/95 mm Hg and BP ≥140/90 mm Hg if associated with gestational hypertension, subclinical organ damage, or if associated with symptoms.
  - Women with hypertension with childbearing potential should not receive renin-angiotensin system (RAS) blockers.
  - Methyldopa and nifedipine should be initial therapy for hypertension. Labetalol and nitroprusside are the intravenous drugs of choice.
- Hypertension goal with CAD, diabetes, and nephropathy.
  - SBP goal <140 mm Hg should be considered.

Source
- Williams et al. *Eur Heart J.* 2018;39:3021-3104.

Population
- Hypertension in pregnancy.

Recommendations
▶ 2014 AHA/ASA
- Risk factors of pregnancy-induced hypertension: obesity, age >40-y-old, chronic HTN, personal or family history of preeclampsia, gestational HTN, nulliparity, multiple pregnancy, preexisting vascular disease, collagen vascular disease, diabetes, renal disease.
- Severe hypertension per JNC VII: BP ≥160/110 mm Hg (high risk of stroke and eclampsia).
- BP goal during pregnancy: 130–155/80–105 mm Hg.
- Prevention of eclampsia:
  - Women with chronic primary or secondary hypertension, or previous pregnancy-related hypertension, should take low-dose aspirin from the 12th week of gestation until delivery.
  - Calcium supplementation (of at least 1 g/d, orally) should be considered for women with low dietary intake of calcium (<600 mg/d) to prevent preeclampsia.

–Treatment of hypertension in pregnancy and postpartum recommendations:
- Severe hypertension in pregnancy should be treated with safe and effective antihypertensive medications such as methyldopa, labetalol, and nifedipine, with consideration of maternal and fetal side effects.
- Atenolol, ARBs, and direct renin inhibitors are contraindicated in pregnancy and should not be used.
- Because of the increased risk of future hypertension and stroke 1 to 30 y after delivery in women with a history of preeclampsia it is reasonable to:
  - Consider evaluating all women starting 6 mo to the 1 y postpartum, as well as those who are past childbearing age, for a history of preeclampsia/eclampsia, and document their history of preeclampsia/eclampsia as a risk factor.
  - Evaluate and treat for cardiovascular risk factors including hypertension, obesity, smoking, and dyslipidemia.
- After giving birth, women with chronic hypertension should be continued on their antihypertensive regimen, with dosage adjustments to reflect the decrease in volume of distribution and glomerular filtration rate that occurs following delivery. They should also be monitored carefully for the development of postpartum preeclampsia.

Source
–Bushnell C, McCullough LD, Awad IA, et al. Guidelines for the prevention of stroke in women: a statement for healthcare professionals from the American Heart Association/American Stroke Association. *Stroke*. 2014;45. doi: 10.1161/01.str.0000442009.06663.48.

PERIPHERAL ARTERIAL DISEASE

Population
–Adults with lower extremity peripheral arterial disease (PAD).

Recommendations
▶ ACC/AHA 2016, NICE 2012
- In patients with history or physical examination findings suggestive of PAD, use the resting ankle-brachial index (ABI) to establish the diagnosis.
- Report resting ABI results as abnormal (ABI ≤ 0.90), borderline (ABI 0.91–0.99), normal (1.00–1.40), or noncompressible (ABI > 1.40).
- Measure toe-brachial index (TBI) to diagnose patients with suspected PAD when the ABI > 1.40 (noncompressible).

- Use duplex ultrasound, CTA, or MRA of the lower extremities to diagnose anatomic location and severity of stenosis for patients with symptomatic PAD if revascularization is being considered.
- Use antiplatelet therapy with aspirin alone (range 75–325 mg/d) or clopidogrel alone (75 mg/d), smoking cessation, a statin, and good glycemic control to reduce MI, stroke, and vascular death in patients with symptomatic PAD.
- Use cilostazol to improve symptoms and increase walking distance in patients with claudication.
- Give patients with PAD an annual influenza vaccination.
- Recommend a supervised exercise program for patients with claudication to improve functional status and quality of life and to reduce leg symptoms.
- Counsel patients with PAD and diabetes mellitus about self–foot examination and healthy foot behaviors.
- Endovascular procedures are effective as a revascularization option for patients with lifestyle-limiting claudication and hemodynamically significant aortoiliac occlusive disease.
- Endovascular procedures establish in-line blood flow to the foot in patients with nonhealing wounds or gangrene.
- When surgical revascularization is performed, choose a bypass to the popliteal artery with autogenous vein rather than prosthetic graft material.
- In patients with critical limb ischemia, perform revascularization when possible and construct bypass to the popliteal or infrapopliteal arteries (ie, tibial, pedal) with suitable autogenous vein.
- In patients with acute limb ischemia (ALI), give systemic anticoagulation with heparin immediately unless contraindicated.
- Monitor and treat patients with ALI (eg, fasciotomy) for compartment syndrome after revascularization.
- Perform amputation as the first procedure in patients with a nonsalvageable limb.

Sources

- 2016 AHA/ACC Guideline on the Management of Patients with Lower Extremity Peripheral Artery Disease: executive summary. *Circulation.* 2017;135:e686–e725.
- https://guidelines.gov/summaries/summary/38409

Comments

1. Recommend bare metal stents when stenting people with intermittent claudication.
2. Prefer autologous vein bypass when possible for infrainguinal bypass surgery.

3. Prefer bypass surgery over stenting for aortoiliac or femoropopliteal stenosis causing intermittent claudication or critical limb ischemia.
4. Stenting is an option for complete aortoiliac occlusion.

PREOPERATIVE CLEARANCE

Population
–Asymptomatic population without cardiac history.

Recommendation
▶ Choosing Wisely 2014, ACC 2014

–Do not obtain stress cardiac imaging or advanced noninvasive imaging as a preoperative assessment in patients scheduled to undergo low-risk noncardiac surgery.

Source
–http://www.choosingwisely.org/societies/american-college-of-cardiology/

VALVULAR HEART DISEASE

Population
–Adults with aortic stenosis.

Recommendation
▶ ACC/AHA 2014

–Obtain transthoracic echocardiogram (TTE) as initial evaluation with known or suspected aortic stenosis to establish the diagnosis and to determine the severity of the stenosis.
–Exercise treadmill testing is rarely indicated but helpful to evaluate patients who have discordant echo/clinical findings (ie, moderate or severe stenosis in the absence of expected symptoms). Previously undetected symptoms of chest pain, shortness of breath, exertional dizziness, or syncope may be identified to prevent sudden death.
–Treat hypertension in the presence of significant AS.
–Statin therapy does not prevent the progression of the AS.
–No medical therapy is available to address symptoms or disease progression.

–Aortic valve replacement (AVR) is indicated in symptomatic patients with a mean gradient >40 mm Hg; aortic valve replacement is indicated in asymptomatic patients with decreased systolic function (EF 50%) and mean gradient >40 mm Hg (valve gradient is underestimated with systolic dysfunction).

–Consider transcatheter aortic valve replacement (TAVR) in patients with a high surgical risk, marked frailty, associated comorbidities, and minimal associated coronary artery disease who have the same indication for AVR and have a 12-mo life expectancy.

–Percutaneous aortic balloon dilation procedure should be considered a "bridging therapy" to AVR or TAVR therapy.

Population

–Adults with aortic insufficiency.

Recommendation

▶ ACC/AHA 2014

–Use transthoracic echocardiogram as initial evaluation with known or suspected aortic insufficiency to establish the diagnosis and to determine the severity if there is insufficiency.

–Cardiac magnetic resonance (CMR) is an alternative form of evaluation if the TTE is nondiagnostic or suboptimal.

–Treat hypertension to keep SBP <140 mm Hg with nondihydropyridine calcium channel blocker, ACE inhibitor, or ARB agent.

–Aortic valve replacement: symptomatic person with severe AI regardless of the systolic function; asymptomatic patient with severe AI and systolic dysfunction <50% or with end systolic volume (ESD) >50 mm.

Population

–Adults with mitral regurgitation.

Recommendations

▶ ACC/AHA 2017

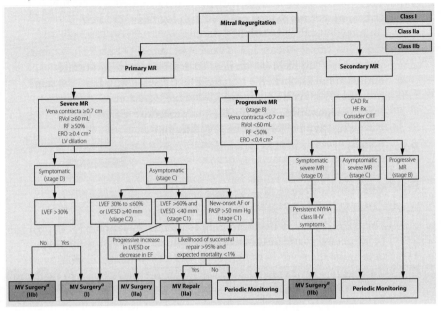

^aMV repair is preferred over MV replacement when possible.

AF, atrial fibrillation; CAD, coronary artery disease; CRT, cardiac resynchronization therapy; EF, ejection fraction; ERO, effective regurgitant orifice; HF, heart failure; LV, left ventricular; LVEF, left ventricular ejection fraction; LVESD, left ventricular end-systolic diameter; MR, mitral regurgitation; MV, mitral valve; NYHA, New York Heart Association; PASP, pulmonary artery systolic pressure; RF, regurgitant fraction; RVol, regurgitant volume; Rx, therapy.

▶ ACC/AHA 2014

– Obtain transthoracic echocardiogram as initial evaluation with known or suspected mitral regurgitation to establish the diagnosis and to determine the severity if there is insufficiency, left atrial and ventricular size, and right ventricular function.

– Cardiac magnetic resonance (CMR) is an alternative form of evaluation if the TTE is nondiagnostic or suboptimal.

– Mitral valve replacement or repair is indicated in a symptomatic patient with severe regurgitation if the systolic function (EF) is >30%.

– Mitral valve replacement is indicated in an asymptomatic patient with severe mitral regurgitation if the systolic function (EF) is between 30% and 60% or the left ventricular end systolic dimension (LVESD) >40%.

Population

–Adults with mitral regurgitation related to infective endocarditis.

Recommendations

▶ ACC/AHA 2017

–Valve surgery during initial hospitalization before completion of full course of antibiotics is indicated for infective endocarditis (IE) associated with:
  • Valve dysfunction resulting in symptoms of HF.
  • Left-sided IE caused by *S. aureus*, fungal, or other highly resistant organisms.
  • Complicated by heart block, annular or aortic abscess, or destructive penetrating lesions.

–Evidence of persistent infection as manifested by persistent bacteremia or fevers lasting longer than 5 to 7 d after onset of appropriate antimicrobial therapy.

–Surgery is recommended for patients with prosthetic valve endocarditis and relapsing infection (defined as recurrence of bacteremia after a complete course of appropriate antibiotics and subsequently negative blood cultures) without other identifiable source for portal of infection.

–Complete removal of pacemaker or defibrillator systems, including all leads and the generator, is indicated as part of the early management plan in patients with IE with documented infection of the device or leads.

Population

–Adults with mitral stenosis.

Recommendations

▶ ACC/AHA 2014

–Use transthoracic echocardiogram as initial evaluation with known or suspected mitral stenosis to establish the diagnosis and to determine the severity if there is stenosis.

–Consider transesophageal echocardiogram (TEE) prior to sending the patient for percutaneous mitral balloon commissurotomy (PMBC) to exclude the presence of left atrial thrombus.

–Give warfarin to patients with mitral stenosis and atrial fibrillation, prior embolic event, or intracardiac thrombus.

–Control heart rate control in atrial fibrillation to allow optimal diastolic filling time across the stenotic valve.

–Balloon commissurotomy is indicated in symptomatic patients with severe mitral stenosis (MVA <1.5 cm^2) with no atrial thrombus and no or minimal mitral insufficiency.

–Mitral valve replacement is indicated if balloon commissurotomy is contraindicated in a patient with severe symptoms and severe mitral stenosis.

Sources

–Nishimura RA, Otto CM, Bonow RO. 2014 AHA/ACC guidelines for the management of patients with valvular heart disease: a report of the American College of Cardiology/American Heart Association Task Force on Practice Guidelines. *J Am Coll Cardiol.* 2014;63(22):e57. doi:10.1016/jack.2014.02.536.

–2017 AHA/ACC focused update of the 2014 AHA/ACC guideline for the management of patients with valvular heart disease: a report of the American College of Cardiology/American Heart Association Task Force on Clinical Practice Guidelines. *Circulation.* 2017;135:e1159–e1195.

Care of the Older Adult

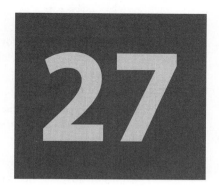

DEMENTIA, FEEDING TUBES

Population

–Patients with advanced dementia.

Recommendations

▶ American Geriatrics Society 2013

–Percutaneous feeding tubes are not recommended for older adults with advanced dementia.

–Careful hand-feeding should be offered.

Source

–http://americangeriatrics.org/health_care_professionals/clinical_ practice/clinical_guidelines_recommendations/

Comment

1. Careful hand-feedings and tube-feedings have identical outcomes of death, aspiration pneumonia, functional status, and patient comfort. In addition, tube-feeding is associated with agitation, increased use of physical and chemical restraints, and worsening pressure ulcers.

DEMENTIA, ALZHEIMER DISEASE

Population

–Adults.

Recommendations

▶ NICE 2018

–Donepezil, galantamine, and rivastigmine are options for mild-to-moderate Alzheimer disease.

–Memantine is an option for moderate Alzheimer disease in patients who cannot tolerate acetylcholinesterase inhibitors, or in severe Alzheimer disease.

Source

–*NICE Guidance: Dementia: Assessment, Management and Support for People Living with Dementia and Their Carers.* NICE guideline (NG97); June 2018.

Comments

1. Common adverse effects of acetylcholinesterase inhibitors include diarrhea, nausea, vomiting, muscle cramps, bradycardia, and insomnia.
2. Common adverse effects of memantine are dizziness, headache, constipation, somnolence, and hypertension.
3. Reassess the efficacy of the pharmacological intervention. If the desired clinical effect (eg, stabilization of cognition) is not perceived by 12 wk or so, discontinue the medication (AGS, 2015).
4. Ineffective medications include statins, NSAID, ginkgo, omega-3 fatty acids (AAFP 2017).

▶ American Geriatrics Society 2015

–Avoid antipsychotics as first-line agents to treat behavioral and psychological symptoms of dementia.

Source

–American Geriatrics Society. *Choosing Wisely Campaign.* 2015.

Comments

1. Antipsychotics have limited and inconsistent benefit while posing risks including increased fall, strokes, and mortality, oversedation, and cognitive worsening.
2. Use should be limited to cases where nonpharmacologic measures have failed, and the patients pose an imminent danger to themselves or others. First aim to identify and treat the underlying cause of the behavior change.
3. Use may be considered in patient with dementia who are experiencing agitation, hallucinations, or delusions that are severely distressing. (NICE, 2018)

DEMENTIA

Population
–Adults with non-Alzheimer dementia.

Recommendations
▶ NICE 2018
–Offer donepezil or rivastigmine in patients with mild-to-moderate dementia with Lewy bodies. Consider galantamine if donepezil/rivastigmine is not tolerated.
–Consider memantine for patient with Lewy bodies if AChE inhibitors are not tolerated or are contraindicated.
–Only consider AChE inhibitors or memantine for people with vascular dementia if they have suspected comorbid Alzheimer dementia, Parkinson's disease dementia, or dementia with Lewy bodies.
–AChE inhibitors and memantine are not recommended for patients with frontotemporal dementia or cognitive impairment caused by multiple sclerosis.

Source
–*NICE Guidance: Dementia: Assessment, Management and Support for People Living with Dementia and Their Careers.* NICE guideline (NG97); June 2018.

DELIRIUM, POSTOPERATIVE

Population
–Older adults at risk for or who have postoperative delirium.

Recommendations
▶ AGS 2015
–Institutions should enact multi-component intervention programs to manage delirium.
–Consider regional anesthesia at the time of surgery to improve postoperative pain control and reduce delirium risk.
–Avoid inappropriate medications postoperatively in older adults. Optimize postoperative pain control, preferably with nonopioid pain medication.
–Use antipsychotics at the lowest effective dose and for the shortest duration possible to treat severe agitated delirium.
–Do not newly prescribe prophylactic cholinesterase inhibitors in the perioperative setting to prevent or treat delirium.

–Avoid benzodiazepines for postoperative delirium.

–Avoid pharmacologic therapy for hypoactive delirium.

–Avoid use of physical restraints.

Source

–*J Am Geriatr Soc.* 2015;63(1):124-150.

Comment

1. Inappropriate medications include benzodiazepines, anticholinergics (eg, cyclobenzaprine, paroxetine, tricyclic antidepressants, diphenhydramine), H2-receptor blockers, sedative-hypnotics, and meperidine.

PALLIATIVE CARE OF DYING ADULTS

Population

–Dying adults.

Recommendations

▶ NICE 2017, NCCN 2019

–Care of the dying patient should be aligned with the patient's goals and wishes and cultural values.

–Symptom management should address physical, emotional, social, and spiritual needs.

–Determine who should be the surrogate decision maker if they cannot make their own decisions.

–Establish if the patient has a preferred care setting.

–Medical management of symptoms:

- Pain is typically managed with opioids.
- Breathlessness can be managed with opioids or benzodiazepines +/– oxygen. Nonpharmacologic therapies include fans, cooler temperatures, stress management, relaxation therapy, and physical comfort measures.
- Nausea can be managed with sublingual ondansetron or promethazine suppositories. Haloperidol, metoclopramide, and dexamethasone are options if nausea is refractory.
- Anxiety can be managed with benzodiazepines.
- Delirium or agitation can be managed with antipsychotics.
- Secretions can be managed with a scopolamine patch.

Sources

–*NICE.* 2015 (Guideline), 2017 (Quality Standard. Care of Dying Adults in the Last Days of Life).

–NCCN Guidelines Version 2. 2019 Palliative Care.

Comment

1. Recognize and treat opioid-induced neurotoxicity, including myoclonus and hyperalgesia.

PALLIATIVE AND END-OF-LIFE CARE: PAIN MANAGEMENT	
Principles of Analgesic Use	
By the mouth	The oral route is the preferred route for analgesics, including morphine.
By the clock	Persistent pain requires round-the-clock treatment to prevent further pain. As-needed (PRN) dosing is irrational and inhumane; it requires patients to experience pain before becoming eligible for relief. Relief is accomplished with long-acting delayed-release preparations (fentanyl patch, slow-release morphine, or oxycodone).
By the WHO ladder	If a maximum dose of medication fails to adequately relieve pain, move up the ladder, not laterally to a different drug in the same efficiency group. Severe pain requires immediate use of an opioid recommended for controlling severe pain, without progressing sequentially through Steps 1 and 2. When using a long-acting opioid, the dose for breakthrough pain should be 10% of the 24-h opioid dose (ie, if a patient is on 100 mg/d of an extended-release morphine preparation, their breakthrough dose is 10 mg of morphine or equivalent every 1–2 h until pain relief is achieved).
Individualize treatment	The right dose of an analgesic is the dose that relieves pain with acceptable side effects for a specific patient.
Monitor	Monitoring is required to ensure the benefits of treatment are maximized while adverse effects are minimized.
Use adjuvant drugs	For example, a nonsteroidal anti-inflammatory drug (NSAID) is often helpful in controlling bone pain. Nonopioid analgesics, such as NSAIDs or acetaminophen, can be used at any step of the ladder. Adjuvant medications also can be used at any step to enhance pain relief or counteract the adverse effects of medications. Neuropathic pain should be treated with gabapentin, duloxetine, nortriptyline, or pregabalin. Moderate- to high-dose dexamethasone is effective as an adjunct to opioids in a pain crisis situation.

Source: Adapted from *Pocket Guide to Hospice/Palliative Medicine.*

Disorders of the Head, Eye, Ear, Nose, and Throat

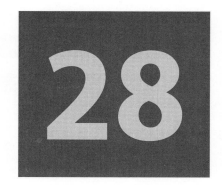

BRONCHITIS, ACUTE

Population
–Adults age ≥18 y.

Recommendations

▶ CDC 2017
  –Avoid chest x-ray if all the following are present:
  - Heart rate <100 beats/min.
  - Respiratory rate <24 breaths/min.
  - Temperature <100.4°F (38°C).
  - No exam findings consistent with pneumonia (consolidation, egophony, fremitus).
  –Avoid routine use of antibiotics regardless of duration of cough.

Source
  –https://www.cdc.gov/antibiotic-use/community/for-hcp/outpatient-hcp/adult-treatment-rec.html

Comments
1. Primary clinical goal is to exclude pneumonia.
2. Consider antitussive agents for short-term relief of coughing.
3. Avoid routine beta-2 agonists or mucolytic agents to alleviate cough.

CATARACT

CATARACT IN ADULTS: EVALUATION AND MANAGEMENT ALGORITHM

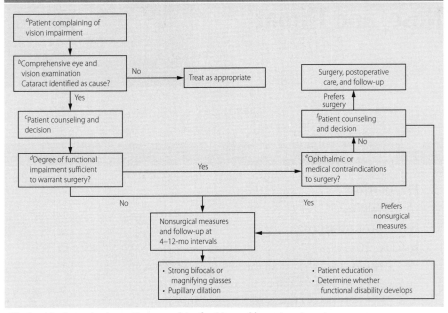

[a]Begin evaluation only when patients complain of a vision problem or impairment.

[b]Essential elements of the comprehensive eye and vision exam:

- Patient history: Consider cataract if acute or gradual onset of vision loss; vision problems under special conditions (eg, low contrast, glare); difficulties performing various visual tasks. Ask about refractive history, previous ocular disease, amblyopia, eye surgery, trauma, general health history, medications, and allergies. It is critical to describe the actual impact of the cataract on the person's function and quality of life. There are several instruments available for assessing functional impairment related to cataract, including VF-14, Activities of Daily Vision Scale, and Visual Activities Questionnaire.
- Ocular examination includes Snellen acuity and refraction; measurement of intraocular pressure; assessment of pupillary function; external exam; slit-lamp exam; and dilated exam of fundus.
- Supplemental testing: May be necessary to assess and document the extent of the functional disability and to determine whether other diseases may limit preoperative or postoperative vision. Most elderly patients presenting with visual problems do not have a cataract that causes functional impairment. Refractive error, macular degeneration, and glaucoma are common alternative etiologies for visual impairment.

[c]Once cataract has been identified as the cause of visual disability, patients should be counseled concerning the nature of the problem, its natural history, and the existence of both surgical and nonsurgical approaches to management. The principal factor that should guide decision making with regard to surgery is the extent to which the cataract impairs the ability to function in daily life. The findings of the physical examination should corroborate that the cataract is the major contributing cause of the functional impairment, and that there is a reasonable expectation that managing the cataract will positively impact the patient's functional activity. Preoperative visual acuity is a poor predictor of postoperative functional improvement: The decision to recommend cataract surgery should not be made solely on the basis of visual acuity.

^dPatients who complain of mild-to-moderate limitation in activities due to a visual problem, those whose corrected acuities are near 20/40, and those who do not yet wish to undergo surgery may be offered nonsurgical measures for improving visual function. Treatment with nutritional supplements is not recommended. Smoking cessation retards cataract progression. Indications for surgery: Cataract-impaired vision no longer meets the patient's needs; evidence of lens-induced disease (eg, phacomorphic glaucoma, phacolytic glaucoma); necessary to visualize the fundus in an eye that has the potential for sight (eg, diabetic patient at risk of diabetic retinopathy).

^eContraindications to surgery: The patient does not desire surgery; glasses or vision aids provide satisfactory functional vision; surgery will not improve visual function; the patient's quality of life is not compromised; the patient is unable to undergo surgery because of coexisting medical or ocular conditions; a legal consent cannot be obtained; or the patient is unable to obtain adequate postoperative care. Routine preoperative medical testing (12-lead EKG, CBC, measurement of serum electrolytes, BUN, creatinine, and glucose), while commonly performed in patients scheduled to undergo cataract surgery, does not appear to measurably increase the safety of the surgery.

^fPatients with significant functional and visual impairment due to cataract who have no contraindications to surgery should be counseled regarding the expected risks and benefits of and alternatives to surgery.

Sources: American Academy of Ophthalmology Preferred Practice Pattern: Cataract in the Adult Eye. 2006. (http://www.aao.org); American Optometric Association Consensus Panel on Care of the Adult Patient with Cataract. Optometric Clinical Practice Guideline: Care of the Adult Patient with Cataract. 2004. (http://www.aoa.org).

Population

–Adults with cataracts.

Recommendations

▶ AAO 2018

–Obtain initial history of symptoms, ocular history, systemic history, assessment of visual functional status, and medications currently used.

–Include the following elements in the initial physical exam: The visual acuity with current correction, external examination, ocular alignment and motility, pupil reactivity and function, measurement of intraocular pressure, slit-lamp exam, and dilated examination with ophthalmology.

–Remove cataracts when visual function no longer meets the patient's needs and cataract surgery provides a reasonable likelihood of quality-of-life improvement.

–Remove cataracts when there is evidence of lens-induced disease or when it is necessary to visualize the fundus in an eye that has the potential for sight.

–Avoid surgery under the following circumstances:
   • Tolerable refractive correction provides vision that meets the patient's needs and desires; surgery is not expected to improve visual function, and no other indication for lens removal exists.
   • The patient cannot safely undergo surgery because of coexisting medical or ocular conditions.
   • Appropriate postoperative care cannot be arranged.
   • Patient or patient's surrogate decision-maker is unable to give informed consent for nonemergent surgery.

Comment

1. Routine preoperative medical testing does not appear to measurably increase the safety of the surgery.

Sources

–*American Academy of Ophthalmology Preferred Practice Pattern: Cataract/Anterior Segment Summary Benchmark.* 2018. http://www.aao.org

–American Optometric Association Consensus Panel on Care of the Adult Patient with Cataract. *Optometric Clinical Practice Guideline: Care of the Adult Patient with Cataract.* 2004. http://www.aoa.org

CERUMEN IMPACTION

Population

–Children and adults.

Recommendations

▶ AAO-HNS 2017

–Strongly recommended treating cerumen impaction when it is symptomatic or prevents a needed clinical examination.
–Treat cerumen impaction with an appropriate intervention:
  • Ceruminolytic agents.
  • Irrigation.
  • Manual removal.

Source

–https://www.entnet.org//content/clinical-practice-guideline-cerumen-impaction

Comments

1. Ceruminolytic agents include water or saline, Cerumenex, addax, Debrox, or dilute solutions of acetic acid, hydrogen peroxide, or sodium bicarbonate.
2. Ear candling is not recommended for treatment or prevention of cerumen impaction.
3. Removal of cerumen is not necessary if the patient is asymptomatic and adequate clinical exam is possible.

HEADACHE

Population
–Adults

Recommendations
▶ ACR 2019

–Do not perform imaging for uncomplicated headaches.

–Neuroimaging for diagnosis:

- In patients with sudden, severe headache or worst headache of their life, obtain CT head without IV contrast for initial imaging.
- In patients with new headache and optic disc edema, consider MRI head without and with IV contrast, MRI head without IV contrast, or CT head without IV contrast for the initial imaging. These procedures are equivalent alternatives (ie, only one procedure will be ordered to provide the clinical information to effectively manage the patient's care).
- In patients with new or progressively worsening headache with one or more of the following "red flags" of subacute head trauma, related activity or event (sexual activity, exertion, position), neurological deficit, known or suspected cancer, immunosuppressed or immunocompromised state, age 50 y or older, consider CT head without IV contrast, MRI head without and with IV contrast, or MRI head without IV contrast for the initial imaging. Pregnancy is also considered a "red flag" condition, with separate considerations for radiation and contrast exposure. These procedures are equivalent alternatives.
- Avoid imaging for the initial imaging of patients with new primary migraine or tension-type headache, with normal neurologic examination.
- In patients with new primary headache of suspected trigeminal autonomic origin, obtain MRI head without and with IV contrast for the initial imaging.
- Avoid imaging in the initial assessment of patients with chronic headache, without new features or neurologic deficit.
- In patients with chronic headache presenting with new features or increasing frequency, consider MRI head without and with IV contrast or MRI head without IV contrast for the initial imaging. These procedures are equivalent alternatives.

-Patients with emergent red flag symptoms require immediate emergency room evaluation:
  • Onset of severe headache that is sudden (seconds to a minute to a peak onset of intensity).
  • Headache with fever and neck stiffness.
  • Papilledema with altered level of consciousness and/or focal neurological signs.
-Urgent red flag symptoms require prompt evaluation:
  • Signs of systemic illness in the patient with new-onset headache.
  • New headache in patients over 50 y of age with symptoms of temporal arteritis.
  • Papilledema in an alert patient without focal neurological signs.
  • Elderly patient with new headache and subacute cognitive change.
-Consider imaging or specialty consultation for patients with the following:
  • Atypical headaches and changes in headache pattern.
  • Unexplained focal signs in the patient with a headache.
  • Headache precipitated by exertion, postural change, cough, or valsalva.
  • New-onset cluster headache or another trigeminal autonomic cephalgia, hemicrania continua, or new daily persistent headache.

Sources
-https://acsearch.acr.org/docs
-http://www.choosingwisely.org/societies/american-college-of-radiology/

HEADACHE, MIGRAINE PROPHYLAXIS

Population
-Adults.

Recommendations
▶ AAN 2012
-The following medications have **established efficacy** for migraine prophylaxis:
  • Divalproex sodium.
  • Sodium valproate.
  • Topiramate.
  • Metoprolol.
  • Propranolol.
  • Timolol.

–Frovatriptan is effective for menstrual migraine prophylaxis.

–The following medications are **probably effective** for migraine prophylaxis:

- Amitriptyline.
- Venlafaxine.
- Atenolol.
- Nadolol.

Source

–http://www.neurology.org/content/78/17/1337.full.pdf+html

Comment

1. Lamotrigine and clomipramine are ineffective for migraine prevention.

HEADACHE DIAGNOSIS ALGORITHM—ICSI 2011

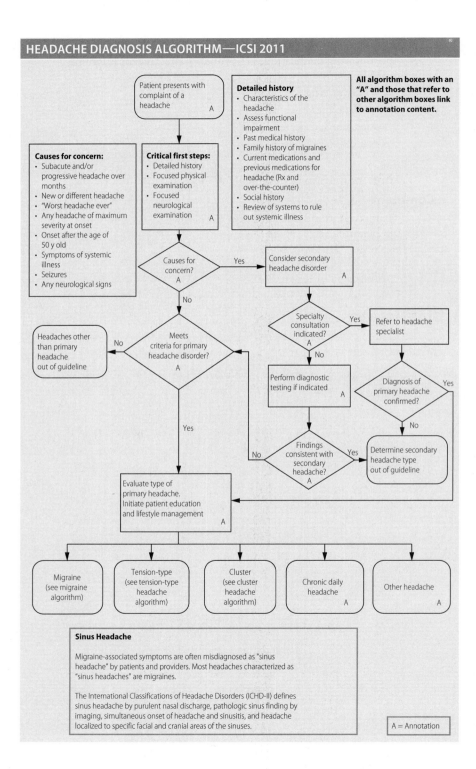

Patient presents with complaint of a headache A

Detailed history
- Characteristics of the headache
- Assess functional impairment
- Past medical history
- Family history of migraines
- Current medications and previous medications for headache (Rx and over-the-counter)
- Social history
- Review of systems to rule out systemic illness

All algorithm boxes with an "A" and those that refer to other algorithm boxes link to annotation content.

Causes for concern:
- Subacute and/or progressive headache over months
- New or different headache
- "Worst headache ever"
- Any headache of maximum severity at onset
- Onset after the age of 50 y old
- Symptoms of systemic illness
- Seizures
- Any neurological signs

Critical first steps:
- Detailed history
- Focused physical examination
- Focused neurological examination A

Causes for concern? A
— Yes → Consider secondary headache disorder A

No

Specialty consultation indicated? A
— Yes → Refer to headache specialist

No

Headaches other than primary headache out of guideline
— No — Meets criteria for primary headache disorder? A

Perform diagnostic testing if indicated A

Diagnosis of primary headache confirmed?
— Yes

No

Findings consistent with secondary headache? A
— No / Yes → Determine secondary headache type out of guideline

Yes

Evaluate type of primary headache. Initiate patient education and lifestyle management A

Migraine (see migraine algorithm)

Tension-type (see tension-type headache algorithm)

Cluster (see cluster headache algorithm)

Chronic daily headache A

Other headache A

Sinus Headache

Migraine-associated symptoms are often misdiagnosed as "sinus headache" by patients and providers. Most headaches characterized as "sinus headaches" are migraines.

The International Classifications of Headache Disorders (ICHD-II) defines sinus headache by purulent nasal discharge, pathologic sinus finding by imaging, simultaneous onset of headache and sinusitis, and headache localized to specific facial and cranial areas of the sinuses.

A = Annotation

MIGRAINE TREATMENT ALGORITHM—ICSI 2011

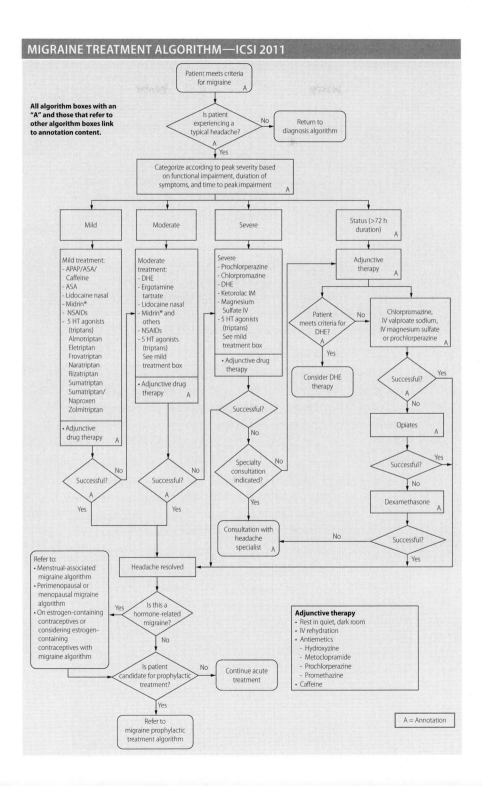

All algorithm boxes with an "A" and those that refer to other algorithm boxes link to annotation content.

TENSION-TYPE HEADACHE ALGORITHM—ICSI 2011

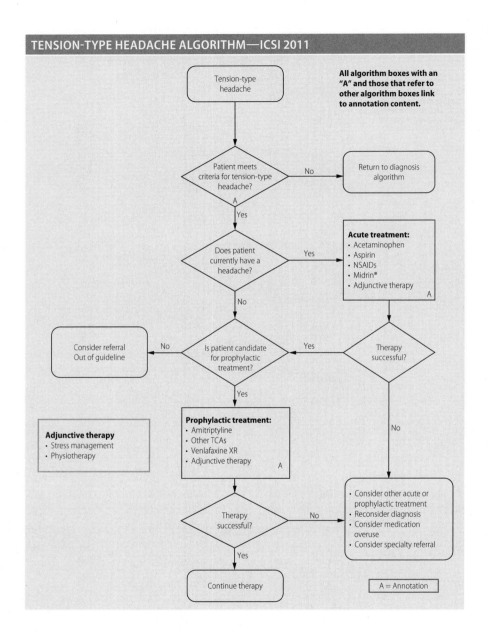

Tension-type headache

All algorithm boxes with an "A" and those that refer to other algorithm boxes link to annotation content.

Patient meets criteria for tension-type headache?
A

No → Return to diagnosis algorithm

Yes

Does patient currently have a headache?

Yes → **Acute treatment:**
- Acetaminophen
- Aspirin
- NSAIDs
- Midrin®
- Adjunctive therapy
A

No

Is patient candidate for prophylactic treatment?

No → Consider referral Out of guideline

Yes ← Therapy successful?

Yes

No

Adjunctive therapy
- Stress management
- Physiotherapy

Prophylactic treatment:
- Amitriptyline
- Other TCAs
- Venlafaxine XR
- Adjunctive therapy
A

Therapy successful?

No →
- Consider other acute or prophylactic treatment
- Reconsider diagnosis
- Consider medication overuse
- Consider specialty referral

Yes

Continue therapy

A = Annotation

CLUSTER HEADACHE ALGORITHM—ICSI 2011

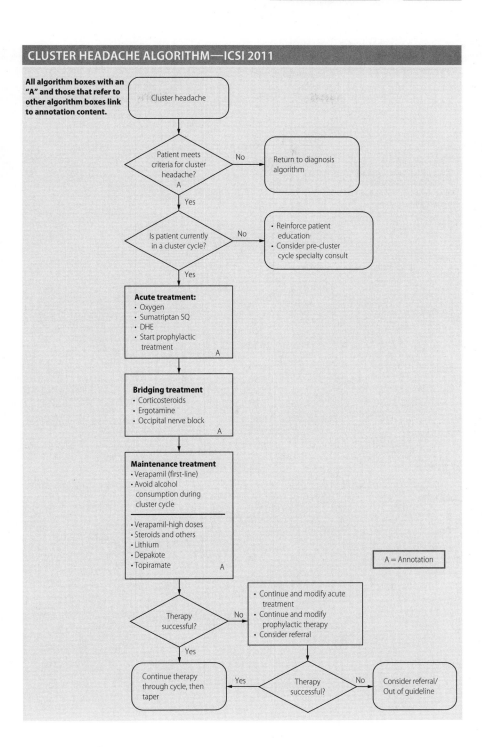

All algorithm boxes with an "A" and those that refer to other algorithm boxes link to annotation content.

Cluster headache

Patient meets criteria for cluster headache?
A

No → Return to diagnosis algorithm

Yes

Is patient currently in a cluster cycle?

No →
- Reinforce patient education
- Consider pre-cluster cycle specialty consult

Yes

Acute treatment:
- Oxygen
- Sumatriptan SQ
- DHE
- Start prophylactic treatment
A

Bridging treatment
- Corticosteroids
- Ergotamine
- Occipital nerve block
A

Maintenance treatment
- Verapamil (first-line)
- Avoid alcohol consumption during cluster cycle

- Verapamil-high doses
- Steroids and others
- Lithium
- Depakote
- Topiramate
A

A = Annotation

Therapy successful?

No →
- Continue and modify acute treatment
- Continue and modify prophylactic therapy
- Consider referral

Yes

Therapy successful?

Yes → Continue therapy through cycle, then taper

No → Consider referral/Out of guideline

MENSTRUAL-ASSOCIATED MIGRAINE ALGORITHM—ICSI 2011

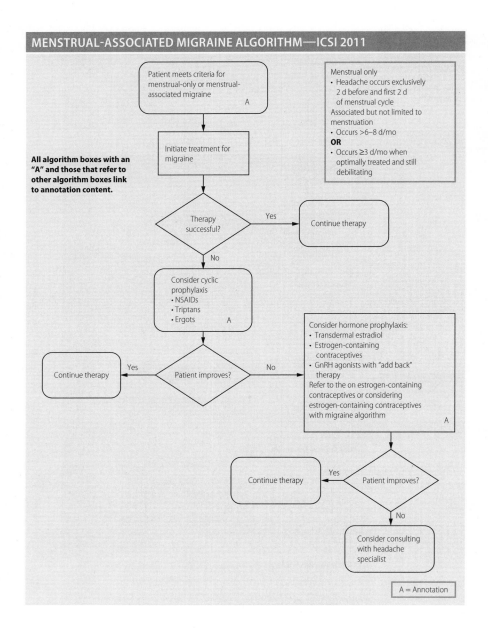

All algorithm boxes with an "A" and those that refer to other algorithm boxes link to annotation content.

Patient meets criteria for menstrual-only or menstrual-associated migraine   A

Menstrual only
• Headache occurs exclusively 2 d before and first 2 d of menstrual cycle
Associated but not limited to menstruation
• Occurs >6–8 d/mo
OR
• Occurs ≥3 d/mo when optimally treated and still debilitating

Initiate treatment for migraine

Therapy successful? — Yes → Continue therapy

No

Consider cyclic prophylaxis
• NSAIDs
• Triptans
• Ergots   A

Patient improves? — Yes → Continue therapy

No →

Consider hormone prophylaxis:
• Transdermal estradiol
• Estrogen-containing contraceptives
• GnRH agonists with "add back" therapy
Refer to the on estrogen-containing contraceptives or considering estrogen-containing contraceptives with migraine algorithm   A

Patient improves? — Yes → Continue therapy

No

Consider consulting with headache specialist

A = Annotation

PERIMENOPAUSAL OR MENOPAUSAL MIGRAINE ALGORITHM—ICSI 2011

All algorithm boxes with an "A" and those that refer to other algorithm boxes link to annotation content.

Perimenopausal or menopausal with active migraine history and is a potential candidate for HT
A

HT: newer terminology for HRT. In this guideline, HT indicates treatment with one of several available estrogens, with or without progestin.

Patient is willing to start HT? → No → Attempt treatment with migraine prophylactic treatment algorithm

Yes ↓

Hormone therapy
- Oral, transvaginal or transdermal estrogen
- Progestin if indicated
- Estrogen-containing contraceptives

Refer to the on estrogen-containing contraceptives or considering estrogen-containing contraceptives with migraine algorithm

Continue therapy ← Yes ← Successful?

Successful? A → No → Consider changing delivery system or formulation of estrogen and progestin A

Yes ↓

Continue with therapy and follow-up ← Yes ← Successful? → No →
- Specialty consultation
- Return to migraine treatment algorithm

No ↓ (from Successful?)

A = Annotation

ON ESTROGEN-CONTAINING CONTRACEPTIVES OR CONSIDERING ESTROGEN-CONTAINING CONTRACEPTIVES WITH MIGRAINE ALGORITHM—ICSI 2011

All algorithm boxes with an "A" and those that refer to other algorithm boxes link to annotation content.

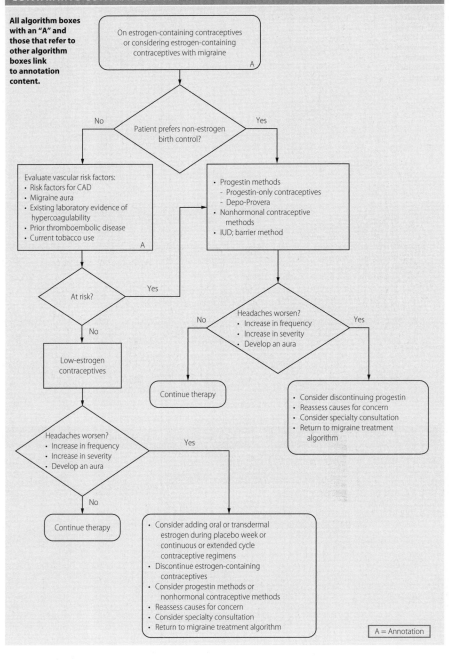

On estrogen-containing contraceptives or considering estrogen-containing contraceptives with migraine
A

Patient prefers non-estrogen birth control?

No → Evaluate vascular risk factors:
- Risk factors for CAD
- Migraine aura
- Existing laboratory evidence of hypercoagulability
- Prior thromboembolic disease
- Current tobacco use
A

Yes →
- Progestin methods
  - Progestin-only contraceptives
  - Depo-Provera
- Nonhormonal contraceptive methods
- IUD; barrier method

At risk?

Yes →

No → Low-estrogen contraceptives

Headaches worsen?
- Increase in frequency
- Increase in severity
- Develop an aura

No → Continue therapy

Yes →

Headaches worsen?
- Increase in frequency
- Increase in severity
- Develop an aura

No → Continue therapy

Yes →
- Consider adding oral or transdermal estrogen during placebo week or continuous or extended cycle contraceptive regimens
- Discontinue estrogen-containing contraceptives
- Consider progestin methods or nonhormonal contraceptive methods
- Reassess causes for concern
- Consider specialty consultation
- Return to migraine treatment algorithm

Yes →
- Consider discontinuing progestin
- Reassess causes for concern
- Consider specialty consultation
- Return to migraine treatment algorithm

A = Annotation

MIGRAINE PROPHYLACTIC TREATMENT ALGORITHM—ICSI 2011

All algorithm boxes with an "A" and those that refer to other algorithm boxes link to annotation content.

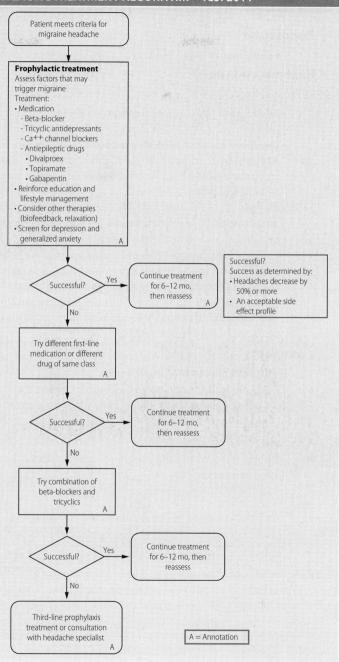

Patient meets criteria for migraine headache

Prophylactic treatment
Assess factors that may trigger migraine
Treatment:
• Medication
  - Beta-blocker
  - Tricyclic antidepressants
  - Ca++ channel blockers
  - Antiepileptic drugs
    • Divalproex
    • Topiramate
    • Gabapentin
• Reinforce education and lifestyle management
• Consider other therapies (biofeedback, relaxation)
• Screen for depression and generalized anxiety   A

Successful?   Yes →   Continue treatment for 6–12 mo, then reassess   A

No ↓

Successful?
Success as determined by:
• Headaches decrease by 50% or more
• An acceptable side effect profile

Try different first-line medication or different drug of same class   A

Successful?   Yes →   Continue treatment for 6–12 mo, then reassess

No ↓

Try combination of beta-blockers and tricyclics   A

Successful?   Yes →   Continue treatment for 6–12 mo, then reassess

No ↓

Third-line prophylaxis treatment or consultation with headache specialist   A

A = Annotation

HEARING LOSS, SUDDEN

Population
–Adults age 18 y and older.

Recommendations

▶ AAO-HNS 2019
–Distinguish hearing loss between sensorineural and conductive hearing loss.
–Diagnose idiopathic sudden sensorineural hearing loss (ISSNHL) when audiometry confirms a 30 decibel hearing loss at three consecutive frequencies and an underlying condition cannot be identified by history and physical.
–Evaluate patients with ISSNHL for retrocochlear pathology by obtaining an MRI of the internal auditory canal, auditory brainstem responses, and an audiology exam.
–Consider treatment of ISSNHL with incomplete hearing recovery with systemic or intratympanic steroids within 14 d. Hyperbaric oxygen therapy is considered only as an adjunct to steroids.
–In patients with ISSNHL, recommend against antivirals, thrombolytics, vasodilators, or antioxidants for treatment and against CT scanning of the head or routine lab testing.

Comments
1. Prompt diagnosis is important.
2. Obtain audiometric testing as soon as possible and within 14 d.
3. Counsel patients with incomplete recovery of hearing about the benefits of hearing aids.

Source
–https://www.entnet.org//content/aao-hnsf-clinical-practice-guideline-sudden-hearing-loss

HOARSENESS

Population
–Persons with hoarseness.

Recommendations
▶ AAO-HNS 2018
–Most but not all hoarseness is benign or self-limited; some of the most common causes are URI and voice overuse.
–Begin assessment with history and physical to identify underlying causes and factors that may modify management.
–If hoarseness fails to resolve or improve within 4 wk, refer for laryngoscopy.
–Recommends against screening neck imaging (CT or MRI scanning) for chronic hoarseness prior to laryngoscopy.
–Recommends against the routine use of antibiotics or steroids to treat hoarseness.
–Recommends against routine use of antireflux medications unless the patient exhibits signs or symptoms of gastroesophageal reflux disease.
–Recommends voice therapy for all patients with hoarseness and a decreased voice-related quality of life.
–Consider surgery for possible laryngeal CA, benign laryngeal soft-tissue lesions, or glottis insufficiency.
–Consider botulinum toxin injections for spasmodic dysphonia.

Source
–https://www.entnet.org//content/clinical-practice-guideline-hoarseness-dysphonia

Comment
1. Nearly one-third of Americans will have hoarseness at some point in their lives.

LARYNGITIS, ACUTE

Population
–Adults.

Recommendation
▶ Cochrane Database Systematic Reviews 2015
–Insufficient evidence to support the use of antibiotics for acute laryngitis.

Source
–http://www.cochrane.org/CD004783/ARI_antibiotics-to-treat-adults-with-acute-laryngitis

Comment
1. Many methodological flaws in studies evaluated.

OTITIS EXTERNA, ACUTE (AOE)

Population
–Children age 2 y or older and adults.

Recommendations
▶ AAO-HNS 2014
–Recommends against systemic antimicrobials as initial therapy for diffuse, uncomplicated acute otitis externa (AOE).
–Recommends topical antibiotics for initial therapy of AOE.
–In the presence of a perforated tympanic membrane or tympanostomy tubes, prescribe a non-ototoxic topical antibiotic.

Source
–https://www.entnet.org//content/clinical-practice-guideline-acute-otitis-externa

Comment
1. Recommends reassessment of the diagnosis if the patient fails to respond within 72 h of topical antibiotics.

OTITIS MEDIA, ACUTE (AOM)

Population
–Children age 3 mo to 18 y.

Recommendations

▶ **AAP 2013**

–Make diagnosis with pneumatic otoscopy.
–Use a wait-and-see approach for 48–72 h with children at low risk.[a]
–Give symptomatic relief with acetaminophen or ibuprofen and warm compresses to the ear.
–Educate caregivers about prevention of otitis media: encourage breast-feeding, feed child upright if bottle fed, avoid passive smoke exposure, limit exposure to groups of children, careful handwashing prior to handling child, avoid pacifier use >10 mo, ensure immunizations are up to date.
–Amoxicillin is the first-line antibiotic for low-risk children.
–Use alternative medication if failure to respond to initial treatment within 72 h; penicillin allergy; presence of a resistant organism found on culture.
–Refer to an ear, nose, and throat (ENT) specialist for a complication of otitis media: mastoiditis, facial nerve palsy, lateral sinus thrombosis, meningitis, brain abscess, or labyrinthitis.
–Do not schedule routine rechecks at 10–14 d in children feeling well.
–Management of otitis media with effusion:
  • Educate that effusion will resolve on its own.
  • Do not offer antihistamines or decongestants.
  • Try antibiotics for 10–14 d prior to referral for tympanostomy tubes.

Source
–*Pediatrics.* 2013;131:e964-e999.

▶ **AAFP 2013**

–Do not prescribe antibiotics to children age 2–12 y with nonsevere AOM when observation is an option.

Source
–http://www.choosingwisely.org/societies/american-academy-of-family-physicians/

---

[a]Children older than age 2 y without severe disease (temperature >102°F [39°C] and moderate-to-severe otalgia), otherwise healthy, do not attend daycare, and have had no prior ear infections within the last month.

Comments

1. Amoxicillin is first-line therapy for low-risk children:
   a. 40 mg/kg/d if no antibiotics used in last 3 mo.
   b. 80 mg/kg/d if child is not low risk.
2. Alternative antibiotics:
   a. Amoxicillin-clavulanate.
   b. Cefuroxime axetil.
   c. Ceftriaxone.
   d. Cefprozil.
   e. Loracarbef.
   f. Cefdinir.
   g. Cefixime.
   h. Cefpodoxime.
   i. Clarithromycin.
   j. Azithromycin.
   k. Erythromycin.

Population

–Children 6 mo to 12 y.

Recommendations

▶ AAP 2013

–**Diagnosis of AOM**
  • Moderate-to-severe bulging of the tympanic membrane.
  • New-onset otorrhea not due to otitis externa.
  • Mild bulging of an intensely red tympanic membrane and new otalgia <48 h duration.

–**Treatment of AOM**
  • Analgesics and antipyretics.
  • Indications for antibiotics:
    ◦ Children <24 mo old with bilateral AOM.
    ◦ Symptoms that are not improving or worsening during a 48-h to 72-h observation period.
    ◦ AOM associated with severe symptoms (extreme fussiness or severe otalgia).
  • Observe for 48–72 h in the absence of severe symptoms and fever <102.2°F.

–Consider tympanostomy tubes for recurrent AOM (3 episodes in 6 mo or 4 episodes in 1 y).

Source

–http://www.guidelines.gov/content.aspx?id=43892

Comments

1. AOM is **not** present in the absence of a middle ear effusion based on pneumatic otoscopy or tympanometry.
2. Amoxicillin is the preferred antibiotics if the child has not received amoxicillin in the last 30 d.
3. Augmentin is the preferred antibiotic if the child has received amoxicillin in the last 30 d.

PHARYNGITIS, ACUTE

APPROACH TO ACUTE PHARYNGITIS

Symptoms of possible streptococcal pharyngitis: close exposure to strep throat; sudden onset of sore throat; exudative tonsillitis; tender anterior cervical adenopathy; fever; absence of rhinorrhea, cough, hoarseness, oral ulcers; headache and abdominal pain may be present with other symptoms in pt >3 y[a]

Obtain a rapid strep test and backup strep culture

Negative and low likelihood of bacterial pharyngitis[b]

Negative and high likelihood of bacterial pharyngitis

Educate and offer home remedies

Send throat strep culture → Positive

Symptoms improved at 1 wk?

Negative

Start penicillin or amoxicillin if rapid strep test is positive (clindamycin or azithromycin if PCN-allergic)

Symptoms improved at 48–72 h?

Yes / No

No / Yes

Continue symptomatic therapy

Reevaluate and consider testing for mononucleosis

Reevaluate for complications:
- Lemierre's syndrome
- Peritonsillar or retropharyngeal abscess
- Intracranial extension of infection
- Mono testing (if appropriate)

Complete 10 d antibiotic course

[a]Diagnostic studies for GAS is not indicated for children <3 y because acute rheumatic fever is very rare in this age group.
[b]Low likelihood of GAS if rhinorrhea, cough, hoarseness, or oral ulcers.

Source: IDSA 2012 guidelines on group A Streptococcus (GAS) pharyngitis.

RHINITIS

MANAGEMENT OF NONINFECTIOUS RHINITIS

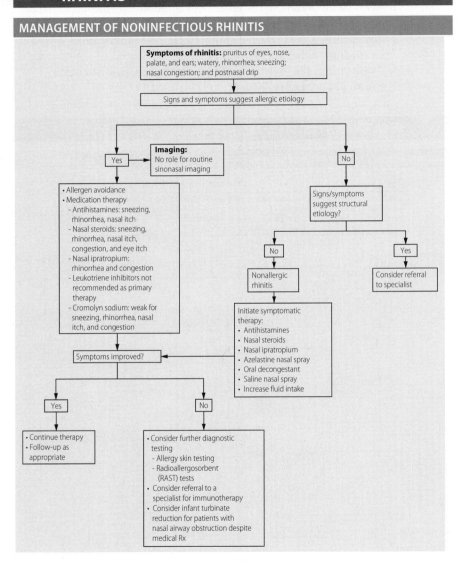

Sources
–ICSI, JAN 2011; AAO-HNSF, FEB 2015.
–https://www.entnet.org//content/clinical-practice-guideline-allergic-rhinitis

SINUSITIS

Population
–Children age 1–18 y.

Recommendation
▶ ACEP 2013

–Avoid prescribing antibiotics in the ER for patients presenting with uncomplicated acute sinusitis.

Source
–http://www.choosingwisely.org/societies/american-college-of-emergency-physicians/

Comment
1. Improvement of symptoms should occur within 72 h of antibiotic initiation.

SINUSITIS, ACUTE BACTERIAL

Population
–Children age 1–18 y with acute bacterial sinusitis.

Recommendations
▶ AAP 2013

–Presumptive acute sinusitis if child with acute URI and one of the following:
  • Nasal discharge or persistent cough lasting more than 10 d.
  • Worsening course.
  • Severe onset with fever $\geq 102.2°F$ and purulent nasal discharge for at least 3 d.
–Recommend against imaging studies for uncomplicated sinusitis.
–Contrast-enhanced CT scan of sinuses for any suspicion of orbital or CNS involvement.
–Recommend antibiotics for any sinusitis with a severe onset or worsening course.
  • Amoxicillin +/– clavulanate is first-line therapy.
  • Persistent cough or rhinorrhea in the absence of severe symptoms may be managed with ongoing observation.

Source
–https://guidelines.gov/summaries/summary/46939

SINUSITIS

Population
  –Adults.

Recommendations
▶ AAO-HNS APRIL 2015
    –**ACUTE RHINOSINUSITIS (ARS)**
      • Up to 4 wk of purulent nasal drainage (anterior, posterior, or both) accompanied by nasal obstruction, facial pain/pressure/fullness, or both.
    –**VIRAL RHINOSINUSITIS (VRS)**
      • Acute rhinosinusitis that is caused by, or is presumed to be caused by, viral infection. Diagnose viral rhinosinusitis when symptoms or signs of acute rhinosinusitis are present <10 d and the symptoms are not worsening.
    –**SYMPTOMATIC RELIEF OF VRS**
      • Clinicians may recommend analgesics, topical intranasal steroids, and/or nasal saline irrigation for symptomatic relief of VRS.
    –**ACUTE BACTERIAL RHINOSINUSITIS (ABRS)**
      • Acute rhinosinusitis that is caused by, or is presumed to be caused by, bacterial infection. Diagnose acute bacterial rhinosinusitis when
        ◦ Symptoms or signs of acute rhinosinusitis fail to improve within 10 d or more beyond the onset of upper respiratory symptoms.
        ◦ Symptoms or signs of acute rhinosinusitis worsen within 10 d after an initial improvement (double worsening).
    –**ABRS—INITIAL MANAGEMENT**
      • Offer watchful waiting (without antibiotics) or prescribe initial antibiotic therapy for adults with uncomplicated ABRS.
      • Offer watchful waiting only when there is assurance of follow-up such that antibiotic therapy is started if the patient's condition fails to improve by 7 d after ABRS diagnosis or if it worsens at any time.
    –**ABRS—CHOICE OF ANTIBIOTIC**
      • If a decision is made to treat ABRS with an antibiotic agent, prescribe amoxicillin with or without clavulanate as first-line therapy for 5–10 d for most adults.
    –**ABRS—TREATMENT FAILURE**
      • If the patient's condition worsens or fails to improve with the initial management option by 7 d after diagnosis or worsens during the initial management, reassess the patient to confirm ABRS, exclude other causes of illness, and detect complications.

- If ABRS is confirmed in the patient initially managed with observation, begin antibiotic therapy.
- If the patient was initially managed with an antibiotic, change the antibiotic.

–ABRS—SYMPTOMATIC RELIEF

- Consider recommending analgesics, topical intranasal steroids, and/or nasal saline irrigation for symptomatic relief of ABRS.

–DIFFERENTIAL DIAGNOSIS

- Distinguish presumed ABRS from ARS caused by viral upper respiratory infections and noninfectious conditions.
- Diagnose ABRS when
  - Symptoms or signs of ARS (purulent nasal drainage accompanied by nasal obstruction, facial pain/pressure/fullness, or both) persist without evidence of improvement for at least 10 d beyond the onset of upper respiratory symptoms.
  - Symptoms or signs of ARS worsen within 10 d after an initial improvement (double worsening).

–RADIOGRAPHIC IMAGING

- Do not obtain radiographic imaging for patients who meet diagnostic criteria for ARS, unless a complication or alternative diagnosis is suspected.

–CHRONIC RHINOSINUSITIS (CRS)

- Twelve weeks or longer of 2 or more of the following signs and symptoms:
  - Mucopurulent drainage (anterior, posterior, or both).
  - Nasal obstruction (congestion).
  - Facial pain/pressure/fullness.
  - Decreased sense of smell.
- AND inflammation is documented by one or more of the following findings:
  - Purulent (not clear) mucus or edema in the middle meatus or anterior ethmoid region.
  - Polyps in nasal cavity or the middle meatus.
  - Radiographic imaging showing inflammation of the paranasal sinuses.

–RECURRENT ACUTE RHINOSINUSITIS

- Four or more episodes per year of acute bacterial rhinosinusitis without signs or symptoms of rhinosinusitis between episodes, provided each episode of acute bacterial rhinosinusitis meets diagnostic criteria for ARS.

–**CRS OR RECURRENT ARS—DIAGNOSIS**
  • Distinguish CRS and recurrent ARS from isolated episodes of ABRS and other causes of sinonasal symptoms.
–**CRS—OBJECTIVE CONFIRMATION**
  • Confirm a clinical diagnosis of CRS with objective documentation of sinonasal inflammation, which may be accomplished using anterior rhinoscopy, nasal endoscopy, or computed tomography.
–**CRS—TOPICAL INTRANASAL THERAPY**
  • Recommend saline nasal irrigation, topical intranasal corticosteroids, or both for symptom relief of CRS.
–**CRS—ANTIFUNGAL THERAPY**
  • Do not prescribe topical or systemic antifungal therapy for patients with CRS.

Source
  –https://www.entnet.org//content/clinical-practice-guideline-adult-sinusitis

TINNITUS

Population
  –Adults and children.

Recommendations
▶ **AAO-HNS 2014, American Speech-Language-Hearing Association 2018**
  –Recommend a thorough history and exam on patients with tinnitus. Elicit features such as unilateral or pulsatile tinnitus which may suggest more insidious etiology.
  –Refer for a comprehensive audiologic examination for unilateral or persistent tinnitus or any associated hearing impairment.
  –Obtain imaging studies only for unilateral tinnitus, pulsatile tinnitus, asymmetric hearing loss, or focal neurological abnormalities.
  –Refer for a hearing aid for tinnitus with hearing loss.
  –Consider cognitive behavioral therapy or sound therapy for persistent, bothersome tinnitus.
  –Recommend against medical or herbal therapy or transcranial magnetic stimulation for tinnitus (ASHA: "remain current" in the evidence or lack thereof for these approaches).

Sources
  –https://www.entnet.org//content/clinical-practice-guideline-tinnitus
  –https://www.asha.org/Practice-Portal/Clinical-Topics/Tinnitus-and-Hyperacusis/

TONSILLECTOMY

Population
–Children.

Recommendations

▶ AAO-HNS 2019

–Recommends against routine perioperative antibiotics for tonsillectomy.
–Tonsillectomy indicated for:
  • Tonsillar hypertrophy with sleep-disordered breathing.
  • Recurrent throat infections for ≥7 episodes of recurrent throat infection in last year; ≥5 episodes of recurrent throat infection per year in last 2 y; or at least 3 episodes per year for 3 y with documentation in the medical record for each episode of sore throat and ≥1 of the following: temperature >38.3°C (101°F), cervical adenopathy, tonsillar exudate, or positive test for group A beta-hemolytic streptococcus.
–Give post-tonsillectomy pain control, but do not use codeine in children less than age 12.

Source
–https://www.entnet.org/content/clinical-practice-guideline-tonsillectomy-children-update

TYMPANOSTOMY TUBES

Population
–Children 6 mo to 12 y.

Recommendations

▶ AAO 2013

–Do not insert tympanostomy tubes for children with:
  • A single episode of otitis media with effusion (OME) of <3 mo duration.
  • Recurrent acute otitis media without effusion.
–Obtain a hearing test if OME persists for at least 3 mo or if tympanostomy tube insertion is being considered.
–Offer bilateral tympanostomy tube insertion to children with:
  • Bilateral OME for at least 3 mo **AND** documented hearing impairment.
  • Recurrent acute otitis media with effusions.

• Tympanostomy tube insertion is an option for chronic symptomatic OME associated with balance problems, poor school performance, behavioral problems, or ear discomfort thought to be due to OME.

Source
–http://www.guideline.gov/content.aspx?id=46909

Comment
1. No need for prophylactic water precautions (avoidance of swimming or water sports or use of earplugs) for children with tympanostomy tubes.

VERTIGO, BENIGN PAROXYSMAL POSITIONAL (BPPV)

Population
–Adults.

Recommendations
▶ AAO-HNS March, 2017
–Recommends the Dix–Hallpike maneuver to diagnose posterior semicircular canal BPPV.
–Recommends treatment of posterior semicircular canal BPPV with a particle repositioning maneuver.
–If the Dix–Hallpike test result is negative, recommends a supine roll test to diagnose lateral semicircular canal BPPV.
–Recommends offering vestibular repositioning exercises such as the Epley maneuver for the initial treatment of BPPV.
–Observation is an acceptable initial management for patients with BPPV.
–Recommends against post-procedural postural restrictions for posterior canal BPPV.
–Recommends evaluating patients for an underlying peripheral vestibular or central nervous system disorder if they have an initial treatment failure of presumed BPPV.
–Recommends against routine radiologic imaging for patients with BPPV.
–Recommends against routine vestibular testing for patients with BPPV.
–Recommends against routine use of antihistamines or benzodiazepines for patients with BPPV.

Source
–https://www.entnet.org//content/clinical-practice-guideline-benign-paroxysmal-positional-vertigo-bppv

Comment
1. BPPV is the most common vestibular disorder in adults, afflicting 2.4% of adults at some point during their lives.

Disorders of the Skin, Breast, and Musculoskeletal System

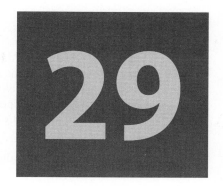

ANKYLOSING SPONDYLITIS AND SPONDYLOARTHRITIS

Population
–Adults with ankylosing spondylitis (AS) or nonradiographic spondyloarthritis.

Recommendations

▶ ACR/Spondylitis Association of America/Spondyloarthritis Research and Treatment Network 2015

–**Recommendations for treatment of ankylosing spondylitis**
  • Scheduled NSAIDs.
  • Tumor necrosis factor inhibitor (TNFi) therapy.
  • Recommends addition of slow-acting anti-rheumatic drugs when TNFi medications contraindicated.
  • Local parenteral corticosteroids for active sacroiliitis, active enthesitis, or peripheral arthritis for symptoms refractory to NSAIDs.
  • Avoid systemic corticosteroid use.
  • Refer to an ophthalmologist for concomitant iritis.
  • Recommend TNFi monoclonal antibody therapy for AS with inflammatory bowel disease.
  • Physical therapy program.
  • Screen for fall risk, osteoporosis.
–**Recommendations for treatment of nonradiographic axial spondyloarthritis**
  • NSAIDs.
  • Tumor Necrosis Factor inhibitor (TNFi) therapy.

Source

–Ward MM, Deodhar A, Akl EA, et al. American College of
Rheumatology/Spondylitis Association of America/Spondyloarthritis
Research and Treatment Network 2015 Recommendations for the
treatment of ankylosing spondylitis and nonradiographic axial
spondyloarthritis. *Arthritis Rheumatol.* 2016;68(2):282-298.

Comment

1. An update to the 2015 guidelines is expected in 2019.

ATOPIC DERMATITIS (AD)

Population

–Adults and children.

Recommendations

▶ AAD 2014

–Generous application of skin moisturizers after bathing.

–Recommend limited use of hypoallergenic non-soap cleansers.

–Consider wet-wrap therapy with topical corticosteroids for moderate-
to-severe AD during flares.

–Twice-daily topical corticosteroids are the first-line therapy for AD.

–Topical calcineurin inhibitors (tacrolimus or pimecrolimus) can be
used for maintenance AD therapy.

–Recommend against topical antihistamine therapy for AD.

–Phototherapy is second-line treatment for refractory cases.

–Consider systemic immunomodulating agents for severe cases that are
refractory to topical agents and phototherapy.

Sources

–http://www.guideline.gov/content.aspx?id=48409

–http://www.guideline.gov/content.aspx?id=48410

Comment

1. Systemic immunomodulating agents that have been studied in AD are
azathioprine, cyclosporine, or methotrexate.

▶ AAD 2018

–Do not use oral antibiotics in atopic dermatitis unless there is clinical
evidence of infection.

–Do not use systemic (oral or injected) corticosteroids for long-term
treatment of dermatitis.

–Do not use skin prick tests or blood tests (eg, radioallergosorbent test)
for the routine evaluation of atopic dermatitis.

Source
  –American Academy of Dermatology. Choosing Wisely. 2018.

Comment
  1. Skin prick tests and RAST-type blood tests are useful to identify causes of allergic reactions, but not for diagnosing dermatitis or eczema. When testing for suspected allergies is indicated, patch testing with ingredients of products that come in contact with the patient's skin is recommended.

BACK PAIN, LOW

Population
  –Adults.

Recommendations

▶ ACP 2017
  –Consider nonpharmacologic treatments for acute or subacute low-back pain including superficial heat, massage, acupuncture, or spinal manipulation.
  –If pharmacologic treatments needed, start with NSAIDs or skeletal muscle relaxants.
  –For chronic low-back pain, start a trial of nonpharmacologic treatments including exercise, multidisciplinary rehabilitation, acupuncture, mindfulness-based stress reduction, tai chi, yoga, biofeedback, cognitive behavioral therapy, or spinal manipulation.
  –For persistent chronic low-back pain, pharmacologic therapy with NSAIDs as first-line therapy and tramadol or duloxetine as second-line therapy.
  –Use opiates for chronic low-back pain only if patients have failed all other therapies and only if the potential benefits outweigh the risks of dependency, addiction, overdose, and misuse.

Sources
  –http://guidelines.gov/summaries/summary/50781/noninvasive-treatments-for-acute-subacute-and-chronic-low-back-pain-a-clinical-practice-guideline-from-the-american-college-of-physicians?q=back+pain
  –Qaseem A, Wilt TJ, McLean RM, Forciea MA, Clinical Guidelines Committee of the American College of Physicians. Noninvasive treatments for acute, subacute, and chronic low-back pain: a clinical practice guideline from the American College of Physicians. *Ann Intern Med.* 2017;166(7):514-530.

▶ NICE 2009
    –Educate patients and promote self-management of low-back pain.
    –Recommends offering one of the following treatment options:
      • Structure exercise program.
      • Manual therapy.[a]
      • Acupuncture.
    –Consider a psychology referral for patients with a high disability and/or who experience significant psychological distress from their low-back pain.
    –Recommends against routine lumbar spine x-rays.
    –Recommends an MRI scan of lumbar spine only if spinal fusion is under consideration.
    –Consider a referral for surgery in patients with refractory, severe nonspecific low-back pain who have completed the programs above and would consider spinal fusion.

    Source
    –http://www.nice.org.uk/nicemedia/live/11887/44343/44343.pdf

▶ ICSI 2018
    –For patients with acute and subacute low-back pain, a biopsychosocial assessment should be performed.
    –Routine imaging (x-ray, CT, MRI) should not be recommended in patients with nonspecific or radicular low-back pain without red flag symptoms.
    –Appropriate education and treatment and recovery expectations are recommended for all patients with acute and subacute low-back pain.
    –Both heat and cold therapy can be used for pain relief.
    –Recommend staying active and continuing activities of daily living within the limits permitted by the patient's symptoms.
    –Consider spinal manipulation as an early intervention for acute and subacute low-back pain.
    –Consider acupuncture for subacute low-back pain.
    –NSAIDs and muscle relaxants can be used for short-term relief with acute and subacute low-back pain. Acetaminophen is also an option.
    –Generally avoid opioids for acute and subacute low-back pain.
    –Consider epidural steroid injections as an adjunct for acute and subacute low-back pain with a radicular component.

    Source
    –ICSI. *Adult Acute and Subacute Low Back Pain*. March 2018.

---

[a]Manual therapy includes spinal manipulation, spinal mobilization, and massage.

Comments

1. When using pharmacologic therapy, consider and counsel the patients on potential side effects.
2. Muscle relaxants should not be used for >1 wk.

LUMBAR DISC HERNIATION

Population

–Adults.

Recommendations

▶ North American Spine Society 2012

–TNFα inhibitors do not provide benefit (grade B).
–Insufficient evidence to recommend for or against the use of IV glucocorticoids, 5-ht receptor inhibitors, gabapentin, amitriptyline, and agmatine sulfate.
–Insufficient evidence to recommend for or against PT/exercise programs as a stand-alone treatment modality, but it is an option for patients with mild-to-moderate symptoms. There is insufficient evidence for traction therapy.
–Spinal manipulation is an option for symptomatic relief (grade C).
–Transforaminal epidural steroid injection is recommended for short-term (2–4 wk) pain relief in selected patients (grade A).

Source

–North American Spine Society. *Clinical Guidelines for Multidisciplinary Spine Care Diagnosis and Treatment of Lumbar Disc Herniation with Radiculopathy.* 2012.

ROTATOR CUFF TEARS

Population

–Adults.

Recommendations

▶ AAOS 2019

–Small-to-medium tears
  • Physical therapy and operative treatment both result in significant improvement in patient-reported outcomes.
  • Do not use routine acromioplasty as a concomitant treatment.

–A single injection of corticosteroids with local anesthetic provides short-term improvement in pain and function. Avoid multiple steroid injections, as they may compromise the rotator cuff integrity and affect subsequent repair attempts.

–Limited evidence for the use of hyaluronic acid injections and platelet-rich plasma.

Source

–AAOS. *Management of Rotator Cuff Injuries Clinical Practice Guideline.* 2019.

BREAST CANCER FOLLOW-UP CARE

Population

–Early-stage women with curable breast cancer.

Recommendation

▶ American Society of Clinical Oncology (ASCO) 2013

–**Mode of Surveillance**

- Careful history and physical examination every 3–6 mo for first 3 y after primary therapy (with or without adjuvant treatment), then every 6–12 mo for next 2 y, and then annually.
- Counsel patients about symptoms of recurrence including new lumps, bone pain, chest pain, dyspnea, abdominal pain, or persistent headaches.
- High-risk women for familial breast CA syndromes should be referred for genetic counseling—high-risk criteria include Ashkenazi Jewish heritage, history of ovarian CA at any age in the patient or any first-degree relatives; any first-degree relative with breast CA before age 50; two or more first- or second-degree relatives diagnosed with breast CA at any age; patient or relative with bilateral breast CA; and history of breast CA in male relative.
- All women should be counseled to perform monthly self-breast examinations.
- Mammography—women treated with breast-conserving therapy should have first posttreatment mammogram no earlier than 6 mo after radiation. Subsequent mammograms every 6–12 mo for surveillance (yearly preferred if stability of mammogram achieved).
- Regular gynecology follow-up with pelvic examination. Tamoxifen increases risk of uterine cancer, and therefore patients should be advised to report any vaginal bleeding if they are taking tamoxifen.
- Coordination of care: Risk of recurrence continues through more than 15 y (especially in woman who are hormone receptor

positive). Continuity of care by physicians experienced in surveillance of patients and in breast examination is recommended. Follow-up by a primary care physician (PCP) leads to the same outcome as specialist follow-up. If the patient desires transfer of care to PCP, 1 y after definitive therapy is appropriate.

Sources
–*NCCN Guidelines.* 2015;BINV-16:27.
–*J Clin Oncol.* 2013;31:961-965.

Comments

1. **Reduce Routine Investigative Testing**
   The following routine studies are NOT recommended for routine breast cancer surveillance:
   a. CBC and automated chemistry studies.
   b. Routine chest x-ray.
   c. Bone scans.
   d. Liver ultrasound.
   e. Routine CT scanning.
   f. Routine FDG-PET scanning.
   g. Breast MRI (unless patient has BRCA1 or BRCA2 mutation or previous mediastinal radiation at young age).
   h. Tumor markers including CA27.29, CA15-3, or CEA are not recommended for routine surveillance. (*JAMA.* 1994;27:1587-1592)

2. Although studies have shown no survival benefit for routine surveillance testing, many oncologists will do routine blood studies including tumor markers especially in higher risk women. The most important follow-up strategy is to make certain patients know and report early signs or symptoms that may reflect recurrent disease.

3. There is a significant difference in the behavior of hormone receptor (HR) positive vs. hormone receptor negative disease. HR-negative disease tends to recur earlier (2–3 y) than HR-positive breast cancer (>50% of relapses occur after 5 y).

4. There is also a 3- to 4-fold increase in risk of brain metastasis in HR-negative women vs. HR-positive women.

5. Overexpression of Her2 is found in 20% of breast cancer patients and targeted therapy in this group has significantly improved prognosis. Her2 overexpressed patients, however, are also at increased risk for brain metastasis.

6. HR-positive patients have a 4-fold increased risk of bone metastasis compared to HR-negative patients in whom metastases to liver, lung, and brain are more common. (*N Engl J Med.* 2007;357:39)

GOUT, ACUTE ATTACKS

Population
- –Adults.

Recommendations

▶ ACR 2012

- –Therapy options for acute gout attacks.
  - Mild-to-moderate attacks involving 1–2 joints.
    - ○ NSAIDs: full-dose naproxen, sulindac, or indomethacin is preferred.
    - ○ Colchicine 1.2 mg PO × 1, then 0.6 mg 1 h later, then 0.6 mg daily bid.
    - ○ Corticosteroids: prednisone or prednisolone 0.5 mg/kg PO daily for 5–10 d.
  - Severe attacks or polyarticular gout.
    - ○ Colchicine + NSAIDs.
    - ○ Colchicine + steroids.
  - Expert opinion to continue urate-lowering therapy (eg, allopurinol) during acute attacks.
  - Ice applied to affected joints can help.
- –Pharmacologic urate-lowering therapy.
  - Allopurinol.
    - ○ Starting dose should not exceed 100 mg/d.
    - ○ Uptitrate dose every 2–4 wk to max of 800 mg/d, unless renal impairment exists.
    - ○ Desire uric acid level of <6 mg/dL.
  - Consider adding a uricosuric agent (eg, probenecid) for refractory hyperuricemia despite urate-lowering therapy.
  - Initiate allopurinol after an acute gout attack has resolved and continue prophylactic anti-inflammatory agents for 3 mo beyond achieving urate level <6 mg/dL.
    - ○ Colchicine 0.6 mg daily bid.
    - ○ Naproxen 250 mg PO bid.

Sources
- –http://www.guideline.gov/content.aspx?id=38624
- –http://www.guideline.gov/content.aspx?id=38625

Comment

1. Consider HLAB*5801 testing prior to the initiation of allopurinol for patients at particularly high risk of allopurinol hypersensitivity reaction.

a. Highest risk group are those of Korean, Han Chinese, or Thai descent, especially if Stage 3 or higher CKD is present.

Population

1. Adults with suspected gout.

Recommendation

▶ American College of Physicians 2017

–Clinicians should use synovial fluid analysis when diagnostic testing is necessary in patients with possible gout.

Sources

–http://guidelines.gov/summaries/summary/50607/diagnosis-of-acute-gout-a-clinical-practice-guideline-from-the-american-college-of-physicians?q=gout

–Qaseem A, McLean RM, Starkey M, Forciea MA; Clinical Guidelines Committee of the American College of Physicians. Diagnosis of acute gout: a clinical practice guideline from the American College of Physicians. *Ann Intern Med*. 2017;166(1):52-57.

Population

–Adults >18 y with acute or recurrent gout.

Recommendations

▶ American College of Physicians 2017

–Options for treatment of acute gout include corticosteroids, NSAIDs, or colchicine (low-dose recommended).

–Corticosteroids should be considered first-line therapy in patients without contraindications. Prednisolone 35 mg orally for 5 d.

–Recommends against using long-term urate-lowering therapy in most patients with infrequent attacks (<3 attacks per year).

–Febuxostat and allopurinol are equally effective at decreasing serum urate levels.

Sources

–http://guidelines.gov/summaries/summary/50608/management-of-acute-and-recurrent-gout-a-clinical-practice-guideline-from-the-american-college-of-physicians?q=gout

–Qaseem A, Harris RP, Forciea MA; Clinical Guidelines Committee of the American College of Physicians. Management of acute and recurrent gout: a clinical practice guideline from the American College of Physicians. *Ann Intern Med*. 2017;166(1):58-68.

HIP FRACTURES

Population
–Elderly patients with hip fractures.

Recommendations
▶ AAOS 2014
-Recommends preoperative pain control in patients with hip fractures.
-Insufficient evidence to support preoperative traction in hip fractures.
-Recommends hip fracture surgery within 48 h of admission.
-Do not delay hip fracture surgery for patients on aspirin +/– clopidogrel.
-Recommends operative fixation for nondisplaced femoral neck fractures.
-Recommends unipolar or bipolar hemiarthroplasty for displaced femoral neck fractures.
-Recommends prolonged thromboprophylaxis to prevent venous thromboembolism after hip fracture surgery.
-Recommends intensive physical therapy post-discharge to improve functional outcomes.
-Recommends evaluation for osteoporosis in all patients who have sustained a hip fracture.

Source
-http://www.guideline.gov/content.aspx?id=48518

MULTIPLE SCLEROSIS (MS)

Population
–Adults.

Recommendations
▶ AAN 2014, 2015, 2018
-Patients with newly diagnosed MS should be counseled on specific treatment options with disease modifying therapy (DMT) at a dedicated treatment visit, with a clinician who has expertise with DMTs.
-Weekly home or outpatient physical therapy (8 wk) may improve balance, disability, and gait, but not upper-extremity dexterity.
-Motor and sensory balance training or motor balance training (3 wk) may improve static and dynamic balance.

-Consider oral cannabis extract and THC in patients with MS with spasticity and pain (excluding central neuropathic pain).
-Consider Sativex oromucosal cannabinoid spray to reduce MS-related spasticity, pain, and urinary frequency.
-Ineffective therapies include: gingko biloba for improving cognitive function; a low-fat diet with ω-3 fatty acid or lofepramine use or bee venom therapy for relapses, depression, or fatigue.
-Reflexology may benefit paresthesia and reduce fatigue but not depression.

Sources
-AAN. *Complementary and Alternative Medicine in Multiple Sclerosis.* 2014.
-AAN. *Comprehensive Systemic Rehabilitation in Multiple Sclerosis.* 2015.
-AAN. *Practice Guideline: Disease-modifying Therapies for Adults with Multiple Sclerosis.* 2018.

MUSCLE CRAMPS

Population
-Patients with idiopathic muscle cramps.

Recommendations

▶ AAN 2010

-Data are insufficient on the efficacy of calf stretching in reducing the frequency of muscle cramps.
-AAN recommends that although quinine is likely effective, it should not be used for routine treatment of cramps. Quinine derivatives should be reserved for disabling muscle cramps.
-Quinine derivatives are effective in reducing the frequency of muscle cramps, although the magnitude of benefit is smaller than the serious side effects.

Source
-Katzberg HD, Khan AH, So YT. Assessment: symptomatic treatment for muscle cramps (an evidence-based review): report of the Therapeutics and Technology Assessment Subcommittee of the American Academy of Neurology. *Neurology.* 2010;74(8):691-696.

OSTEOARTHRITIS (OA)

Population
–Adults.

Recommendations

▶ ACR 2012

–Nonpharmacologic recommendations for the management of hand OA:
- Evaluate ability to perform activities of daily living (ADLs).
- Instruct in joint-protection techniques.
- Provide assistive devices to help perform ADLs.
- Instruct in use of thermal modalities.
- Provide splints for trapeziometacarpal joint OA.

–Nonpharmacologic recommendations for the management of knee or hip OA–Pharmacologic options for OA:
- Participate in aquatic exercise.
- Lose weight.
- Start aerobic exercise program.
- Instruct in use of thermal modalities.
- Consider for knee OA:
  ◦ Medially directed patellar taping.
  ◦ Wedged insoles for either medial or lateral compartment OA.
- Topical capsaicin.
- Topical or PO NSAIDs.
- Acetaminophen.
- Tramadol.
- Intraarticular steroids are an option for refractory knee or hip OA.

Source
–http://www.rheumatology.org/practice/clinical/guidelines/PDFs/ACR_OA_Guidelines_FINAL.pdf

Comment
1. The following should *not* be used for OA:
   a. Chondroitin sulfate.
   b. Glucosamine.
   c. Opiates (if possible).

Population
–Adults with osteoarthritis.

Recommendations

▶ NICE 2014

- Exercise is a core treatment to include muscle strengthening and general aerobic fitness.
- Recommends weight loss for people who are obese.
- Recommends against acupuncture, glucosamine, chondroitin, or intraarticular hyaluronan for OA.
- Recommends against arthroscopic lavage and debridement unless knee OA with mechanical locking.
- Recommended oral analgesics include acetaminophen and/or topical NSAIDs first line.
  - Oral NSAIDs or COX-2 inhibitors at the lowest effective dose for breakthrough pain.
  - Topical capsaicin can be used as an adjunct for knee or hand OA.
- Consider referral for joint surgery for people with OA and severe joint symptoms refractory to nonsurgical treatments.

Source

- https://guidelines.gov/summaries/summary/47862

Comment

1. For chronic NSAID use, consider concomitant therapy with a proton pump inhibitor to prevent NSAID-induced ulcers.

Recommendations

▶ AAOS 2017 (Hip OA)

- NSAIDs improve short-term pain, function, or both in patients with symptomatic hip OA.
- Avoid glucosamine sulfate for improving function, reducing stiffness, and decreasing pain associated with hip OA.
- Offer intraarticular corticosteroids to improve function and reduce pain in the short-term for symptomatic hip OA.
- Do not offer intraarticular hyaluronic acid to improve function, reducing stiffness, and reducing pain associated with hip OA.
- Recommend physical therapy to improve function and reduce pain in hip OA associated with mild-to-moderate symptoms.
- Recommend postoperative physical therapy to improve early function for those who have undergone total hip arthroplasty.

OSTEOPOROSIS

Population
–Adults at risk for osteoporosis or who have confirmed osteoporosis.

Recommendations

▶ ICSI 2011, ACP 2017
–Evaluate all patients with a low-impact fracture for osteoporosis.
–Advise smoking cessation and alcohol moderation (≤2 drinks/d).
–Advise 1500-mg elemental calcium daily for established osteoporosis, glucocorticoid therapy, or age >65 y.
–Assess for vitamin D deficiency with a 25-hydroxy vitamin D level.
  • Treat vitamin D deficiency if present.
–Treatment of osteoporosis.
  • Bisphosphonate therapy.
  • Consider estrogen therapy in menopausal women <50 y of age.
  • Consider parathyroid hormone in women with very high risk for fracture.
  • Treat osteoporotic women with pharmacologic therapy for 5 y. Do not monitor bone density during this time.
  • Offer pharmacologic treatment with bisphosphonates to reduce vertebral fracture risk in men with clinically recognized osteoporosis.
–Fall prevention program.
  • Home safety evaluation.
  • Avoid medications that can cause sedation and orthostatic hypotension or affect balance.
  • Assistive walking devices as necessary.

Sources
–https://www.icsi.org/_asset/vnw0c3/Osteo.pdf
–*ACP. Treatment of Low Bone Density or Osteoporosis to Prevent Fractures in Men and Women: A Clinical Practice Guideline Update from the American College of Physicians.* 2017.

Comments
1. All patients should have serial heights and observed for kyphosis.
2. Obtain a lateral vertebral assessment with DXA scan or x-ray if height loss exceeds 4 cm.
3. DXA bone mineral densitometry should be repeated no more than every 12–24 mo.

Population

–Postmenopausal women.

Recommendations

▶ NAMS 2010, AACE 2010, ACOG 2012, ACP 2017

- –Recommend maintaining a healthy weight, eating a balanced diet, avoiding excessive alcohol intake, avoiding cigarette smoking, and utilizing measures to avoid falls.
- –Recommend supplemental calcium 1200 mg/d and vitamin D_3 800–1000 international units (IU)/d.
- –Recommend an annual check of height and weight, and assess for chronic back pain.
- –DXA of the hip, femoral neck, and lumbar spine should be measured in women age ≥65 y or postmenopausal women with a risk factor for osteoporosis.[b]
- –Recommend repeat DXA testing every 1–2 y for women taking therapy for osteoporosis and every 2–5 y for untreated postmenopausal women.
- –Recommend against measurement of biochemical markers of bone turnover.
- –Recommend drug therapy for osteoporosis for:
  - Osteoporotic vertebral or hip fracture.
  - DXA with T score ≤−2.5.
  - DXA with T score ≤−1 to −2.4 and a 10-y risk of major osteoporotic fracture of ≥20% or hip fracture ≥3% based on FRAX calculator, available at http://www.shef.ac.uk/FRAX/
- –Consider the use of hip protectors in women at high risk of falling.
- –Avoid menopausal estrogen therapy, estrogen + progesterone therapy, or raloxifene for osteoporosis treatment.

Sources

- –http://www.guidelines.gov/content.aspx?id=15500
- –https://www.aace.com/files/osteo-guidelines-2010.pdf
- –http://www.guidelines.gov/content.aspx?id=38413

Comments

1. Options for osteoporosis drug therapy:
   a. Bisphosphonates:
      i. First-line therapy.
      ii. Options include alendronate, ibandronate, risedronate, or zoledronic acid.
      iii. Potential risk for jaw osteonecrosis.

[b]Previous fracture after menopause, weight <127 lb, BMI <21 kg/m², parent with a history of hip fracture, current smoker, rheumatoid arthritis, or excessive alcohol intake.

b. Denosumab:
   i. Consider for women at high fracture risk.
c. Raloxifene:
   i. Second-line agent in younger women with osteoporosis.
d. Teriparatide is an option for high fracture risk when bisphosphonates have failed:
   i. Therapy should not exceed 24 mo.
e. Calcitonin:
   i. Third-line therapy for osteoporosis.
   ii. May be used for bone pain from acute vertebral compression
   fractures.
2. Vitamin D therapy should maintain a 25-OH vitamin D level between
   30 and 60 ng/mL.

OSTEOPOROSIS, GLUCOCORTICOID-INDUCED

Population
–Glucocorticoid-induced osteoporosis.

Recommendations

▶ ACR 2017

–All patients receiving glucocorticoid therapy should receive education
and assess risk factors for osteoporosis annually.
–FRAX calculator should be used to place patients at low risk, medium
risk, or high risk for major osteoporotic fracture. Use FRAX with BMD
testing every 1–3 y if never treated for osteoporosis, every 2–3 y
during treatment if on very high-dose glucocorticoids, osteoporosis
fracture at least 18 mo after osteoporosis treatment, poor medication
compliance, or other osteoporosis risk factors present, and every 2–3 y
after completion of osteoporosis treatment.
–If glucocorticoid treatment is expected to last >3 mo, recommend:
   • Weight-bearing or resistance training exercises.
   • Smoking cessation.
   • Limit alcoholic drinks to 1–2 per day.
   • Calcium 1000–1200 mg/d.
   • Vitamin D 600–800 IU/d.
   • Fall risk assessment.
   • Annual 25-OH vitamin D.
   • Baseline and annual height measurement.
   • Assessment of prevalent fragility fractures.
   • X-rays of spine.

- Assessment of degree of osteoporosis medication compliance, if applicable.
–For adults ≥40 y + glucocorticoid use >3 mo:
  - Low-risk group.
    ◦ Optimize calcium/vitamin D intake and lifestyle modifications over treatment with bisphosphonates, teriparatide, denosumab, or raloxifene.
  - Moderate- and high-risk groups.
    ◦ Treat with oral bisphosphonate over calcium/vitamin D alone. Oral bisphosphonate preferred over IV bisphosphonates, teriparatide, denosumab, or raloxifene.
–For adults <40 y + glucocorticoid use >3 mo:
  - Low-risk group.
    ◦ Optimize calcium/vitamin D intake and lifestyle modifications over bisphosphonates.
  - Moderate-to-high-risk groups.
    ◦ Treat with an oral bisphosphonate over calcium/vitamin D alone, or IV bisphosphonates, teriparatide, or raloxifene.

Source
–ACR. American College of Rheumatology Guideline for the Prevention and Treatment of Glucocorticoid-Induced Osteoporosis. *Arthritis Rheumatol.* 2017;69:1521-1537.

Comments

1. Clinical factors that may increase the risk of osteoporotic fracture estimated by FRAX calculator:
   a. BMI <21 kg/m².
   b. Parental history of hip fracture.
   c. Current smoking.
   d. ≥3 alcoholic drinks/d.
   e. Higher glucocorticoid doses or cumulative dose.
   f. IV pulse glucocorticoid use.
   g. Declining central bone mineral density measurement.
2. In women of childbearing potential, first line in those indicated for osteoporosis treatment is oral bisphosphonates. Second line is teriparatide.

PRESSURE ULCERS

Population
–Adults at risk for pressure ulcers.

Recommendations
▶ NICE 2014
–Regular documentation of ulcer size.
–Debride any necrotic tissue if present with sharp debridement or autolytic debridement.
–Nutritional supplementation for patients who are malnourished.
–Recommend a pressure-redistributing foam mattress.
–Negative pressure wound therapy, electrotherapy, or hyperbaric oxygen therapy is not routinely recommended.
–Antibiotics are only indicated for superimposed cellulitis or underlying osteomyelitis.

Source
–http://www.guideline.gov/content.aspx?id=48026

Population
–Patients with pressure ulcers.

Recommendations
▶ ACP 2015
–Recommends nutritional supplementation with protein and amino acids to reduce wound size.
–Use hydrocolloid or foam dressings to reduce wound size.
–Use electrical stimulation as adjunctive therapy to accelerate wound healing.

Source
–https://guidelines.gov/summaries/summary/49050

Comment
1. Moderate-quality evidence supports the addition of electrical stimulation to standard therapy to accelerate healing of Stage II–IV ulcers.

PSORIASIS, PLAQUE-TYPE

Population
–Adults.

Recommendations

▶ AAD 2009

Topical Therapies
–Topical therapies are most effective for mild-to-moderate disease.
–Topical corticosteroids daily—bid:
- Cornerstone of therapy.
- Limit Class I topical steroids to 4 wk maximum.

–Topical agents that have proven efficacy when combined with topical corticosteroids:
- Topical vitamin D analogues.
- Topical tazarotene.
- Topical salicylic acid.

–Emollients applied 1–3 times daily are a helpful adjunct.

Source
–http://www.aad.org/File%20Library/Global%20navigation/
Education%20and%20quality%20care/Guidelines-psoriasis-sec-3.pdf

Comments
1. Approximately 2% of population has psoriasis.
2. Eighty percent of patients with psoriasis have mild-to-moderate disease.
3. Topical steroid toxicity:
   a. Local: skin atrophy, telangiectasia, striae, purpura, or contact dermatitis.
   b. Hypothalamic–pituitary–adrenal axis may be suppressed with prolonged use of medium- to high-potency steroids.

Recommendations

▶ AAD-NPF 2009

–Systemic Therapies
- Indicated for severe, recalcitrant, or disabling psoriasis.
- Methotrexate (MTX):
  ○ Dose: 7.5–30 mg PO weekly.
  ○ Monitor CBC and liver panel monthly.
- Cyclosporine:
  ○ Initial dose: 2.5–3 mg/kg divided bid.
  ○ Monitor for nephrotoxicity, HTN, and hypertrichosis.

- Acitretin:
  - Dose: 10–50 mg PO daily.
  - Monitor: liver panel.

Source
  - http://www.aad.org/File%20Library/Global%20navigation/
    Education%20and%20quality%20care/Guidelines-psoriasis-sec-4.pdf

Comments

1. MTX contraindications: pregnancy, breast-feeding, alcoholism, chronic liver disease, immunodeficiency syndromes, cytopenias, hypersensitivity reaction.
2. Cyclosporine contraindications: CA, renal impairment, uncontrolled HTN.
3. Acitretin contraindications: pregnancy, chronic liver, or renal disease.

PSORIASIS AND PSORIATIC ARTHRITIS

Population
  - Adults.

Recommendations

▶ AAD 2010, AAD-NPF 2019
  - Treatment options for patients with limited plaque-type psoriasis.
    - First-line therapy:
      - Topical corticosteroids.
      - Topical calcipotriene/calcitriol.
      - Topical calcipotriene/steroid.
      - Topical tazarotene.
      - Topical calcineurin inhibitors (flexural surfaces and face).
      - Targeted phototherapy.
    - Second-line therapy:
      - Systemic agents.
  - Treatment of extensive plaque-type psoriasis.
    - First-line therapy:
      - UVB phototherapy ± acitretin.
      - Topical PUVA.
    - Second-line therapy:
      - Acitretin + biologic.
      - Cyclosporine + biologic.
      - Cyclosporine + methotrexate.
      - Methotrexate + biologic.
      - UVB + biologic.

–Treatment of palmoplantar psoriasis.
- First-line therapy:
  ◦ Topical corticosteroids.
  ◦ Topical calcipotriene/calcitriol.
  ◦ Topical calcipotriene/steroid.
  ◦ Topical tazarotene.
- Second-line therapy:
  ◦ Acitretin.
  ◦ Targeted UVB.
  ◦ Topical PUVA.
- Third-line therapy:
  ◦ Adalimumab.
  ◦ Alefacept.
  ◦ Cyclosporine.
  ◦ Etanercept.
  ◦ Infliximab.
  ◦ Methotrexate.
  ◦ Ustekinumab.
–Treatment of erythrodermic psoriasis.
- Acitretin.
- Adalimumab.
- Cyclosporine.
- Infliximab.
- Methotrexate.
- Ustekinumab.
–Treatment of psoriatic arthritis.
- First-line therapy:
  ◦ Adalimumab.
  ◦ Etanercept.
  ◦ Golimumab.
  ◦ Infliximab.
  ◦ Methotrexate.
  ◦ Tumor necrosis factor (TNF) blocker + methotrexate.
- Second-line therapy:
  ◦ Ustekinumab and methotrexate.
–Considerations for comorbidities:
- Consider early and more frequent cardiovascular screening (obesity, HTN, HLD, DM, metabolic syndrome) in patients with psoriasis requiring systemic or phototherapy treatments, or psoriasis involving >10% of BSA.

- Recommend screening for anxiety and depression in patients with psoriasis.
- Recommend smoking cessation and limiting alcohol intake.
- If a concern for comorbid IBD arises, refer the patient back to their PCP or to a gastroenterologist. Avoid IL-17 inhibitor therapy in patients with IBD.

Sources
  –http://www.guideline.gov/content.aspx?id=15650
  –http://www.aad.org/File%20Library/Global%20navigation/
  Education%20and%20quality%20care/Guidelines-psoriasis-sec-2.pdf
  –AAD-NPF. Joint AAD-NPF guidelines of care for the management and treatment of psoriasis with awareness and attention to comorbidities. *J Am Acad Dermatol.* 2019;90:1073-1113.

Comment
  1. Use of potent topical corticosteroids should be limited to 4 wk duration.

RHEUMATOID ARTHRITIS (RA), BIOLOGIC DISEASE-MODIFYING ANTIRHEUMATIC DRUGS (DMARDs)

Population
  –Adults.

Recommendations
▶ ACR 2015
  –DMARDs (biologics or tofacitinib) and tuberculosis (TB) screening:
  - Check a TB skin test or IGRA before initiating these medications.
  - Any patient with latent TB needs at least 1 mo treatment prior to the initiation of a biologic or tofacitinib.
  –Symptomatic early RA:
  - If the disease activity is low, and the patient is naïve to DMARD therapy, use DMARD monotherapy (MTX preferred) over double or triple therapy.
  - If the disease activity is moderate or high, and the patient is naïve to DMARD therapy, use DMARD monotherapy over double or triple therapy.
  - If the disease activity remains moderate or high despite DMARD monotherapy (with or without glucocorticoids), use combination DMARDs, a TNFi, or a non-TNF biologic (all with or without MTX).

- If disease flares, add short-term glucocorticoids at the lowest dose and for the shortest duration possible.
  –Established RA:
    - If disease activity is low and the patient is naïve to DMARD, use DMARD monotherapy (MTX preferred), over TNFi.
    - If disease activity is moderate to high and the patient is naïve to DMARD, use DMARD monotherapy (MTX preferred), over tofacitinib and combination DMARD therapy.
    - If disease activity remains moderate or high despite DMARD monotherapy, use combination DMARDs, add a TNFi, non-TNF biologic, or tofacitinib (all with or without MTX).

Comments

1. Anti-TNFα agents, abatacept, and rituximab all contraindicated in:
   a. Serious bacterial, fungal, and viral infections, or with latent TB.
   b. Acute viral hepatitis or Child's B or Child's C cirrhosis.
   c. Instances of a lymphoproliferative disorder treated ≤5 y ago; decompensated congestive heart failure (CHF); or any demyelinating disorder.
   d. CBCD, LFTs, and Cr should be monitored every 2–4 wk during the first 3 mo, every 8–12 wk during the next 3–6 mo, and every 12 wk thereafter for patients on leflunomide, methotrexate, and sulfasalazine. Only baseline levels are recommended for hydroxychloroquine.
   e. Live attenuated vaccines, if indicated, can be given prior to initiating therapy with TNFi biologics or non-TNF biologics. A 2-wk waiting period is recommended before starting biologics. Live attenuated vaccines are not recommended during therapy with biologics.

Source

–ACR. American College of Rheumatology Guideline for the Treatment of Rheumatoid Arthritis. *Arthritis Care Res.* 2015.

POLYMYALGIA RHEUMATICA

Population

–Adults diagnosed with PMR.

Recommendations

▶ ACR 2015

–Choose glucocorticoid therapy over NSAIDs to treat PMR.
–Initiate glucocorticoids at a minimum dose of 12.5–25 mg prednisone equivalent daily as initial treatment. Avoid doses ≤7.5 mg/d or >30 mg/d.

–Duration of glucocorticoids will be individualized, but a minimum of 12 mo of therapy is assumed. Tapering schedules should be customized based on regular monitoring of disease activity, lab markers, and adverse effects.

–Consider addition of methotrexate (MTX) in patients at high risk of relapse, prolonged therapy, or glucocorticoid-related adverse events (due to comorbidities, concomitant medications).

–Avoid TNFα-blocking agents.

–Consider an individualized exercise program targeting maintenance of muscle mass/function and reducing fall risk.

–Avoid the use of Chinese herbal preparations Yanghe and Biqi.

Source

–ACR. Recommendations for the management of polymyalgia rheumatica. *Arthritis Rheumatol.* 2015(67):2569-2580.

SYSTEMIC LUPUS ERYTHEMATOSUS (SLE, LUPUS)

Population

–Adults.

Recommendations

▶ British Society for Rheumatology (BSR) 2017

–Diagnose lupus in patients with 4 or more of the following symptoms/findings, with at least 1 serological finding and 1 clinical finding, either contemporaneously or sequentially at any time:

- Malar rash.
- Discoid rash.
- Photosensitivity.
- Oral or nasal ulcers.
- Inflammatory arthritis.
- Serositis (ie, pleural effusion, pericardial effusion, pericarditis).
- Renal dysfunction (ie, proteinuria >500 mg/d, cellular casts).
- Neurologic dysfunction (ie, severe headache, altered mental status, seizures, psychosis, mononeuritis multiplex, myelitis, peripheral or cranial neuropathy).
- Hematologic dysfunction (ie, hemolytic anemia, WBC <4000, lymphocytes <1500, platelets <100,000).
- Autoimmune dysfunction (ie, positive anti-DNA Ab, anti-Sm Ab, Lupus Anticoagulant test, or false-positive syphilis FTA).
- Antinuclear antibody (ANA) positivity.

–Mild disease (SLEDAI-2K <6, BILAG C) is characterized by fatigue, malar rash, diffuse alopecia, oral ulcers, arthralgias, myalgias, or platelets 50,000–150,000.
  - Acute treatment: Prednisone ≤20 mg daily, hydroxychloroquine ≤6.5 mg/kg/d, methotrexate 7.5–15 mg/wk, and/or NSAIDs.
  - Maintenance treatment: Prednisone ≤7.5 mg/d, hydroxychloroquine 200 mg/d, and/or methotrexate 10 mg/wk.
–Moderate disease (SLEDAI-2K 6–12, BILAG B) represents potential permanent damage, with fever, rash up to 22% of body surface area, cutaneous vasculitis, alopecia with scalp inflammation, arthritis, pleurisy, pericarditis, hepatitis, or platelets 25,000–50,000.
  - Acute treatment: Prednisone ≤0.5 mg/kg/d AND (azathioprine 1.5–2.0 mg/kg/d OR methotrexate 10–25 mg/wk OR mycophenolate mofetil 2–3 g/d OR cyclosporin ≤2.0 mg/kg/d).
  - Maintenance treatment: Prednisone ≤7.5 mg/d AND azathioprine 50–100 mg/d) OR methotrexate 10 mg/wk OR mycophenolate mofetil 1 g/d OR (cyclosporin 50–100 mg/d AND hydroxychloroquine 200 mg/d).
–Severe disease (SLEDAI-2K >12 or BILAG A) represents organ or life-threatening disease, with rash involving more than 22% of body surface area, myositis, severe pleurisy, and/or pericarditis with effusion, ascites, enteritis, myelopathy, psychosis, acute confusion, optic neuritis, or platelets <25,000.
  - Acute treatment: Prednisone ≤0.5 mg/kg/d and/or IV methylprednisolone 500 mg × 1–3 OR Prednisone ≤0.75–1 mg/kg/d and Azathioprine 2–3 mg/kg/d OR mycophenolate mofetil 2–3 g/d OR cyclosporin 2.5 mg/kg/d.
  - Maintenance treatment: Prednisone 7.5 mg/d AND mycophenolate mofetil 1.0–1.5 g/d OR azathioprine 50–100 mg/d OR cyclosporin 50–100 mg/d and hydroxychloroquine 200 mg/d.
–Consider rituximab and belimumab in patients who do not respond to the regimens above. Consider rituximab especially for patients with severe renal or CNS flare (SLEDAI ≥10). Belimumab is specifically approved for use with antibody positive SLE (anti-dsDNA).
–IVIG and plasmapheresis may be considered in patients with refractory cytopenias, thrombotic thrombocytopenia purpura (TTP), rapid deteriorating acute confusional state, and catastrophic antiphospholipid antibody syndrome.
–Aim to reduce and stop drugs except hydroxychloroquine eventually when in stable remission.
–Test for TPMT (thiopurine S-methyltransferase) activity prior to starting azathioprine:

- • Very low levels of TPMT activity are associated with life-threatening bone marrow toxicity.
- –Assess blood counts weekly as azathioprine doses are increased.
- –Measure serum immunoglobulins prior to starting mycophenolate mofetil, cyclosporin, and rituximab, 3–6 mo later and then annually.
- –Screen for chronic infections (tuberculosis, hepatitis B, hepatitis C, HIV, and HPV) prior to starting immunosuppressive therapy.
- –Encourage high-SPF UV-A and UV-B sunscreen use for patients with photosensitivity symptoms.
- –In patients with stable/low-activity disease, assess the following every 6–12 mo:
  - • Vital signs, vaccination status, modifiable risk factors (hypertension, hyperlipidemia, diabetes, obesity, tobacco use).
  - • Blood count, renal function, liver function, vitamin D3, anti-dsDNA titer, C3/C4 level, urinalysis.
  - • Disease activity using standardized questionnaire (eg, BILAG, SLEDAI, or SLICCC/ACR scores).
  - • Quality of life using standardized questionnaire (eg, Short-form 36 or LupusQoL).
- –In patients with active disease, assess the following every 1–3 mo:
  - • Blood count, renal function, liver function, creatine, anti-dsDNA titer, C3/C4 level, urinalysis.
- –Check anti-Ro and anti-La antibodies prior to pregnancy as these are associated with neonatal lupus.

Comments

1. 5% of the general population will have a positive ANA; 95% of patients with SLE will have a positive ANA.
2. Do not routinely test for ANA or other autoimmune antibodies unless the patient has other signs/symptoms of SLE and a positive result would therefore be diagnostic.
3. Be aware that leukopenia and neutropenia are common in SLE and may therefore be indicative of active disease or a medication side effective.
4. Cyclosporin and tacrolimus may be particularly useful in patients with cytopenias as these medications have this side effect less frequently.
5. Infections, cardiovascular disease, and malignancy are the leading causes of death in patients with SLE.
6. Consider the etiology of an acute flare when treating it. Common causes include medication nonadherence, exposure to sunlight, concurrent or recent infection, hormonal changes, or recent medication changes.

7. CRP is often normal or only mildly elevated in SLE, even with arthritis or serositis. ESR is more sensitive but also not specific.
8. Rising anti-dsDNA antibodies and falling, low complement levels are associated with an acute flare.
   a. 40% of patients with SLE however don't have positive anti-dsDNA antibodies.
9. ANA, anti-Sm, and anti-RNP antibodies do not fluctuate with disease intensity.

Source

–*Rheumatology.* 2018;57(1):e1-e45. https://doi.org/10.1093/rheumatology/kex286

Endocrine and Metabolic Disorders

30

ADRENAL INCIDENTALOMAS

Population
–Adults.

Recommendations

▶AACE 2009

–Evaluate clinically, biochemically, and radiographically for evidence of hypercortisolism, aldosteronism, the presence of pheochromocytoma or a malignant tumor.

–Reevaluate patients who will be managed expectantly at 3–6 mo and then annually for 1–2 y.

Source

–https://www.aace.com/files/adrenal-guidelines.pdf

Comments

1. A 1-mg overnight dexamethasone suppression test can be used to screen for hypercortisolism.
2. Measure plasma-fractionated metanephrines and normetanephrines to screen for pheochromocytoma.
3. Measure plasma renin activity and aldosterone concentration to assess for primary or secondary aldosteronism.

ANDROGEN DEFICIENCY SYNDROME (SEE HYPOGONADISM, MALE)

CUSHING'S SYNDROME (CS)

Population
–Pediatric and adult patients with Cushing's syndrome.

Recommendations
▶ Endocrine Society 2015
- –Treatment goals for Cushing's syndrome
  - Normalize cortisol levels to eliminate the signs and symptoms of CS.
  - Monitor and treat cortisol-dependent comorbidities.
- –Recommend vaccinations against influenza, herpes zoster, pneumococcus.
- –Recommend perioperative thromboprophylaxis for venous thromboembolism.
- –Recommend surgical resection of primary adrenal or ectopic focus underlying CS.
- –Assess postoperative serum cortisol levels.

Source
- –www.endocrine.org/guidelines-and-clinical-practice/clinical-practice-guidelines/treatment-of-cushing-syndrome

DIABETES MELLITUS (DM), TYPE 1

Population
–Children and adults with Type I DM.

Recommendations
▶ ADA 2019
- –Use intensive insulin therapy with >3 injections daily using either basal and prandial insulin or an insulin pump.
- –Patients using multiple insulin injections should self-monitor blood glucose at least 4 times daily.
- –Continuous glucose monitoring in both children and adults results in lower HbA1c levels.
- –Assess psychological and social situation.

–Advise all patients not to smoke.

–Begin screening at age 10, at onset of puberty, or after 5 y with Type 1 DM, whichever is earlier:
  - Urine albumin-to-creatinine ratio annually.
  - Dilated funduscopic exam q 1–2 y.
  - Monofilament screening for diabetic neuropathy annually.
  - Comprehensive foot examination at least annually.

–Screen for other autoimmune conditions at time of diagnosis of Type 1 DM:
  - Celiac disease: IgA tissue transglutaminase antibodies. If negative, rescreen 2 and 5 y after DM diagnosis.
  - Thyroid dysfunction: TSH, thyroperoxidase and thyroglobulin antibodies.

–Fasting lipid panel at age 10 or at onset of puberty, whichever is earlier (consider as early as age 2 y for a strong family history of hyperlipidemia).
  - Repeat annually if results are abnormal or every 5 y if results are acceptable (LDL <100 mg/dL).

–Consider statin therapy if age ≥10 y and LDL ≥160 mg/dL, or LDL ≥130 mg/dL and one or more CVD risk factors.

–Aspirin 75–162 mg/d for adults with:
  - 10-y risk of CVD >10% (primary prevention).
  - Pre-existing CVD (secondary prevention).

Source
–http://care.diabetesjournals.org/content/41/Supplement_1/S126

Comment
1. Glycemic control recommendations for children and adolescents:
   a. Before meals, capillary blood glucose (CPG) 90–130 mg/dL.
   b. Bedtime, CPG 90–150 mg/dL.
   c. HgbA1c <7.5%.

Population
–Adults with type 1 diabetes.

Recommendations
▶ NICE 2016

–Do *not* routinely confirm diagnosis of Type 1 DM by checking C-peptide levels or auto-antibody testing. Consider doing so only if diagnosis is uncertain.

–Provide all adults with DM 1 a structured education program.

–Offer carbohydrate counting education.

–Offer peer support groups.

–Counsel women of childbearing potential on implications for pregnancy and family planning.

–Measure glycohemoglobin every 3–6 mo.

- Fructosamine level is an alternative test for anemic patients.

–Recommend self-glucose monitoring at least 4 times daily.

–Glucose targets are:

- 90–126 mg/dL fasting.
- 72–126 mg/dL before meals.
- 90–162 mg/dL 90 min after meals.
- HbA1c ≤6.5%.

–Basal insulin

- Insulin detemir BID is preferred.
- Daily insulin glargine is acceptable if BID detemir isn't acceptable or tolerated.

–Recommend rapid-acting prandial insulin analogs (vs. human or animal insulin) before meals.

–Educate patients on prevention and management of hypoglycemia and hyperglycemia, including DKA.

–Consider referral for islet cell transplantation in those with recurrent severe hypoglycemia.

–Screen adults with low BMI for celiac disease.

–Measure a TSH annually.

–Recommend therapy with ACEI or ARB for patients with hypertension or diabetic nephropathy.

–Offer digital retinopathy screening annually.

–Offer men with DM 1 and erectile dysfunction a phosphodiesterase-5 inhibitor.

–Do *not* offer aspirin for primary prevention of CVD to adults with Type 1 DM.

Source

–https://nice.org.uk/guidance/ng17

DIABETES MELLITUS (DM), TYPE 2

Population

–Nonpregnant adults.

Recommendations

▶ AACE/ACE 2018

–Lifestyle optimization is essential for all patients with diabetes but should not delay starting pharmacotherapy.

–Weight loss: reduced-calorie meal plan, physical activity, behavioral intervention, consider weight-loss medication.

–HbA1c target ≤6.5% is optimal, but higher targets may be appropriate for patients who are older and with other serious illness.

–Individualize medication regimens and blood glucose targets (fasting and postprandial) based on patient-specific factors (likely adherence, cost, and comorbidities such as heart, kidney, and liver disease).

–Minimize the risks of hypoglycemia, weight gain, and other adverse drug reactions.

–Control lipids and blood pressure.

–Metformin is first-line medication but combination therapy is usually necessary. Choose agents with complementary mechanisms of action.

–Monitor therapy Q 3 mo until stable (HbA1c, self-monitor blood glucose records, weight, BP, lipids).

Source

–https://www.aace.com/sites/all/files/diabetes-algorithm-executive-summary.pdf

▶ ADA 2019

–Use a multidisciplinary team-based model (including physicians, nurses, dietitians, exercise specialists, dentists, podiatrists, mental health, etc.). Assess barriers to care including food, housing, and financial insecurity as well as literacy and numeracy. Refer to available community resources.

–Perform a complete medical evaluation at initial visit to confirm dx and classify type, evaluate for complications and comorbidities, review previous treatment, and develop a collaborative care plan.

–On follow-up, address interval medical history, medication adherence, side effects, lab evaluation, nutrition, psychosocial health, routine health maintenance screening, and immunizations.

–Provide diabetes self-management education and support (DSMES) at appropriate intervals including education about hypoglycemia management and adjustments during illness.

–Check HgbA1c every 3 mo if therapy has changed or if blood glucose control is inadequate. Check A1c at least twice a year in well-controlled patients. Reassess glycemic targets over time based on patient-specific criteria.

–Glycemic control recommendations:
  • Preprandial glucose: 70–130 mg/dL.
  • Postprandial glucose: <180 mg/dL (1–2 h postmeals).
  • HgbA1c <7%.
  • Less (>8%) or more stringent (<6.5%) goals may be appropriate for select patients.

–Assess for symptomatic/asymptomatic hypoglycemia (BG <70 mg/dL) at each visit.

–Reevaluate treatment regimen and glycemic targets if hypoglycemia unawareness or level 3 hypoglycemia (altered mental/physical functioning requiring assistance).

–Prescribe glucagon to patients at high risk of level 2 hypoglycemia (BG <54 mg/dL).

–Prescribe metformin as initial pharmacological agent and continue as long as tolerated.

–Initiate dual therapy if A1c is more than 1.5% above target. Individualize medication regimen based on comorbidities, cost, hypoglycemia risk, weight effect, and patient preference.

–Consider initiating insulin if ongoing catabolic weight loss, symptomatic hyperglycemia, A1c >10% or BG >300 mg/dL.

–Recommend ACEI or ARB for patients with hypertension and diabetes with urinary albumin-to-creatinine ratio >30 mg/g creatinine or eGFR <60 mL/min/1.73 m^2.

–Optimize BP and glycemic control to prevent progression of diabetic kidney disease and use antihyperglycemic agents demonstrated to reduce CKD progression.

–Refer patients with any evidence of diabetic retinopathy to ophthalmologist.

–Treat diabetic neuropathic pain with pregabalin, duloxetine, or gabapentin.

–Perform foot examination at every visit for high-risk patients, and annually for lower risk patients.

–Additionally, recommend the following:
  • Immunizations:
    ◦ Annual influenza vaccination if age ≥6 mo.
    ◦ Pneumococcal polysaccharide vaccine if age >2 y.
    ◦ Revaccinate with pneumococcal polysaccharide vaccine when age ≥65 y *and* >5 y since the first dose.
    ◦ Hepatitis B vaccination if unvaccinated and age 19–59 y.

- Recommend at least 150 min/wk of moderate aerobic physical activity.
- Advise against tobacco use and provide smoking cessation counseling/treatment.
- Weight loss:
  - Recommend weight loss >5% for all overweight or obese diabetic patients.
  - Individualize diet and exercise regimen to achieve 500–750 kcal/d energy deficit.
  - Provide resources to maintain long-term weight-loss goals.
  - Recommend bariatric surgery for good surgical candidates with BMI ≥40 kg/m^2 (≥37.5 kg/m^2 in Asian-Americans), or ≥35 kg/m^2 without durable weight loss and poor diabetes control with nonsurgical methods.
- Blood pressure control:
  - Monitor blood pressure at every visit.
  - Target BP <130/80 mm Hg if 10-y ASCVD risk >15% or existing ASCVD, and <140/90 for lower risk patients.
  - Initiate lifestyle therapies, weight loss, DASH diet for BP >120/80.
  - Recommend single-agent pharmacotherapy for BP >140/90 and two drug therapy for BP <160/100.
  - Use agents demonstrated to reduce cardiovascular events in patients with diabetes.
- Lipid control:
  - High-intensity statin therapy if diabetes plus existing ASCVD or 10-y ASCVD risk >20%.
  - Moderate-intensity statin therapy if >40 y and no ASCVD, or <40 y with ASCVD risk.
  - Add LDL-lowering therapy if LDL >70 mg/dL on max statin with existing CVD.
- ASA 75–162 mg/d if:
  - Primary prevention of ASCVD if 10-y risk of CAD >10%.
  - Secondary prevention of existing ASCVD.
- Check annually:
  - Urine albumin-to-creatinine ratio.
  - eGFR and serum creatinine.
  - Fasting lipid profile.
  - Dilated funduscopic exam.
  - Monofilament screening for diabetic neuropathy.
  - Comprehensive foot exam

–Consider assessing patients for the following comorbidities that are increased with DM:
- Hearing impairment.
- Obstructive sleep apnea.
- Fatty liver disease.
- Low testosterone in men.
- Periodontal disease.
- Cognitive impairment.

Source
–https://clinical.diabetesjournals.org/content/37/1/11

Comments

1. Metformin may cause vitamin B12 deficiency; consider periodic monitoring of vitamin B12 levels especially in patients with anemia or neuropathy. Avoid if eGFR <30 mL/min or unstable CHF.
2. Several SGLT2 inhibitors and GLP1 receptor agonists have demonstrated cardiovascular benefit and reduced risk of diabetic kidney disease progression.
   a. Recommend addition of SGLT2 inhibitors and GLP1 receptor agonists with demonstrated benefit to patients with ASCVD or CKD as second-line agent after metformin.
   b. SGLT2 inhibitors are preferred in patients with heart failure.
   c. Consider GLP1 receptor agonist as first-line injectable medication before insulin.
3. ACEIs or ARBs are first-line antihypertensives. Second-line antihypertensives are dihydropyridine calcium channel blockers, thiazide diuretic if GFR $\geq$30 mL/min/1.73 m² or a loop diuretic if GFR <30 mL/min/1.73 m².

▶ ACP 2017, 2018

–Prescribe metformin as initial therapy for improved glycemic control.
–Add either a sulfonylurea, a thiazolidinedione, an SGLT-s inhibitor, or a DPP-4 inhibitor to metformin when a second agent is required, based on discussion of benefits, adverse effects, and cost.
–Personalize goals for glycemic control to patient's preferences regarding benefits and harms of therapy, treatment burden, costs, and life expectancy.
–Aim for HbA1c between 7% and 8%.
–De-intensify therapy if HbA1c <6.5%.
–Avoid targeting HbA1c level in patients with life expectancy <10 y due to age (80 and older), residence in nursing home, or

chronic conditions[a]; rather, treat to minimize symptoms related to hyperglycemia.

Sources
−*Ann Intern Med.* 2017;166:279-290.
−*Ann Intern Med.* 2018;168:569-576.

▶ International Diabetes Federation 2017
- −General target for HbA1c in Type 2 diabetes (T2D) is <7%; up to 8% may be appropriate in patients with <10-y life expectancy.
- −Self-monitored blood glucose (SMBG) is mandatory for patients using insulin, and useful when adjusting medications, during acute illness, as an education tool for self-care.
- −Patient education is a cornerstone to diabetes management and should, at a minimum, involve the PCP, a trained diabetic educator, and a structured education program.
- −Lifestyle recommendations include: weight loss, exercise (150 min/wk), a high-fiber, low-glycemic index foods diet, and smoking cessation.
- −Consider anti-obesity drugs in T2D patients with BMI ≥27 kg/m².
- −Encourage smoking cessation and limiting alcohol intake.
- −Consider referral to bariatric surgery in T2D patients with BMI ≥35 kg/m², or BMI 30–35 kg/m² who have not responded to regular treatment.
- −Pharmacotherapy:
  - Metformin is preferred choice for monotherapy.[b]
  - Considering starting two agents if the HbA1c is 1%–2% or more above target.
    - Combination therapy should be metformin plus sulfonylurea (SU),[c] DPP4 inhibitor, SGLT2 inhibitor,[d] or GLP1 receptor agonist.[e]
- −BP goal is 130–140/80; SBP of 130 is recommended in younger patients and those with CV risk or microvascular disease.
  - Start with an ACEI or ARB; add a calcium channel blocker or a thiazide diuretic if needed.
  - An ACEI or ARB should also be started if the patient has microalbuminuria in the absence of high BP.

---

[a]In patients with dementia, cancer, ESRD, and severe COPD or CHF, intensive HbA1c-directed antihyperglycemic therapy resulted in harms outweighing benefits (UKPDS Trial).
[b]Titrate metformin from 500 to 2000 mg/d to minimize GI side effects.
[c]When starting an SU, the patient must learn how to prevent, recognize, and treat hypoglycemia.
[d]SGLT2 inhibitors reduce major cardiovascular events in patients with T2D and are preferred in patients with CVD.
[e]GLP1 RA can be used if weight loss is a priority and the drug is affordable.

–Prescribe a high-intensity statin for patients with:

- T2D and established CVD (secondary prevention).
- T2D without CVD who are >40 y with LDL >100 mg/dL (primary prevention).

–Start low-dose aspirin (75–350 mg/d) in patients with T2D and CVD (secondary prevention).

–Additional recommendations:

- Screen for depression (eg, PHQ-2).
- Retina screening every 1–2 y with retinal photography.
- Annual urine microalbumin-to-creatinine ratio.
  - Annual serum creatinine and eGFR if albuminuria or HTN is present.
- Annual monofilament foot exam for peripheral neuropathy.
- Frequent foot exams at office visits.
- Screen for peripheral vascular disease by checking foot pulses and/or calculating the ankle/brachial index.
- Routine screening for CAD is not recommended for asymptomatic patients.
- T2D patients who observe Ramadan should interrupt their fast if SMBG is <70 or >300. High-risk patients are advised not to fast at all.

Source

–International Diabetes Federation. *Recommendations for Managing Type 2 Diabetes in Primary Care.* 2017. www.idf.org/managing-type2-diabetes

Comments

1. Metformin, smoking cessation, blood pressure control, and statins consistently improve cardiovascular outcomes.
2. Glycemic control is a staple of care, but controversy exists regarding optimal A1c goals for ambulatory adults. Advocates of tighter control (ie, <7) rely on data from several trials (ACCORD, ADVANCE, UKPDS, VADT) that show improvements in surrogate markers (ie, nerve conduction velocity) but not patient-oriented outcomes (ie, painful neuropathy or mortality) with tighter control. Advocates of more permissive control (ie, <8%) point to potential harm from medication burden and hypoglycemia and the absence of evidence for patient-oriented benefit in tighter control of type 2 DM.
3. The largest trials for glycemic control do not include SGLT2 inhibitors or GLP-1 receptor agonists, which may provide some cardiovascular benefit apart from glycemic reduction.

Population
–Hospitalized adults older than 18 y.

Recommendations

AAFP 2017
–Avoid intensive insulin therapy in hospitalized patients (even in ICU).
–Target blood glucose level of 140–180 mg/dL if insulin therapy is used in hospitalized patients, especially those who are critically ill.
–Either basal insulin or basal plus bolus correctional insulin may be used in the treatment of hospitalized patients; sliding scale regimens are no longer recommended.

Source
–https://www.aafp.org/journalpdfrestricted/afp/2017/1115/p648.pdf

Comment
1. Intensive insulin therapy in SICU/MICU patients does not improve mortality but has a 5-fold increased risk of hypoglycemia.

Population
–Children and adolescents with newly diagnosed DM2.

Recommendations

▶AAP 2013
–Initiate insulin therapy for children with:
  • Diabetic ketoacidosis.
  • HbA1c >9%.
  • Random glucose >250 mg/dL.
–Diet, exercise, and metformin are initial therapy for other situations.
–Recommend moderate-to-vigorous exercise for 60 min daily.
–Limit nonacademic screen time to <2 h/d.
–Monitor HbA1c every 3 mo.
–Desire HbA1c <7%.

Source
–pediatrics.aappublications.org/content/131/2/364.full.pdf

ORAL DIABETES MELLITUS TYPE 2 AGENTS—CPG 2015

Category	Metformin	DPP-4I	GLP-1 RA	TZD	AGI	Colesevelam	BCR-QR	SU/MGN	Insulin	SGLT-2	Pramlintide
Hypoglycemia	Neutral	Neutral	Neutral	Neutral	Neutral	Neutral	Neutral	Moderate/severe/mild	Moderate/severe	Neutral	Neutral
Weight	Slight loss	Neutral	Loss	Gain	Neutral	Neutral	Neutral	Gain	Gain	Loss	Loss
Renal/GU	CI if Crt >1.4 (W) Crt >1.5 (M) CrCl <50 mL/min	Dose adjust if CrCl <30 mL/min	CI if CrCl <30 mL/min	Fluid retention	Neutral	Neutral	Neutral	Renal impairment increases hypoglycemia	Renal impairment increases hypoglycemia	Infection; CI if CrCl <45 mL/min	Neutral
Gastrointestinal[a]	Moderate	Neutral	Moderate	CI in cirrhosis	Moderate	Mild	Moderate	Neutral	Neutral	Neutral	Moderate
CHF	Neutral	Neutral	Neutral	Moderate	Neutral	Neutral	Neutral	Neutral	Neutral	Neutral	Neutral
CVD	Benefit	Neutral	Neutral	Slight risk	Neutral	Neutral	Neutral	Unclear	Neutral	Orthostasis in elderly	Neutral
Bone loss	Neutral	Neutral	Neutral	Moderate	Neutral	Neutral	Neutral	Neutral	Neutral	Small	Neutral
Miscellaneous	B_{12} deficiency	–	–	–	–	–	–	SIADH/headaches	–	–	Avoid with gastroparesis; headache

AGI, alphaglucosidase inhibitors; BCR-QR, bromocriptine quick release; CI, contraindicated; CVD, cardiovascular disease; DPP-4I, dipeptidyl peptidase-4 inhibitor; GLP-1 RA, glucagon-like peptide-1 receptor antagonist; GU, genitourinary; MGN, meglitinides; SIADH, syndrome of inappropriate antidiuretic hormone; SGLT-2, salt glucose contransporter 2; SU, sulfonylurea; TZD, thiazolidinediones.

[a]GI symptoms can include nausea, vomiting, flatulence, diarrhea, anorexia, and pancreatitis (for GLP-1 RA).

Source: Garber A, et al. *Endocr Pract.* 2013;19:327. Reprinted with permission from American Association of Clinical Endocrinologists © 2013 AACE.

INJECTABLE MEDICATIONS FOR DM 2

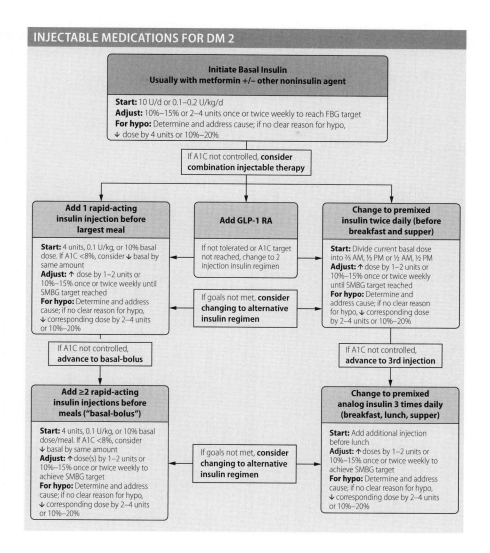

Initiate Basal Insulin
Usually with metformin +/− other noninsulin agent

Start: 10 U/d or 0.1–0.2 U/kg/d
Adjust: 10%–15% or 2–4 units once or twice weekly to reach FBG target
For hypo: Determine and address cause; if no clear reason for hypo,
↓ dose by 4 units or 10%–20%

If A1C not controlled, **consider combination injectable therapy**

Add 1 rapid-acting insulin injection before largest meal

Start: 4 units, 0.1 U/kg, or 10% basal dose. If A1C <8%, consider ↓ basal by same amount
Adjust: ↑ dose by 1–2 units or 10%–15% once or twice weekly until SMBG target reached
For hypo: Determine and address cause; if no clear reason for hypo, ↓ corresponding dose by 2–4 units or 10%–20%

Add GLP-1 RA

If not tolerated or A1C target not reached, change to 2 injection insulin regimen

If goals not met, **consider changing to alternative insulin regimen**

Change to premixed insulin twice daily (before breakfast and supper)

Start: Divide current basal dose into ⅔ AM, ⅓ PM or ½ AM, ½ PM
Adjust: ↑ dose by 1–2 units or 10%–15% once or twice weekly until SMBG target reached
For hypo: Determine and address cause; if no clear reason for hypo, ↓ corresponding dose by 2–4 units or 10%–20%

If A1C not controlled, **advance to basal-bolus**

If A1C not controlled, **advance to 3rd injection**

Add ≥2 rapid-acting insulin injections before meals ("basal-bolus")

Start: 4 units, 0.1 U/kg, or 10% basal dose/meal. If A1C <8%, consider ↓ basal by same amount
Adjust: ↑ dose(s) by 1–2 units or 10%–15% once or twice weekly to achieve SMBG target
For hypo: Determine and address cause; if no clear reason for hypo, ↓ corresponding dose by 2–4 units or 10%–20%

If goals not met, **consider changing to alternative insulin regimen**

Change to premixed analog insulin 3 times daily (breakfast, lunch, supper)

Start: Add additional injection before lunch
Adjust: ↑ doses by 1–2 units or 10%–15% once or twice weekly to achieve SMBG target
For hypo: Determine and address cause; if no clear reason for hypo, ↓ corresponding dose by 2–4 units or 10%–20%

DIABETES MELLITUS TYPE 2 MANAGEMENT

Start with Monotherapy unless:

A1C is greater than or equal to 9%, consider Dual Therapy.

A1C is greater than or equal to 10%, blood glucose is greater than or equal to 300 mg/dL, or patient is markedly symptomatic, consider Combination Injectable Therapy.

	Monotherapy	Metformin					Lifestyle Management
EFFICACY		high					
HYPO RISK		low risk					
WEIGHT		neutral/loss					
SIDE EFFECTS		GI/lactic acidosis					
COSTS		low					

If A1C target not achieved after approximately 3 mo of monotherapy, proceed to 2-drug combination (order not meant to denote any specific preference—choice dependent on a variety of patient- and disease-specific factors):

Dual Therapy

Metformin +

| | Lifestyle Management |

	Sulfonylurea	Thiazolidinedione	DPP-4 inhibitor	SGLT2 inhibitor	GLP-1 receptor agonist	Insulin (basal)
EFFICACY	high	high	intermediate	intermediate	high	highest
HYPO RISK	moderate risk	low risk	low risk	low risk	low risk	high risk
WEIGHT	gain	gain	neutral	loss	loss	gain
SIDE EFFECTS	hypoglycemia	edema, HF, fxs	rare	GU, dehydration, fxs	GI	hypoglycemia
COSTS	low	low	high	high	high	high

If A1C target not achieved after approximately 3 mo of dual therapy, proceed to 3-drug combination (order not meant to denote any specific preference—choice dependent on a variety to patient- and disease-specific factors):

Triple Therapy

Metformin +

| | Lifestyle Management |

Sulfonylurea +	Thiazolidinedione +	DPP-4 inhibitor +	SGLT2 inhibitor +	GLP-1 receptor agonist+	Insulin (basal) +
TZD	SU	SU	SU	SU	TZD
or DPP-4-i	or DPP-4-i	or TZD	or TZD	or TZD	or DPP-4-i
or SGLT2-i	or SGLT2-i	or SGLT2-i	or DPP-4-i	or SGLT2-i	or SGLT2-i
or GLP-1-RA	or GLP-1-RA	or Insulin³	or GLP-1-RA	or Insulin³	or GLP-1-RA
or Insulin³	or Insulin³		or Insulin³		

If A1C target not achieved after approximately 3 mo of triple therapy and patient (1) on oral combination, move to basal insulin or GLP-1 RA, (2) on GLP-1 RA, add basal insulin, or (3) on optimally titrated basal insulin, add GLP-1 RA or mealtime insulin. Metformin therapy should be maintained, while other oral agents may be discontinued on an individual basis to avoid unnecessarily complex or costly regimens (ie, adding a fourth antihyperglycemic agent).

Combination Injectable Therapy

Sources
- –https://professional.diabetes.org/sites/professional.diabetes.org/files/media/dc_40_s1_final.pdf and Inzucchi SE, et al. *Diabetes Care.* 2015;38:140-149.
- –Qaseem A, Barry MJ, Humphrey LL, Forciea MA; Clinical Guidelines Committee of the American College of Physicians. Oral pharmacologic treatment of type 2 diabetes mellitus: a clinical practice guideline update from the American College of Physicians. *Ann Intern Med.* 2017;166(4):279-290.

HYPOGONADISM, MALE

Population
- –Adults.

Recommendations
▶ Endocrine Society 2018
- –Obtain an AM total testosterone level for men with symptoms and signs of androgen deficiency.[f]
- –Confirm diagnosis with a second AM total testosterone level.
- –Measure a serum luteinizing hormone (LH) and follicular stimulating hormone (FSH) in all men with testosterone deficiency to distinguish between primary and secondary hypogonadism.
- –Obtain a dual-energy x-ray absorptiometry (DEXA) scan for all men with severe androgen deficiency.
- –Testosterone therapy is indicated for androgen deficiency syndromes unless contraindications exist.[g]

Source
- –https://academic.oup.com/jcem/article/103/5/1715/4939465

▶EAU 2018
- –Consider testosterone testing in men with:
  - • Pituitary masses.
  - • Obesity.
  - • Metabolic syndrome.
  - • Moderate-to-severe COPD.

---

[f]Lethargy, easy fatigue, lack of stamina or endurance; reduced libido, decreased spontaneous erections; male infertility; mood changes; gynecomastia, loss of body hair, small testes; osteopenia/osteoporosis.

[g]Breast cancer, prostate cancer, hematocrit >50%, PSA >4 ng/mL, desire for fertility in the near term, MI or CVA within last 6 mo, untreated severe obstructive sleep apnea, severe obstructive urinary symptoms, or uncontrolled heart failure.

- Infertility.
- Osteoporosis.
- HIV infection.
- DM type 2.
- Chronic use of corticosteroids and/or opiates.
- Signs and symptoms of hypogonadism:
  - Reduced testis volume.
  - Gynecomastia.
  - Decreased lean body mass and muscle strength.
  - Decreased body/facial hair.
  - Erectile dysfunction.
  - Reduced libido.
  - Changes in mood and/or cognitive function.
  - Fatigue, decreased stamina/endurance.

–Diagnose hypogonadism if morning total testosterone level is less than 300 mg/dL on two separate occasions.
- Measure LH and FSH to differentiate between primary and secondary hypogonadism.

–Indications for testosterone treatment are patients with low testosterone and:
- Symptoms of hypogonadism.
- Delayed puberty.
- Klinefelter syndrome.
- Sexual dysfunction not responding to PDE5Is.
- Low bone mass.
- Hypopituitarism.

–Contraindications to testosterone use:
- Locally advanced or metastatic prostate cancer.
  - May consider treatment in men with symptomatic hypogonadism, treated for localized prostate cancer with no evidence of active disease.
- Male breast cancer.
- Men who desire fertility in the near term.
- Hematocrit >54%.
- Severe CHF (NYHA Class IV).

–Monitor clinical response to therapy, testosterone level, PSA, digital prostate exam, and hematocrit 3, 6, and 12 mo after starting therapy, and annually thereafter.

Source
–https://uroweb.org/guideline/male-hypogonadism/

▶AUA 2018

–Diagnose hypogonadism when morning total testosterone level is less than 300 mg/dL on two separate occasions *and* patient has symptoms of hypogonadism.

–Measure luteinizing hormone (LH) if testosterone level is low.

• If LH is low/low-normal in the setting of low testosterone, check a prolactin level.

–Measure serum estradiol in testosterone-deficient patients who present with breast symptoms or gynecomastia prior to the commencement of testosterone therapy.

–Obtain a hemoglobin and hematocrit (and PSA in men over 40 y) prior to initiating testosterone therapy.

• Educate patients about the risk of polycythemia.

–Testosterone therapy should not be commenced for a period of 3–6 mo in patients with a history of cardiovascular events.

–Adjust testosterone therapy dosing to achieve a total testosterone level in the middle tertile of the normal reference range.

–Educate patients on the risk of transference with topical testosterone gels/creams.

–Consider stopping testosterone therapy after 3–6 mo in patients who normalized total testosterone levels but fail to achieve improvement in clinical signs or symptoms.

Source

–http://www.auanet.org/guidelines/testosterone-deficiency-(2018)#x7697

Comment

1. Testosterone therapy options: (treatment goal is to obtain a total testosterone level in mid-normal range)

a. Testosterone enanthate or cypionate: 150–200 mg IM every 2 wk, or 75–100 mg IM weekly.

b. Testosterone transdermal patch: 4–6 mg daily.

c. Testosterone 1% gel: 50–100 mg daily.

d. Testosterone 2% gel: 10–70 mg daily.

e. Testosterone 2% solution: 60–120 mg (2–4 pumps or twists) applied to the axillae daily.

f. Testosterone buccal bioadhesive tablets: 30 mg to buccal mucosa q12h.

g. Testosterone nasal gel: 11 mg (2 pump actuations, 1 actuation per nostril) TID.

MENOPAUSE

Population
–Menopausal women.

Recommendations

▶AACE 2017

–Indications for menopausal hormone therapy:
- Severe menopausal symptoms.
- Severe vulvovaginal atrophy.
- Treatment of osteoporosis.

–Cautions with menopausal hormone therapy:
- Avoid unopposed estrogen use in women with an intact uterus.
- Micronized progesterone is considered the safer alternative for women needing progesterone.
- Consider transdermal or topical estrogens which may reduce the risk of VTE.
- Use hormonal therapy in the lowest effective dose for the shortest duration possible.
- Custom-compounded bioidentical hormone therapy is *not* recommended.
- Hormone replacement is *not* appropriate for prevention or treatment of dementia, diabetes, or cardiovascular disease (CVD).
- Avoid if at high risk for VTE.

–Contraindications of menopausal hormone therapy:
- History of breast CA.
- Suspected estrogen-sensitive malignancy.
- Undiagnosed vaginal bleeding.
- Endometrial hyperplasia.
- History of VTE.
- Untreated hypertension.
- Active liver disease.
- Porphyria cutanea tarda.

Source
www.aace.com/files/position-statements/ep171828ps.pdf

Comments
1. Use of hormone therapy should always occur after a thorough discussion of the risks, benefits, and alternatives of this treatment with the patient.

    2. SSRIs or gabapentin may offer relief of menopausal symptoms for women at high risk from hormone replacement therapy.

        a. Do not use paroxetine or fluoxetine in breast cancer patients as they inhibit the effect of tamoxifen.

Recommendations

▶NICE 2015

    −Consider short-term (<5 y) hormone replacement therapy (HRT) for:

      • Severe vasomotor symptoms.

      • Menopause-related depression.

      • Poor libido.

      • Urogenital atrophy.

    −Consider adjuvant testosterone therapy for decreased libido despite HRT.

    −Offer vaginal estrogen cream for urogenital atrophy (even if already on systemic estrogen).

Source

    −https://www.nice.org.uk/guidance/ng23/chapter/Recommendations#managing-short-term-menopausal-symptoms

Comments

    1. Review risks of HRT before initiating:

        a. Venous thromboembolism (VTE): the risk is greater for oral than transdermal preparations.

        b. HRT with estrogen and progestrogen may slightly increase risk of breast cancer but declines after stopping HRT.

    2. Review benefits of HRT:

        a. Risk of fragility fracture is decreased while taking HRT but this benefit decreases once treatment stops.

Recommendations

▶Endocrine Society 2015

    −Offer HRT for severe vasomotor symptoms in women less than 60 y who do not have excess cardiovascular or breast cancer risk.

    −Offer nonhormonal remedies for women at high risk of CVD or breast cancer.

      • Options include an SSRI, SNRI, gabapentin, or pregabalin.

      • Clonidine is an option for women with severe vasomotor symptoms who do not respond to or tolerate nonhormonal modalities.

    −For women at moderate risk of CVD, recommend transdermal estradiol and micronized progesterone for severe vasomotor symptoms.

–Offer vaginal estrogen cream for urogenital atrophy unless history of a hormone-dependent cancer.

–Consider ospemifene trial for moderate-to-severe dyspareunia (except in women with a history of breast cancer).

Source
–https://www.endocrine.org/guidelines-and-clinical-practice/clinical-practice-guidelines/treatment-of-menopause

OBESITY

MANAGEMENT OF OBESITY IN MATURE ADOLESCENTS AND ADULTS

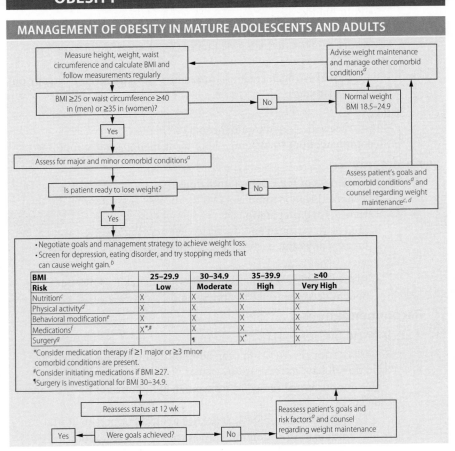

[a]**Minor comorbid conditions:** cigarette smoking; hypertension; LDL cholesterol >130 mg/dL; HDL cholesterol <40 mg/dL (men) or <50 mg/dL (women); glucose intolerance; family history of premature CAD; age ≥65 y (men) or ≥55 y (women).

Major comorbid conditions: waist circumference ≥40 in. (men) or ≥35 in. (women); CAD; peripheral vascular disease; abdominal aortic aneurysm; symptomatic carotid artery disease; type 2 diabetes; and obstructive sleep apnea.

[b]Sulfonylureas; thiazolidinediones; olanzapine, clozapine; risperidone, quetiapine; lithium; paroxetine, citalopram, sertraline; carbamazepine; pregabalin; corticosteroids; megestrol acetate; cyproheptadine; tricyclic antidepressants; monoamine oxidase inhibitors; mirtazapine; valproic acid; and gabapentin.

[c]Encourage a healthy, balanced diet including daily intake of ≥5 servings of fruits/vegetables; 35 g fiber; <30% calories from fat; eliminate takeout, fast foods, soda, and desserts; dietitian consultation for a calorie reduction between 500 and 1000 kcal/kg/d to achieve a 1–2 lb weight reduction per week.

[d]Recommend 30–60 min of moderate activity at least 5 d/wk.

[e]Identify behaviors that may contribute to weight gain (stress, emotional eating, boredom) and use cognitive behavioral counseling, stimulus control, relapse prevention, and goal setting to decrease caloric intake and increase physical activity.

[f]Medications that are FDA approved for weight loss: phentermine; orlistat; lorcaserin phendimetrazine; diethylpropion; and benzphetamine can be used for up to 3 mo as an adjunct for weight loss. Avoid phentermine and diethylpropion in patients with uncontrolled HTN or a history of heart disease.

[g]Bariatric surgery is indicated for patients at high risk for complications. They should be motivated, psychologically stable, have no surgical contraindications, and must accept the operative risk involved.

Source: Adapted from the ICSI Guideline on the Prevention and Management of Obesity; available at http://www. icsi.org/obesity/obesity_3398.html and from pharmacologic management of obesity: an Endocrine Society CPG available at https://academic.oup.com/jcem/article/100/2/342/2813109/Pharmacological-Management-of-Obesity-An-Endocrine.

POLYCYSTIC OVARY SYNDROME

Population
–Women diagnosed with PCOS.

Recommendations
▶ACOG 2018

-Recommend increase in exercise combined with dietary change to reduce diabetes risk and promote weight loss.

-Prescribe combination low-dose hormonal contraceptives for primary treatment of menstrual disorders.

-Screen women with PCOS for cardiovascular risk, metabolic syndrome, and type 2 diabetes (fasting glucose followed by 2-h GTT after 75-g glucose load).

-Consider addition of insulin-sensitizing agent (such as metformin) to decrease androgen levels, improve ovulation rate, improve glucose tolerance, and reduce cardiovascular risk.

-Prescribe letrozole as first-line therapy for ovulation induction in women with PCOS who desire to conceive.

Comments

1. Letrozole has shown increased live birth rate compared with clomiphene citrate.
2. There may be higher pregnancy rates with clomiphene citrate in addition to metformin than with clomiphene alone, particularly in obese women with PCOS.
3. Second-line intervention for failure of pregnancy with letrozole or clomiphene is exogenous gonadotropins or laparoscopic ovarian surgery.
4. Women in ethnic groups at higher risk of nonclassical congenital adrenal hyperplasia should be screened with a fasting 17-hydroxyprogesterone level (normal <2–4 ng/mL).
5. Lower BMI is associated with improved pregnancy rates, decreased hirsutism, and lower risk for metabolic syndrome.
6. There is no clear primary treatment for hirsutism in PCOS, but the addition of eflornithine to laser treatment is superior to laser alone.

Source
–https://journals.lww.com/greenjournal/Fulltext/2018/06000/ACOG_Practice_Bulletin_No__194___Polycystic_Ovary.54.aspx

THYROID DISEASE, HYPERTHYROIDISM

Population
–Nonpregnant adults.

Recommendations

▶American Thyroid Association 2016, AACE 2013

–Determine etiology of thyrotoxicosis. If the diagnosis is not apparent, consider obtaining a thyroid receptor antibody level (TRAb) +/– determination of the radioactive iodine uptake (RAIU).
–Use beta-adrenergic blockade in all patients with symptomatic thyrotoxicosis.
–Treat patients with overt Graves' hyperthyroidism with either radioiodine (RAI) therapy, antithyroid drugs (ATDs), or thyroidectomy.
–Obtain a pregnancy test within 48 h prior to treatment in any woman with childbearing potential who is to be treated with RAI.
–Recheck a T4, T3, and TSH level in 4–8 wk after RAI therapy.
–Prior to initiating ATD therapy obtain a baseline complete blood count with differential (CBCD) and a liver profile.

–Obtain a CBCD for patients on ATD therapy with a febrile illness or a sore throat.

–If near-total or total thyroidectomy is chosen as treatment for GD, render patients euthyroid prior to the procedure with ATD pretreatment and beta-adrenergic blockade. Give potassium iodide in the immediate preoperative period.

–Wean beta-blockers following thyroidectomy.

–Treat thyroid multinodular goiters or thyroid adenomas with hyperthyroidism with surgery or RAI.

–Treat subclinical hyperthyroidism in all individuals ≥65 of age, and in patients with cardiac disease, osteoporosis, or symptoms of hyperthyroidism when the TSH is persistently <0.1 mU/L.

Source

–2016 American Thyroid Association guidelines for diagnosis and management of hyperthyroidism and other causes of thyrotoxicosis. *Thyroid.* 2016;26(10):1343-1421.

▶AACE 2013

–RAI therapy:
  • Assess patients 1–2 mo after ^{131}I therapy with a free T_4 and total triiodothyronine (T_3) level; repeat q 4–6 wk if thyrotoxicosis persists.
  • Consider retreatment with ^{131}I therapy if hyperthyroidism persists 6 mo after ^{131}I treatment.

–Antithyroid drug therapy:
  • Methimazole is the preferred antithyroid drug except during the first trimester of pregnancy.
  • Educate patients on the signs and symptoms of agranulocytosis and hepatic injury.
  • Recommend measurement of TSH receptor antibody level prior to stopping antithyroid drug therapy.

–Thyroidectomy:
  • Indicated for toxic multinodular goiter or toxic adenoma.
  • Follow serial calcium or intact PTH levels postoperatively.
  • Start levothyroxine 1.6 µg/kg/d immediately postoperatively.
  • Check a serum TSH level 6–8 wk postoperatively.

–Treat thyroid storm in the ICU with beta-blockers, antithyroid drugs, inorganic iodide, corticosteroid therapy, volume resuscitation, and aggressive cooling with acetaminophen and cooling blankets.

Source
   –https://www.aace.com/files/hyperguidelinesapril2013.pdf

THYROID DISEASE, HYPOTHYROIDISM

Population
   –Nonpregnant adults.

Recommendations

▶AACE 2012
   –Replacement dosing of levothyroxine is 1.6 μg/kg/d.
   • Initiate replacement at lower dose of 50 μg/d in patients over
     50–60 y without CAD.
   –Check antithyroid peroxidase antibodies (TPOAb) in patients with
   subclinical hypothyroidism or recurrent miscarriages.
   –Treat hypothyroid patients with levothyroxine if:
   • TSH >10 mIU/L.
   • TSH <10 mIU/L and:
   ○ Symptomatic.
   ○ Positive TPOAb.
   ○ History of ASCVD or at high risk for these conditions.
   –Avoid overtreatment with levothyroxine to minimize risk of
   cardiovascular, skeletal, or affective disturbances.
   –Monitor TSH 4–8 wk after starting levothyroxine or adjusting dose,
   then q 6–12 mo once euthyroid.
   –Use levothyroxine monotherapy.
   –Do *not* use levothyroxine to treat obesity or depression in euthyroid
   patients.

Source
   –https://www.aace.com/files/hypothyroidism_guidelines.pdf

THYROID NODULES

MANAGEMENT OF THYROID NODULES

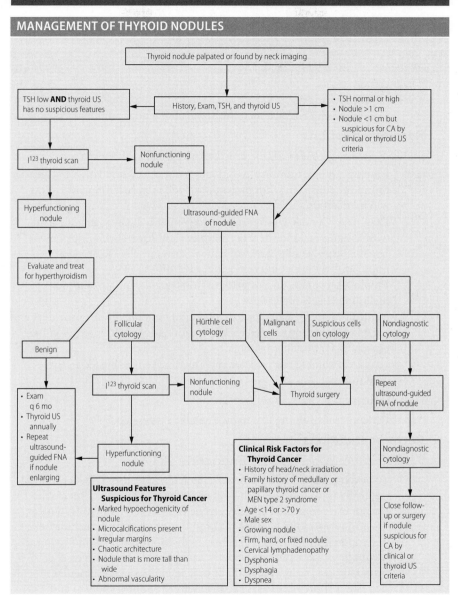

FNA, fine-needle aspiration; MEN, multiple endocrine neoplasia; TSH, thyroid-stimulating hormone; US, ultrasound.

Sources
–AACE. 2010. https://www.aace.com/files/thyroid-guidelines.pdf
–ATA. 2015. https://www.ncbi.nlm.nih.gov/pmc/articles/PMC4739132/

TRANSGENDER HEALTH CARE

Population
–Genderqueer, gender nonconforming, and gender nonbinary people.

Recommendations
▶UCSF 2016, WPATH 2012, Endocrine 2017

–Employ cultural humility. Avoid judgment or editorializing. Use gender pronouns consistent with patients' self-identity. Ask for clarification when uncertain.

–Diagnose "Gender Dysphoria" when gender identity is incongruent with assignment and there is clinically significant social impairment. Use the term "gender nonconformity" to represent the broader population with incongruent gender identities.

–Employ informed consent prior to initiating hormone therapy, including effects on fertility.

–Multidisciplinary team approach including mental health providers and clinicians is recommended to inform and guide treatment modalities, especially for younger patients.

–Assess for suicide risk. Suicide rates are markedly elevated in this community.

Population
–Patients transitioning to a female gender expression.

Recommendations
▶UCSF 2016, WPATH 2012, Endocrine 2017

–To develop female secondary sex characteristics, use 17-beta estradiol (typically transdermal patch, oral or sublingual tablet, or injectable). Do not use conjugated equine estrogens because of difficulty. Do not use ethinyl estradiol because of thrombotic risk. Effects include breast development (to Tanner stage 2–3), redistribution of fat, reduction of muscle mass, reduction of body hair, possible arrest/reversal of scalp hair loss, reduced erectile function, and reduced testicular size. There is an increased risk of venous thromboembolism and hypertriglyceridemia, and possibly of hypertension.

–To suppress male secondary sex characteristics, use spironolactone (monitor for hyperkalemia; max dose 200 mg BID). If contraindicated or unable to tolerate, use 5-alpha reductase inhibitors instead. Titrate dose to clinical effect and testosterone levels <55 ng/dL.

–Screen for breast cancer q2 years if age >50 and 5–10 y of feminizing hormone use. Prostate and testicular cancer risk is reduced by feminizing hormones but not eliminated; individualize screening.

–Hair removal can be achieved through various methods including laser, electrolysis, waxing, plucking, and shaving.

–Patients may consider "tucking" (employ tight-fitting underwear to locate the testicles in the inguinal canal and the penis in the perineal region) and "binding" (tight-fitting bras/shirts/wraps/binders) to disguise male anatomical characteristics.

–If considering breast augmentation ("top surgery"), 24 mo of preoperative hormone therapy are recommended, as breast tissue will continue to develop.

–If considering vaginoplasty ("bottom surgery"), requirements include two assessments by a mental health provider, 12 mo of hormone therapy, and 12 mo of living in a gender role congruent with gender identity.

Population

–Patients transitioning to a male gender expression.

Recommendations

▶UCSF 2016, WPATH 2012, Endocrine 2017

–To develop male secondary sex characteristics, give testosterone (IM, SQ, or transdermal) and titrate to bioavailable level >72 ng/dL. Effects include development of facial hair, voice changes, fat redistribution, increase in muscle mass, increase in body hair, hairline recession, increase in libido, clitoral growth, vaginal dryness, and cessation of menses. There is an increased risk of polycythemia and possibly of hyperlipidemia.

–Discuss contraceptive options, as hormone therapy does not reliably cause infertility and testosterone is teratogenic.

–Screen for breast and cervical cancer according to current guidelines for cis-gendered women. Do not routinely screen for endometrial cancer but explore the possibility if unexplained vaginal bleeding.

–Patients may consider "packing" (use of a penile prosthesis) to provide a male physical appearance.

–If considering mastectomy ("top surgery"), an assessment by a mental health provider is required.

–If considering gonadectomy or hysterectomy ("bottom surgery"), 12 mo of preoperative hormone therapy are required.

–If considering phalloplasty or metoidioplasty, requirements include two assessments by a mental health provider, 12 mo of hormone therapy, and 12 mo of living in a gender role congruent with gender identity.

Population

–Gender nonconforming children and adolescents.

Recommendations

▶UCSF 2016, WPATH 2012, Endocrine 2017

–Suppression of endogenous puberty may represent an opportunity to avoid distressing gender dysphoria and the high rate of suicide that accompanies it.

–Adolescents are candidates for puberty suppression if a long-lasting pattern of gender nonconformity or dysphoria exists, dysphoria emerges or worsens with the onset of puberty, their ability to adhere to treatment is intact, and the adolescent and their parents/guardians have consented to the treatment.

–Do not offer hormonal treatment to prepubertal persons.

–If suppression is desired, use GnRH analogues before the patient has reached Tanner stages 2–3 with frequent monitoring of clinical and lab parameters.

Comments

1. Outcomes data is generally lacking for this population, so most guidelines are based on expert opinion from experienced practitioners.
2. Terminology may be fluid and highly individualized. Approach conversations with humility and open-ended questions.
3. Employ a stepwise approach to therapies. Encourage hormone therapy before surgical intervention for most patients. Informed consent is essential, as every therapy will have reversible and irreversible effects.
4. For patients considering surgical options, refer to surgeon comfortable with the treatment of gender dysphoria. While top surgeries are often well-tolerated, bottom surgeries are relatively complex with higher complication rates and significant post-procedure care. Informed consent is essential and should include the various techniques available, realistic expectations of outcomes, and inherent risks and complications.
5. Dosing of hormones, surveillance regimens, and common adverse effects are detailed in the cited guidelines.

Sources

–AACE. 2010. https://www.aace.com/files/thyroid-guidelines.pdf

–*Guidelines for the Primary and Gender-Affirming Care of Transgender and Gender Nonbinary People*, 2nd ed. University of California, San

Francisco Center of Excellence for Transgender Health. 2016. http://www.transhealth.ucsf.edu/guidelines

–*Standards of Care for the Health of Transsexual, Transgender, and Gender-Nonconforming People*, 7th ed. World Professional Association for Transgender Health. 2012. http://wpath.org

–Guidelines on Gender-Dysphoric/Gender-Incongruent Persons. *J Clin Endocrinol Metab*. 2017;102(11):3869-3903.

VITAMIN DEFICIENCIES

Population
–All patients with or suspected of having serum cobalamin and folate deficiency.

Recommendations
▶BCSH 2014
–Serum cobalamin <200 ng/L is consistent with cobalamin deficiency.
–Patients with normal cobalamin level but high suspicion of cobalamin and/or folate deficiency should have their methylmalonic acid (MMA) and total homocysteine (tHC) levels measured.
–Patients with cobalamin deficiency or unexplained anemia, neuropathy, or glossitis (regardless of cobalamin level) should have an anti-intrinsic factor antibody test to rule out pernicious anemia.
–Initial therapy for cobalamin deficiency is vitamin B_{12} 1 mg IM TIW for 2 wk and then maintenance therapy.
–Maintenance therapy is either 1 mg IM every 3 mo (if no neurologic symptoms) or every 2 mo (if neurologic symptoms) or vitamin B_{12} 2 mg PO daily.
–Serum folate level <7 nmol/L (<3 μg/L) indicates folate deficiency.
–Treatment of folate deficiency is 1–5 mg PO daily for 1–4 mo, or until folate level normalizes.

Source
–onlinelibrary.wiley.com/doi/full/10.1111/bjh.12959

Comments
1. Do not use anti-parietal cell antibody to test for pernicious anemia.
2. Both MMA and tHC will be elevated in cobalamin deficiency; normal MMA and elevated tHC are consistent with folate deficiency.

TABLE I: COMPARISON OF RECOMMENDED HEMOGLOBIN A1C TARGETS

Organization	Recommended A1c Target
American Diabetes Association (2019)	<7%; less (>8%) or more stringent (<6.5%) goals may be appropriate for select patients
American Academy Clinical Endocrinologists (2018)	6.5%; consider higher targets if older or with comorbidities
American College of Physicians (2017)	7%–8%; de-intensify therapy if <6.5%; de-emphasize A1c if life expectancy <10 y
International Diabetes Federation (2017)	<7%; <8% if life expectancy <10 y

Gastrointestinal Disorders

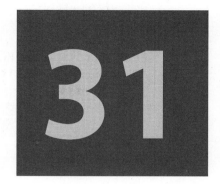

ABNORMAL LIVER CHEMISTRIES

Recommendations
American College of Gastroenterology 2017

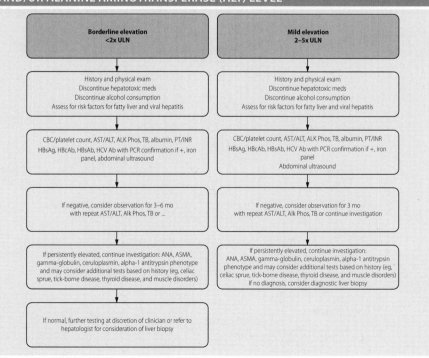

ALGORITHM FOR EVALUATION OF ASPARTATE AMINOTRANSFERASE (AST) AND/OR ALANINE AMINOTRANSFERASE (ALT) LEVEL

Borderline elevation <2x ULN	Mild elevation 2–5x ULN
History and physical exam Discontinue hepatotoxic meds Discontinue alcohol consumption Assess for risk factors for fatty liver and viral hepatitis	History and physical exam Discontinue hepatotoxic meds Discontinue alcohol consumption Assess for risk factors for fatty liver and viral hepatitis
CBC/platelet count, AST/ALT, ALK Phos, TB, albumin, PT/INR HBsAg, HBcAb, HBsAb, HCV Ab with PCR confirmation if +, iron panel, abdominal ultrasound	CBC/platelet count, AST/ALT, ALK Phos, TB, albumin, PT/INR HBsAg, HBcAb, HBsAb, HCV Ab with PCR confirmation if +, iron panel Abdominal ultrasound
If negative, consider observation for 3–6 mo with repeat AST/ALT, Alk Phos, TB or ...	If negative, consider observation for 3 mo with repeat AST/ALT, Alk Phos, TB or continue investigation
If persistently elevated, continue investigation: ANA, ASMA, gamma-globulin, ceruloplasmin, alpha-1 antitrypsin phenotype and may consider additional tests based on history (eg, celiac sprue, tick-borne disease, thyroid disease, and muscle disorders)	If persistently elevated, continue investigation: ANA, ASMA, gamma-globulin, ceruloplasmin, alpha-1 antitrypsin phenotype and may consider additional tests based on history (eg, celiac sprue, tick-borne disease, thyroid disease, and muscle disorders) If no diagnosis, consider diagnostic liver biopsy
If normal, further testing at discretion of clinician or refer to hepatologist for consideration of liver biopsy	

HCV, hepatitis C virus.

Source
–ACG Clinical Guideline: Evaluation of Abnormal Liver Chemistries. *Am J Gastroenterol.* 2017;112:1835.

ALGORITHM FOR EVALUATION OF ELEVATED SERUM ALKALINE PHOSPHATASE

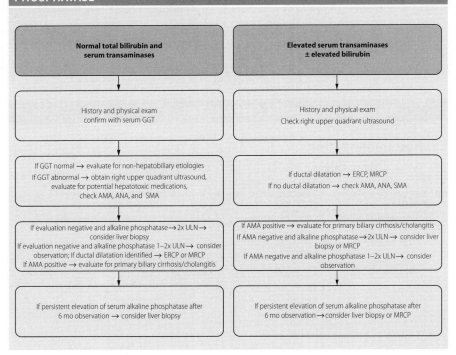

ALGORITHM FOR EVALUTION OF ELEVATED SERUM TOTAL BILIRUBIN

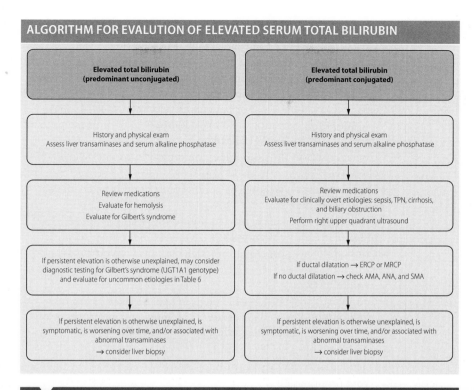

Elevated total bilirubin (predominant unconjugated)	Elevated total bilirubin (predominant conjugated)
History and physical exam. Assess liver transaminases and serum alkaline phosphatase	History and physical exam. Assess liver transaminases and serum alkaline phosphatase
Review medications. Evaluate for hemolysis. Evaluate for Gilbert's syndrome	Review medications. Evaluate for clinically overt etiologies: sepsis, TPN, cirrhosis, and biliary obstruction. Perform right upper quadrant ultrasound
If persistent elevation is otherwise unexplained, may consider diagnostic testing for Gilbert's syndrome (UGT1A1 genotype) and evaluate for uncommon etiologies in Table 6	If ductal dilatation → ERCP or MRCP. If no ductal dilatation → check AMA, ANA, and SMA
If persistent elevation is otherwise unexplained, is symptomatic, is worsening over time, and/or associated with abnormal transaminases → consider liver biopsy	If persistent elevation is otherwise unexplained, is symptomatic, is worsening over time, and/or associated with abnormal transaminases → consider liver biopsy

ASCITES, FROM CIRRHOSIS

Population
–Adults with cirrhosis.

Recommendations

▶ AASLD 2013, EASL 2018
–Perform diagnostic paracentesis for all patients with new-onset ascites.
–Do not routinely give platelets or fresh frozen plasma prior to a paracentesis.
–Ascitic fluid analysis:
  • Cell count with differential.
  • Albumin.
  • Protein.
  • Bedside inoculation of aerobic and anaerobic culture bottles.
–Management of cirrhotic ascites:
  • Alcohol cessation.
    ◦ Consider baclofen to reduce alcohol craving and alcohol consumption.

- Recommend low sodium diet.[a]
- Give furosemide and spironolactone in a 2:5 ratio.
- During the first episode of ascites, start spironolactone at 100 mg/d and increase q3 d in 100-mg steps until at 400 mg/d if no response to lower dosage. If not responding to spironolactone alone (defined as <2 kg/wk weight loss or patients developing hyperkalemia) add furosemide starting at 40 mg/d increasing in 40-mg steps to a maximum of 160 mg/d (EASL).
- Consider substituting other loop diuretics if furosemide is not effective (EASL).
- Target maximum weight loss per day of 0.5 kg/d if no edema or 1 kg/d if edema.
- Restrict fluid intake if serum sodium is low (AASLD <125 mmol/L; EASL <130 mmol/L).
- Consider liver transplantation for all patients with cirrhosis and ascites.
- Avoid NSAIDs.
- Cautious use of ACEI, ARB, and even beta-blockers. If used, monitor blood pressure carefully as an independent predictor of survival in patients with cirrhosis.
- Avoid aminoglycosides (EASL).

–Management of refractory cirrhotic ascites:

- Avoid propranolol.
- Avoid ACEI or ARB.
- Consider oral midodrine.
- Consider serial therapeutic paracentesis.
- Consider transjugular intrahepatic portosystemic shunt (TIPSS) in carefully selected patients.
- Give albumin for large volume paracentesis (AASLD: give 6–8 g/L of ascitic fluid removed if >5 L; EASL: give 8 g/L ascitic fluid removed and consider even when <5 L).

–Management of spontaneous bacterial peritonitis (SBP):

- Give cefotaxime 2 g IV q8h for 5–7 d.
- Alternative is ofloxacin 400 mg PO bid.
- For locations with high bacterial resistance piperacillin/tazobactam or carbapenem should be used (EASL).
- Repeat paracentesis in 48 h to assess for reduction in leukocyte count of >25% (EASL).
- Add albumin 1.5 g/kg/d on day 1 and 1 g/kg/d on day 3 if creatinine >1 mg/dL, BUN >30 mg/dL, or bilirubin >4 mg/dL.

[a]2 g sodium/d is recommended by AASLD. EASL recommends 4.6–6.9 g/d which is equivalent to a no salt-added and no processed food diet.

- Consider diagnosis of secondary bacterial peritonitis and obtain CT scan of abdomen and early surgery if high neutrophil count in ascitic fluid, multiple cultured organisms, or high ascitic protein count (EASL).

–SBP prophylaxis:

- Give cefotaxime or oral norfloxacin for 7 d to anyone with cirrhosis admitted for upper gastrointestinal bleed (regardless of the presence of ascites).
- Give long-term oral trimethoprim-sulfamethoxazole or norfloxacin to any patient with a history of SBP. EASL: stop prophylaxis if long-term improvement with disappearance of ascites.
- Consider SBP prophylaxis if ascitic fluid protein <1.5 g/dL in association with creatinine >1.2 mg/dL or sodium <130 mmol/L or bilirubin >3 mg/dL.
- Consider liver transplant after first episode of SBP due to poor long-term survival (EASL).
- Only use PPIs in those with clear indication due to possible increased risk for SBP (EASL).

–Hepatorenal syndrome options for treatment:

- Midodrine + SQ Octreotide + albumin.
- Norepinephrine infusion + albumin.
- Consider terlipressin over the use of norepinephrine since norepinephrine requires a central line with possible ICU admission. Albumin 20% in doses of 20–40 g/d should be used (EASL).
- Treatment should bring the serum creatinine to within 0.3 mg/dL of baseline. If hepatorenal syndrome recurs after treatment, repeat the course. Consider renal replacement therapy in severe illness.
- Refer for liver transplantation.

–Hepatic hydrothorax:

- Do not place chest tube.
- Restrict dietary sodium and give diuretics. EASL: perform therapeutic thoracentesis if dyspnea.
- Consider TIPS for refractory cases.

–Avoid percutaneous gastrostomy tube placement in patients with ascites.

Sources

–AASLD. 2013. https://www.aasld.org/sites/default/files/guideline_documents/AASLDPracticeGuidelineAsciteDuetoCirrhosisUpdate2012 Edition4_.pdf

–EASL. 2018. https://doi.org/10.1016/j.jhep.2018.03.024

OTHER COMPLICATIONS OF CIRRHOSIS

Population
  –Adults with cirrhosis.

Recommendations

▶ EASL 2018

  –Portal hypertensive gastropathy and intestinopathy (PHG):
  • Use nonselective beta-blockers, iron supplementation, and/or blood transfusion as first-line therapy for chronic hemorrhage from PHG.
  • Consider TIPS for transfusion-dependent patients.
  • Acute PHG bleeding can be treated similarly to variceal bleeding, but there is limited data on efficacy of treatment.

  –Renal impairment:
  • Categorize renal disease as either CKD, AKD, or AKI.
  • Remove diuretics, NSBB, and nephrotoxic drugs immediately when impairment suspected.
  • Replace fluid losses as needed.
  • For AKI stage >1A (based on KDIGO criteria), or from infection-induced AKI, give 20% albumin at 1 g/kg for 2 d. Maximum dose of 100 g/d.
  • In patients with AKI and tense ascites, perform paracentesis and replace albumin regardless of the volume removed.

  –Acute-on-chronic liver failure:
  • Acute-on-chronic liver failure has no particular therapy.
  • Seek precipitating factors and treat.
  • Expedite consideration for liver transplant.
  • Suggest withdrawal of ongoing intensive care support if four or more organs are failing after 1 wk of adequate intensive treatment.

  –Relative adrenal insufficiency (RAI):
  • There is no recommended current treatment for RAI in cirrhosis.

  –Cardiopulmonary complications:
  • Assess systolic function with cardiac echo with dynamic stress testing (pharmacologic or exercise).
  • Diastolic dysfunction may occur as an early sign of cardiomyopathy.
  • Evaluate for prolonged QTc and discontinue medications as appropriate.

  –Hepatopulmonary syndrome (HPS):

- Assess for HPS in patients with tachypnea, digital clubbing, and/or cyanosis. Screen initially with pulse oximetry, and if SpO2 <96% obtain ABG and further workup as indicated.
- Characterize HPS with contrast (microbubble) echocardiography. Consider transesophageal study to exclude intracardiac shunts.
- Treat patients with HPS and severe hypoxemia with long-term oxygen therapy. It is unclear how this treatment effects survival.
- Liver transplant is the only proven effective treatment for HPS.
- Perform ABG every 6 mo to prioritize liver transplant recipients since severe hypoxemia (PaO2 <45–50 mm Hg) predicts increased mortality post–liver transplant.

–Portopulmonary hypertension (PPHT):
- Screen for PPHT with transthoracic echocardiogram and grade as mild, moderate, and severe based on mean pulmonary arterial pressure (mPAP).
- If there is evidence of PPHT, obtain a right heart catheterization.
- Stop beta-blockers and manage varices with endoscopic tools.
- Do not perform TIPS in patients with PPHT.

Sources
–AASLD. 2013. https://www.aasld.org/sites/default/files/guideline_documents/AASLDPracticeGuidelineAsciteDuetoCirrhosisUpdate2012Edition4_.pdf
–EASL. 2018. https://doi.org/10.1016/j.jhep.2018.03.024

BARRETT ESOPHAGUS

Population
–Patients with biopsy diagnosis of Barrett esophagus (metaplastic columnar epithelium in distal esophagus).

Recommendations
▶ AGA 2011

Perform endoscopic surveillance in patients with Barrett esophagus at intervals that vary with grade of dysplasia found in the metaplastic epithelium.

–No dysplasia
- Endoscopic surveillance (ES) every 3–5 y.

–Low-grade dysplasia
- ES every 6–12 mo—consider radiofrequency ablation (RFA)—90% complete eradication of dysplasia.

–High-grade dysplasia
- ES every 3 mo if no eradication therapy.

–Eradication therapy
- RFA, photodynamic therapy (PDT), or endoscopic mucosal resection (EMR) is preferred over ES in high-grade dysplasia (strong recommendation).

Two practice updates have been released since the publication of this AGA position statement. The first is specifically regarding low-grade dysplasia in Barrett esophagus, while the second refines recommendations regarding long-term use of PPIs.

–Low-grade dysplasia
- The AGA recommends very specific biopsy techniques to determine grade of dysplasia. It is important that patients with a confirmed histologic diagnosis of LGD should be referred to an endoscopist with expertise in managing Barrett esophagus–related neoplasia, practicing at centers equipped with high-definition endoscopy, and capable of performing endoscopic resection and ablation.
- If confirmed, repeat upper endoscopy using high-definition/high-resolution white-light endoscopy under maximal acid suppression (twice daily PPI) in 8–12 wk.
- After complete eradication of intestinal metaplasia, patients should undergo surveillance in 2 y, then every 3 y thereafter.
- Patients who have not achieved complete eradication should undergo surveillance every 6 mo for 1 y after the last endoscopy, then annually for 2 y, then every 3 y thereafter.

–Long-term use of proton pump inhibitors:
- Patients with Barrett esophagus should take a long-term PPI even if asymptomatic.
- However, patients with symptomatic GERD who respond to short-term PPIs should subsequently attempt to stop or reduce them.
- Long-term PPI users should not routinely use probiotics to prevent infection.
- Long-term PPI users should not routinely raise their intake of calcium, vitamin B12, or magnesium beyond the Recommended Dietary Allowance.
- Long-term PPI users should not routinely screen or monitor bone mineral density, serum creatinine, magnesium, or vitamin B12.

Sources

–https://www.gastrojournal.org/article/S0016-5085(11)00084-9/fulltext
–https://www.gastrojournal.org/article/S0016-5085(16)35137-X/fulltext
–https://www.gastrojournal.org/article/S0016-5085(17)30091-4/fulltext

Comments

Clinical facts:

1. In patients with Barrett esophagus without dysplasia, 0.12% develop esophageal cancer per year compared to 0.5% with low-grade dysplasia.
2. Progression from high-grade dysplasia to cancer is 6% per year. (*N Engl J Med.* 2011;365:1375)
3. Esophagectomy for high-grade dysplasia is an option, but less morbidity with ablation therapy. (*N Engl J Med.* 2009;360:2277)
4. Forty percent of patients with Barrett esophagus and esophageal cancer have no history of chronic GERD symptoms.
5. Long-term high-dose PPIs or antireflux therapy have been shown to decrease risk of neoplastic progression in patients with Barrett esophagus; however, dose frequency more than once daily is not recommended. (*Clin Gastroenterol Hepatol.* 2013;11:382)
6. Risk of developing cancer is higher among men, older patients (>65 y) and patients with long segments of Barrett mucosa or dysplasia. (*Am J Gastroenterol.* 2011;106:1231) (*Gut.* 2016;65:196)

CELIAC DISEASE

Population

–Children and adults with celiac disease.

Recommendations

▶ NICE 2017

–Serological testing for suspected celiac disease:
  • Test for total IgA and IgA tissue transglutaminase (tTG).
  • Use IgA endomysial antibody test if IgA tTG is weakly positive.
  • Other immunoassays regarded as good are the IgA-transglutaminase 2 (TG2) test or IgG-deamidated gliadin peptide (DGP) test.

–Refer individuals with positive serological tests to a GI specialist for endoscopic duodenal biopsy to confirm the diagnosis.

–After diagnosis, monitoring, including antibody tests, is recommended every 3–6 mo in the first year and once a year thereafter in stable patients responding to the gluten-free diet.

–For refractory celiac disease despite strict adherence to gluten-free diet:
  • Review certainty of diagnosis.

- Consider coexisting conditions such as irritable bowel syndrome, lactose intolerance, microscopic colitis, or inflammatory bowel disease.

Source
  –https://www.nice.org.uk/guidance/qs134

Comments
1. The incidence has been increasing over the last 20 y.
2. The highest incidence of celiac disease seroconversion is between 12 and 36 mo of age.

COLITIS, CLOSTRIDIUM DIFFICILE

Population
  –Adults and children.

Recently, the IDSA and SHEA have updated previously published practice guidelines. While many of the recommendations remain the same, there are a few key changes that the update has addressed. These include:
  –Inclusion of specific pediatric guidelines.
  –Discussion on laboratory-guided diagnosis in adults.
  –Removal of metronidazole for first-line therapy in adults.
  –Discussion on fecal transplantation utilization.
  –Consideration of prophylaxis techniques.

Recommendations
▶ IDSA SHEA 2017
  –Diagnosis of *C. difficile* infection
- Updated guidelines provide a much clearer algorithm for laboratory testing, though initial step of this algorithm is centered upon each institution's practice.
- In general, Nucleic Acid Amplification Test (NAAT) is preferred to Enzyme Immunoassay (EIA or toxin testing).
- If the institution uses only specimens from patients who are not taking laxatives and have at least 3 or more unformed stools in a 24-h period, then using the NAAT alone is satisfactory.
- Stool toxin test may be used in a multistep algorithm with glutamate dehydrogenase (GDH) to satisfy the recommendation.
- If toxin test is negative, algorithm still recommends follow-up with the NAAT.
- Testing for *C. difficile* or its toxins should be performed only on diarrheal stool (3 or more unformed stool in 24-h period).

- Testing of stool on asymptomatic patients should be avoided.
- Repeat testing (within 7 d) during same episode of diarrhea is not recommended.

–Treatment of *C. difficile* infection:

- Discontinue inciting antibiotic agent as soon as possible.
- Avoid antiperistaltic agents.
- New guidelines recommend vancomycin and fidaxomicin, instead of metronidazole, as first-line treatments for *C. difficile*.
- Metronidazole can still be considered as first-line treatment in situations where accessibility to vancomycin and fidaxomicin is limited and in mild-to-moderate disease.
- Initial *C. difficile* infection: vancomycin 125 mg orally 4 times per day or fidaxomicin 200 mg twice daily for 10 d.
- Initial *C. difficile* infection, fulminant[b]: vancomycin 500 mg 4 times per day by mouth or by nasogastric tube. If ileus, consider adding rectal instillation of vancomycin. Intravenously administered metronidazole (500 mg every 8 h) should be administered together with oral or rectal vancomycin particularly if ileus is present.
- First recurrence, if metronidazole was used for the initial episode: vancomycin 125 mg given 4 times daily for 10 d.
- First recurrence, if standard regimen was used: a prolonged tapered and pulsed vancomycin regimen (eg, 125 mg 4 times per day for 10–14 d, 2 times per day for a week, once per day for a week, and then every 2 or 3 d for 2–8 wk) or fidaxomicin 200 mg twice daily for 10 d.
- Second or subsequent recurrence: prolonged tapered and pulsed vancomycin regimen, or vancomycin 125 mg given 4 times daily for 10 d followed by rifaximin 400 mg 3 times daily for 20 d, or fidaxomicin 200 mg twice daily for 10 d, or fecal microbiota transplantation.

Source

–https://academic.oup.com/cid/article/66/7/e1/4855916

Comments

1. Probiotics such as *Lactobacillus* and *Saccharomyces boulardii* have been associated with some reduction in *C. difficile* recurrence; however, significant results demonstrating efficacy in controlled clinical trials have yet to be seen. Thus, standard utilization of probiotics in the setting of *C. difficile* is not currently supported.

[b]Fulminant *C. difficile* infection, previously referred to as severe, complicated CDI, is characterized by hypotension or shock, ileus, or megacolon.

2. Perform hand hygiene before and after contact with patient. Handwashing with soap and water is preferred if there is direct contact.
3. Use disposable patient equipment when possible and ensure that reusable equipment is thoroughly cleaned and disinfected, preferentially with a sporicidal disinfectant.
4. With regards to antibiotic stewardship in order to control increasing rates of *C. difficile*, the guidelines stress attempts to minimize the frequency and duration of high-risk antibiotic therapy and the number of antibiotic agents prescribed.

Population
–Children.

Recommendations
▶ IDSA SHEA 2017

–Pediatric diagnosis of *C. difficile*:
- Because of the high prevalence of asymptomatic carriage of toxigenic *C. difficile* in infants, testing for CDI should never be routinely recommended for neonates or infants ≤12 mo of age with diarrhea.
- Colonization rates decrease with increasing age. By 2–3 y of age, approximately 1%–3% of children are asymptomatic carriers of *C. difficile* (a rate similar to that observed in healthy adults).
- In children ≥2 y of age, *C. difficile* testing is recommended for patients with prolonged or worsening diarrhea and risk factors (underlying inflammatory bowel disease, immunocompromising conditions, presence of a gastrostomy or jejunostomy tube) or relevant exposures (contact with the health care system or recent antibiotics).

–Pediatric treatment of *C. difficile*:
- Discontinue inciting antibiotic agent as soon as possible.
- Avoid antiperistaltic agents.
- Either metronidazole or vancomycin is recommended for the treatment of children with an initial episode or first recurrence of nonsevere *C. difficile* infection.
- Initial *C. difficile* infection, nonsevere: metronidazole po for 10 d (7.5 mg/kg/dose tid or qid) or vancomycin po for 10 d (10 mg/kg/dose qid).
- Initial *C. difficile* infection, severe/fulminant: vancomycin po/pr for 10 d (10 mg/kg/dose qid). Consider addition or IV metronidazole for 10 d (10 mg/kg/dose tid).

- First recurrence, nonsevere: metronidazole po for 10 d (7.5 mg/kg/ dose tid or qid) or vancomycin po for 10 d (10 mg/kg/dose qid).
- Second or subsequent recurrence: prolonged tapered and pulsed vancomycin regimen,[c] or vancomycin for 10 d (10 mg/kg/dose qid) followed by rifaximin[d] for 20 d, or fecal microbiota transplantation.

Source
  –https://academic.oup.com/cid/article/66/7/e1/4855916

Population
  –Adult patients with *C. difficile*–associated disease.

Recommendations
▶ EAST 2014
  –If surgery is indicated, recommend a subtotal or total colectomy.
  –For severe CDAD, patients should undergo surgery prior to the development of shock and need for vasopressors.

Source
  –https://www.east.org/education/practice-management-guidelines/ clostridium-difficile-associated-disease---timing-and-type-of-surgical- treatment

COLORECTAL CANCER FOLLOW-UP CARE

Population
  –Adults with nonmetastatic colorectal cancer (Stages II and III).

Recommendations
▶ American Society of Clinical Oncology Cancer Care Ontario (CCO) 2013
  –At time of diagnosis:
    - Emphasis on importance of complete high-quality colonoscopy to exclude synchronous tumors and find and resect polyps in patients with diagnosis of CRC. Perioperative colonoscopy should be meticulous, with the goal of detecting both synchronous cancers and precancerous lesions.

[c]10 mg/kg with max of 125 mg 4 times per day for 10–14 d, then 10 mg/kg with max of 125 mg 2 times per day for a week, then 10 mg/kg with max of 125 mg once per day for a week, and then 10 mg/kg with max of 125 mg every 2 or 3 d for 2–8 wk.
[d]No pediatric dosing for rifaximin given as it is not approved by the US Food and Drug Administration for use in children.

–Follow-up for recurrence:

- Surveillance guided by risk of recurrence and functional status of the patient. Early detection of relapse would lead to treatment including surgery for possible cure.
- Highest risk of recurrence during first 4 y after diagnosis; 95% of relapses occur in first 5 y.
- Medical history, physical exam, and CEA testing every 3–6 mo for 5 y. The higher the risk, the more frequent the follow-up.
- Abdominal and chest CT scan is recommended annually for 3 y. Highest risk patients (Stage III, >4 nodes+) should consider imaging every 4–6 mo.
- Routine PET scan not recommended for surveillance.
- Patients with rectal cancer should also have pelvic CT annually for 3–5 y.
- A surveillance colonoscopy should be performed 1 y after initial surgery. If normal, repeat colonoscopy every 5 y. If complete colonoscopy not performed before diagnosis, perform it as soon as the patient recovers from adjuvant therapy.
  ○ Any new or persistent worsening of symptoms warrant consideration of recurrence.
- There is insufficient evidence to recommend routine use of FIT or fecal DNA for surveillance after CRC resection.

Sources

–*J Clin Oncol.* 2013;31:4465-4470.
–https://www.ncbi.nlm.nih.gov/pmc/articles/PMC4445789/

Comments

Clinical correlation:

1. Stage I colon cancer with very low risk of recurrence. Colonoscopy follow-up every 5 y but CEA and imaging not needed.
2. Colon cancer with >90% to liver as the first site of metastasis. In rectal cancer, 50% of first metastasis is to lung and 50% to liver. (*CA Cancer J Clin.* 2015;65:5)
3. Patients found to have resectable metastatic disease (liver, lungs) or local recurrence who are rendered disease free by surgical or radiofrequency ablation (RFA) should be followed with frequent surveillance. Ten-year survival is in the 30%–40% range. (*J Clin Oncol.* 2010;28:2300)
4. BRAF mutation prognostic for early relapse and chemotherapy resistance with shortened survival. (*PLoS One.* 2013;8:eb5995)
5. Patients with CRC younger than 50 y or with significant family history should be evaluated for Lynch syndrome with microsatellite instability and immune histochemistry testing. (*N Engl J Med.* 2009;361:2449)

6. Patients with Stage II CRC with microsatellite instability will have a shorter survival if given adjuvant 5-fluorouracil compared to placebo. (*Clin Genet.* 2009;76:1)
7. Uncertainty remains regarding use of cyclooxygenase inhibitor to reduce risk of recurrence but aspirin is now approved to decrease risk of CRC.
8. Exercise (>150 min/wk), weight loss for high BMI, smoking cessation, and healthy diet advised—evidence suggests a decrease in disease recurrence.

CONSTIPATION, IDIOPATHIC

Population
–Children age ≤18 y.

Recommendations

▶ NICE 2010 (updated 2017)
–Assess all children for fecal impaction.
–If evidence of poor growth, test for celiac disease and hypothyroidism.
–Recommends polyethylene glycol (PEG) as first-line agent for oral disimpaction.
–Add a stimulant laxative if PEG therapy is ineffective after 2 wk.
–Recommends sodium citrate enemas for disimpaction only if all oral medications have failed.
–Recommends a maintenance regimen with PEG for several months after a regular bowel pattern has been established.
–Recommends gradually tapering maintenance dose over several months as bowel pattern allows.
–Recommends adequate fluid intake.

Source
–https://www.nice.org.uk/guidance/cg99

Comment
1. Minimal fluid intake for age

Age (y)	Volume (mL)
1–3	1300
4–8	1700
9–13	2200
14–18	2500

Population

–Adults.

Recommendations

▶ AGA 2013

–Digital examination to evaluate resting sphincter tone.

–Discontinue all medications that can cause constipation.

–Assess for hypercalcemia, hypothyroidism.

–Trial of laxatives and fiber:

- Bisacodyl.
- Milk of magnesia.
- Polyethylene glycol.
- Senna.

–Refractory constipation may require biofeedback or pelvic floor retraining.

- Severe cases of refractory slow transit constipation may require a total colectomy with ileorectal anastomosis.

Source

–http://www.gastrojournal.org/article/S0016-5085%2812%2901545-4/fulltext

CONSTIPATION, OPIATE INDUCED

Population

–Adults.

Recommendations

▶ AGA 2018

–Use laxatives as first-line agents.

–For patients with laxative refractory opiate-induced constipation, use one of three peripherally acting μ-opioid receptor antagonists (PAMORAs):

- Naldemedine (high-quality evidence).
- Naloxegol (moderate-quality evidence).
- Methylnatrexone (low-quality evidence).

–No recommendation for or against using lubiprostone (intestinal secretagogue) or prucalopride (selective 5-HT agonist). Currently there is not enough evidence.

Source

–https://doi.org/10.1053/j.gastro.2018.07.016

Comment

1. Traditional laxatives are divided into osmotic, stimulant, detergent/surfactant, or lubricant. Examples from each category are: PEG/lactulose/magnesium citrate, bisacodyl/senna/sodium picosulfate, docusate, mineral oil.

DIARRHEA, ACUTE

Population

–Adults with acute diarrheal illness.

Recommendations

APPROACH TO EMPIRIC THERAPY AND DIAGNOSTIC-DIRECTED MANAGEMENT OF THE ADULT PATIENT WITH ACUTE DIARRHEA (SUSPECT INFECTIOUS ETIOLOGY)

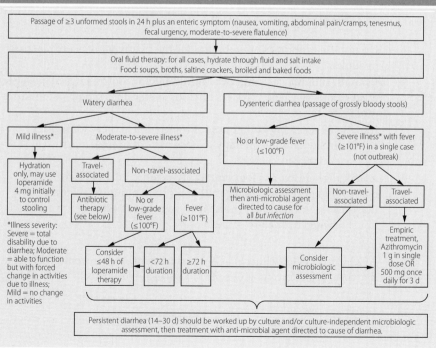

ACUTE DIARRHEA ANTIBIOTIC TREATMENT RECOMMENDATIONS

Antibiotic[a]	Dose	Treatment duration
Levofloxacin	500 mg by mouth	Single dose[b] or 3-d course
Ciprofloxacin	750 mg by mouth or	Single dose[b]
	500 mg by mouth	3-d course
Ofloxacin	400 mg by mouth	Single dose[b] or 3-d course
Azithromycin[c,d]	1000 mg by mouth or	Single dose[b]
	500 mg by mouth	3-d course[d]
Rifaximin[e]	200 mg by mouth 3 times daily	3-d

ETEC, Enterotoxigenic *Escherichia coli*.

[a]Antibiotic regimens may be combined with loperamide, 4 mg first dose, and then 2 mg dose after each loose stool, not to exceed 16 mg in a 24-h period.
[b]If symptoms are not resolved after 24 h, complete a 3-d course of antibiotics.
[c]Use empirically as first line in Southeast Asia and India to cover fluoroquinolone-resistant *Campylobacter* or in other geographical areas if *Campylobacter* or resistant ETEC are suspected.
[d]Preferred regimen for dysentery or febrile diarrhea.
[e]Do not use if clinical suspicion for *Campylobacter*, *Salmonella*, *Shigella*, or other causes of invasive diarrhea.

- –Do not use probiotics or prebiotics for the treatment of acute diarrhea in adults.
- –Bismuth subsalicylates can be administered to control rates of passage of stool and may help travelers function better during bouts of mild-to-moderate illness.
- –In patients receiving antibiotics for traveler's diarrhea, administer adjunctive loperamide therapy to decrease duration of diarrhea and increase chance for a cure.
- –Discourage antibiotics for community-acquired diarrhea, as epidemiological studies suggest that most community-acquired diarrhea is viral in origin (norovirus, rotavirus, and adenovirus) and is not shortened by the use of antibiotics.

Source
- –ACG Clinical Guideline: Diagnosis, treatment, and prevention of acute diarrheal infections in adults. *Am J Gastroenterol.* 2016;111:602-622.

DYSPEPSIA

▶ American College of Gastroenterology/Canadian Association of Gastroenterology 2017

Population

- –Adults with dyspepsia.
- –Avoid routine motility studies for patients with functional dyspepsia unless there is a strong suspicion for gastroparesis in which case a motility study is indicated.

WORKUP OF UNDIAGNOSED DYSPEPSIA

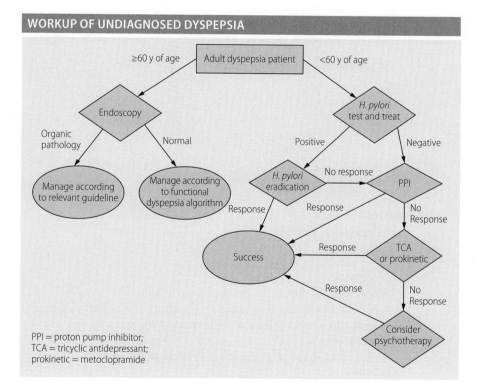

Source

- –ACG and CAG Clinical Guideline: Management of dyspepsia. *Am J Gastroenterol.* 2017;112(7):988-1013.

MANAGEMENT OF FUNCTIONAL DYSPEPSIA

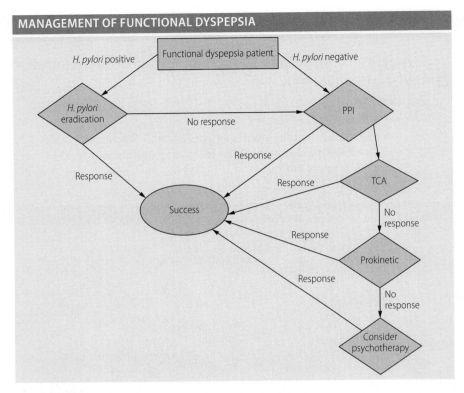

Population

–Adults with GERD and dyspepsia.

Recommendations

▶ NICE 2014

–Recommend smoking cessation and weight reduction.
–Consider discontinuation of offending medications (calcium channel blockers, nitrates, theophylline, bisphosphonates, steroids, and NSAIDs).
–Consider testing for *H. pylori* after a 2-wk washout off proton pump inhibitors.
–Empiric trial of proton pump inhibitor therapy.
–Consider laparoscopic fundoplication for patients who do not wish to continue with acid suppressive therapy long term.
–Consider specialist referral for:
  • Dyspepsia refractory to meds.
  • Consideration of surgery.
  • Refractory *H. pylori* infection.
  • Barrett esophagus.

DYSPHAGIA

Population
  –Adults with dysphagia, role of endoscopy.

Recommendations
▶ ASGE 2014
  –Recommend endoscopic dilation for benign esophageal strictures or eosinophilic esophagitis.
  –Recommend through-the-scope balloon dilation for complex esophageal strictures.
  –Concomitant antisecretory therapy with dilation for peptic strictures.
  –Reserve esophageal stents for refractory esophageal strictures.
  –Options for endoscopic management of achalasia include pneumatic dilation or botulinum toxin injections.

Source
  –https://www.asge.org/docs/default-source/education/practice_guidelines/doc-3c0fc1c6-37ac-4906-9301-74f813979375.pdf?sfvrsn=6

GALLSTONES

Population
  –Adults with or suspected of having gallstones.

Recommendations
▶ NICE 2014, EASL 2014
  –Prevention
    • In general gallstones cannot be prevented. However, a healthy lifestyle and diet, regular physical activity, and maintenance of an ideal body weight might prevent cholesterol gallbladder stones and symptomatic gallstones.
    • In situations that are associated with rapid weight loss (eg, very-low-calorie diet, bariatric surgery), temporary ursodeoxycholic acid (at least 500 mg/d until body weight has stabilized) may be recommended in obese patients.
    • Physicians who prescribe hormone replacement therapy should be aware of the increased risk for gallstones. However, currently there is no indication for pharmacological or surgical stone prevention during hormone replacement therapy.

–Diagnosis
- Obtain liver function tests and ultrasound if suspected gallstone disease.
- Acute cholecystitis should be suspected in a patient with fever, severe pain located in the right upper abdominal quadrant lasting for several hours, and right upper abdominal pain and tenderness on palpation.
- Consider magnetic resonance cholangiopancreatography (MRCP) if ultrasound has not detected common bile duct stones but the:
    ◦ Common bile duct is dilated.
    ◦ Liver function tests are abnormal.

–Treatment
- Offer cholecystectomy for symptomatic gallstones or acute cholecystitis.
- Litholysis using bile acids alone or in combination with extracorporeal shock wave lithotripsy is not recommended for gallbladder stones.
- Offer percutaneous cholecystostomy for acute cholecystitis or gallbladder empyema if surgery is contraindicated.
- Options for choledocholithiasis:
    ◦ Cholecystectomy and intraoperative clearance of CBD stones.
    ◦ ERCP prior to cholecystectomy.

Sources
–https://www.nice.org.uk/guidance/cg188
–http://www.easl.eu/medias/cpg/Prevention-diagnosis-and-treatment-of-gallstones/English-report.pdf

GASTROINTESTINAL BLEEDING, LOWER

Population
–Adults with suspected lower GI bleeding.

Recommendations
▶ ACG 2016
–Platelet transfusion should be considered to maintain a platelet count of 50,000 in patients with severe bleeding and those requiring endoscopic hemostasis.
–Reversal of anticoagulation should be considered before endoscopy in patients with an INR >2.5.

Source
–ACG clinical guideline: management of patients with acute lower gastrointestinal bleeding. *Am J Gastroenterol.* 2016;111:459-474.

ALGORITHM FOR THE MANAGEMENT OF PATIENTS PRESENTING WITH ACUTE LGIB STRATIFIED BY BLEEDING SEVERITY

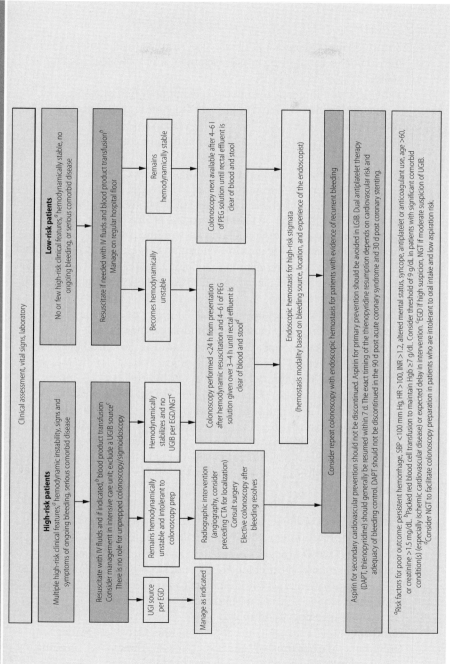

CTA, computed tomographic angiography; DAPT, dual antiplatelet therapy; EGD, esophagogastroduodenoscopy; LGIB, lower gastrointestinal bleeding; NGT, nasogastric tube; PEG, polyethylene glycol; UGIB, upper gastrointestinal bleeding.

Source: Strate LL, Gralnek IM. ACG clinical guideline: management of patients with acute lower gastrointestinal bleeding. *Am J Gastroenterol.* 2016;111:459-474, Fig. 1.

Recommendations

▶ BSG 2019

–Stratify as unstable or stable. Stable bleeds can be further subdivided into major vs minor using a risk assessment tool such as the Oakland score.

–Patients with a minor self-limited bleed and no other indication for hospitalization may be discharged home for urgent outpatient investigation.

–Patients with major bleed should be admitted for colonoscopy as soon as possible.

–In patients who are unstable or have a shock index >1 (heart rate/ systolic BP) after initial resuscitation or are having ongoing active bleeding, CT angiography is the fastest and least invasive method to localize the site of blood loss. If no source is identified on CT angiography, perform an upper endoscopy immediately as LGIB with hemodynamic instability may indicate an upper gastrointestinal bleed.

–In centers with 24/7 interventional radiology services, consider catheter angiography with the intent to embolize the site of bleeding prior to endoscopic investigation.

–Defer emergency laparotomy unless all effort has been made to localize the bleeding using radiological and endoscopic modalities.

–If transfusion is required, use a restrictive transfusion threshold of 7 g/dL and target of 7–9 g/dL. If history of cardiovascular disease, the threshold is 8 g/dL with a target of 8–10 g/dL.

–Stop warfarin therapy at presentation. For low thrombotic risk patients, consider resuming in 7 d and for high-risk thrombotic patients (ie, prosthetic heart valve in mitral location, atrial fibrillation with prosthetic valve or mitral stenosis, <3 mo after venous thromboembolism) begin low-molecular-weight heparin after 48 h. If unstable from bleeding, reverse with prothrombin complex concentrate and vitamin K.

–Patients with lower GI bleeds should stop aspirin for primary prophylaxis of cardiovascular events permanently. Aspirin for secondary prevention may be restarted after hemostasis is achieved.

–For patients with coronary stents in situ and on dual antiplatelet therapy, discuss with cardiology but do not stop routinely. For unstable hemorrhage patients, aspirin should be continued but P2Y12 receptor antagonist stopped. P2Y12 receptor antagonist therapy can be restarted in 5 d after bleeding is controlled.

–Stop direct oral anticoagulants at presentation. Consider treating with inhibitors (idarucizumab or andexanet) for life-threatening bleeding. Medication can be restarted in 7 d after hemorrhage.

–All hospitals should have agreed-upon pathways for management of GI bleeding. Those who admit patients with on-site colonoscopy and endoscopic therapy should have availability 7 d/wk as well as access to 24/7 interventional radiology (either on site or via referral pathway).

Source
–http://dx.doi.org/10.1136/gutjnl-2018-317807

GASTROINTESTINAL BLEEDING, UPPER (UGIB)

Population
–Adults, 16 y or older.

Recommendations
▶ NICE 2012 (updated in 2016), EASL 2018
–Recommend a formal risk assessment for patients with a UGIB:
  • Blatchford score at first assessment.
  • Rockall score after endoscopy.
–Avoid platelet transfusions in patients who are not actively bleeding and are hemodynamically stable.
–For UGIB, give FFP if:
  • Fibrinogen <100 mg/dL.
  • Partial thromboplastin time >1.5× normal.
–Prothrombin complex concentrate (PCC) indicated for UGIB on warfarin.
–Timing of endoscopy:
  • Immediately for unstable patients.
  • Within 24 h for stable patients.
–Management of nonvariceal bleeding:
  • Surgical clips.
  • Thermal coagulation.
  • Epinephrine injection.
  • Fibrin or thrombin glue.
  • Recurrent bleeding can be assessed by repeat endoscopy or by interventional radiology angioembolization.
  • Proton pump inhibitors.
–Management of variceal bleeding:
  • Esophageal variceal band ligation (EASL: within 12 h of admission).
  • Terlipressin or octreotide infusions.
  • Prophylactic third-generation cephalosporin.

- Transjugular intrahepatic portosystemic shunt for recurrent esophageal variceal bleeding or gastric variceal bleeding.
- Blood transfusion if necessary (EASL: use restrictive transfusion strategy with threshold of 7 g/dL and target of 7–9 g/dL).
- Use balloon tamponade only as bridge therapy to definitive treatment and for a maximum of 24 h.
- Stop beta-blockers and vasodilators and consider using lactulose to prophylaxis for hepatic encephalopathy.

–Prevention and treatment of variceal hemorrhage:
- Primary prophylaxis for varices is indicated for high-risk varices— small varices with red signs, medium or large varices, or small varices in Child-Pugh C patients.
- After banding and stabilization, initiate nonselective beta-blockers used to decrease risk.
- Use propranolol or nadolol. Do not use carvedilol. Use caution in patients with ascites.
- Patients intolerant to beta-blockers should be considered for TIPS.

–Gastric varices:
- Use nonselective beta-blockers as primary prevention.
- Give medical therapy for acute gastric variceal hemorrhage as for esophageal variceal hemorrhage. During endoscopy, choose cyanoacrylate as sclerosing agent.
- Consider TIPS or selective embolization thru interventional radiology.

Sources
–NICE. 2012. https://www.nice.org.uk/Guidance/cg141
–EASL. 2018. https://doi.org/10.1016/j.jhep.2018.03.024

Comments

1. Patients should stop NSAIDs.
2. Alcohol cessation if a factor.
3. Low-dose aspirin can be resumed if needed for secondary prevention of vascular events once hemostasis has been achieved.
4. Ongoing use of thienopyridine agents (eg, clopidogrel, ticagrelor, or prasugrel) should be only after discussion with appropriate specialist.

HELICOBACTER PYLORI INFECTION

Population
–Adults.

Recommendations

▶ American College of Gastroenterology 2017

–Screen the following patients for *Helicobacter pylori* (*H. pylori*) infection—active peptic ulcer disease (PUD), a past history of PUD (unless previous cure of *H. pylori* infection has been documented), low-grade gastric mucosa-associated lymphoid tissue (MALT) lymphoma, undiagnosed dyspepsia: patients who are under the age of 60 y, patients initiating chronic treatment with a nonsteroidal anti-inflammatory drug (NSAID), unexplained iron deficiency anemia, idiopathic thrombocytopenic purpura, or a history of endoscopic resection of early gastric cancer (EGC) should be tested for *H. pylori* infection.

–Treat all patients who test positive for *H. pylori*.

–Choice of therapy depends on prior antibiotic exposure.

–Consider clarithromycin triple therapy consisting of a PPI, clarithromycin, and amoxicillin or metronidazole for 14 d in regions where *H. pylori* resistance to clarithromycin is known to be <15% and in patients with no previous history of macrolide exposure for any reason.

–Consider bismuth quadruple therapy consisting of a PPI, bismuth, tetracycline, and a nitroimidazole for 10–14 d. Bismuth quadruple therapy is particularly attractive in patients with any previous macrolide exposure or who are allergic to penicillin.

–Consider levofloxacin triple therapy consisting of a PPI, levofloxacin, and amoxicillin for 10–14 d.

–Consider concomitant therapy consisting of a PPI, clarithromycin, amoxicillin, and a nitroimidazole for 10–14 d.

–Whenever *H. pylori* infection is identified and treated, perform testing to prove eradication using a urea breath test, fecal antigen test- or biopsy-based testing at least 4 wk after the completion of antibiotic therapy and after PPI therapy has been withheld for 1–2 wk.

–Bismuth quadruple therapy or levofloxacin salvage regimens are the preferred treatment options if a patient received a first-line treatment containing clarithromycin.

Sources
- –ACG clinical guideline: treatment of *Helicobacter pylori* infection. *Am J Gastroenterol.* 2017;112:212-238.
- –http://gi.org/guideline/treatment-of-helicobacter-pylori-infection/

▶ Cochrane Database Systematic Reviews 2013
- –Recommends using longer duration therapy for PPI-based *H. pylori* therapy.

Source
- –http://www.cochrane.org/CD008337/UPPERGI_ideal-length-of-treatment-for-helicobacter-pylori-h.-pylori-eradication

HEPATITIS B VIRUS (HBV)

Population
- –Adults and children with HBV infection.

Recommendations

▶ AASLD 2016 (with 2018 guidance update)
- –Screening, Counseling, and Prevention
  - The presence of HBsAg establishes the diagnosis of hepatitis B. Chronic versus acute infection is defined by the presence of HBsAg for at least 6 mo.
  - HBV is transmitted by perinatal, percutaneous, sexual exposure and by close person-to-person contact.
  - Perinatal transmission is an important cause of chronic infection.
  - Recommend HBV immunoglobulin and HBV vaccine to all infants born to HBsAg-positive women.
  - High-risk individuals should be screened for HBV infection and immunized if seronegative. These include:
    - ○ Persons born in regions of high or intermediate HBV endemicity (HBsAg prevalence of >2%).
    - ○ US-born persons not vaccinated as an infant whose parents were born in regions with high HBV endemicity (>8%).
    - ○ Persons who have ever injected drugs.
    - ○ Men who have sex with men.
    - ○ Persons needing immunosuppressive therapy, including chemotherapy, immunosuppression related to organ transplantation, and immunosuppression for rheumatologic or gastroenterologic disorders.
    - ○ Individuals with elevated ALT or AST of unknown etiology.
    - ○ Donors of blood, plasma, organs, tissues, or semen.

- Persons with end-stage renal disease.
- All pregnant women.
- Infants born to HBsAg-positive mothers.
- Persons with chronic liver disease, eg, HCV.
- Persons with HIV.
- Household, needle-sharing, and sexual contacts of HBsAg-positive persons.
- Persons seeking evaluation or treatment for a sexually transmitted disease.
- Health care and public safety workers at risk for occupational exposure to blood or blood-contaminated body fluids.
- Travelers to countries with intermediate or high prevalence of HBV infection.
- Inmates of correctional facilities.
- Unvaccinated persons with diabetes who are aged 19 through 59 y.

–Screening should be performed using both HBsAg and anti-HBs
- HBsAg-positive persons should be counseled regarding prevention of transmission of HBV to others.
- Other than practicing universal precautions, no special arrangements are indicated for HBV-infected children unless they are prone to biting.
- Abstinence or only limited use of alcohol is recommended in HBV-infected persons.

–All pregnant women should be screened for HBsAg:
- HBV vaccination is safe in pregnancy, and pregnant women who are not immune to or infected with HBV should receive this vaccine series.
- Women who meet standard indications for HBV therapy should be treated. Women without standard indications but who have HBV DNA >200,000 IU/mL in the second trimester should consider treatment to prevent mother-to-child transmission.
- Breastfeeding is not prohibited.
- HBV vaccines have an excellent safety record and are given as a 3-dose series at 0, 1, and 6 mo.
- Sexual and household contacts of HBV-infected persons who are negative for HBsAg and anti-HBs should receive HBV vaccination.
- Newborns of HBV-infected mothers should receive HBIG and HBV vaccine at delivery and complete the recommended vaccination series. Infants of HBsAg-positive mothers should undergo postvaccination testing at 9–15 mo of age.

–Diagnosis
- Diagnostic criteria of chronic hepatitis B
  ◦ HBsAg present for 6 mo.
  ◦ Subdivided into HBsAg positive and negative. HBV-DNA levels are typically >20,000 IU/mL in HBsAg-positive CHB, and lower values (2000–20,000 IU/mL) are often seen in HBsAg-negative CHB.
  ◦ Normal or elevated ALT and/or AST levels.
  ◦ Liver biopsy results show chronic hepatitis with variable necroinflammation and/or fibrosis.
- Quantitative HBV-DNA testing is essential to guide treatment decisions.
- HBV genotyping can be useful in patients being considered for peg-IFN therapy, otherwise not recommended.
- Testing for viral resistance in treatment-naive patients is not recommended. Resistance testing can be useful in patients with past treatment experience, those with persistent viremia, or those who experience virological breakthrough during treatment.

–Treatment
- Recommend antiviral therapy for adults and alanine transaminase (ALT) >2× normal, moderate-to-severe hepatitis on biopsy, compensated cirrhosis or advanced fibrosis and HBV DNA >20,000 IU/mL; or for reactivation of chronic HBV after chemotherapy or immunosuppression.
- Recommend antiviral therapy in children for ALT >2× normal and HBV DNA >20,000 IU/mL for at least 6 mo.
- Patients who do not meet criteria for treatment require regular monitoring to assess the need for future therapy.
  ◦ HBsAg-positive patients with persistently normal ALT should have ALT tested every 3–6 mo.
  ◦ Patients who are HBsAg positive with HBVDNA levels >20,000 IU/mL and ALT levels less than 2 times the ULN should undergo testing to evaluate histological disease severity:
    ▫ Liver biopsy, elastography, or liver fibrosis biomarkers (FIB-4 or FibroTest).
  ◦ All HBsAg-positive patients with cirrhosis should be screened with US examination with or without AFP every 6 mo.

Source
–https://www.aasld.org/sites/default/files/HBVGuidance_Terrault_et_al-2018-Hepatology.pdf

HEPATITIS B VIRUS INFECTION—TREATMENT SPECIFICS

Population
–Adults.

Recommendations

▶ AASLD 2016 (with 2018 guidance update)

–Offer antiviral therapy to adults to decrease the risk of liver-related complications, if:
- Without a liver biopsy to adults with a transient elastography score ≥11 kPa.
- HBV DNA >2000 IU/mL and ALT >30 IU/mL (males) or >19 IU/mL (females).
- Cirrhosis and detectable HBV DNA.

–Initial antiviral options for HBV infection:
- Peginterferon α-2a.
- Entecavir.
- Tenofovir disoproxil.
  ◦ Tenofovir alafenamide fumarate (TAF) has also been approved as a preferred treatment. It has decreased renal and bone toxicity.
  ◦ Test for HIV and baseline Cr before treatment initiation.

–Coinfection with HBV and HCV:
- All HBsAg-positive patients should be tested for HCV infection.
- HCV treatment is indicated for patients with HCV viremia.
- HBV treatment is determined by HBV-DNA and ALT levels.
- Peginterferon alfa-2a and ribavirin.

Population
–Children and young adults.

Recommendations

▶ AASLD 2016 (with 2018 guidance update)

–Consider liver biopsy if HBV DNA >2000 IU/mL and ALT >30 IU/mL (males) or >19 IU/mL (females).
–Initial antiviral options:
- Peginterferon α-2a.
- Interferon alpha, nucleos(t)ide analogues (NAs).

Comments

1. Consider a liver biopsy to confirm fibrosis for a transient elastography score 6–10 kPa.

2. Monitor CBC, liver panel, and renal panel at 2, 4, 12, 24, 36, and 48 wk while on interferon therapy.
3. Monitor CBC, liver panel, and renal panel at 4 wk and every 3 mo while on tenofovir therapy.

Population

–Pregnant women.

Recommendations

AASLD 2016 (with 2018 guidance update)

–The only antivirals studied in pregnant women are lamivudine, telbivudine, and tenofovir disoproxil.
–Of these 3 options, TDF is preferred to minimize the risk of emergence of viral resistance during treatment. Interim studies show high efficacy of TDF in preventing mother-to-child transmission.
–Consider tenofovir disoproxil if HBV DNA >107 IU/mL in the third trimester.

Source

–https://www.aasld.org/sites/default/files/HBVGuidance_Terrault_et_al-2018-Hepatology.pdfc

HEPATITIS C VIRUS (HCV)

Population

–Adults and children with HCV infection.

Recommendations

▶ AASLD 2018

Adults
–Recommends education on methods to avoid transmission to others.
–As of May 1, 2018 there are 11 single-drug or coformulated direct-acting antivirals (DAA) available to treat hepatitis C infection. Options are based on genotype and in general, trend away from interferon, peginterferon, and ribavirin toward DAA agents.
–Two of the most useful tools for clinicians treating HCV are:
  • https://www.HCVGuidelines.org for updated guidelines
  • https://www.hep-druginteractions.org for drug–drug interaction checking
–Indications depend on the HCV genotype/subtype, the severity of liver disease, and/or prior therapy.
–There is very limited evidence for treating patients with mixed genotypes (ie, multiple genotypes of HCV infection concurrently).

Utilization of a pangenotypic regimen should be considered and if the optimal regimen or duration is unclear, a specialist should be consulted.
- Recommends antiviral treatment for:
  - Bridging fibrosis or compensated cirrhosis (Child-Pugh A).
  - During acute HCV infection if treatment must be given in the first 6 mo, use a similar regimen that would be given for a chronic infection. Twenty to 50% of acute HCV cases will resolve spontaneously in the first 6 mo so monitoring for 12–16 is recommended prior to starting treatment.
- If patient coinfected with HIV, hepatitis B (HBV), or prior HBV, refer the patient for treatment.
- For patients with renal impairment (CKD) stages 1 thru 3, follow standard treatment protocols; CKD stages 4 and 5 are based on genotype.
- Test quantitative HCV RNA before treatment and at 12 wk of therapy.
- Patients who lack antibodies for hepatitis A and B viruses should receive vaccination.
- Abstain from alcohol consumption.
- Insufficient evidence to recommend herbal therapy.

Children and adolescents
- Patients >3-y-old can be treated if a DAA regimen is available for their genotype and age range. If the child has cryoglobulinemia, rashes, and glomerulonephritis, as well as advanced fibrosis then treatment should be started as soon as possible.
- Avoid interferon-based treatment regimens in children and adolescents.

Perinatal exposure
- All children born to HCV-infected women should be tested for HCV using an antibody-based test at or after 18 mo of age.
- HCV RNA assay testing can be used in the first year of life but optimal timing is unknown.
- If positive at 18 mo with antibody-based HCV test then an HCV RNA assay should be used at 3 y of age to confirm chronic HCV infection.
- Any siblings in the family born from the same mother should be tested for HCV.

Counseling parents who have HCV-infected children
- HCV is not transmitted through casual contact, so HCV-infected children do not pose a risk to other children. They can participate in school, sports, athletics, and regular childhood activities without restriction.

–Universal precautions should be used at school and in the home. Family members should not share toothbrushes, razors, nail clippers, and should use gloves and dilute bleach to clean up blood.

Pregnancy

–All pregnant women should be screened for HCV infection at the start of prenatal care.

–All women with HCV infection should be offered treatment prior to becoming pregnant to reduce the risk of vertical transmission.

–Do not treat during pregnancy.

–HCV RNA and routine liver function tests are recommended at the start of pregnancy to help assess disease severity.

–There is no known way to reduce mother-to-child-transmission risk for HCV-infected women.

–In HCV-infected pregnant women with pruritus or jaundice, intrahepatic cholestasis of pregnancy should be suspected and worked up.

–HCV-infected women with cirrhosis should be managed by a maternal-fetal medicine (ie, high-risk pregnancy) obstetrician.

–Breastfeeding is not contraindicated in HCV-infected mothers other than when the mother has cracked, damaged, or bleeding nipples or if co-infected with HIV.

–Women with HCV infection should be reassessed after delivery with an HCV-RNA assay to see if they have spontaneously cleared.

HCV infection management in injection drug users

–At least annual testing should be offered to any person who injects drugs. This includes those who have spontaneously cleared or had prior treatment but continue to inject drugs. Testing can be more frequent dependent on risk factors.

–Substance use disorder and/or needle/syringe exchange programs should offer opt-out HCV antibody testing with reflex or immediate confirmation HCV RNA testing and linkage to care.

–Provide counseling to reduce risky behaviors and referral to needle/syringe exchange programs.

–Active or recent drug use or a concern for reinfection is not a contraindication to treatment.

HCV infection management in men who have sex with men (MSM)

–Annual HCV testing is recommended for all sexually active adolescent and adult MSM. This includes HIV-positive, HIV-negative, starting HIV PreP therapy, spontaneously cleared HCV infections or prior treated. Testing can be more frequent dependent on risk factors.

–All MSM should be counseled on high-risk sexual and drug use practices that increase the risk for HCV infection and measures to prevent transmission.

–Couple HCV treatment with ongoing counseling to reduce reinfection.

HCV infection management in jail settings

–Jails should implement opt-out HCV testing encompassing HCV antibody with reflex to HCV RNA confirmation testing.

–Chronically infected should be linked with community health care organizations that can help with treatment and assessment of liver disease when released.

–If a person is jailed for a long enough time to receive treatment, they should have it provided in jail. If a person is jailed while on treatment, it should be continued while in jail. After treatment they may be linked with community health care organizations for further care.

–Jails should provide counseling on harm reduction and substance use disorders to decrease HCV reinfection/progression of liver disease.

Source

–https://doi.org/10.1093/cid/ciy585

▶ AGA 2017

Outreach and screening

–Screen for hepatitis C in all persons born between 1945 and 1965 and anyone who is high risk.

–Treatment teams should be patient centered with four distinct roles of hepatitis C provider, care coordinator, clinical pharmacist, and mental health/substance abuse provider.

Initial/Subsequent evaluations

–Initial visits:

- History:
  - HCV exposure risk factors and timing of exposure.
  - Symptoms of advanced liver disease such as: jaundice, ascites, variceal bleeding, fatigue, pruritus, confusion.
  - Extrahepatic manifestations.
  - Prior HCV treatment.
  - Other medical issues: diabetes, CVA, anemia, CKD, HIV, hepatitis B coinfection, depression, solid organ transplant recipient.
  - Family history of cirrhosis, liver cancer, alcohol dependence.
  - Social history of past and current alcohol use, current illicit drug use.
- Labs:
  - HCV quantitative PCR.
  - HCV genotype (unless done previously).
  - CBC.
  - Serum: Creatinine, sodium, potassium, chloride, albumin, total protein, total bilirubin, ALT, AST, alkaline phosphatase, glucose, protime (INR).

○ Resistance-associated variant testing in patients with HCV genotype 1a who are using grazoprevir/elbasvir or prior treatment with a direct acting antiviral agent.

○ Hepatic fibrosis testing.

○ Hepatic ultrasound.

–Subsequent visits:

- For hepatic fibrosis stage 3 or 4 patient should have

○ EGD evaluation for esophageal varices.

○ Alpha fetoprotein.

○ Hepatic ultrasound (or, if images inadequate, CT scan of abdomen with contrast).

○ Risk reduction/mitigation:

▫ Hepatitis A and B vaccinations if not immune.

▫ Age-appropriate vaccinations and cancer screening.

▫ Counseling on alcohol abstinence.

▫ Counseling on transmission/reinfection of HCV.

▫ Management of comorbid conditions.

▫ Counseling on adherence and consequences of treatment failure if being treated.

Important considerations prior to selecting a treatment regimen

–If patient has ever received prior treatment.

–If cirrhotic whether compensated or decompensated.

–HCV genotype.

–HIV coinfection.

–Renal impairment (eGFR <30 or dialysis).

–Postliver transplant.

–Medications to assess for drug–drug interactions.

–Should reassess labs within 12 wk of starting treatment which include: CBC, INR, Hepatic Function Panel (Albumin, Tot and Dir Bilirubin, ALT/AST, Alk Phos), Renal Function (eGFR).

Treatment monitoring for 8, 12, and 16 wk regimens

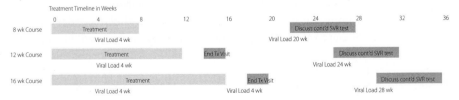

Long-term follow-up

–Patients with advanced cirrhosis, multiple treatment failures, coinfection with HIV or hepatitis B should be referred to hepatology clinic for proper management.

–Patients with hepatic fibrosis scores of stage 3 or 4 should receive:
- Hepatocellular carcinoma screening every 6 mo with:
  - Hepatic ultrasound or equivalent imaging study.
  - Alpha-fetoprotein levels.
  - Hepatic function panel.
  - Renal function panel.
  - Protime (INR).
- Annual visit with hepatology for continued management and possible referral for liver transplant if worsening liver dysfunction.

–For patients who are NOT treated due to refusal, financial issues, drug–drug interactions, ongoing substance use, or other issues should be reassessed yearly to see if they qualify for treatment.

–For patients who are successfully treated with
- Fibrosis score 0–2 need no further monitoring and should be counseled on reinfection risk, HIV prevention.
- Fibrosis score 3–4 they require ongoing HCC monitoring described above and yearly visits with hepatology.

Source
–https://doi.org/10.1053/j.gastro.2017.03.039

Comment
1. High-risk patients are defined as "history of injection drug use, transfusion or organ transplant before 1992, received clotting factors before 1987, history of long-term dialysis, HIV infection, persistently elevated liver enzymes, healthcare and public safety workers after needle sticks, sharps, or mucosal exposure to HCV-positive blood, and children born to HCV-positive women."

▶ EASL 2018

Diagnosis of acute and chronic hepatitis C
–Anyone suspected of HCV infection should have an antibody test performed first and if positive, reflex to an HCV RNA confirmation test. In immunocompromised or chronic dialysis patients, HCV RNA should be the first-line test.

–For low- and middle-income countries and specific settings in high-income countries, qualitative HCV RNA assays with detection limits of ≤1000 IU/mL may be used or HCV core antigen can replace HCV RNA testing to diagnose acute or chronic infection if cost is prohibitive.

–Antibody-positive HCV but HCV RNA–negative individuals should be retested for HCV RNA in 12 and 24 wk to confirm definite clearance.

–Whole blood sampled on dried blood spots can be used in place of serum of venipuncture.

Goals and endpoints of HCV therapy C

–Goal of therapy is cure to prevent chronic liver disease complications, improve quality of life, and prevent further transmission.

–HCV treatment is considered successful if HCV RNA is undetectable in a sensitive assay (lower limit ≤15 IU/mL) at 12 wk or 24 wk after the end of treatment. HCV core antigen and a qualitative HCV RNA assay are acceptable alternatives to quantitative HCV RNA.

–For patients with advanced fibrosis (F3) or cirrhosis (F4), hepatocellular carcinoma (HCC) screening is still required after successful treatment.

Pretherapeutic assessment

–Assess and treat any comorbid conditions.

–Assess liver disease severity as patients with advanced fibrosis (F3) or cirrhosis (F4) require special treatment and HCC surveillance.

–Fibrosis is assessed noninvasively if possible with liver biopsy if uncertain.

–Renal function and extrahepatic manifestations should be documented.

–Vaccinate for hepatitis B and hepatitis A if not protected.

HCV RNA or HCV core antigen detection/quantification

–As above, HCV RNA detection and quantification is preferred with a lower limit of ≤15 IU/mL. If not available, HCV core antigen or qualitative HCV RNA with a lower limit of ≤1000 IU/mL may be used.

–HCV genotype 1 (subtypes 1a or 1b) effect treatment choices.

–If genotype is not available, a pangenotypic regimen can be used.

–HCV resistance testing is not recommended but may be required if treatment optimization is needed and the resistance test is available (NS5A resistance testing spanning amino acids 24–93).

Contraindications to therapy

–Cytochrome P450–inducing agents are contraindicated with all regimens (such as carbamazepine and phenytoin).

–Protease inhibitors should not be used in patients with Child-Pugh B or C decompensated cirrhosis or if a previous episode of decompensation.

–For eGFR <30 mL/min/1.73 m^2 sofosbuvir should be avoided unless no alternative.

Indications for treatment

–All patients with HCV infection should be considered for treatment.

–Patients with decompensated (Child-Pugh B or C) cirrhosis and an indication for liver transplant with MELD score of ≥18–20 should receive a liver transplant first and treatment afterwards. If waiting time for a liver is >6 mo, treatment can be considered but clinical benefit is not well established.

–Do not treat if limited life expectancy from nonliver-related issues.

General guidelines for treatment

–Always start with a direct antiviral agent (DAA) for HCV-infected patients who do not have cirrhosis or with compensated cirrhosis (Child-Pugh A).

–Drug–drug interactions should always be considered at treatment start. For medications that may interact, either stop them for the treatment duration, find an alternative, or pick a different HCV treatment regimen.

–Use the same treatment regimens for HIV-coinfected patients as those without HIV infections while adjusting dosages based on interactions with HIV antiretroviral drugs.

–Where possible (same length of treatment and SVR rates) use 2 drug regimens over 3 drug regimens.

–Genotype-specific treatment regimens will not be covered other than:
  • Pangenotypic regimen sofosbuvir/velpatasvir (Epclusa) can be used for treatment of naive and experienced patients with compensated (Child-Pugh A) cirrhosis or no cirrhosis for 12 wk.
  • Pangenotypic regimen gelcaprevir/pibrentasvir (Mavyret) can be used for treatment of naive and experienced patients without cirrhosis for 8 wk. For patients with compensated cirrhosis (Child-Pugh A) a 12-wk course is needed.

Treatment of patients with severe liver disease with or without indication for liver transplant

–Interferon regimens are the only option for HCV infected or HIV/HCV infected with decompensated cirrhosis.

–Do not use protease inhibitor–containing regimens with decompensated cirrhotic patients.

–Referral to hepatology is highly recommended given treatment regiments are complex, liver transplantation may be required, and decompensation can worsen on treatment.

Postliver transplantation recurrence

–All patients posttransplant with recurrence should be considered for HCV treatment.

–Coordination with hepatology is advised.

HBV coinfection

–HBV-HCV-coinfected patients should receive the same regimens as monoinfected HCV patients.

–Coinfected patients meeting treatment criteria should receive nucleoside/nucleotide analogue treatment according to EASL 2017 clinical practice guidelines.

–Patients with HBs antigen-positive should receive nucleoside/nucleotide analogue prophylaxis at least until 12 wk post anti-HCV therapy and monitored month if HBV treatment is stopped.

–In HBs antigen-negative patients who have anti-HBc antibodies, serum ALT levels need to be drawn monthly. If ALT levels do not normalize or rise then HBs antigen and HBV DNA should be tested and HBV treatment started if present.

Treatment in renal impairment

–Patients with eGFR of $\geq$30 mL/min/1.73 m^2 can receive standard treatment with no dose adjustment. Careful monitoring is recommended.

–Patients with eGFR <30 mL/min/1.73 m^2 or with end-stage renal disease on hemodialysis need to be treated in expert centers with close monitoring.

Nonhepatic solid organ transplant recipients

–Treatment of HCV can occur before or after transplantation, provided the recipient appears to have a life expectancy exceeding 1 y.

–Discussion with transplant team and timing of treatment should be determined on a case-by-case basis.

Recipients of an HCV-positive organ transplant

–HCV-positive patients may receive HCV-positive organs.

–HCV-negative patients may receive HCV-positive organs, provided it is legal and extensive informed consent has been performed with assurance of rapid posttransplant DAA treatment.

People who inject drugs (PWID) and patients on opioid substitution therapy

–PWID should be screened for HCV with antibody and RNA-based tests at least annually and more often if high-risk behaviors are identified.

–Harm reduction can be achieved with opiate substitution therapy (methadone or buprenorphine) and clean needle exchange.

–All PWID infected with HCV should be offered treatment. If accepted then pretherapy counseling on harm reduction/reducing transmission should be provided.

–DAA-based anti-HCV therapy does not require dose adjustment to methadone or buprenorphine.

–Following SVR, biannual surveillance or at a minimum annual HCV RNA testing should be used to detect reinfection.

–If reinfected, retreatment should be offered.

Hemoglobinopathies and bleeding disorders

–HCV treatment indications are the same for patients with hemoglobinopathies and bleeding disorders. Use the same treatment regimens for patients without hemoglobinopathies or bleeding disorders.

Adolescents and children

–For adolescents $\geq$12-y-old infected with genotypes 1, 4, 5, or 6 who do not have decompensated cirrhosis, use a 12-wk regimen of sofosbuvir/

ledipasvir (400 mg/90 mg). If infected with genotype 2 or 3 without decompensated cirrhosis, treat with a regimen approved for adults with caution as there is little safety data in this population.

–Defer treatment for children <12 y until DAAs are approved for this age group.

Retreatment of nonsustained virological responders

–Patients who fail an initial regimen of DAA should be referred to hepatology for consideration of resistance testing and optimal retreatment strategy.

Treatment of acute hepatitis C

–Patients with acute HCV infection can use a pangenotypic regimen after confirmation of chronic ongoing infection or if requiring treatment immediately.

–SVR should be assessed at 12 and 24 wk as late relapses have been reported.

–There is no indication for postexposure prophylaxis without documented HCV transmission.

Treatment monitoring and safety

–HCV RNA-based tests with lower limit of ≤15 IU/mL are preferred when available but HCA RNA assays with a lower limit of ≤1000 IU/mL or HCV core antigen levels can be used as an alternative if necessary.

–HCV RNA levels or HCV core antigen levels should be measured at baseline and then at 12 and 24 wk after the end of therapy (SVR12 and SVR24).

–For some places with high SVR12 rates expected with DAA-based treatment it can be skipped except in patients with high-risk behaviors or risk for reinfection.

–Patients should be assessed for clinical side effects at each visit.

–ALT levels should be assessed at baseline and at 12 and 24 wk or more frequently if suggestive symptoms.

–Monitoring of indirect bilirubin, renal function, and labs may be indicated based on the treatment being used.

–Treatment should be stopped if having severe adverse events or if ALT flare with levels >10 times the upper limit of normal.

Improving treatment adherence

–When possible a multidisciplinary team should be used to deliver HCV treatment.

–Importance of adherence to treatment should be stressed.

–Services recommended to improve compliance are: social services support, peer-based support, and patient activation assessment.

–Harmful alcohol consumption during treatment should be screened for and treated.

Posttreatment follow-up for patients with SVR

–Patients with SVR and fibrosis scores of:

- F0–F2 and no ongoing risky behavior for reinfection may be discharged.
- F3 requires HCC surveillance every 6 mo with ultrasound.
- F4 (cirrhosis) requires HCC surveillance as well as endoscopic surveillance for esophageal varices if seen on pretreatment endoscopy.

–Remind patients of the risk of reinfection and monitoring for reinfection should be carried out in high-risk group (ie, injection drug users, men who have sex with men) biannually preferred but annually at a minimum.

–Retreat as needed if reinfected.

Follow-up for untreated patients and treatment failures

–Untreated and treatment failures should be followed regularly with continued surveillance for liver fibrosis every 1 to 2 y.

–HCC surveillance is every 6 mo indefinitely for all patients with advanced fibrosis (F3) and cirrhosis (F4).

▶ WHO 2016

–All adults and children with chronic HCV infection, including people who inject drugs, should be assessed for antiviral treatment.

–It is now recommended that DAA regimens be used for the treatment of persons with hepatitis C infection rather than regimens with pegylated interferon/ribavirin.

–For patients with HCV genotype 3 infection with cirrhosis, and patients with genotypes 5 and 6 infection with and without cirrhosis, an interferon-based regimen (sofosbuvir/pegylated interferon/ribavirin) is still recommended as an alternative treatment option.

–The use of boceprevir—or telaprevir—containing regimens is no longer recommended for the treatment of persons with hepatitis C infection.

–None of the DAAs have been approved for use among children; thus, the only approved treatment for children remains pegylated interferon/ribavirin, which is recommended for children older than 2 y.

Source

–http://www.who.int/hepatitis/publications/hepatitis-c-guidelines-2016/en/

HEREDITARY HEMOCHROMATOSIS (HH)

Recommendations

▶ American Association for the Study of Liver Disease (AASLD) 2011

  –Clinical Features

  - Asymptomatic patients with abnormal iron studies (increased ferritin and iron saturation) should be evaluated for hemochromatosis.
  - All patients with liver disease should be evaluated for hemochromatosis. (*Ann Intern Med.* 2006;145:209)

  –Diagnosis

  - Combination of transferrin saturation (TS) and ferritin should be done—if either is abnormal (TS >45% or ferritin >upper limit of normal), the HFE mutation analysis is indicated.
  - Screening (iron studies and HFE mutation studies) is recommended for first-degree relatives. (*Ann Intern Med.* 2009;143:522)
  - Liver biopsy is recommended for diagnosis and prognosis in patients with phenotypic markers of iron overload who are not C282Y homozygotes or compound heterozygotes (C282Y, H63D).
  - Liver biopsy to stage the degree of liver disease in C282Y homozygote or compound heterozygotes if liver enzymes elevated or ferritin >1000 µg/L.

  –Treatment of Hemochromatosis

  - Therapeutic phlebotomy weekly until ferritin level 50–100 µg/L.
  - C282Y homozygotes who have an elevated ferritin (but <1000 µg/L) should proceed to phlebotomy without liver biopsy.
  - Patients with end-organ damage due to iron overload should undergo regular phlebotomy to keep ferritin between 50 and 100 µg/L.
  - Vitamin C and iron supplements should be avoided but other dietary adjustments not necessary.
  - Patients should be monitored on a regular basis for reaccumulation of iron and undergo maintenance with targeted ferritin levels of 50–100 µg/L.
  - Use of iron chelation with deferoxamine or deferasirox is not recommended in hemochromatosis. (*Blood.* 2010;116:317-325) (*Blood.* 2008;111:3373-3376) (*Hepatology.* 2011;54:328-343)

Source

  –Practice guidelines. *Hepatology.* 2011;54:328-343.

Comments

Problems in Hemochromatosis

1. Symptoms besides liver function abnormalities include skin pigmentation, pancreatic dysfunction with diabetes, arthralgias, impotence, and cardiac involvement with ECG changes and heart failure.

2. Other rare mutations causing phenotypic hemochromatosis include transferrin receptor 2 mutation, ferroportin mutation, and H ferritin mutation.

3. The most devastating complication of hemochromatosis is a 20-fold increase in the risk of hepatocellular carcinoma (HCC). Less than 1% of patients whose ferritin has never been >1000 µg/L develop HCC, while the risk rises considerably in patients with cirrhosis and ferritin level >1000 µg/L. These patients should be screened with hepatic ultrasound every 6 mo. Alfa fetoprotein (AFP) is elevated in only 60% of patients with HCC and should not be used as a single screening test. (*Liver Cancer.* 2014;3:31)

4. Patients with hemochromatosis are at increased risk for certain bacterial infections whose virulence is increased in the presence of iron overload. These include *Listeria monocytogenes* (most common in renal dialysis patients), *Yersinia enterocolitica*, and *Vibrio vulnificus* (uncooked seafood is a common source). Infections are made more virulent by iron overload of macrophages impairing their antibacterial activity.

5. Secondary iron overload (most commonly secondary to a transfusion requirement due to blood or bone marrow disease) is best managed by iron chelation beginning when the ferritin rises above 1000 µg/L. In contrast to HH, excess iron is deposited primarily in the reticuloendothelial system, although visceral iron overload does occur over time. (*Blood.* 2014;124:1212)

INFLAMMATORY BOWEL DISEASE, CROHN'S DISEASE

Population

–Children, young adults, and adults with Crohn's disease.

Recommendations

▶ NICE 2012 (updated in 2016)

–Inducing remission in Crohn's disease.
- Glucocorticoids are recommended for a single exacerbation in a 12-mo period.
  - Prednisolone, methylprednisolone, or IV hydrocortisone.

- Add azathioprine or mercaptopurine to steroids if steroids cannot be tapered or ≥2 exacerbations in last 12 mo.
  - Assess thiopurine methyltransferase (TPMT) activity before offering azathioprine or mercaptopurine. Do not offer azathioprine or mercaptopurine if TPMT activity is deficient.
  - Monitor for neutropenia.
- Consider adding methotrexate in people who cannot tolerate azathioprine or mercaptopurine.
- Infliximab or adalimumab is indicated with active fistulizing refractory to conventional therapy.
  - Given for maximum of 12 mo at a time, or until treatment failure (ie, need for surgery).
- Maintaining remission.
  - Azathioprine.
  - Mercaptopurine.
  - Do not offer a conventional glucocorticosteroid or budesonide to maintain remission.
- Managing strictures.
  - Balloon dilation is an option for single stricture that is short, straight, and accessible by colonoscopy.
- Recommend routine surveillance for osteopenia or osteoporosis.

Source
- https://www.nice.org.uk/Guidance/cg152

Comments
The American College of Gastroenterology (ACG) updated its clinical guideline for the management of Crohn's disease in adults in 2018. Recommendations are generally in line with the above. New updates include:

1. Fecal calprotectin is a helpful diagnostic test to differentiate the presence of IBD from irritable bowel syndrome.
2. NSAIDs may exacerbate disease activity and should be avoided.
3. Oral mesalamine has not consistently been demonstrated to be effective for induction of remission and achieving mucosal healing in patients with active Crohn's disease.
4. Natalizumab is more effective than placebo and should be considered to be used for induction of symptomatic response and remission in patients with active Crohn's disease.
5. Other treatments such as Ustekinumab, novel anti-integrin therapy (with vedolizumab), and diet may be helpful.
6. Surgery is required to treat enteric complications of Crohn's disease; a resection of a segment of diseased intestine is the most common surgery.
7. If a patient has risk factors, it may be helpful to take postoperative prophylaxis with anti-TNF agents.

INFLAMMATORY BOWEL DISEASE, ULCERATIVE COLITIS

Population
–Children, young adults, and adults.

Recommendations

▶ AGA 2019

–Mild-to-moderate proctitis and proctosigmoiditis to achieve and maintain remission:
  • Start treatment with mesalamine enemas (or suppositories) rather than oral mesalamine or rectal corticosteroids.
  • For patients with proctitis, use mesalamine suppositories. If suppositories are ineffective then use rectal corticosteroids.
–Mild-to-moderate extensive, left-sided:
  • Add rectal mesalamine to oral 5-ASA for treatment.
–Mild-to-moderate extensive, pan colonic:
  • Use standard-dose mesalamine (2–3 g/d) or diazo-bonded 5-ASA rather than low-dose mesalamine, sulfasalazine, budesonide MMX, or no treatment.
  • If suboptimal response to standard-dose mesalamine or diazo-bonded 5-ASA or with moderate disease activity patients should be increased to high-dose mesalamine (>3 g/d) with rectal mesalamine.
  • For patients on oral mesalamine once daily dosing is recommended to increase compliance.
–Mild-to-moderate ulcerative colitis, refractory:
  • For patients with refractory disease that are optimized on oral and rectal 5-ASA, regardless of extent of disease, use oral prednisone or budesonide MMX.

Source
–https://doi.org/10.1053/j.gastro.2018.12.009

Comments

1. Patients with prominent arthritic symptoms may reasonably choose to use sulfasalazine 2–4 g/d if alternatives are cost-prohibitive.
2. Patients who place a higher value on convenience and lower value on effectiveness may use oral rather than rectal administration.
3. Patients who place a higher value on avoiding issues with the mesalamine enemas and do not mind lower effectiveness may use rectal corticosteroid foam preparations.

Population

–Children, young adults, and adults.

Recommendations

▶ NICE 2013

–Mild-to-moderate proctitis and proctosigmoiditis to achieve and maintain remission.
- Aminosalicylate suppository or enemas.
- Oral aminosalicylate.
- Topical corticosteroid.

–Mild-to-moderate extensive left-sided colitis.
- Induction dose oral aminosalicylate.
- Consider adding oral tacrolimus to oral prednisolone if remission not achieved after 4 wk of prednisolone therapy.
- Maintain remission with low-dose aminosalicylate.

–Severe acute ulcerative colitis.
- IV methylprednisolone.
- Consider IV cyclosporine for those in whom steroids cannot be used or have not improved after 72 h of steroid therapy.
- Consider a colectomy for:
  ◦ Persistent diarrhea >8 bowel movements/d.
  ◦ Fevers.
  ◦ Hemodynamic instability.
  ◦ Toxic megacolon.
  ◦ CRP >4.5 mg/dL.

Source

–https://www.nice.org.uk/Guidance/cg166

Comments

1. Oral prednisolone is an adjunct to aminosalicylates for proctitis or colitis if remission is not attained within 4 wk.
2. Consider adding oral azathioprine or oral mercaptopurine to maintain remission if not maintained by aminosalicylates alone.
3. Monitor bone health in children and young adults with chronic active disease or who require frequent steroid therapy.

INFLAMMATORY BOWEL DISEASE, ULCERATIVE COLITIS, SURGICAL TREATMENT

Population
–Patients with UC.

Recommendation

▶ American Society of Colon and Rectal Surgeons 2014
–Indications for surgery in UC:
- Patients with acute colitis and actual or impending perforation.
- Chronic UC refractory to medical therapy.
- Presence of carcinoma or high-grade dysplasia in colon.
- Development of a colonic stricture.
- Consider a second-line agent or surgery for acute colitis that is worsening after 96 h of first-line medical therapy.

Source
–https://www.fascrs.org/sites/default/files/downloads/publication/practice_parameters_for_the_surgical_treatment_of.3.pdf

Comments
1. Procedure of choice for emergency surgery is a total or subtotal colectomy with end ileostomy.
2. Procedure of choice for elective surgery is a total proctocolectomy with ileostomy or ileal pouch-anal anastomosis.
3. Patient with severe diarrhea (>8 stools/d) in absence of *C. difficile* colitis and a c-reactive protein >4.5 mg/dL despite medical therapy for 72 h has an 85% chance of requiring a colectomy.

IRRITABLE BOWEL SYNDROME (IBS)

Population
–Adults with symptoms of IBS.

Recommendations

▶ NICE 2015
–Consider IBS for any adult with any of these symptoms for at least 6 mo.
- Abdominal pain.
- Bloating.
- Change in bowel habit.

–Assess all patients with possible IBS for red flag indicators that argue against IBS.
- Unintentional weight loss.
- Rectal bleeding.
- Anemia.
- Abdominal mass.
- Change in bowel habit to looser and more frequent stools if over 60 y.

–Recommend for all patients with suspected IBS.
- Complete blood count.
- ESR.
- C-reactive protein.
- Anti-endomysial antibody and anti-tissue transglutaminase antibody to rule out celiac disease.

–Lifestyle recommendations for IBS.
- Eat regular meals.
- Drink at least 8 cups of non-caffeinated beverage daily.
- Limit intake of tea, coffee, and alcohol.
- Reduce intake of "resistant starch."
- Avoid sorbitol, an artificial sweetener, for diarrhea-predominant IBS.

–Pharmacologic therapy for IBS.
- Consider laxatives as needed (except lactulose) for constipation.
- Consider linaclotide for refractory constipation for longer than 12 mo.
- Consider antispasmodic agents as needed for pain.
- Loperamide is the antimotility agent of choice for diarrhea.
- Consider low-dose tricyclics (TCAs) as second-line treatment if antispasmodics or antimotility agents have not helped.
- Consider SSRI therapy if TCAs are ineffective.
- Consider cognitive behavioral therapy or hypnotherapy for IBS refractory to above therapies.

Source
–https://www.nice.org.uk/guidance/qs114

LIVER DISEASE, ALCOHOLIC

Population
- Adults.

Recommendations
▶ EASL 2018
- Public Health Policies to Reduce Alcoholic Liver Disease (ALD)
  - Address excess alcohol consumption using pricing-based policies and regulation of availability.
  - Ban advertising or marketing of alcohol.
  - Screen for harmful alcohol consumption in primary care and emergency settings.
  - Screen for alcoholic liver disease in high-risk populations (rehabilitation clinics or patients identified with excessive alcohol consumption).
  - Give identified patients a brief intervention and referral to a multidisciplinary team for treatment.
- Alcohol use disorder (AUD)
  - Alcohol use disorder (defined by DSM-V criteria) is the preferred term in place of alcoholic, alcohol abuse, alcohol dependence, or risky drinker.
  - Screen for AUD using AUDIT or AUDIT-C.
  - Evaluate patients with AUD for concurrent psychiatric disorders and other addictions.
  - Use benzodiazepines to treat alcohol withdrawal syndrome (AWS) but for no more than 10–14 days due to potential abuse and/or encephalopathy.
  - Access to effective psychosocial therapies is important while treating patients with AUD.
  - Patients who have both AUD and ALD should receive pharmacotherapy for cessation.
- Management of alcoholic hepatitis (AH)
  - Suspect AH in patients with recent onset of jaundice and excessive alcohol consumption.
  - Identify severe forms of AH who are at risk of early mortality using prognostic calculators.
  - If no infection, give prednisolone 40 mg/d or methylprednisolone 32 mg/d for patients with severe AH to reduce short-term mortality. Medium- and long-term survival do not change.

- Assess response at 7 d and if no response, stop steroids. If non-responder highly, selected patients can be considered for liver transplant.
- Consider N-acetylcysteine (for 5 d IV) as adjunct to corticosteroids in patients with severe AH.
- Provide nutrition orally to maintain ≥35–40 kcal/kg body weight and 1.2–1.5 g/kg protein per day.
- Alcohol-related fibrosis and cirrhosis
  - Complete abstinence from alcohol is recommended for patients with alcohol-related cirrhosis as it reduces liver-related complications and death.
  - Identify and manage cofactors including obesity and insulin resistance, malnutrition, cigarette smoking, iron overload, and viral hepatitis.
  - Screening and management of complications from cirrhosis are managed similarly for alcohol-related cirrhosis.
- Liver transplantation
  - Liver transplant for patients with Child-Pugh C or MELD ≥15 confers a survival benefit.
  - Do not use a 6-mo sobriety criterion alone for consideration of liver transplant and instead include degree of liver-insufficiency, addiction and psychological profile, and supportive relatives.
  - Patients on the liver transplant list should be regularly checked for abstinence.
  - A multidisciplinary approach evaluating medical and psychological suitability for transplant is mandatory.
  - An addiction medicine specialist may reduce relapses in heavy drinking patients.
  - Early liver transplant may be proposed in a minority of patients with severe AH and not responding to treatments.
  - All liver transplant candidates should be screened for cardiovascular, neurological, psychiatric disorders, and neoplasms before and after liver transplant.
  - Risk factors for cancer should be aggressively targeted such as cigarette smoking, and early reduction in calcineurin inhibitor therapy can be considered to decrease the risk for de novo cancers after liver transplant.

Source
- https://doi.org/10.1016/j.jhep.2018.03.018

LIVER DISEASE, NONALCOHOLIC (NAFLD)

Population
–Children and adults.

Recommendations

▶ AASLD 2017

Adults

–Patients suspected of having NAFLD must have competing etiologies excluded: significant alcohol consumption, hepatitis C, medications, parenteral nutrition, Wilson's disease, autoimmune liver disease, and severe malnutrition.

–Do not screen routinely for NAFLD in high-risk groups such as diabetic or obesity clinics or in family members of patients with NAFLD.

–Ongoing or recent alcohol consumption >21 standard drinks per week for men and >14 standard drinks per week for women is considered significant alcohol consumption, and patients should be evaluated for NAFLD.

–Patients with an incidental finding of hepatic steatosis (HS) on imaging should be managed:

- If LFTs are normal then metabolic risk factors should be assessed (obesity, diabetes mellitus, dyslipidemia) and other causes of HS sought such as significant alcohol consumption or medications.
- If signs/symptoms attributable to liver disease or abnormal LFTs, evaluate for NAFLD.

–Clinicians should have a high index of suspicion for NAFLD or nonalcoholic steatohepatitis (NASH) in type 2 diabetic patients and those with metabolic syndrome. A clinical decision tool such as the NFS or fibrosis-4 index can help identify those at low or high risk for advanced fibrosis. Alternatives are using vibration-controlled transient elastography or MR elastography to assess fibrosis.

–Consider liver biopsy in patients:

- With high ferritin and high iron saturation liver to determine the extent of iron accumulation in the liver.
- At increased risk of steatohepatitis and/or advanced fibrosis.
- All patients with a competing etiology for hepatosteatosis which requires a liver biopsy to exclude.

–Pharmacological treatment aimed to improve liver disease is limited to those with biopsy-proven NASH and fibrosis.

–Weight loss is first-line therapy to reduce hepatosteatosis. Weight loss of 3%–5% of body weight improves steatosis; however, weight loss of

7%–10% of body weight is needed to improve liver fibrosis. Bariatric surgery can be considered in select patients to help with weight loss but is not an established first-line therapy.

–Metformin is not recommended to treat NASH.

–Pioglitazone improves NASH histology in patients with and without type 2 diabetes. It may be used to treat patients with biopsy-proven NASH after risks and benefits have been discussed. It should not be used in patients with suspected NASH.

–GLP-1 agonists should not be used to treat NAFLD or NASH patients.

–Vitamin E at 800 IU/d in nondiabetic biopsy-proven NASH patients improves liver histology. It should not be used with diabetics, NAFLD without liver biopsy, NASH cirrhosis, or cryptogenic cirrhosis.

–Ursodeoxycholic acid, omega-3 fatty acids are not recommended to treat NAFLD or NASH.

–NAFLD patients are at high risk for cardiovascular disease and should have aggressive lifestyle modifications and pharmacotherapy. NAFLD and NASH do not have increased risk of liver injury from statins and they should be prescribed when appropriate.

–Patients with NASH cirrhosis should be screened for esophageal varices and HCC with the same frequency/modalities used for other types of cirrhosis. Non-cirrhotic NASH patients do not require screening.

Children

–Children with fatty liver disease who are very young or not overweight should prompt testing for chronic liver disease related to fatty acid oxidation defects, lysosomal storage diseases, and peroxisomal disorders in addition to the usual causes found in adults.

–Do not screen for NAFLD in children.

–A liver biopsy should be obtained before starting pharmacotherapy in children.

–Intensive lifestyle modifications are first-line treatment in children.

–Metformin is not recommended.

–Vitamin E 800 IU/d in biopsy-proven NASH patients has been shown to improve liver histology. Long-term use of vitamin E in children is unknown and should be discussed prior to starting treatment.

Source
–https://doi.org/10.1002/hep.29367

PANCREATITIS, ACUTE (AP)

Population

–Individuals with acute pancreatitis.

Recommendations

ACG 2013

–Diagnosis of acute pancreatitis
- Includes the presence of 2 of the 3 following criteria:
  ◦ abdominal pain consistent with the disease,
  ◦ serum amylase and/or lipase greater than 3 times the upper limit of normal, and/or
  ◦ characteristic findings from abdominal imaging.
- Recommend a contrast-enhanced CT scan or MRI of the pancreas if the diagnosis is unclear or if symptoms are not improving within 72 h.
- A gallbladder ultrasound should be performed in all patients with AP.
- All patients without a history of alcohol abuse or gallstones should have a serum triglyceride level checked.
- Consider ICU or intermediate-level monitoring for any organ dysfunction.

–Initial management
- Aggressive isotonic fluids at 250–500 mL/h.
- ERCP indicated for AP associated with choledocholithiasis.
- In the absence of cholangitis or jaundice, recommend MRCP or endoscopic ultrasound to screen for choledocholithiasis.
- Prophylactic antibiotics for severe necrotizing AP is not recommended.
- In patients with infected necrosis, antibiotics known to penetrate pancreatic necrosis, such as carbapenems, quinolones, and metronidazole, may be useful in delaying or sometimes totally avoiding intervention, thus decreasing morbidity and mortality.
- In mild AP, oral feedings with clear liquids or low-fat diet can be started immediately if there is no nausea and vomiting, and the abdominal pain has resolved.
- In severe AP, enteral nutrition is recommended to prevent infectious complications. Parenteral nutrition should be avoided, unless the enteral route is not available, not tolerated, or not meeting caloric requirements.
- Nasogastric delivery and nasojejunal delivery of enteral feeding appear comparable in efficacy and safety.

- In patients with mild AP, found to have gallstones in the gallbladder, a cholecystectomy should be performed before discharge to prevent a recurrence of AP.
  - In a patient with necrotizing biliary AP, in order to prevent infection, cholecystectomy is to be deferred until active inflammation subsides and fluid collections resolve or stabilize.
  - In stable patients with infected necrosis, surgical, radiologic, and/or endoscopic drainage should be delayed preferably for more than 4 wk to allow liquefaction of the contents and the development of a fibrous wall around the necrosis (walled-off necrosis).

Source
  –https://gi.org/guideline/acute-pancreatitis/

Population
  –Adults with acute pancreatitis.

Recommendations

▶ AGA 2018
  –Use judicious goal-directed therapy for fluid management for resuscitation.
  –Do not use hydroxyethyl starch (HES) fluids.
  –Start oral feeding early (within 24 h) as tolerated rather than nil per os (NPO).
  –If patients are unable to feed orally, use enteral nutrition rather than parenteral.
  –For patients with predicted severe acute pancreatitis and necrotizing pancreatitis:
    - Do not give prophylactic antibiotics.
    - If requiring enteral tube feeding, use the nasogastric or nasojejunal route.
  –For patients with acute biliary pancreatitis and no cholangitis:
    - Do not obtain urgent ERCP.
    - Perform cholecystectomy during the initial admission rather than after discharge.
  –For patients with acute alcoholic pancreatitis, give a brief alcohol intervention and counseling.

Source
  –https://doi.org/10.1053/j.gastro.2018.01.032

PARACENTESIS

Population
–Adults with ascites.

Recommendations
▶ AASLD 2012

–Diagnostic abdominal paracentesis should be performed in inpatients and outpatients with clinically apparent new-onset ascites.
–The initial laboratory investigation of ascitic fluid should include an ascitic fluid cell count and differential, ascitic fluid total protein, and serum-ascites albumin gradient.
–Do not routinely administer fresh frozen plasma prior to a paracentesis.

Source
–https://www.aasld.org/sites/default/files/guideline_documents/ AASLDPracticeGuidelineAsciteDuetoCirrhosisUpdate2012Edition4_.pdf

ULCERS, STRESS

Recommendation
▶ SHM 2013

–Do not prescribe medications for stress ulcer prophylaxis to medical inpatients unless they are at high risk for GI complications.

Source
–https://www.shmabstracts.com/abstract/evaluation-of-stress-ulcer-prophylaxis-for-patients-with-coagulopathy-secondary-to-chronic-liver-disease/

Genitourinary Disorders

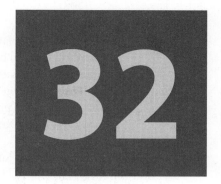

BENIGN PROSTATIC HYPERPLASIA (BPH)

Population

–Adult men age >45 with lower urinary tract symptoms (LUTS) from prostatic enlargement.

Recommendations

▶ AUA 2010

–Do not routinely measure serum creatinine in men with BPH.

–Do not recommend dietary supplements or phytotherapeutic agents for LUTS management.

–Patients with LUTS and no signs of bladder outlet obstruction by flow study should be treated for detrusor overactivity.

- Alter fluid intake.
- Behavioral modification.
- Anticholinergic medications.

–Options for moderate-to-severe LUTS from BPH (AUA symptom index score ≥8).

- Watchful waiting.
- Medical therapies.
  ○ Alpha-blockers.[a]
  ○ 5-Alpha-reductase inhibitors.[b]
  ○ Anticholinergic agents.
  ○ Combination therapy.
- Transurethral needle ablation.
- Transurethral microwave thermotherapy.

---

[a]Alfa-blockers: alfuzosin, doxazosin, tamsulosin, and terazosin. All have equal clinical effectiveness.
[b]5-Alfa-reductase inhibitors: dutasteride and finasteride.

- Transurethral laser ablation or enucleation of the prostate.
- Transurethral incision of the prostate.
- Transurethral vaporization of the prostate.
- Transurethral resection of the prostate.
- Laser resection of the prostate.
- Photoselective vaporization of the prostate.
- Prostatectomy.

–Surgery is recommended for BPH causing renal insufficiency, recurrent urinary tract infections (UTIs), bladder stones, gross hematuria, or refractory LUTS.

Source
　–http://www.guidelines.gov/content.aspx?id=25635&search=aua+2010+bph

Comments

1. Combination therapy with alpha-blocker and 5-alpha-reductase inhibitor is effective for moderate-to-severe LUTS with significant prostate enlargement.
2. Men with planned cataract surgery should have cataract surgery before initiating alpha-blockers.
3. 5-Alpha-reductase inhibitors should not be used for men with LUTS from BPH without prostate enlargement.
4. Anticholinergic agents are appropriate for LUTS that are primarily irritative symptoms, and if patient does not have an elevated post-void residual (>250 mL).
5. The choice of surgical method should be based on the patient's presentation, anatomy, surgeon's experience, and patient's preference.

ERECTILE DYSFUNCTION (ED)

Population
　–Adult men.

Recommendations
▶ EAU 2018, Endocrine Society 2018
　–Perform a medical and psychosexual history on all patients.
　–Perform a focused physical examination to assess CV status, neurologic status, prostate disease, penile abnormalities, and signs of hypogonadism.
　–Recommend exercise and decreased BMI.

–Check a fasting glucose, lipid profile, and morning fasting total testosterone levels.

–Refer for psychosexual therapy if psychogenic ED.

–Offer testosterone therapy for androgen deficiency if no contraindications are present.[c]

–Selective phosphodiesterase 5 (PDE5) inhibitors are first-line therapy for idiopathic ED.

–If PDE5 fail, consider intercavernosal injections or penile prosthesis.

Sources

–*J Clin Endocrinol Metab.* 2018;103(5):1-30.

–https://uroweb.org/guideline/male-sexual-dysfunction/

Comments

1. Selective PDE5 inhibitors:
   a. Sildenafil (100 mg, half-life 2–4 h).
   b. Tadalafil (20 mg, half-life 18 h).
   c. Vardenafil (20 mg, half-life 4 h).
   d. Avanafil (200 mg, half-life 6–17 h).
2. Avoid nitrates and use alpha-blockers with caution when prescribing a selective PDE5 inhibitor.

HEMATURIA

Population

–Adults with microscopic hematuria.

Recommendation

▶ AUA 2012

–Workup and management of microscopic hematuria.

Source

–Davis R, Jones JS, Barocas DA, et al. *Diagnosis, Evaluation and Follow-up of Asymptomatic Microhematuria (AMH) in Adults: AUA Guideline.* American Urological Association Education and Research, Inc., 2012:1-30.

[c]Prostate CA, breast CA, signs of prostatism, men who intend fertility in short term, PSA >4 ng/mL or >3 ng/mL and high-risk, or comorbidities that would be a contraindication.

ALGORITHM FOR THE DIAGNOSIS AND MANAGEMENT OF INCIDENTALLY DISCOVERED MICROSCOPIC HEMATURIA

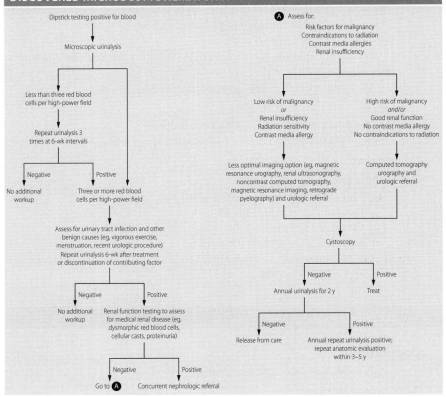

INDWELLING URINARY CATHETERS OR INTERMITTENT CATHETERIZATION

Recommendation
▶ AUA 2015
  - Avoid empiric antibiotics unless the patient has symptoms of a urinary tract infection.

Source
  - http://www.choosingwisely.org/clinician-lists/american-urological-association-antimicrobials-indwelling-or-intermittent-bladder-catheterization/

INFERTILITY, MALE

Population
  - Adults.

Recommendations
▶ EAU 2018
  - Assessment of male infertility includes:
    • Semen analysis.
  - Scrotal ultrasound:
    • If semen analysis is abnormal, check FSH, LH, and testosterone levels.
  - Refer patients with abnormal screens to a specialist in male infertility for potential treatments that may include clomiphene citrate, tamoxifen, human chorionic gonadotropin (hCG), dopamine agonists, or surgical treatments depending on the underlying etiology.

Source
  - https://uroweb.org/guideline/male-infertility/#4

Comment
1. Infertility is defined as the inability of a sexually active couple not using contraception to conceive in 1 y.

OVARIAN CANCER FOLLOW-UP CARE

Population

–Women treated for ovarian cancer with complete response (Stages I–IV).

Recommendation

▶ NCCN 2015

–**Follow-up plan**

- Office visits every 2–4 mo for 2 y, then 3–6 mo for 3 y, then annually after 5 y.
- Physical exam including pelvic exam and measurement of CA-125 with each visit.
- Refer for genetic risk evaluation if not previously done.
- Chest/abdominal/pelvic CT, MRI, PET-CT, or PET as clinically indicated due to symptoms or rising CA-125.

Source

–https://www/nccn.org/professionals/physician_gls/pdf/ovarian/pdf

Comments

–**Clinical Points**

1. All patients with ovarian cancer should be screened for BRCA 1 and 2 mutations. Ten percent of patients with Lynch syndrome will develop ovarian cancer.
2. Around 23,000 new cases of ovarian cancer are reported in the United States, with 14,000 deaths; 5-y survival is related to stage:
   a. Stage I: 86% alive at 5 y.
   b. Stage II: 68%.
   c. Stage III: 38%.
   d. Stage IV: 19%.
3. Relapsed ovarian cancer is rarely curable, but sequential treatments and intraperitoneal chemotherapy have extended survival to 50–60 mo.

PAP SMEAR, ABNORMAL

ABNORMAL PAP SMEAR ALGORITHM

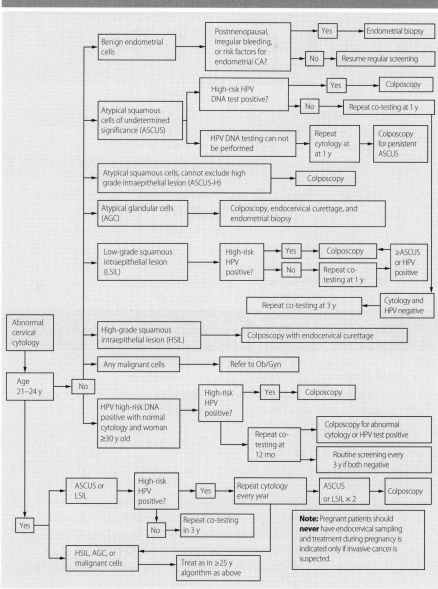

Source: Modified from the ASCCP 2013 Updated Consensus Guidelines for Managing Abnormal Cervical Cancer Screening Tests and Cancer Precursors at http://www.asccp.org/ConsensusGuidelines/tabid/7436/Default.aspx.

POLYCYSTIC OVARY SYNDROME

Population

–Adolescent and adult women.

Recommendations

▶ Endocrine Society 2013

–Diagnosis if 2 of 3 criteria are met:
- Androgen excess.
- Ovulatory dysfunction.
- Polycystic ovaries.

–Treatment
- Hormonal contraceptives for menstrual irregularities, acne, and hirsutism.
- Exercise and diet for weight management.
- Clomiphene citrate recommended for infertility.
- Recommends against the use of metformin, inositols, or thiazolidinediones.

Source
–http://www.guideline.gov/content.aspx?id=47899

PROSTATE CANCER: ACTIVE SURVEILLANCE (AS) FOR THE MANAGEMENT OF LOCALIZED DISEASE

Population

–Men with early clinically localized prostate cancer (Stages T_1 and T_2 and Gleason score less than or equal to 7).

Recommendations

▶ CCO 2016, ASCO 2016

–For most patients with low-risk (Gleason score 6 or less) localized prostate cancer with a PSA <10, employ active surveillance (AS).

–If younger age, high-volume Gleason 6 cancer, patient preference, and/or African-American ethnicity, consider definitive therapy.

–For patients with limited life expectancy (<5 y) and low-risk cancer, consider watchful waiting rather than active surveillance.

–Offer active treatment (radical prostatectomy [RP] or radiation therapy [RT]) for most patients with intermediate-risk (Gleason score 7) localized prostate cancer. For select patients with low-volume, intermediate-risk (Gleason score $3 + 4 = 7$) localized prostate cancer, consider active surveillance.

–Active surveillance consists of:
- PSA test every 3–6 mo.
- Direct rectal exam at least once a year.
- At least a 12-core confirmatory transrectal ultrasound-guided biopsy (including anterior-directed cores) within 6–12 mo and then serial biopsy every 2–5 y thereafter or more frequently if clinically warranted. Men with limited life expectancy may transition to watchful waiting and avoid further biopsies.

–For patients undergoing AS who are reclassified to a high-risk category (Gleason score now 7 or greater and/or significant increase in volume of Gleason 6 tumor consideration) should be given active therapy (RP or RT).

Comments

1. There are other ancillary tests that may make a difference in deciding when definitive therapy is indicated. The multiparametric MRI (mpMRI) and genomic testing of the malignant prostate cancer may reveal larger tumor size or unfavorable mutations that put the patient in a higher risk category which will need definitive therapy.

2. Data at 10-y follow-up from both observational and randomized trials show a very similar survival, although patients on surveillance had an increase in frequency of metastatic disease and clinical progression. (*N Engl J Med.* 2016;375:1415)

3. This approach is especially beneficial to patients older than 65 who have comorbidities and higher risk of complications. Active surveillance also significantly avoids over-treatment and therapy-related morbidity. A recent 10-y follow-up comparing monitoring, surgery, and radiation therapy treatment outcomes resulted in very similar overall survival.

Sources

–ASCO. *J Clin Oncol.* 2016;34:2182-2190.
–*N Engl J Med.* 2016;375:1415.
–*N Engl J Med.* 2014;370:932.
–*Eur Urol.* 2015;67:233.

PROSTATE CANCER FOLLOW-UP CARE

Population
–Prostate cancer survivors.

Recommendations

▶ ASCO 2015

–**Surveillance for prostate cancer patient recurrence**
- Measure serum PSA (prostate-specific antigen) every 4–12 mo (depending on recurrence risk) for the first 5 y then recheck annually thereafter.
- Evaluate survivors with elevated or rising PSA levels as soon as possible by their primary treating specialist.
- Perform an annual direct rectal examination.
- Adhere to ASCO screening and early detection guidelines for 2nd cancers (increased risk of bladder and colon cancer after pelvic radiation).

–**Assessment and management of physical and psychosocial effects of PC and treatment**
- Anemia related to androgen deprivation therapy (ADT).
- Bowel dysfunction and symptoms especially rectal bleeding.
- Cardiovascular and metabolic effects for men receiving ADT—follow USPSTF guidelines for evaluation and screening for cardiovascular risk factors.
- Assess for distress and depression and refer to appropriate specialist.
- Osteoporosis and fracture risk in men on ADT—do baseline DEXA (dual energy x-ray absorptiometry) scan and support with calcium, vitamin D, and bisphosphonates as indicated.
- Sexual dysfunction—phosphodiesterase type 5 inhibitors may help—refer to appropriate specialist.
- Urinary dysfunction (incontinence and leakage)—refer to urology specialist.
- Vasomotor symptoms (hot flushes) in men receiving ADT—selective serotonin or noradrenergic reuptake inhibitors or gabapentin may be helpful. Low-dose progesterone may be helpful in refractory patients.

Source
–Prostate cancer survivorship care guidelines. *J Clin Oncol.* 2015;33: 1078-1085.

Comments

General health promotion can be helpful

1. Counsel survivors to achieve and maintain a healthy weight by limiting consumption of high-caloric food and beverages.
2. Counsel survivors to engage in at least 150 min/wk of physical activity.
3. Improve dietary pattern with more fruits and vegetables and whole grains.
4. Encourage intake of at least 600 IU of vitamin D per day as well as sources of calcium not to exceed 1200 mg/d.
5. Counsel survivors to avoid or limit alcohol consumption to no more than 2 drinks/d.
6. Counsel survivors to avoid tobacco products.

Rising PSA in patients with nonmetastatic PC

1. A PSA ≥0.2 ng/mL on 2 consecutive tests is reflective of recurrent prostate cancer. These patients are treated with pelvic radiation with improvement in 10-y survival and freedom from recurrence. The earlier radiation is started after a PSA rise, the better the outcome. Patients who have had previous radiation to the prostate occasionally undergo surgery but most are treated with ADT or cryoablation (*JCO.* 2009;27:4300-4305). A recent trial adding ADT to radiation in this setting increased disease-free progression. (*Eur Urol.* 2016;69:802)
2. Routine CT or bone scanning is not indicated but evaluate new symptoms even if PSA is not rising (transformation to small cell carcinoma in 5% of patients).
3. In newly relapsed patients with visceral metastasis and/or more than 4 separate bone lesions, a combination of concurrent androgen deprivation and taxotere chemotherapy is associated with a 15%–20% increased survival at 5 y vs. sequential therapy. (*N Engl J Med.* 2015;373:737. *Lancet.* 2016;387:1163)

URINARY INCONTINENCE, OVERACTIVE BLADDER

Population

–Adults.

Recommendations

▶ American Urologic Association 2014

–Rule out a urinary tract infection.

–Recommend checking a post-void residual to rule out overflow incontinence.

–First-line treatments:
- Bladder training.
- Bladder control strategies.
- Pelvic floor muscle training.

–Second-line treatments:
- Antimuscarinic meds.

–Darifenacin, fesoterodine, oxybutynin, solifenacin, tolterodine, or trospium.

–Contraindicated with narrow-angle glaucoma or gastroparesis.

–Third-line treatments:
- Sacral neuromodulation.
- Peripheral tibial nerve stimulation.
- Intradetrusor botulinum toxin A.

–Recommend against indwelling urinary catheters.

Source
–http://www.guideline.gov/content.aspx?id=48226

URINARY INCONTINENCE, STRESS

Population
–Adult women.

Recommendations
▶ AUA 2017

AUA SUI ALGORITHM 2017

Female Stress Urinary Incontinence: AUA/SUFU Evaluation and Treatment Algorithm

EVALUATION (INDICATIONS)

Initial evaluation
The initial evaluation of patients desiring to undergo surgical intervention should include the following components:
- History
- Physical exam
- Demonstration of SUI
- PVR assessment
- Urinalysis

Cystoscopy
Should not be performed unless there is a concern for lower urinary tract abnormalities

Urodynamics
May be omitted when SUI is clearly demonstrated

Additional evaluation
Additional evaluation **should** be performed in the following scenarios:
- Lack of definitive diagnosis
- Inability to demonstrate SUI
- Known/suspected NLUTD
- Abnormal urinalysis
- Urgency-predominant MUI
- Elevated PVR
- High-grade POP (if SUI not demonstrated with POP reduction)
- Evidence of significant voiding dysfunction

Additional evaluation **may** be performed in the following scenarios:
- Concomitant OAB symptoms
- Failure of prior anti-incontinence surgery
- Prior POP surgery

In patients who wish to undergo treatment, physicians should counsel regarding the availability of observation, pelvic floor muscle training, other non-surgical options, and surgical interventions. Physicians should counsel patients on potential complications specific to the treatment options.

TREATMENT

Non-Surgical
- Continence pessary
- Vaginal inserts
- Pelvic floor muscle exercises

Surgical
- Bulking agents
- Midurethral sling (synthetic) - - - - - -
- Autologous fascia pubovaginal sling
- Burch colposuspension

If a midurethral sling surgery is selected, either the retropubic or transobturator midurethral sling may be offered. A single-incision sling may be offered to index patients if they are informed as to the immaturity of evidence regarding their efficacy and safety. Physicians must discuss the specific risks and benefits of mesh as well as alternatives to a mesh sling.

SPECIAL CASES

1. Fixed immobile urethra
- Pubovaginal sling
- Retropubic midurethral sling
- Urethral bulking agents

2. Concomitant surgery for POP repair and SUI
Any incontinence procedure

3. Concomitant NLUTD
Surgical treatment following appropriate evaluation and counseling

4. Child-bearing, diabetes, obesity, geriatric
Surgical treatment following appropriate evaluation and counseling

MUI, mixed urinary incontinence; NLUTD, neurogenic lower urinary tract dysfunction; OAB, overactive bladder; POP, pelvic organ prolapse; PVR, post-void residual; SUI, stress urinary incontinence.

Source: http://www.auanet.org/guidelines/stress-urinary-incontinence

▶ ACP 2014

–Recommends pelvic floor muscle training and bladder training for urinary incontinence in women.

Source

–http://www.guideline.gov/content.aspx?id=48543

INITIAL MANAGEMENT OF URINARY INCONTINENCE IN MEN: EAU 2011

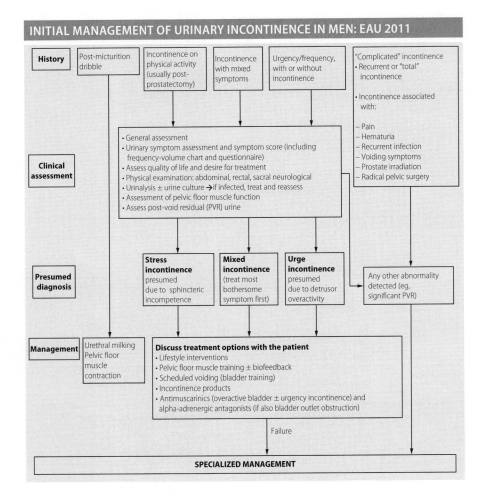

INITIAL MANAGEMENT OF URINARY INCONTINENCE IN WOMEN: EAU 2011

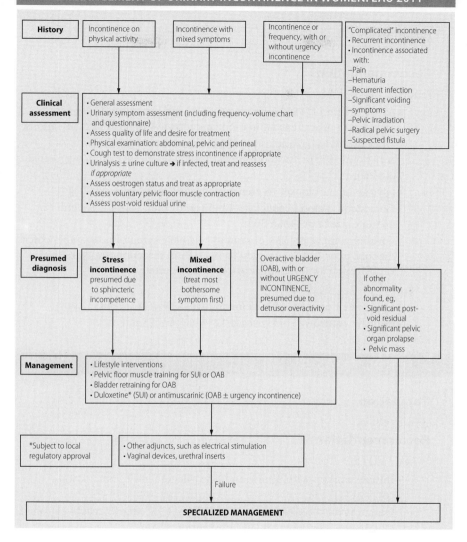

History

- Incontinence on physical activity
- Incontinence with mixed symptoms
- Incontinence or frequency, with or without urgency incontinence
- "Complicated" incontinence
  - Recurrent incontinence
  - Incontinence associated with:
    - Pain
    - Hematuria
    - Recurrent infection
    - Significant voiding
    - symptoms
    - Pelvic irradiation
    - Radical pelvic surgery
    - Suspected fistula

Clinical assessment

- General assessment
- Urinary symptom assessment (including frequency-volume chart and questionnaire)
- Assess quality of life and desire for treatment
- Physical examination: abdominal, pelvic and perineal
- Cough test to demonstrate stress incontinence if appropriate
- Urinalysis ± urine culture → if infected, treat and reassess if appropriate
- Assess oestrogen status and treat as appropriate
- Assess voluntary pelvic floor muscle contraction
- Assess post-void residual urine

Presumed diagnosis

- **Stress incontinence** presumed due to sphincteric incompetence
- **Mixed incontinence** (treat most bothersome symptom first)
- Overactive bladder (OAB), with or without URGENCY INCONTINENCE, presumed due to detrusor overactivity
- If other abnormality found, eg,
  - Significant post-void residual
  - Significant pelvic organ prolapse
  - Pelvic mass

Management

- Lifestyle interventions
- Pelvic floor muscle training for SUI or OAB
- Bladder retraining for OAB
- Duloxetine* (SUI) or antimuscarinic (OAB ± urgency incontinence)

*Subject to local regulatory approval

- Other adjuncts, such as electrical stimulation
- Vaginal devices, urethral inserts

Failure

SPECIALIZED MANAGEMENT

▼ URINARY TRACT SYMPTOMS, LOWER

Population
–Adult men.

Recommendations
▶ NICE 2010, EAU 2011

–All men with LUTS should have a thorough history and exam, including a prostate examination, and a review of current medications.
–Offer supervised bladder training exercises and consider anticholinergic medications for symptoms suggestive of an overactive bladder.
–Give an alpha-blocker to men with moderate-to-severe LUTS.[d]
–Consider a 5-alpha-reductase inhibitor for men with LUTS and prostate size larger than 30 g.
–For men with refractory obstructive urinary symptoms despite medical therapy, offer 1 of 3 surgeries: transurethral resection, transurethral vaporization, or laser enucleation of the prostate.

Sources
–http://www.nice.org.uk/nicemedia/live/12984/48557/48557.pdf
–http://www.uroweb.org/gls/pdf/12_Male_LUTS.pdf

▼ UROLITHIASIS

Population
–Adults.

Recommendations
▶ EAU 2018

–Initiate workup with ultrasound if febrile; otherwise obtain non-contrast CT.
–Obtain urine dipstick, serum chemistries, CBC, and C-reactive protein.
–Obtain coagulation testing if intervention planned.
–Obtain stone analysis for first episode or for recurrent stones despite drug therapy.
–Use NSAIDs and acetaminophen for pain control. Opioids are less effective but may be used.
–Refer for ureteral stent or nephrostomy tube if decompression required (sepsis with obstructing stones).

[d]Alfuzosin, doxazosin, tamsulosin, or terazosin.

–If intervention not pursued, offer medical therapy with alpha-blockers (tamsulosin), calcium channel blockers (nifedipine), and phosphodiesterase type 5 inhibitors (tadalafil) to improve clearance of stones. Tamsulosin has the best data to support use.

Source
–https://uroweb.org/guideline/urolithiasis/#3

Population
–Adults and children with kidney stone disease.

Recommendations
▶ AUA 2014
–Obtain noncontrast CT urogram for patients with acute flank pain.
–Evaluate renal colic by obtaining:
  • Urinalysis.
  • Serum CBC, creatinine, uric acid, calcium, and albumin +/– intact parathyroid hormone.
  • Stone analysis by x-ray crystallography or infrared spectroscopy.
–Obtain 24-h urine analysis for complicated calcium stone disease: calcium, oxalate, citrate, creatinine, urate, magnesium, phosphate, sodium, and potassium.
–Treat patients with hypercalciuria with a thiazide diuretic.
–Treat with an alkaline citrate for hypocitraturia, type 1 renal tubular acidosis (RTA), hypercalciuria, and hyperoxaluria.
–Advise adults with a history of urinary stones to drink sufficient water to maintain a urine output >2.5 L/d.
–Consider use of an alpha-receptor blocker to facilitate spontaneous passage of ureteral stones <10 mm.
–Consider active ureteral stone removal for persistent obstruction, failure of spontaneous passage, or the presence of severe, unremitting colic.
  • Options include shockwave lithotripsy or ureteroscopy.
–For calcium stones and hypercalciuria:
  • Limit sodium intake and consume 1–2 g/d of dietary calcium.
  • Thiazide diuretic.
–For calcium oxalate stones:
  • If high urinary oxalate, limit intake of oxalate-rich foods and maintain normal calcium consumption.
  • If hyperuricosuria, treat with allopurinol.
–For uric acid stones and high urinary uric acid, limit intake of nondairy animal protein.

−For struvite stones refractory to surgical management, consider acetohydroxamic acid therapy.

−For uric acid or cystine stones, consider potassium citrate therapy to raise urinary pH to optimal level.

Sources
−http://www.uroweb.org/gls/pdf/18_Urolithiasis.pdf
−http://www.guideline.gov/content.aspx?id=48229

Comment

1. Patients at high risk for recurrent stone formation:
   a. ≥3 stones in 3 y.
   b. Infection stones.
   c. Urate stones.
   d. Children and adolescents with stones.
   e. Cystinuria.
   f. Primary hyperoxaluria.
   g. Type 1 RTA.
   h. Cystic fibrosis.
   i. Hyperparathyroidism.
   j. Crohn's disease.
   k. Malabsorption syndromes.
   l. Nephrocalcinosis.
   m. Family history of kidney stone disease.

Population

−Adults with kidney stone disease.

Recommendations

▶ EAU 2013

−Recommended evaluation for renal colic:
  • Sodium, potassium.
  • CRP.
  • PT, PTT (if intervention is likely).

−Contrast-enhanced CT scan recommended if stone removal is planned and the renal anatomy needs to be assessed.

−Hyperoxaluria:
  • Oxalate restriction.
  • Pyridoxine.

−Renal colic analgesia:
  • NSAIDs.
  • Opiates.
  • Alpha-blockers.

  –Management of sepsis with obstructed kidney:
  - Requires urgent decompression with a ureteral stent or percutaneous nephrostomy tubes.
  - Start antibiotics immediately.
  –Indications for active kidney stone treatment:
  - Stone growth.
  - Acute or chronic pain.
  - Kidney infection.
  - Kidney obstruction.
  –Stop antiplatelets and anticoagulation before stone removal.
  –Goal is to drink water to maintain a urine output >2.5 L/d.
  –Struvite and infection stones:
  - Surgical removal of stones.
  - Antibiotics.
  - Urinary acidification.
  - Urease inhibition.
  –Cystine stones.
  - Potassium citrate.
  –Tiopronin.

Source
  –http://www.guideline.gov/content.aspx?id=45324

Population
  –Children with kidney stone disease.

Recommendations
▶ EAU 2013
  –Recommend a complete metabolic workup based on stone analysis.
  –Ultrasound is the preferred imaging method in children.
  –Percutaneous nephrolithotripsy is recommended for treatment of renal pelvic or calyceal stones with a diameter >20 mm.

Source
  –http://www.guideline.gov/content.aspx?id=45324

Hematologic Disorders

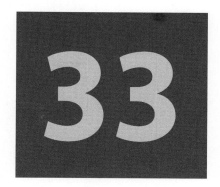

ANEMIA

Population
–Adults and children.

Recommendations
▶ British Society of Gastroenterology 2011
–Initial evaluation should include a complete blood count, including Hb and mean corpuscular volume, as well as a reticulocyte count, ferritin level, total iron-binding capacity, and transferrin saturation, permitting the calculation of a reticulocyte index and Mentzer index.

Comment
1. Iron deficiency anemia (IDA) and anemia of chronic disease (ACD), sometimes called anemia of inflammation, are the two most common causes of anemia. ACD is often underrecognized, with some hospital-based studies in the United States estimating the prevalence as high as 70%.

ANEMIA, CHEMOTHERAPY ASSOCIATED

Population
–Adults with cancer and anemia.
▶ ASH 2019

Recommendations
–Offer erythrocyte-stimulating agents (ESAs) to patients with chemotherapy-associated anemia whose cancer treatment is intended to cure and whose Hb has declined to <10 g/dL. RBC transfusion is

TABLE I: COMMON CAUSES OF ANEMIA						
Cause	MCV	Ferritin Level	RDW	Hb Electrophoresis	Iron/TIBC	Mentzer Index[a]
Iron deficiency anemia (IDA)	Low	<30	High	Normal	<10%	>13
Anemia of chronic disease (ACD)	Normal/Decreased	High	Normal/High	Normal	>15%	>13
IDA + ACD	Normal	<100	High	Normal	<20%	>13
Beta thalassemia	Low	Normal	Normal	↑A_2, F hemoglobin	~20%	<13
Alpha thalassemia	Low	Normal	Normal	Normal	~20%	<13
Hemoglobin E	Low	Normal	Normal	↑HgbE	~20%	<13
B_{12}/Folate deficiency	High	Normal	High	Normal	Normal	<13

[a]Mentzer index = MCV divided by red blood cell number (RBC) in millions.
RDW, red cell distribution of width; TIBC, total iron binding capacity.

also an option, depending on the severity of the anemia or clinical circumstances.

–Do not offer ESAs to most patients with cancer not on chemotherapy who have anemia. It may be offered to patients with lower risk myelodysplastic syndromes and a serum erythropoietin <500 IU/L.

–In patients with myeloma, non-Hodgkin lymphoma, or chronic lymphocytic leukemia (CLL), clinicians should observe the hematologic response to cancer treatment before considering an ESA.

–Counsel patients on the thromboembolic risks associated with ESAs prior to initiation.

–Epoetin beta and alfa, darbepoetin, and biosimilar epoetin alfa have equivalent safety and efficacy.

–Discontinue ESAs if no response within 6–8 wk.

–Consider iron replacement to improve Hb response and reduce RBC transfusions. See "Anemia of Chronic Disease" section for iron store assessment in inflammatory states.

Comment

1. FDA-approved starting dose of epoetin is 150 U/kg 3 times/wk or 40,000 U weekly. For darbepoetin the dose is 2.25 µg/kg weekly or 500 µg every 3 wk subcutaneously.

ANEMIA, HEMOLYTIC (HA)

Population

–Adults.

Recommendations

▶ BSH 2016

–Diagnose when there is evidence of hemolysis (anemia, jaundice, elevated LDH, decreased haptoglobin, elevated reticulocyte index), a positive direct antiglobulin test, and clinical evaluation has excluded an alternative cause. Categorize into primary autoimmune hemolytic anemia (AIHA), secondary AIHA, and drug-induced autoimmune hemolytic anemia (DIIHA).

–Give prednisolone 1 mg/kg/d for primary AIHA or secondary AIHA not responding to other treatments.

–Often, in secondary AIHA, treating the associated condition may improve the AIHA.

  • Eg, rituximab with or without chemotherapy for non-Hodgkin lymphoma, anti-lymphoma therapy for Hodgkin lymphoma (HL), splenectomy for splenic marginal zone lymphoma.

–If DIIHA is suspected, stop the offending medication. Improvement usually occurs within 1–2 wk. The addition of steroids is of uncertain benefit though it is frequently used.

–CMV reactivation and parvovirus B_{12} infection should be excluded in the evaluation of AIHA associated with hematologic malignancy.

–Patients presenting with AIHA during remission of HL should be assessed for recurrence. If remission is confirmed, treatment should be for primary AIHA.

–Azathioprine, danazol, mycophenolate mofetil, and rituximab may be considered in AIHA due to systemic lupus erythematosus not responding to steroids.

–In metastatic malignancy, AIHA can respond to disease control or to corticosteroids.

–Assess for thromboprophylaxis, given association between hemolysis and thrombosis.

–Transfuse for life-threatening anemia with ABO, Rh, and Kell-matched RBCs rather than waiting for full compatibility testing.

–Consider intravenous immunoglobulin (IVIG) as a rescue option in patients with AIHA.

Comments

1. HA is caused by the host's immune system acting against its own red cell antigens.
2. Incidence is 1 per 100,000/y. Approximately half are secondary to an associated disorder. Of these, half are associated with malignancy, a third due to infection, and one-sixth to collagen vascular disorders.
3. Most cases of AIHA are warm agglutinins, but cold hemagglutinin diseases (CHAD) are also reported.
4. AIHA occurs in 5%–10% of patients with CLL.
5. Secondary causes of warm AIHA include neoplasms (CLL, lymphoma, solid organ tumors), infections (hepatitis C, HIV, CMV, VZV, pneumococcal infection, leishmaniasis, tuberculosis), and immune dysregulation (SLE, Sjögren, scleroderma, ulcerative colitis, primary biliary cirrhosis, sarcoidosis, posttransplantation).
6. Secondary causes of cold AIHA include neoplasms (CLL, NHL, solid organ tumors), infections (mycoplasma, viral infections including infectious mononucleosis), autoimmune diseases, and postallogenic hematopoietic stem cell transplant.
7. The most frequent benign associations to AIHA are ovarian teratoma and thymoma. Resection of the tumor consistently resolves the AIHA.
8. Case reported causes of DIIHA include anti-infectives (ceftriaxone and other cephalosporins, beta-lactamase inhibitors, piperacillin, ciprofloxacin, doxycycline, amoxicillin), anti-neoplastics (fludarabine,

oxaliplatin, chlorambucil), pain medications (diclofenac, acetaminophen, ibuprofen), antihypertensives (hydrochlorothiazide, amlodipine, ramipril, enalapril), and omeprazole.

9. AIHA associated with solid organ tumors tends to be less steroid responsive.

10. Watch out for Evan's syndrome: autoimmune thrombocytopenia plus autoimmune hemolytic anemia, occurring either concurrently or consecutively. Neutropenia is also a common feature. Generally chronic, affects both children and adults. Treatment is largely the same as for AIHA (first line: prednisone 1–2 mg/kg/d; second line: IVIG; third line: cyclosporin, MMF, azathioprine, danazol, ribuximab, and splenectomy).

ANEMIA, IRON DEFICIENCY

Population
–Adults.

Recommendations
▶ British Society of Gastroenterology 2011

Evaluation

–Screen with upper and lower endoscopy for postmenopausal females and all male patients with confirmed IDA unless there is a history of recent significant non-GI blood loss.

–Screen all patients with IDA for celiac disease and *H. pylori*, but do not defer colonoscopy if the patient is >50-y-old, has marked anemia, or has a significant family history of colorectal cancer.

–Screen all patients for hematuria and work up accordingly.

–Fecal occult blood testing is of no benefit and rectal exam is seldom contributory in IDA.

–If the patient has undergone gastrectomy and has IDA, obtain upper and lower endoscopy if >40-y-old.

–If there is no response to iron replacement, perform an iron absorption test: check a baseline iron level and then a second iron level 2–4 h after ingesting a single 325-mg ferrous sulfate tablet with water. An increase in the iron level of at least 100 µg/dL indicates adequate absorption.

–If upper and lower GI tracts are normal, obtain small bowel visualization if the patient has symptoms of small bowel disease and/or continued anemia despite iron replacement.

–Iron deficiency without significant anemia should also be worked up with GI evaluation in postmenopausal women and men >40-y-old.

Treatment

–Ferrous sulfate 200 mg (65-mg elemental iron) administered twice per day is the classic treatment of IDA; however, new data suggests that every other day dosing may be superior to BID dosing. Ferrous fumarate, gluconate, and suspensions are noninferior and may be better tolerated. Taking iron 15–30 min before a meal with orange juice or 500 mg of vitamin C may enhance absorption. Continue treatment for 4–8 mo to fully replete iron stores.

–If intolerant of iron, noncompliant, or not improving despite oral therapy, give intravenous iron sucrose (dose 200 mg once or twice a week until the calculated iron deficit is administered), ferric carboxymaltose (dose 1000 mg once weekly). Hemoglobin levels can take 8–10 wk to normalize. Reserve transfusion of RBC for cardiovascular instability or persistent symptomatic anemia despite IV iron therapy.

Comments

1. Symptoms of IDA: weakness, headache, irritability, fatigue, exercise intolerance, and restless leg syndrome. Symptoms may occur without anemia in patients with iron depletion (ferritin < 30 ng/mL). As many as 40% of patients with IDA will experience pica (appetite for clay, starch, and paper products) and/or pagophagia (craving for ice) which resolves rapidly with iron repletion.

2. Rarely, in severe prolonged iron deficiency, dysphagia with esophageal webs (Plummer–Vinson syndrome), koilonychias (spoon nails), glossitis with decreased salivary flow, and alopecia can occur.

3. Common causes of non-occult IDA: menstruation and blood donation.

4. Common causes of occult IDA: aspirin/NSAID use, colonic carcinoma, gastric carcinoma, benign gastric ulcerations, angiodysplasia, and celiac disease. Less common causes include *H. pylori* infection, gastrectomy, esophagitis, hematuria, gastric antral vascular ectasias, and small bowel tumors. Infrequent causes of IDA include *Ancylomasta duodenale* infection, epistaxis, intravascular hemolysis (especially paroxysmal nocturnal hemoglobinuria and microangiopathic hemolytic anemia), pulmonary hemosiderosis, autoimmune gastritis, and congenital IDA (germline mutation in the *TMPRSS6* gene which leads to a reduction in iron absorption and mobilization).

5. 20%–25% of patients will have dose-dependent GI side effects from oral iron including abdominal pain, nausea, constipation, and diarrhea.

ANEMIA OF CHRONIC DISEASE

Population
–Adults and children.

Recommendations
▶ BJH 2011, NICE 2015
- –Treat the underlying inflammatory or malignant process.
- –Test for concomitant iron deficiency and determine potential responsiveness to iron therapy and long-term iron requirements every 3 mo (every 1–3 mo for people receiving hemodialysis):
  - Percentage of hypochromic cells >6%, reticulocyte hemoglobin content <29 pg, or transferrin saturation <20%, and serum ferritin <100 mg/L are consistent with iron deficiency.
  - The ratio of the serum transferrin receptor (sTFR) to the log of the serum ferritin can also be used to establish the presence of IDA. A ratio <1 makes ACD likely, whereas a ratio >2 suggests that iron stores are deficient, with or without ACD.
- –Do not order transferrin saturation or serum ferritin alone to assess iron deficiency in people with ACD or chronic kidney disease (CKD).
- –In people with anemia of CKD, treat clinically relevant hyperparathyroidism to improve the management of the anemia.
- –In people treated with iron, serum ferritin levels should not rise above 800 mcg/L.
- –Do not initiate erythropoietic-stimulating agent (ESA) therapy in the presence of absolute iron deficiency without also managing the iron deficiency.
- –Offer treatment with ESAs to patients with ACD/anemia of CKD who are likely to benefit in terms of quality of life and physical function. ESA should not be used if hemoglobin >10 g/dL. The main benefit of ESA is to reduce transfusion need.
- –ESA is not to be used in patients with curable malignancies or in patients with cancer not on chemotherapy. Side effects of thrombosis and potentially increased cancer growth should be discussed with the patient.
- –Goal Hb is typically 10–12 g/dL for adults, young people, and children 2 y and older, and between 9.5 and 11.5 g/dL for children younger than 2 y of age. Rate of rise goal is typically 1–2 g/dL/mo.
- –Avoid blood transfusions in people with anemia of CKD in whom kidney transplant is a treatment option due to antibody formation. Blood transfusion should be reserved for severe or life-threatening anemia in the context of ACD.

–For patients with anemia of CKD who are iron deficient and not on ESA therapy, consider a trial of oral iron before offering intravenous iron therapy. If intolerant of oral iron or target Hb levels are not reached within 3 mo, offer IV iron therapy. If the patients are receiving hemodialysis, offer IV iron.

–For patients who are iron deficient, receiving ESA therapy, and receiving hemodialysis, offer IV iron.

Comments

1. Frequent causes of ACD include infections (viral, bacterial, parasitic, fungal), malignancies, autoimmune diseases (rheumatoid arthritis, systemic lupus erythematosus, vasculitis, sarcoidosis, inflammatory bowel disease), CKD, and heart failure.
2. IDA frequently occurs concomitantly with ACD.
3. Classically ACD has a mild-to-moderate anemia, normochromic and normocytic, with a low reticulocyte index. Inflammation is typically evident through inflammatory markers such as the white blood cell count, platelet count, C-reactive protein, or erythrocyte sedimentation rate.
4. Routine measurement of erythropoietin is not recommended.
5. Epoetin and darbepoetin are equal in efficacy. FDA-approved starting dose of epoetin is 150 U/kg 3 times/wk or 40,000 U weekly. For darbepoetin the dose is 2.25 μg/kg weekly or 500 μg every 3 wk subcutaneously.
6. When patients stop chemotherapy for any reason, stop ESAs and substitute transfusion therapy according to FDA guidelines.
7. In people treated with iron, serum ferritin levels should not rise above 800 mcg/L.

COBALAMIN (B_{12}) AND FOLATE (B_9) DEFICIENCY

Population

–Adults ≥ 19 y of age.

Recommendations

▶ BJH 2014

–There is no gold standard test for the diagnosis of cobalamin deficiency. Serum cobalamin lacks sensitivity and specificity (a cutoff of 200 ng/L results in a sensitivity of 95% but specificity of 50%).

–Consider cobalamin or folate deficiency when CBC shows oval macrocytes or hyper-segmented neutrophils in the presence of an elevated MCV.

–Cobalamin and folate assays should be assessed concurrently.

–Consider plasma total homocysteine (tHcy) and/or plasma methylmalonic acid (MMA) as supplementary tests if there is clinical suspicion of cobalamin deficiency but intermediate cobalamin level. Both are elevated in cobalamin deficiency. tHcy is a sensitive marker, but MMA is more specific. Holotranscobalamin, the active fraction of plasma cobalamin, may be a suitable assay for assessment of cobalamin status in the future.

–Test all patients with anemia, neuropathy, or glossitis, suspected of having pernicious anemia for anti-intrinsic factor antibodies (IFAB) regardless of cobalamin levels. Do not test for antigastric parietal cell antibodies.

–Test for IFAB in patients with low-serum cobalamin levels in the absence of anemia and who do not have other causes of deficiency. Patients found to have a positive test should have lifelong cobalamin therapy.

–Therapy of cobalamin deficiency is important because neurologic symptoms may be irreversible if treatment is delayed.

–For patients with neurological symptoms, give parenteral cobalamin 1000 mcg IM daily or every other day for 2 wk. Then give 1000 mcg IM q3mo or 1000–2000 mcg PO daily. Oral crystalline cyanocobalamin is as effective as parenteral unless IFAB.

–Retest serum cobalamin levels after 2–4 mo to ensure normalization.

–A serum folate level <7 nmol/L (3 mcg/L) is indicative of folate deficiency. Routine RBC folate testing is not necessary.

–In the presence of strong clinical suspicion of folate deficiency, despite a normal level, an RBC folate assay may be undertaken, having ruled out B_{12} deficiency.

–The dose of folic acid necessary for treatment depends on the cause of the deficiency. Folic acid 0.8 mg PO daily is typically sufficient; however, 5 mg daily is necessary in hemolytic states and patients on hemodialysis.

Comments

1. The interpretation of cobalamin testing should be considered in relation to the clinical circumstances. Falsely low-serum cobalamin levels may be seen in the presence of folate deficiency. Moreover, neurological symptoms due to cobalamin deficiency can occur in the presence of a normal MCV.

2. The most frequently cited causes of cobalamin deficiency include *H. pylori*, *Giardia lamblia*, fish tapeworm, pernicious anemia, gastric resection, celiac disease, tropical sprue, Crohn disease, low dietary intake (ie, Vegan diet), metformin use, and achlorhydria due to atrophic gastritis or proton pump inhibitors.

3. The incidence of B_{12} deficiency in the elderly (>70-y-old) is 5%–10%.

4. Pernicious anemia (the most common cause of B_{12} deficiency) is an autoimmune illness with antibodies to gastric parietal cells and intrinsic factor resulting in gastric atrophy and malabsorption of food-derived B_{12}. It is associated with Hashimoto disease, type 1 diabetes, vitiligo, and hypoadrenalism.

5. Independent of the etiology of B_{12} deficiency, oral B_{12} (1000–2000 mg) daily will correct lower B_{12} levels due to intrinsic-factor independent absorption.

6. Causes of low folic acid levels include poor diet (lack of legumes and green leafy vegetables), goat's milk (as opposed to cow's milk in children), alcoholism, pregnancy, increased RBC turnover (thalassemia, hemolytic anemias, sickle cell anemia), and hemodialysis.

7. Patients with elevated MCV who are folate deficient must have B_{12} deficiency ruled out since treatment with folate in patients with B_{12} deficiency will accelerate peripheral neuropathy.

8. Drugs that can cause folate deficiency and B_{12} deficiency include trimethoprim, pyrimethamine, methotrexate, and phenytoin.

9. When treating B_{12} and folate deficiency, the MCV may decrease due to acquired iron deficiency as iron is incorporated into red cell precursors in response to B_{12} and/or folate therapy.

SICKLE CELL DISEASE

Population
–Adults and children.

Recommendations
▶ NHLBI 2014

–Give oral penicillin prophylaxis to children <5-y-old and older children who have had splenectomy or invasive pneumococcal infection. Dose (125 mg for age <3 y and 250 mg for age >3 y) twice daily. Consider withholding from children with HbSC diseases and HbS-Beta thalassemia who have not had splenectomy.

–Assure that people of all ages with sickle cell disease (SCD) have been vaccinated against *Streptococcus pneumoniae*. All infants with SCD should receive the complete series of the 13-valent conjugate pneumococcal vaccine series beginning shortly after birth and the 23-valent pneumococcal polysaccharide vaccine at 2 y, with a second dose at age 5 y. Give all other vaccines according to ACIP harmonized vaccine schedule.

–Screen annually for proteinuria beginning at age 10. If positive, perform a first morning void urine albumin-creatinine ratio and if abnormal, consult a renal specialist.

–Evaluate patients with symptoms of dyspnea on exertion for possible pulmonary hypertension.

–Refer all patients to an ophthalmologist for annual dilated eye exam beginning at age 10.

–Screen children with SCD annually with transcranial Doppler beginning at age 2 and continuing until at least age 16. Refer children with conditional (170–199 cm/sec) or elevated (>200 cm/sec) transcranial Doppler results. Do not screen patients with genotypes other than SCD.

–Ensure every patient with SCD has a reproductive plan. Provide contraceptive counseling to prevent unintended pregnancy and preconception counseling if pregnancy is desired. Progestin-only contraceptives, levonorgestrel IUDs, and barrier methods have no restrictions for use in women with SCD. If the benefits are considered to outweigh the risk, combined hormonal contraceptives (pills, patches, rings) may be used in women with SCD.

–If a partner of a patient with SCA has unknown SCD or thalassemia status, refer the partner for hemoglobinopathy screening.

–Test women with SCD who have been transfused and are anticipating pregnancy for red cell alloantibodies. If she has red cell alloantibodies, test her partner for the corresponding red cell antigens.

–Use an individualized prescribing and monitoring protocol to promote rapid, effective, and safe analgesic management and resolution of vasoocclusive crises (VOC). Use NSAIDs as an adjuvant analgesic in the absence of contraindications as well as adjunctive nonpharmacologic approaches to treat pain such as local heat application and distraction.

  • In adults and children with SCD and a VOC, do not administer a blood transfusion unless there are other indications for transfusion.
  • In adults and children with SCD and a VOC and an oxygen saturation <95% on room air, administer oxygen.

–Advise that patients seek immediate medical attention for temperatures greater than 101.3°F (38.5°C) due to the risk of severe bacterial infections. Evaluate fevers immediately with a history and physical exam, CBCD, reticulocyte count, blood culture, and urine culture when UTI is suspected.

–In children with SCD and a temperature >101.3 (38.5°C), promptly administer ongoing empiric parenteral antibiotics that provide coverage against *S. pneumoniae* and gram-negative enteric organisms. Subsequent outpatient management using an oral antibiotic is feasible in people who do not appear ill.

–In adults with SCD who have pain that interferes with daily activities and quality of life, treat with hydroxyurea.

–In infants 9 mo of age and older, children, and adolescents with SCD, offer treatment with hydroxyurea regardless of clinical severity to reduce SCD-related complications.

–Discontinue hydroxyurea in females who are pregnant or breastfeeding.

–In people with HbS-Beta thalassemia or HbSC who have recurrent sickle cell–associated pain that interferes with daily activities, consult a sickle cell expert for consideration of hydroxyurea therapy.

–Transfuse RBCs to bring the Hb level to 1 g/dL prior to undergoing a surgical procedure involving general anesthesia.

–Blood transfusion is not indicated for uncomplicated painful crisis, priapism, asymptomatic anemia, recurrent splenic sequestration, and acute kidney injury unless there is multisystem organ failure.

–Chronic transfusion therapy is recommended for a child with TCD >200 cm/sec and adults and children with previous clinically overt stroke.

–Monitor for iron overload in chronic transfusion therapy with liver function tests, serum ferritin levels, liver biopsies, and MRIs.

–Administer iron chelation therapy, in consultation with a hematologist, to patients with SCD with documented transfusion-acquired iron overload.

Comments

1. More than 2 million US residents are estimated to be either heterozygous or homozygous for the sickle cell mutation.

2. Those most affected are of African ancestry of self-identified as Black. A minority are Hispanic, southern European, Middle Eastern, or Asian Indian descent.

3. Clinical improvement with hydroxyurea may take 3–6 mo. Watch for thrombocytopenia and neutropenia with hydroxyurea treatment.

4. RBC units that are to be transfused to individuals with SCD should include matching for C, E, and K antigens.

IMMUNE THROMBOCYTOPENIA (ITP)

Population
- –Adults.

Recommendations

▶ American Society of Hematology (ASH)—Evidence-Based Practice Guidelines for ITP 2011

Diagnosis

–Diagnosis of exclusion:
- There is no reliable diagnostic test (including antiplatelet antibody studies).
- Bone marrow examination not necessary.
- Test for hepatitis C and HIV.
- Test for other underlying illnesses based on history and physical exam (ie, rheumatologic disorders, lymphoproliferative disease, *H. pylori* infection, antiphospholipid syndrome).

–Risk factors:
- Drug induced (trimethoprim-sulfa, rifampin, carbamazepine, vancomycin, quinine derivatives, and many more).
- Systemic lupus/Sjögren syndrome, and other rheumatologic diseases.
- Infections—hepatitis C, HIV, cytomegalovirus (CMV), *H. pylori*, Epstein–Barr virus (EBV), varicella.
- Indolent lymphomas, breast and colon cancer.
- Vaccinations—mostly in children.
- Common variable immunodeficiency—almost exclusively in children.

Treatment

–Newly diagnosed ITP:
- Treat if platelet count <30,000 with or without bleeding.
- First-line therapy: Corticosteroids (Prednisone 0.5–2 mg/kg daily with taper).
- Use IVIG with corticosteroids when a more rapid rise in platelet count is needed (ie, prior to surgery).
- Second-line therapy: Rituximab.
- If corticosteroids are contraindicated: IVIG or anti-D immune globulin (in patients that are Rh(+) and spleen in place).
  - IVIG dose: 1 g/kg as a one-time dose that may be repeated as necessary. (*Lancet Haematol.* 2016;3:e489) (*Blood.* 2016;127:296) (see Table II)

TABLE II: FIRST-LINE THERAPY FOR ITP		
Corticosteroids	**RR**	**% With Sustained Response**
Prednisone 0.5–2 mg/kg/d for 2 wk followed by taper	70%–80%	10-y disease-free—13%–15%
Dexamethasone 40 mg daily for 4 d every 2–4 wk for 1–4 cycles	90%	As high as 50% (2–5 y follow-up)
IV anti-D immune globulin	80%	Usually lasts 3–4 wk, but may persist for months in some patients
50–75 µg/kg—warning regarding brisk hemolysis and rare DIC		
IVIG 0.4 g/kg/d × 5 d or 1 g/kg/d for 1–2 d	80%	Transient benefit lasting 2–4 wk

– Unresponsive or relapse after initial therapy:
  • Splenectomy, either laparoscopic or open, should be done at least 2–4 wk after vaccination with pneumococcal, meningococcal, and *Haemophilus influenzae* b vaccine. Splenectomy is significantly more effective in patients less than 40-y-old compared to the elderly.
  • Thrombopoietin receptor agonists (romiplostim or eltrombopag) are often used in second-line therapy after steroids and IVIG failure or after splenectomy relapse to maintain an adequate platelet count. (*Blood*. 2012;120:960) (*J Thromb Haemost*. 2015;13:457) (*Lancet*. 2008;371:395) (*Blood*. 2013;121:537)
  • Thrombopoietin receptor agonists can be used in patients at risk for bleeding who have failed one line of therapy but have not had a splenectomy. Response rate is 80%–90%. Rituximab may be considered in patients at risk of bleeding who have failed one line of therapy, including splenectomy. (*N Engl J Med*. 2011;366:734) (*Blood*. 2014;124:3228)
– Treatment of ITP after splenectomy:
  • Platelets >30,000, no further treatment indicated in asymptomatic patients.
  • Platelets <30,000, second-line therapy (Rituxan, thrombopoietin receptor agonists, and immunosuppression) should be used (see Table III).
– Treatment of ITP in pregnancy:
  • Corticosteroids or IVIG should be used.
  • Romiplostim and eltrombopag are not approved for use in pregnant women.

TABLE III: SELECTED SECOND-LINE THERAPY OPTIONS IN ADULT ITP	
TPO Receptor Agonist	**RR**
Eltrombopag 25–75 mg orally daily	70%–80%
Romiplostim 1–10 µg/kg SQ weekly	80%–90%
Immunosuppression	
Azathioprine 1–2 mg/kg	40%
Cyclosporine 5 mg/kg/d for 6 d then 2.5–3 m/kg/d to titrate blood levels of 100–200 mg/mL	50%–60%
Cytoxan 1–2 mg/kg orally or IV (0.3–1 g/m²) for 113 doses every 2–4 wk	30%–60%
Rituximab 375 mg/m² weekly × 4	50%–60% respond—sustained >3–5 y in 10%–15%
Uncertain Mechanism	
Danazol 200 mg 2–4× daily (orally)	~50%
Vinca alkaloid 1–2 mg IV weekly to max of 6 mg	~30% variable

- Refractory patients: splenectomy can be performed during second trimester.
- Method of delivery: based upon obstetrical indications, ie, no indication for cesarean section.
  – Treatment of specific forms of secondary ITP (see Table III):
    - HCV-associated: Antiviral therapy should be considered in absence of contraindications. Initial therapy in this setting should be IVIG.
    - HIV-associated: start HAART first unless patient has significant bleeding complications. If ITP therapy is required, use corticosteroids, IVIG, anti-D immune globulin, and romiplostim or eltrombopag. Refractory patients should have a splenectomy.
    - *H. pylori*–associated: Eradication therapy of newly diagnosed active *H. pylori* infection (stool antigen, urea breath test, endoscopic biopsy) will result in resolution of ITP in 25%–35% of patients.

Sources
  – *Blood.* 2016;128:1547.
  – *Blood.* 2011;117:4190-4207.
  – *Blood.* 2010;115:168-186.

Comments

1. Be aware of autosomal-dominant hereditary macrothrombocytopenia. Platelets are large, hypogranular, and misshapen with counts between 30,000 and 60,000. Bleeding is modest but is often confused with ITP. The treatment is with platelet transfusion for significant bleeding. Treatment for ITP is ineffective.

2. TTP (thrombotic thrombocytopenic purpura) should always be excluded. Symptoms: ill appearing, low-grade fever, myalgia, chest pain, and altered mental status. Labs: thrombocytopenia and a hemolytic anemia with red cell fragmentation, elevated reticulocyte count, and significant elevation of lactate dehydrogenase. This is a *medical emergency* and should be treated urgently with plasma exchange. See next section for more details.

3. In the elderly, myelodysplastic syndrome is common, but isolated thrombocytopenia occurs in <10%. ITP is by far the most common cause of isolated thrombocytopenia, even in elderly patients.

4. Be alert to pseudothrombocytopenia caused by platelet clumping in response to ethylenediaminetetraacetic acid (EDTA). Reviewing the peripheral smear or repeating the platelet count in a citrated or heparinized tube is needed to make the diagnosis.

5. In event of life-threatening hemorrhage (usually brain or GI tract), consider platelet transfusion along with standard therapy. The platelet count usually will not rise significantly, but bleeding can be slowed. Do not give prophylactic platelets based on platelet counts or for minor bleeding.

6. Anti-D immune globulin therapy (WinRho) is associated with a small percentage of patients developing disseminated intravascular coagulation (DIC) and resultant death. Close monitoring of patients is required. This therapeutic approach is used much less frequently because of complications and more effective new drugs.

Population

–Pediatric.

Recommendations

▶ American Society of Hematology (ASH) 2011

–**Diagnosis:**

- Bone marrow (BM) examination *unnecessary* in children and adolescents with typical features of ITP (isolated thrombocytopenia, large, morphologically normal platelets, asymptomatic except for bleeding).

- BM examination also not necessary in patients failing intravenous IVIG therapy or before splenectomy.

–**Initial management:**
  - Absent or mild bleeding (bruising, petechiae): observation alone *regardless* of platelet count.
  - Moderate-to-severe bleeding: single dose of IVIG (0.8–1 g/kg) or short-course corticosteroid is first line.
  - Anti-D immune globulin (WinRho): first-line therapy in Rh-positive, nonsplenectomized children needing treatment.
    ○ Not advised in children with a hemoglobin concentration that is decreasing because of bleeding or with evidence of autoimmune hemolysis.

–**Second-line treatment for pediatric ITP:**
  - Rituximab can be considered if bleeding ongoing despite IVIG, anti-D immune globulin, and steroids.
    ○ Can also be considered as an alternative to splenectomy or in patients not responding to splenectomy.
  - High-dose dexamethasone (0.6 mg/kg/d × 4 d q 4 wk) may be considered for patients with bleeding and persistent thrombocytopenia despite initial therapy.

–**Splenectomy:**
  - Recommended for pediatric patients with chronic or persistent ITP who have significant or persistent bleeding and lack of responsiveness or intolerance to other standard therapies.
  - Do not do splenectomy for at least 12 mo after start of ITP treatment unless severe disease with significant serious bleeding risks.
  - Splenectomy in patients over 45 y has a significant risk of recurrence of thrombocytopenia compared to splenectomy in patients younger than 45 y.

–**Immunizations:**
  - Children with a history of ITP who are unimmunized should receive their scheduled first MMR vaccine.
  - If the child displays immunity based on a positive vaccine titer, then no further MMR vaccine should be given. If the child does not have adequate immunity, then the child should be re-immunized with the MMR vaccine at the recommended age.

Sources
–*Pediatr Blood Cancer.* 2009;53:652-654.
–*Blood.* 2010;115:168-186.
–*Blood.* 2013;121:4457-4462.
–*Blood.* 2014;124:3295.

Comments

1. Measurement of immunoglobulin to exclude common variable immune deficiency (CVID) is common practice as ITP can be the presenting feature of CVID.
2. Treatment focuses on severity of bleeding, not platelet cell count. In a study of 505 children with platelets <20,000 and skin bleeding, only 3 patients developed severe bleeding and none had intracranial hemorrhage.
3. The older the child or adolescent, the more likely they are to have chronic ITP (defined as platelet count <150,000 at 6-mo follow-up).
4. Anti-D immune globulin therapy more effective at 75 vs. 50 μg/kg, but increased toxicity including small percentage with DIC. Drop in hemoglobin averages 1.6 g/dL.
5. Response rate to splenectomy is 70%–80%, but unless a child has severe unresponsive disease, delay the splenectomy for at least 12 mo since 20%–30% will have spontaneous remission.
6. Immunize patients undergoing splenectomy at least 2 wk before surgery with pneumococcal, meningococcal, and *H. influenzae* type b vaccine.
7. Rituximab efficacy varies from 30% to 50% in trials. Serious side effects: serum sickness, severe hepatitis in hepatitis B carriers, and rare cases of multifocal leukoencephalopathy.
8. MMR (measles, mumps, rubella) vaccination-induced ITP occurs in 2.6 per 100,000 vaccine doses. ITP following natural measles or rubella infection ranges from 600 to 1200 per 100,000 cases.
9. Thrombopoietin receptor agonists (romiplostim and eltrombopag) are active agents for ITP in adults but have not been adequately studied in children.

HEPARIN-INDUCED THROMBOCYTOPENIA (HIT)

Population

–Adults.

Recommendations

▶ American Society of Hematology 2018

–Screening
- Only screen patients receiving heparin (including unfractionated heparin [UFH] and low-molecular-weight heparin [LMWH]).
- Low risk of HIT (<0.1%), no need to monitor platelet counts to screen for HIT.

- Intermediate risk (0.1%–1.0%) or high risk (>1%) of HIT (see comments for definitions of low, intermediate, and high risk):
  ○ If patient has received heparin in the last 30 d before starting heparin, monitor platelets on day 0 (the day heparin is initiated).
  ○ If no prior heparin in the last 30 d, monitor platelet count from days 4 to 14 or until heparin is stopped.
  ○ In intermediate-risk patients, monitor platelets every 2–3 d.
  ○ In high-risk patients, monitor platelet counts at least every other day.
–Diagnosis
- If platelets drop 30%–50%, suspect HIT and use 4T scoring model (see Table IV) to assess likelhood of HIT.
  ○ If intermediate-to-high probability, treat for HIT and send immunologic (enzyme-linked immunosorbent assay [ELISA]) and functional testing (platelet serotonin release assay).
- Do not test for or empirically treat for HIT in patients with a low-probability 4T score.
–**Management**
- Unless 4T score predicts low probability, discontinue heparin and start nonheparin anticoagulation at therapeutic intensity. Suggested agents include argatroban, bivalirudin, danaparoid, fondaparinux, or a direct oral anticoagulant (DOAC). If patient is at high bleeding risk and 4T score is intermediate, reduce intensity to prophylactic dosing.
  ○ Bivalirudin and argatroban preferred in critical illness or increased bleeding risk due to short half-life.
  ○ Fondaparinux and DOACs reasonable in clinically stable patients with average bleeding risk.
- With negative immunoassay resume heparin in place of the nonheparin anticoagulant.
- If immunoassay is positive in patients at moderate or high-probability 4T score, discontinue heparin and initiate nonheparin anticoagulant at therapeutic intensity.
- Do not give routine antiplatelet medications for isolated HIT or HITT.
- Do not start a vitamin K antagonist (VKA) before platelet count recovery (ie, >150,000/mcL):
  ○ Discontinue VKA and administer IV vitamin K and start nonheparin anticoagulant if patient is already taking VKA at onset of HIT or HITT.
- Avoid platelet transfusion unless life-threatening bleeding.

TABLE IV: DIAGNOSTIC TOOL FOR DIAGNOSIS OF HIT

4Ts	2 Points	1 Point	0 Point
Thrombocytopenia	• Fall in platelet count >50% and nadir of ≥20,000 **AND** • No surgery in preceding 3 d	• >50% fall in platelets but with surgery in preceding 3 d • 30%–50% platelet fall with nadir 10–19,000	• <30% fall in platelets • Any platelet fall with nadir <10,000
Timing of platelet fall	• 5–10 d after start of heparin • Platelet fall <5 d with heparin exposure within past 30 d	• Platelet fall after day 10 • Platelet fall <5 d with heparin exposure in past 100 d	• Platelet fall ≤day 4 without exposure to heparin in last 100 d
Thrombosis or other sequelae	• Confirmed new venous or arterial thrombosis • Skin necrosis at heparin injection sites • Anaphylactoid reaction to IV heparin	• Progressive or recurrent thrombosis while on heparin • Erythematous skin reaction at heparin injection sites	• Thrombosis suspected
Other causes of thrombocytopenia	• No alternative cause of platelet drop evident	• At least one other possible cause of drop in platelet count	Definite or highly likely cause present • Sepsis • Chemotherapy within 20 d • DIC • Drug-induced ITP • Posttransfusion purposes

High probability: 6–8 points; intermediate probability: 4–5 points; low probability: ≤3 points.

- Screen for bilateral lower extremity deep vein thrombosis (DVT) with compression ultrasonography. Include screening for bilateral upper extremity DVT if the patient has an upper extremity central venous catheter. If no DVT, continue anticoagulation until platelets are >150,000/mcL. If DVT present, continue anticoagulation for 3–6 mo.
- In patients with remote history of HIT who require VTE treatment or prophylaxis, use a nonheparin anticoagulant rather than UFH or LMWH.

Comments

1. HIT is an immune-mediated disorder triggered by the formation of antibodies to a heparin/platelet factor 4 antigen complex. The complex binds to platelet FC receptors, causing activation of the platelet microparticle release and increased risk of clotting.
2. Low-risk patients include medical and obstetrical patients receiving LMWH, patients receiving LMWH after minor surgery or minor trauma, and any patients receiving fondaparinux.
3. Intermediate-risk patients include medical and obstetrical patients receiving UFH and patients receiving LMWH after major surgery or major trauma.
4. High-risk populations include surgical and trauma patients receiving postoperative UFH. In this group the HIT prevalence is 0.1%–5%, with 35%–50% developing thrombosis.
5. UFH is 8- to 10-fold more likely to cause HIT compared to LMWH. Low-molecular-weight heparin is equal if not better than UFH. UFH should be used only in patients with significant renal insufficiency.
6. Platelet counts can mildly decrease in the first 4 d after starting heparin but this is not immunologically mediated and is not associated with thrombosis. (*Blood.* 2016;128:348)
7. Both VTE and arterial clotting occur in the HIT syndrome in a ratio of 3:1. Adrenal infarction with shock from arterial thrombosis has been reported.
8. HIT occurs very rarely in patients <40-y-old. HIT increases 2.4-fold in females compared to males.
9. The median platelet count in HIT is 60,000 and seldom falls below 20,000. HIT-associated thrombosis shows a propensity to occur in areas of vessel injury (sites of central venous catheter, arterial line insertion, or other vascular interventions).
10. The development of HIT is not related to the degree of exposure to heparin. A single flush of an IV line or 1 dose of prophylactic heparin can trigger the HIT syndrome. If HIT is not recognized, further administration of heparin will lead to significant increased risk of clot, morbidity, and mortality. (*N Engl J Med.* 2006;355:809-817) (*JAMA.* 2004;164:361-369)

11. The 4T scoring system is most accurate in the low-risk subset, with a negative predictive value of 0.998. (*Blood.* 2012;120:4160-4167)

THROMBOTIC THROMBOCYTOPENIA PURPURA (TTP)

Population
–Acquired TTP in adults and children.

Recommendations

▶ *British Journal of Haematology* 2012

–Classic pentad is microangiopathic hemolytic anemia (MAHA) (jaundice, anemia, schistocytes, low haptoglobin, elevated LDH, increased reticulocyte count), thrombocytopenia (epistaxis, bruising, retinal hemorrhage, hemoptysis), renal impairment (proteinuria, microscopic hematuria), fever (>37.5°C), and neurologic signs (confusion, encephalopathy, coma, headache, paresis, aphasia, dysarthria, visual problems), often with insidious onset.

- Revised diagnostic criteria state that TTP must be suspected even with only thrombocytopenia and MAHA.
- Up to 35% of patients do not have neurologic symptoms. Renal failure requiring hemodialysis on presentation is more indicative of HUS than in TTP. Median platelet count is 10,000–30,000/mcL at presentation.
- Direct Coombs test will be negative.

–If TTP is suspected, order ADAMTS-13 activity prior to starting treatment.

- Treat empirically. Do not wait for confirmatory tests.
- ADAMTS-13 activity <5% with or without the presence of an inhibitor or IgG antibodies confirms the diagnosis.

–Lab tests: ADAMTS-13 assay (activity/antigen and inhibitor/antibody), CBCD, reticulocyte count, haptoglobin, coagulation studies, CMP, cardiac troponins, LDH, urinalysis, Coombs, blood type and antibody screen, TSH, HIV, hepatitis A/B/C viruses, and autoantibodies (ANA/RF/LA/ACLA), stool culture (for pathogenic *E. coli*), CT chest/abdomen pelvis (to look for possible underlying malignancy).

–Check a pregnancy test in women of childbearing age.

–Consider EKG or echocardiogram and brain imaging (CT or MRI).

–TTP is a medical emergency: 3 units of fresh-frozen plasma should be given while a large-bore catheter is placed for plasma exchange, which should begin within 4–8 h of presentation.

–Plasma exchange (TPE) should be started with 40 mL/kg body weight plasma volume (PV) exchanges. The volume of exchange can be reduced to 30 mL/kg body weight as clinical conditions and lab studies improve.

–Consider intensification in frequency of TPE to twice a day if platelet count is not rising and LDH remains high.

–Continue daily TPE for a minimum of 2 d after platelet count >150,000 and then stopped.

–Steroids (eg, IV methylprednisolone 1 g/d × 3 d or oral prednisone 1 mg/kg/d) often administered, although benefits are uncertain.

–In patients with neurologic and/or cardiac pathology (associated with increased mortality), rituximab should be used at a dose of 375 mg/m² weekly for 4 doses.

–Consider cyclosporin or tacrolimus in patients with acute and chronic relapsing TTP.

–Aspirin benefit in TTP is uncertain, but it is safe at a dose of 81 mg/d with a platelet count >50,000.

–In patients who relapse, repeat the plasma exchange protocol and add rituximab weekly.

–Folate supplementation is recommended during active hemolysis.

–Platelet transfusions are CONTRAINDICATED in TTP unless life-threatening hemorrhage (brain or GI tract).

–Thromboprophylaxis with LMWH once platelet count >50,000.

–Caplacizumab is a monoclonal antibody to VWD protein interfering with platelet binding and improves course of TTP.

Comments

1. TTP results from congenital or autoimmune loss of ADAMTS-13 activity. Loss of ADAMTS-13 prevents cleavage of large high-molecular-weight vWF. vWF binds to platelet receptor GPIB and the resulting complex obstructs the microvasculature leading to red cell fragmentation, thrombocytopenia, and organ ischemia.

2. Congenital TTP is rare, with <200 patients described worldwide. Onset usually is in later infancy or childhood. Patients may present as adults, with pregnancy as a common precipitant. Diagnosis is made by ADAMTS-13 activity <5%, with absence of antibody and confirmation of mutations in ADAMTS-13 gene. Treatment is with fresh-frozen plasma administration prophylactically every 10–20 d.

3. Differential diagnosis primarily of thrombocytopenia and MAHA includes autoimmune hemolysis/Evans syndrome, disseminated intravascular coagulation (DIC), pregnancy-associated conditions (eg, HELLP, eclampsia, hemolytic uremic syndrome [HUS]), drugs (quinine, simvastatin, interferon, calcineurin inhibitors), malignant hypertension, infections (cytomegalovirus, adenovirus, herpes simplex virus, meningococcus, pneumococcus, fungal), autoimmune

diseases (lupus nephritis, acute scleroderma), vasculitis, HUS, malignancy, catastrophic antiphospholipid syndrome.

4. Plasma exchange is not a curative therapy but does protect the patient until antibody levels decline either spontaneously or with use of corticosteroids and rituximab.

5. Mortality prior to intervention of plasma exchange in the early 1980s was 85%–90%; today the mortality is 10%–15%.

6. Precipitating factors: drugs (quinine, ticlopidine, clopidogrel, simvastatin, trimethoprim, interferon, and combined oral contraceptive pills), HIV infection, and pregnancy (usually in the second trimester).

7. Removal of the fetus has not been shown to affect the course of TTP in pregnancy.

8. In HIV-associated TTP, remission is dependent on improving the immune status of the patients.

9. Relapse at a rate of 20%–30%, commonly in the first month following successful therapy. Studies show monitoring ADAMTS-13 levels and instituting rituximab proactively can decrease the rate of disease relapse. (*Br J Haematol.* 2007;136-145) (*Blood.* 2011;118:1746)

10. HUS clinically resembles TTP, but has a different pathophysiology, and TPE is of minimal benefit. This illness is commonly caused by bacterial toxins (*Shiga*-like toxin from *E. coli*) or drugs (quinine, gemcitabine, mitomycin C). It is also associated with malignancy and autoimmune disease. In HUS, there is disruption of the endothelium and release of high-molecular-weight vWF that overwhelms the cleaving capacity of ADAMTS-13. An antibody to ADAMTS-13 is not involved. Renal failure dominates the clinical picture and 15%–20% succumb to the disease. (*Br J Haematol.* 2010;148:37) (*N Engl J Med.* 2014;371:654)

TABLE V: GUIDELINES FOR RBC TRANSFUSION

Patient Situation	Transfusion Threshold	Strength of Evidence
Nonsurgical	Hgb 7–8 g/dL	
Symptomatic, continued bleed	Any	
ICU[a]	Hgb ≤7 g/dL	Moderate
Hip fracture and cardiovascular disease	Hgb ≤8 g/dL or symptoms[a]	Moderate
Cardiac surgery	Hgb ≤7.5 g/dL or symptoms[a]	Moderate
Gastrointestinal bleeding (hemodynamically stable)	7 g/dL	Low

[a]Includes chest pain, hypoxia, hypotension and tachycardia, CHF, and ischemic bowel.

TRANSFUSION THERAPY, RED BLOOD CELL (RBC) TRANSFUSION

Population
–General population, male and female.

Recommendations
▶ 2018 Frankfurt Consensus Conference, NICE 2015
- –Transfusion carries risk of infection, immunosuppression, hemolytic transfusion reaction, transfusion-related acute lung injury (TRALI) (see Table VI).
- –Liberal transfusion strategies did not affect mortality, but did show more usage of blood products based on multiple studies in ICU patients, cardiac surgery patients, and orthopedic surgery patients with cardiovascular disease.
- –Patients with pharmacologically treatable anemia such as iron deficiency or B_{12} or folate deficiency should not be transfused unless they are significantly symptomatic.
- –Transfusion of red cells should be given slowly over first 15 min and completed within 4 h.
- –In the absence of acute hemorrhage, RBC transfusions should be given as single units.
- –High-risk situations for transfusion-associated graft versus host disease include:
  - Product donated by family member or HLA-selected donor.
  - Acute leukemia and Hodgkin and non-Hodgkin lymphoma patients on therapy.
  - Allogenic or autologous hemopoietic progenitor cell transplant recipient.
  - Aplastic anemia patients on antithymocyte globulin and/or cyclosporine.
  - Purine analogues and other drugs affecting T-cell count and function—fludarabine, clofarabine, bendamustine, nelarabine, alemtuzumab, and temozolomide.
- –Recommended preventive strategy is 2500 cGy of radiation to product to be transfused. This dose will destroy T cells. Shelf life of irradiated product is 28 d.

Sources
–*Ann Intern Med.* 2012;157:49-58.
–*Blood.* 2012;119:1757-1767.
–*Crit Care Med.* 2009:37(12):3124-3157.

TABLE VI: NONINFECTIOUS COMPLICATIONS OF BLOOD TRANSFUSION

Complication	Incidence	Diagnosis	Rx and Outcome
Acute hemolytic transfusion reaction (AHTR)	1:40,000	Serum-free hemoglobin, Coombs	Fluids to keep urine output >1 mL/kg/h, pressors, treat DIC, fatal in 1:1.8 × 10^6 RBC exposures
Delayed transfusion reaction (HTR)	1:3000–5000	Timing (10–14 d after tx)–(+) Coombs, ↑ LDH, indirect bilirubin, reticulocyte count—Ab often to Kidd or Rh	Identify responsible antigen, transfuse compatible blood if necessary
Febrile non-HTR	0.1%–1%	Exclude AHTR —↓ risk with leucocyte depletion—starts within 2 h of transfusion	Acetaminophen PO, support and reassurance
Allergic (urticarial)	1%–3%	Urticaria, pruritus but no fever—caused by antibody to donor-plasma proteins	Hold tx—give antihistamines and complete tx when symptoms resolve
Anaphylactic	1:20,000–50,000	Hypotension, bronchospasm, urticaria, anxiety, rule out hemolysis	Epinephrine 1:1000—0.2–0.5 mL SQ, steroids, antihistamine
Transfusion-related acute lung injury (TRALI)	1:10,000	HLA or neutrophil antibodies in donor blood hypoxia, bilateral lung infiltrates, and fever within 6 h of transfusion	Supportive care—steroids ineffective mortality—10%–20% (most common cause of transfusion-related fatality)

–*JAMA* 2016;316:1984.
–*N Engl J Med*. 2011;365:2433-2462.

Comments

1. If TA-GVHD does occur, mortality approaches 100%.
2. In immunosuppressed patients and in donating family members with shared genes, targeting T cells from the donor may not be eliminated through immunologic attack. These surviving T cells then interact with host cellular antigens damaging skin, liver, GI tract, and lung with high mortality.
3. Immune-compromised patients needing transfusion should have CMV serology checked and if antibodies not present CMV-negative blood should be given (70%–80% of recipients are antibody positive).

TRANSFUSION THERAPY—ALTERNATIVES TO RED BLOOD CELL TRANSFUSION

Population

–Adults and children over 1 y.

Recommendations

▶ NICE 2015

–Do not routinely offer erythropoietin to reduce the need for blood transfusion in patients having surgery.

TABLE VII: INFECTIOUS COMPLICATIONS OF TRANSFUSION	
Transfusion-Transmitted Organism	**Risk per Unit of Blood Transfused**
HIV	1 in 1,467,000
Hepatitis C	1 in 1,149,000
Hepatitis B	1 in 282,000
West Nile virus	Rare
Cytomegalovirus (CMV)	70%–80% of donors are carriers, leukodepletion ↓ risk but in situation of significant immunosuppression gives CMV-negative blood
Bacterial infection	1 in 3000—5-fold more common in platelet vs. RBC transfusion
Parasitic infection (Babesiosis, malaria, Chagas disease)	Rare

- Exceptions might include patients with anemia who meet criteria for a blood transfusion but decline it for religious reasons or in patients for whom the appropriate blood type is not available.
–Offer oral iron before and after surgery to patients with iron deficiency anemia.
–Intravenous iron can be considered for patients who:
  - Cannot tolerate, absorb, or adhere to an oral iron regimen.
  - Have too short of a time interval before surgery for oral iron to be effective.
–Offer tranexamic acid (TXA) for people undergoing surgery with expected blood loss >500 mL (adults) or >10% blood volume (children).
–Offer cell salvage with TXA for patients undergoing surgery with expected very high volume of blood loss.
  - Do not routinely offer cell salvage without TXA.

Comments

1. Correct coagulopathy, enhance hemostasis, and replete vitamin deficiencies, ie, vitamin K, prothrombin complex concentrations, tranexamic acid, B_{12}, folate, iron.
2. Consider autologous blood donation in advance of surgery, although this has marginal clinical and cost effectiveness.
3. Consider cell salvage therapy for cardiac surgery, complex vascular surgery, major obstetrical procedures, and pelvic reconstruction or scoliosis surgery.
4. Topical medications can be applied intraoperatively, such as collagen gel, cellulose, and thrombin.
5. Have a discussion with the patient and surgeon about techniques to limit blood loss, ie, hemostasis, hypotensive anesthesia, intraoperative hemodilution, blood salvage, and hypothermia.
6. Limit blood draws and use pediatric-sized blood draw tubes.

TRANSFUSION THERAPY, PLATELET TRANSFUSION

Population

–Adults and children.

Recommendations

▶ American Association of Blood Banks (AABB) 2014, NICE 2015, *Br J Haematol* 2016

–Consider platelet transfusion based on World Health Organization (WHO) bleeding score (Table VIII): prophylaxis for Grade 0 or 1 and therapeutic transfusion of >Grade 2.

TABLE VIII: MODIFIED WHO BLEEDING SCORE (Stanworth et al., 2013)	
Grade	**Type of Bleeding**
1	Petechiae/purpura that is localized to 1 or 2 dependent sites, or is sparse/nonconfluent Oropharyngeal bleeding, epistaxis <30-min duration
2	Melena, hematemesis, hemoptysis, fresh blood in stool, musculoskeletal bleeding, or soft tissue bleeding not requiring red cell transfusion within 24 h of onset and without hemodynamic instability Profuse epistaxis or oropharyngeal bleeding >30 min Symptomatic oral blood blisters, ie, bleeding or causing major discomfort Multiple bruises, each >2 cm or any one >10 cm Petechiae/purpura that is diffuse Visible blood in urine Abnormal bleeding from invasive or procedure sites Unexpected vaginal bleeding saturating more than 2 pads with blood in a 24-h period Bleeding in cavity fluids evident macroscopically Retinal hemorrhage without visual impairment
3	Bleeding requiring red cell transfusion specifically for support of bleeding within 24 h of onset and without hemodynamic instability Bleeding in body cavity fluids grossly visible Cerebral bleeding noted on computed tomography (CT) without neurological signs and symptoms
4	Debilitating bleeding including retinal bleeding and visual impairment Nonfatal cerebral bleeding with neurological signs and symptoms Bleeding associated with hemodynamic instability (hypotension, >30 mm Hg change in systolic or diastolic blood pressure) Fatal bleeding from any source

–Prophylactic platelet transfusions are indicated for:
- Platelet counts <10,000 (<20,000 in case of infection).
  ○ Except in cases of ITP, HIT, TTP, and chronic bone marrow failure.
- Elective central venous catheter (CVC) placement: platelet count <20,000.
- Lumbar puncture: platelet count <40,000.
- Major non-neurological surgery or percutaneous liver biopsy: platelet count <50,000.
- Neurosurgery or ophthalmic surgery: platelet count <100,000.

– Platelet transfusions are not recommended for:
- Nonthrombocytopenic patients having cardiopulmonary bypass surgery unless they have perioperative bleeding with thrombocytopenia or evidence of platelet dysfunction.
- Insertion of peripherally inserted central catheters (PICC), bone marrow aspiration, removal of central venous catheters, or cataract surgery.
- Intracranial hemorrhage (traumatic or spontaneous): no evidence-based recommendations.

Sources
–*Ann Intern Med.* 2015;162:205-213.
–*Blood.* 2014;123:1146-1151.
–Estcort L, et al. Guidelines for the use of platelet transfusions. *Br J Haemat.* 2016;176:3.
–Stanworth SJ, Walsh TS, Prescott RJ, Lee RJ, Watson DM, Wyncoll DL. Thrombocytopenia and platelet transfusion in UK critical care: a multicenter observational study. *Transfusion.* 2013;53:1050-1058.
–NICE. 2015. https://guidelines.gov/summaries/summary/49905

Comments

1. These guidelines do not pertain to ITP, TTP, or HIT. Platelet transfusion may worsen these immune-mediated diseases and should not be given unless there is major life-threatening bleeding. (*Blood.* 2015;125:1470)
2. Consider Factor VIIa for Glanzmann thrombasthenia and tranexamic acid + desmopressin in other platelet function disorders.
3. There is currently no strong evidence for platelet transfusion with intracranial bleed in patients taking antiplatelet drugs or in patients undergoing neurosurgery with platelets <100,000, although platelets >100,000 is current clinical practice.
4. Guidelines emphasize that clinical judgment and not a specific platelet count should be paramount in decision making.
5. Beware that the risk of bacterial infection with platelet transfusion is 1 in 3000 (5 times more common than RBC transfusions). (*Transfusion.* 2013;55:1603)

TRANSFUSION THERAPY, FRESH FROZEN PLASMA (FFP)

Population
–Adults and children over 1 y.

Recommendations

▶ NICE 2015, ASH 2018

–Consider FFP transfusion only for patients with clinically significant bleeding, without major hemorrhage, if they have abnormal coagulation test results (eg, prothrombin time or activated partial thromboplastin time ratios above 1.5).

–Do not recommend FFP transfusions to correct abnormal coagulation profiles for patients who:

- Are not bleeding (unless they are having invasive procedures or surgery with a risk of clinically significant bleeding).
- Need reversal of a vitamin K antagonist—Prothrombin complex concentrate (PCC) is preferred to FFP.

–Consider prophylactic FFP for patients with abnormal coagulation profiles who are having invasive procedures with a risk of clinically significant bleeding.

Comments

1. Typical dose of FFP is 15 mL/kg.
2. PCC normalizes the INR much faster than FFP in warfarin-associated bleeding and is associated with reduced incidence of volume overload, though has not been shown to have a mortality difference.

TRANSFUSION THERAPY, CRYOPRECIPITATE

Population

–Adults and children over 1 y.

Recommendations

▶ NICE 2015

–Consider cryoprecipitate transfusions for patients with:

- Fibrinogen level <150 mg/dL and significant bleeding.
- Fibrinogen level <100 mg/dL who require an invasive procedure or surgery with high risk of bleeding.

–Do not offer cryoprecipitate transfusions for patients who are not bleeding and are not having invasive procedures with a risk of clinically significant bleeding.

Comments

1. Use an adult dose of 2 pools when giving cryoprecipitate transfusions.
2. For children, use 5–10 mL/kg up to a maximum of 2 pools as a single dose.
3. Repeat the fibrinogen level and given further doses as needed.

TRANSFUSION THERAPY, PROTHROMBIN COMPLEX CONCENTRATE (PCC)

Population
–Adults and children over 1 y.

Recommendations
▶ NICE 2015, ASH 2018

–Offer immediate PCC transfusions for the emergency reversal of warfarin anticoagulation in patients with:
- Severe bleeding.
- Head injury with suspected intracranial hemorrhage.
- Hemorrhagic stroke.

–Consider PCC transfusions to reverse warfarin anticoagulation in patients having emergency surgery, depending on the level of anticoagulation and bleeding risk.

–Monitor the international normalized ratio (INR) to confirm that warfarin anticoagulation has been adequately reversed and consider further PCC.

Comment
1. Dosing of PCC is individualized according to the INR. Typical dosing of PCC is 25–50 U/kg. Administer with 10 mg IV vitamin K concurrently for major bleeding.

NEUTROPENIA WITHOUT FEVER

Population
–Adults.

Recommendations
▶ NIH 2012, IDSA 2018

–Neutropenia is defined as an ANC <1500 cells/mm^3.
- Mild: 1500–1000 cells/mm^3.
- Moderate: 1000–500 cells/mm^3.
- Severe: <500 cells/mm^3.

–Most commonly due to chemotherapy.

–Other etiologies include solid malignancies with bone marrow invasion, lymphoproliferative malignancies (eg, natural killer cell lymphomas, hair cell leukemia, and CLL), radiation therapy, autoimmune etiologies (eg, SLE, rheumatoid arthritis), viral (eg, CMV,

EBV, HIV), parasitic (eg, malaria), and genetic (eg, aplastic anemia, paroxysmal nocturnal hemoglobinuria, May-Hegglin anomaly).

–Chemotherapy-associated neutropenia is typically managed by chemotherapy dose modification, dose interval delays, and/or prophylaxis with G-CSFs.

–Patients who are at high risk of neutropenia from chemotherapy (>20% risk of developing febrile neutropenia) should receive granulocyte colony stimulating factors (G-CSFs).

–Patients at intermediate risk of neutropenia from chemotherapy (10%–20% risk of developing febrile neutropenia) should receive individualized consideration for the need of G-CSFs.

–Patients at low risk of neutropenia from chemotherapy (<10% risk of febrile neutropenia) do not benefit from routine use of G-CSFs.

–Antibiotic (fluoroquinolone) and antifungal (oral triazole or parenteral echinocandin) prophylaxis are recommended for patients at high risk for febrile neutropenia or profound, protracted neutropenia (defined as ANC <100 for >7 d, eg, most patients with AML/MDS or HSCT treated with myeloablative conditioning regimens).

  • Not routinely recommended for patients with solid tumors.

–HSV seropositive patients undergoing HSCT or leukemia induction therapy should receive HSV prophylaxis (eg, acyclovir, valacyclovir).

–*Pneumocystis jirovecii* prophylaxis (eg, TMP-SMX, dapsone, aerosolized pentamidine, atovaquone) is recommended for patients receiving chemotherapy regimens that are associated with >3.5% risk for pneumonia as a result of this organism (eg, those with >20 mg prednisone equivalents daily for >1 mo or purine analogue usage).

–Treatment with a nucleoside reverse transcription inhibitor (eg, entecavir or tenofovir) is recommended for patients at high risk of hepatitis B virus reactivation.

–Generally, there is no role for corticosteroids or IVIG in the outpatient management of neutropenia in cancer patients.

  • IVIG may be used for some autoimmune and chronic neutropenias unrelated to chemotherapy.

–Yearly influenza vaccination with inactivated vaccine is recommended for all patients receiving chemotherapy and all family and household contacts and health care providers.

–Good hand hygiene and minimizing exposure to pets and live plants are recommended during periods of profound neutropenia.

–A Cochrane review found no benefit to low-bacterial diets in patients with neutropenia.

–Fever and/or abdominal pain should immediately prompt further investigation according to the Infectious Disease section on Neutropenic Fever.

Comments

1. Risk factors for neutropenia include older age, comorbidities, and a history of multiple cytotoxic chemotherapy regimens.
2. Bone marrow transplantation and chemotherapy for hematologic malignancies are associated with a higher incidence of neutropenia than chemotherapy for solid tumor malignancies.

HEMOPHILIA A AND B

Population
–Adults and children.

Recommendations
▶ NHF 2018

–Hemophilia A is a loss of Factor VIII activity. Hemophilia B is a loss of Factor IX activity.
  • Usually congenital, though can develop acquired hemophilia due to cancer, SLE, or other autoimmune diseases.
–Treatment is with the corresponding recombinant (r) or plasma-derived (pd) factor concentrates.
  • No seroconversions to HIV, HBV, or HCV have been reported with third-generation recombinant or plasma-derived concentrations.
  • Human Parvovirus B_{12} and hepatitis A were transmitted by pdFVIII; however, additional changes have been made to the manufacturing process to reduce this risk.
  • There is still a theoretical risk of viral transmission with pdFVIII. Recombinant factors are therefore preferred in patients with inherited bleeding disorders.
–Cryoprecipitate should not be used unless there is a risk of loss of life or limb and no FVIII concentrate is available.
  • 1:1,000,000 risk of HIV or HCV transmission with cryoprecipitate versus theoretically zero with rFVIII.
–Desmopressin (DDAVP, intranasal or parenteral) may be used for patients with mild hemophilia A who have been documented by a DDAVP trial to have a significant rise in fVIII.
  • Not to be used in children under the age of 2 y or those who failed a DDAVP trial.
  • Use with caution in pregnancy.

- Excessive water intake can lead to hyponatremia and seizures while taking DDAVP.
- For patients with hemophilia A or B with high titer inhibitors, immune tolerance induction (ITI) is the best option for inhibitor eradication.
- Treatment for patients with hemophilia with inhibitor antibodies include:
  - FEIBA (activation prothrombin complex concentration [aPCC]) contains activation factors IIa, VIIa, and Xa and is used to bypass an inhibitor to FVIII or FIX. It is plasma derived.
  - NovoSeven RT (recombinant activated factor VII concentrate) contains activated FVIIa and is used to bypass inhibitors to FVIII or FIX.
  - Hemlibra (emicizumab-kxwh) is a bispecific FIXa- and FX-directed monoclonal antibody that bridges FIXa and FX, bypassing the FVIII inhibitor to prevent or treat bleeding in patients with hemophilia A and inhibitors.
  - There is a significant risk of thrombosis with the use of these agents. Do not exceed recommended doses.
- Patients with acquired hemophilia A can be treated with NovoSevenRT or Obizur, a recombinant porcine factor VIII (rpFVIII). Often the human FVIII inhibitor does not cross-react with the porcine FVIII, allowing for cessation of bleeding with Obizur treatment.
- Serologic confirmation of hepatitis A and B immunity is recommended for all patients with hemophilia. Seronegative patients should be immunized.

Comment

1. Do not administer DDAVP more than once every 24 h or use it for more than 3 consecutive days.

VON WILLEBRAND DISEASE

Population
- Adults and children.

Recommendations
▶ NHF 2018, NHLBI 2007
- Von Willebrand disease is an inherited bleeding disorder due to dysfunctional von Willebrand Factor (VWF).
- Suspect in patients with mucous membrane bleeding, excessive bruising or bleeding (eg, excessive menstrual bleeding, history of

postpartum hemorrhage, excessive bleeding after dental work or a surgical procedure).

–Type 1 is autosomal dominant, prevalent in 1% of the population, results in low VWF levels, and accounts for 75% of cases of VWD.

–Diagnosis is based on history and physical examination, CBC, PTT, PT/INR, fibrinogen, PFA-100 (if available), and VWD assays (VWF:Ag, VWF:RCo, and FVIII).

–Persons with type 1, 2A, 2M, 2N VWD should be treated with DDAVP.

- For surgery, trauma, or other serious bleeding episodes, if hemostasis is not achieved with DDAVP, FVIII or recombinant VWF concentrate should be used.

–Persons with type 2B and 3 VWD should be treated with FVIII concentrate or recombinant VFW concentrate.

–IV DDAVP dosing is 0.3 mcg/kg IV over 30 min.

- Peak VWF levels occur in 30–90 min.

–Intranasal dosing is 150 mcg (1 puff) for persons who weight <50 kg and 300 mcg (2 puffs) for persons weighting 50 kg or more of Stimate (1.5 mg/mL DDAVP solution, 0.1-mL puff).

–Management of minor bleeding (eg, epistaxis, simple dental extraction, menorrhagia) with DDAVP can be performed without laboratory monitoring.

–For persons with mild-to-moderate VWD, antifibrinolytics combined with DDAVP are generally effective for oral surgery.

–All major surgeries and bleeding events should be treated in hospitals with 24-h laboratory capability, a hematologist, and a surgeon skilled in the management of bleeding disorders.

–For severe bleeding or prophylaxis of major surgery, target VWF:RCo and FVIII activity levels should be at least 100 IU/dL. Subsequent dosing should maintain VWF/RCo and FVIII levels above a trough of 50 IU/dL.

–VWF concentrate is typically dosed with a 30–60 U/kg loading dose. For minor procedures, 20–40 U/kg every 12–48 h is administered as a maintenance dose. For major procedures, 20–40 U/kg every 8–24 h is administered.

–VWF replacement duration:

- Single VWF Treatment: Cardiac catheterization, cataract surgery, endoscopy without biopsy, liver biopsy, lacerations, simple dental extractions.
- 1–5 d: Breast or cervical biopsy, complicated dental extractions, gingival surgery, central line placement, laparoscopic procedures.
- 7–14 d: Cardiothoracic surgery, cesarean section, craniotomy, hysterectomy, open cholecystectomy, prostatectomy.

–In women who do not desire pregnancy, first-line treatment of menorrhagia in VWD is combined oral contraceptives or the levonorgestrel intrauterine device.

–Women who desire pregnancy with WVD should be offered to speak with a genetic counselor and a pediatric hematologist.

–Women who desire pregnancy can be treated with DDAVP, antifibrinolytics, or VWF concentrate.

–Women with VWD who are pregnant should achieve VWF/RCo and FVIII levels of at least 50 IU/dL before delivery and maintain that level for at least 3–5 d afterwards.

–Cryoprecipitate should not be used except in an emergency situation when none of the above-mentioned products are available due to risk of infection as noted above.

–Adjunctive treatments include aminocaproic acid (4-g loading dose then 6 g q6h, PO or IV) and TXA (10 mg/kg q8h IV or 1300 mg q8h PO).

Comment

1. Do not administer DDAVP more than once every 24 h or use it for more than 3 consecutive days.

▼ THROMBOPROPHYLAXIS

Population

–Adults.

Recommendation

▶ ASCO 2014, ASH 2018

Population	Thromboprophylaxis Recommendation
Hospitalized patients	Pharmacological prophylaxis recommended and preferred over mechanical. Pharmacological or mechanical preferred over combined pharmacological and mechanical. Pneumatic compression devices preferred over graduation compression stockings
Post-hospitalized patients (including skilled nursing facility)	Routine prophylaxis not recommended
Medical outpatients with minor risk factors (eg, immobility, minor injury, illness, infection)	Routine prophylaxis not recommended

Long-distance (>4 h) travelers without risk factors	Routine prophylaxis not recommended
Long-distance (>4 h) travelers with substantial risk factors (eg, recent surgery, hx of VTE, postpartum women, active malignancy, or ≥2 risk factors including OCPs, obesity, or pregnancy)	Graduation compression stocking or prophylactic LMWH recommended. Aspirin acceptable if LMWH or compression stockings are not feasible
Ambulatory patients with cancer	Routine prophylaxis not recommended. Consider in select high-risk patients
Patients with multiple myeloma receiving antiangiogenesis agents with chemotherapy and/or dexamethasone	LMWH or low-dose aspirin recommended
Patients undergoing major cancer surgery	Give prophylaxis starting before surgery and continuing for at least 7–10 d after discharge (30-mg enoxaparin BID). Consider extending to 4 wk in those undergoing major abdominal or pelvic surgery with high-risk features
Patients with end-stage cancer	Do not use anticoagulation to extend survival in the absence of other indications related to the patient's goals of care

Comments

1. VTE is the second leading cause of death among cancer patients. The highest risk cancers related to VTE are stomach and pancreas (15%). Significant risk is also associated with lung cancer, lymphoma, gynecological cancer, bladder, and testis cancer (6%).
2. Prostate and breast cancer have a significantly lower risk of VTE (0.8%–2%). Other risk factors include platelet count greater than 350,000, use of red cell growth factors, white blood cell count greater than 12,000, and BMI 35 kg/m² or higher.
3. Inferior vena cava (IVC) filters should only be used when there is documented DVT but a contraindication to anticoagulation such as active bleed, melanoma, renal cell cancer or choriocarcinoma with untreated brain metastasis, platelets below 30,000 or severe platelet dysfunction. The IVC filter must be removed as soon as anticoagulation is begun.
4. Chemotherapy (1.8-fold risk) and tamoxifen (5.5-fold risk) also predispose to VTE and these patients should be followed closely. In patients who develop clot in a vein with an indwelling venous catheter

are initially managed with anticoagulation with the catheter in place. If there is pain, edema, or progression of the clot, the catheter must be removed.

Sources
–*J Clin Oncol.* 2015;33:654-656.
–*J Clin Oncol.* 2013;31:2189-2204.
–*Ann Oncol.* 2011;22(suppl 6):v85-v92.
–*Blood.* 2013;122:2310-2317.
–*J Thromb Thrombolysis.* 2016;41:81-91.

DEEP VEIN THROMBOSIS (DVT) AND PULMONARY EMBOLISM (PE)

Population
–Adults.

Recommendations

▶ ACCP 2012/2016, ACP 2015

–For suspected initial DVT, use Wells Score for DVT to determine pretest probability and therefore diagnostic algorithm.

TABLE IX: WELLS SCORE FOR DVT	
Symptoms	**Points**
Malignancy, treatment, or palliation within 6 mo	+1
Bedridden recently >3 d or major surgery within 4 wk	+1
Calf swelling >3 cm compared to the other leg	+1
Collateral superficial veins present	+1
Entire leg swollen	+1
Localized tenderness along the deep venous system	+1
Pitting edema, confined to symptomatic leg	+1
Paralysis, paresis, or recent plaster immobilization of the lower extremity	+1
Previously documented DVT	+1
Alternative diagnosis to DVT as likely or more likely	−2

Low—0 (3% risk of DVT), Moderate—1 or 2 (20% risk of DVT), High—3 or greater (75% risk of DVT).
Source: Goldhaber SZ, Bounameaux H. Pulmonary embolism and deep vein thrombosis. *Lancet.* 2012;379:1835.

TABLE X: WELLS SCORE FOR PE	
Symptoms	**Points**
Clinical signs and symptoms of DVT	+3
PE is #1 diagnosis OR equally likely	+3
Heart rate >100	+1.5
Immobilization at least 3 d OR surgery in the previous 4 wk	+1.5
Previous, objectively diagnosed PE or DVT	+1.5
Hemoptysis	+1
Malignancy, treatment, or palliation within 6 mo	+1

Low—less than 2 (2%–3% risk of PE), Moderate—2–6 (20%–30% risk of PE), High—6 or greater (>70% risk of PE).

Source: Goldhaber SZ, Bounameaux H. Pulmonary embolism and deep vein thrombosis. *Lancet.* 2012;379:1835.

–For suspected recurrent lower extremity DVT, use the diagnostic algorithm in Figure IV. (CHEST 2012/CHEST 2016)

–For suspected pulmonary embolism, use Wells Score for PE or Revised Geneva Score for PE, creatinine clearance, and age-adjusted D-dimer to guide diagnostic strategy. (ACP 2015)

–Decision to anticoagulate, anticoagulant selection, and duration of therapy guided by multiple factors, as detailed in Figures I–VI and Tables XI–XII. (CHEST 2012/2016)

–Patients with a low-risk PE and whose home circumstances are adequate should be treated at home or discharged early as opposed to standard discharge after the first 5 d of treatment. (CHEST 2012/CHEST 2016)

–Outpatient management of VTE with rivaroxaban, apixaban, edoxaban, or dabigatran is acceptable if the patient does not have any of the following: >80-y-old, history of cancer, hx of COPD, CHF, pulse >110, BP <100, O_2 sat <90.

–Knee-high GCS (graduated compression stockings) with 30–40 mm Hg pressure at ankles for 2 y will reduce post-thrombotic syndrome risk by 50%.

Population

–Adults with cancer and VTE.

Recommendations

▶ International Society on Thrombosis and Hemostasis 2018

–Employ shared decision making, as overall data is lacking.

Figure 1. Diagnostic algorithm for suspected low pretest probability initial lower extremity DVT.

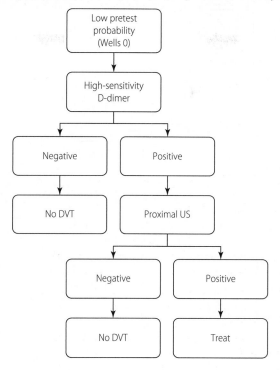

–Consider edoxaban or rivaroxaban as first-line therapy for patients with acute VTE, low bleeding risk, and no drug–drug interactions.

–Otherwise use low-molecular-weight heparins to treat acute VTE in cancer.

Source

–*J Thromb Hemost.* 2018:16(9);1891-1894. https://doi.org/10.1111/jth.14219

Comments

1. Emerging data suggest that use of modern iodinated contrast agents for CTPA is safe at least to a creatinine clearance of 30, if not lower. (*Ann Emerg Med.* 2018;71(1):44-53)
2. Consider catheter-directed thrombolysis for acute iliofemoral DVT <14-d duration, with good functional status, life expectancy of 1 y or more, and a low risk of bleeding.
3. Clinical findings alone are poor predictors of DVT.
4. Early ambulation on heparin is safe.

Figure 2. Diagnostic algorithm for suspected moderate pretest probability initial lower extremity DVT.

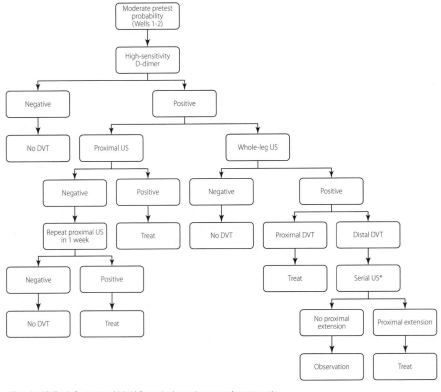

*Treat distal DVT only if patient is at high risk for proximal extension or severely symptomatic.

5. With iliofemoral thrombosis and significant swelling, thrombolysis or surgical thrombectomy not recommended unless significant symptoms.

6. IVC filter indicated if DVT and significant uncontrolled bleeding precluding anticoagulation. (*Chest.* 2016;150:1182)

7. With provoked clot, anticoagulate for 3 mo if precipitating problem is solved.[a]

8. Continue anticoagulation indefinitely if provoking problem continues.

9. In cancer-related clots, continue low-molecular-weight heparin (LMWH), do not transition to warfarin if cancer still active. (*Blood.* 2014;123:3972)

---

[a]Surgery, cancer, hormones, pregnancy, travel, inflammatory bowel disease, nephritic syndrome, hemolytic anemia, immobilization, trauma, CHF, myeloproliferative disorders, stroke, central venous catheter, rheumatologic disorders.

Figure 3. Diagnostic algorithm for suspected high pretest probability initial lower extremity DVT.

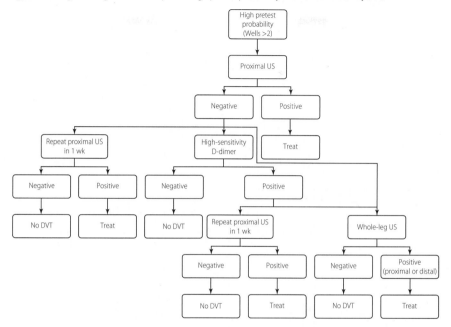

In patients with extensive unexplained leg swelling, if there is no DVT on proximal CUS or whole-leg US and D-dimer testing has not been performed or is positive, the iliac veins should be imaged to exclude isolated iliac DVT.

10. In unprovoked clot, anticoagulate for 3 mo then weigh risk of bleeding to benefit of prolonged anticoagulation to prevent clot; consider thrombophilia evaluation, including hereditary factors and antiphospholipid antibody syndrome. Men have a 50% increase in recurrent clot compared to women, and if first clot is a PE, indefinite anticoagulation is advised because of high risk of the next event being a PE (60% vs. 20%) compared to those with VTE only.

11. Rivaroxaban and other DOACs should not be used in pregnancy or in patients with liver disease.

12. Risk factors for warfarin bleeding—age >65 y, history of stroke, history of GI bleed, and recent comorbidity (MI, Hct <30, creatinine >1.5, diabetes). If all 4 factors present, 40% risk of significant bleed in 12 mo; 0.4% of patients on warfarin die of bleeding yearly. (*Chest.* 2016;149:315) (*Am J Med.* 2011;124:111)

13. Calf and iliofemoral thrombosis have increased incidence of false-negative compression ultrasound—recommend CT or MR venogram or venography for suspected iliofemoral thrombosis, and for calf thrombosis follow-up compression ultrasound (CUS) in 5–7 d is acceptable.

Figure 4. Diagnostic algorithm for suspected recurrent lower extremity DVT.

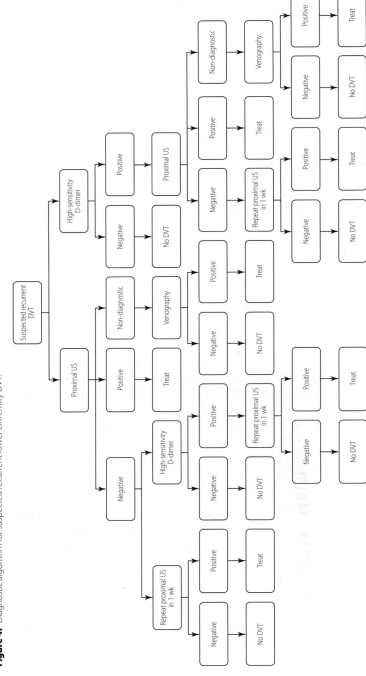

Figure 5. Diagnostic algorithm for suspected pulmonary embolism.

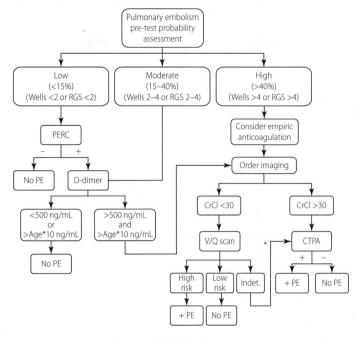

*Consider empiric treatment for PE after risk/benefit analysis.

14. Consider high thrombophilic risk in patients with recurrent VTE or patients with first unprovoked VTE who have the following characteristics:
    a. Age <50-y-old.
    b. Family history of VTE.
    c. Unusual site of thrombosis.
    d. Massive venous thrombosis.
15. In unprovoked VTE 3% of patients are found to have associated malignancy with another 10% diagnosed with cancer over the next 2 y. (*N Engl J Med.* 1998;338:1169) (*Ann Intern Med.* 2008;149:323) (*N Engl J Med.* 2015;373:697)
16. In patients with the antiphospholipid antibody syndrome and a new venous thrombosis, transition to warfarin is superior to using the new oral anticoagulants. (*Am J Hematol.* 2014;89:1017)
17. In patients with unprovoked PE or DVT, elevated D-dimer at the time of discontinuation of warfarin or 2–3 wk after stopping anticoagulants predicts for a 3- to 5-fold increase in risk of clot over the next 12 mo. (*Blood.* 2010;115:481)

Figure 6. Treatment algorithm for confirmed pulmonary embolism.

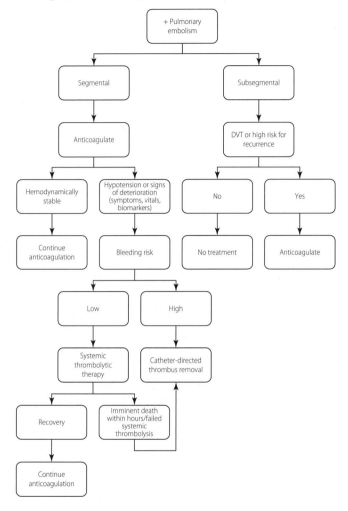

18. The presence of a permanent IVC filter does not mandate continuous anticoagulation unless documented recurrent clot problems.

19. Asymptomatic PE (found incidentally on chest CT) should be treated with same protocol as symptomatic PE. (*Blood*. 2015; 125:1877)

20. The use of aspirin (100 mg PO daily) may reduce the risk of recurrent clot in patients with unprovoked VTE after 6–12 mo of warfarin therapy. (*N Engl J Med*. 2012;366:1959)

TABLE XI: RECOMMENDED ANTICOAGULANT SELECTION AND DURATION OF ANTICOAGULATION BASED ON RISK FACTORS AND LOCATION OF DVT

Limb	Prox vs. Dist	Provoked	Cancer	Bleeding Risk	Anticoagulants	Duration
Upper	Prox	Yes	Yes		No specific recommendations	Indefinite
		No	No		No specific recommendations	3 mo
			No	High	No specific recommendations	3 mo
				Low	No specific recommendations	Indefinite
	Dist[a]	Yes	Yes		No specific recommendations	Indefinite
			No		No specific recommendations	3 mo
		No	No	High	No specific recommendations	3 mo
				Low	No specific recommendations	Indefinite
Lower	Prox	Yes	Yes		LMWH over VKA, direct thrombin, or Xa inhibitors	Indefinite
		No	No		Dabigatran, rivaroxaban, apixaban, or edoxaban over VKA	3 mo
			No	High	Dabigatran, rivaroxaban, apixaban, or edoxaban over VKA	3 mo
				Low	Dabigatran, rivaroxaban, apixaban, or edoxaban over VKA	Indefinite
	Dist[a]	Yes	Yes		LMWH over VKA, direct thrombin, or Xa inhibitors	Indefinite
			No		Dabigatran, rivaroxaban, apixaban, or edoxaban over VKA	3 mo
		No	No	High	Dabigatran, rivaroxaban, apixaban, or edoxaban over VKA	3 mo
				Low	Dabigatran, rivaroxaban, apixaban, or edoxaban over VKA	Indefinite

VKA, vitamin K antagonist.

[a]In general, treatment of isolated distal upper or lower extremity DVT is not recommended unless there are severe symptoms or a high risk for or evidence of proximal extension on ultrasound.

TABLE XII: RECOMMENDED ANTICOAGULANT SELECTION AND DURATION OF ANTICOAGULATION FOR PULMONARY EMBOLISM BASED ON RISK FACTORS AND LOCATION OF PULMONARY EMBOLISM

Location	Provoked	Cancer	Bleeding Risk	Anticoagulants	Duration
Segmental	Yes	Yes		LMWH over VKA, direct thrombin, or Xa inhibitors	Indefinite
	No	No		Dabigatran, rivaroxaban, apixaban, or edoxaban over VKA	3 mo
		No	High	Dabigatran, rivaroxaban, apixaban, or edoxaban over VKA	3 mo
			Low	Dabigatran, rivaroxaban, apixaban, or edoxaban over VKA therapy	Indefinite
Subsegmental[a]	Yes	Yes		LMWH over VKA, direct thrombin, or Xa inhibitors	Indefinite
	No	No		Dabigatran, rivaroxaban, apixaban, or edoxaban over VKA	3 mo
		No	High	Dabigatran, rivaroxaban, apixaban, or edoxaban over VKA	3 mo
			Low	Dabigatran, rivaroxaban, apixaban, or edoxaban over VKA	Indefinite

VKA, vitamin K antagonist.

[a]In general, treatment of a subsegmental PE is not recommended unless there is a concomitant DVT or high risk for recurrence.

TABLE XIII: NEW ORAL ANTICOAGULANTS[a] AND WARFARIN

Agent	Target	Dosing	Monitoring	Half-life	Time to Peak Plasma Concentration	Specific Reversible Agent
Warfarin	Vitamin K epoxide	Once daily	INR–adjusted	40 h	72–96 h	Vitamin K[b] PCC
Dabigatran	Thrombin	Fixed—once or twice daily	None	14–17 h	2 h	Idarucizumab[c]
Rivaroxaban	Factor Xa	Fixed—once or twice daily	None	5–9 h (50-y-old) 9–13 h (elderly)	2.5–4 h	Andexxa[c]
Apixaban	Factor Xa	Fixed twice daily	None	8–15 h	3 h	None[c]
Edoxaban	Factor Xa	Give once daily	None	10–14 h	1–2 h	None[c]

[a]Do not use new oral anticoagulants in patients with mechanical valves. Warfarin is superior.

[b]If significant bleed on warfarin, give vitamin K, and 4-factor prothrombin complex concentrate (PCC/K–centra) or recombinant FVIIa if not controlled.

[c]If significant bleed, aggressively treat source of bleed; consider 4-factor PCC, recombinant FVIIa or Andexxa.

21. Patients with significant risk of recurrent clot, on long-term anticoagulation with reduced dose of a DOAC, have continued protection from clot and reduced risk of bleeding (rivaroxiban— 10 mg/d, apixaban 2.5 mg BID). (*N Engl J Med.* 2017;376:1279, 1211)
22. LMWH has long been preferable to VKA for VTE in cancer (*N Engl J Med* 2003;349:146-153). The convenience and emerging prevalence of DOACs makes them appealing. Few head-to-head trials have shown noninferiority of specific DOACS vs. LMWH (*N Engl J Med.* 2018;378:615-624; *J Clin Oncol.* 2018;36(20):2017-2023), but some have suggested increased bleeding risk.

THROMBOPHILIAS

Population
–Adults.

Recommendations
▶ NICE 2016, ACOG 2018, *J Thromb Thrombol.* 2016, BSH 2012

–The most common thrombophilias include factor V Leiden (FVL), protein C deficiency (PC), protein S deficiency (PS), antithrombin deficiency (AT), prothrombin gene 20210 A/G mutation (PGM), and antiphospholipid syndrome (APS).

–As a general rule, do not perform thrombophilia testing at the time of VTE diagnosis or during the first 3 mo of anticoagulation.
  • Genotype-based tests (FVL, PGM) and antibody titers (cardiolipin and beta-2 glycoprotein I) can be performed at any point.
  • The remaining thrombophilia tests need to be performed 2–4 wk after discontinuation of anticoagulants.

–Only test for thrombophilias when the results will be used to improve or modify management.
  • Do not offer thrombophilia testing to patients who are continuing anticoagulation treatment.
  • Do not offer thrombophilia testing to patients who have had provoked VTE.
  • Consider testing for hereditary thrombophilias or antiphospholipid antibodies in patients who have had unprovoked DVT or PE if it is planned to stop anticoagulation.

–Do not routinely offer thrombophilia testing to first-degree relatives of people with a history of DVT or PE and thrombophilia.
  • This includes patients contemplating estrogen use. Even with a negative thrombophilia screen they still have an elevated risk of VTE. Only do so if the test will change your management.

- An exception would be patients who are pregnant or planning to become pregnant as it could change treatment plans.
- A positive thrombophilia evaluation is not a sufficient basis to offer extended anticoagulation following an episode of provoked VTE where the other provoking factor has resolved.
- Testing for APS requires a dual screening testing (eg, DRVVT and aPTT). If either of these is positive, a confirmatory test is performed (eg, high phospholipid concentration, platelet-neutralizing reagent, or LA-insensitive reagent).
  - Diagnosis is based on the presence of either vascular thrombosis or pregnancy morbidity plus the presence of lupus anticoagulant, anti-cardiolipin IgG and/or IgM, or anti-beta-2 glycoprotein-I.
- Primary thromboprophylaxis is not recommended for incidentally discovered APS.
- Patients <50-y-old with ischemic stroke should be screened for APS.
  - Do not routinely offer APS screening in patients >age 50.
  - Antiplatelet therapy is as effective as warfarin for ischemic stroke associated with a single positive APS test result.
- A baseline PT should be ordered when starting warfarin therapy for APS with thrombosis. If this is prolonged, an alternative PT reagent for which the baseline is normal (ie, not affected by lupus anticoagulant) should be used.
- Women with recurrent pregnancy loss (≥3 losses) before 10 wk gestation with normal fetal anatomy/genomics should be screened for APS.
- Always emphasize improvement in modifiable VTE risk factors: obesity, tobacco use, exogenous estrogen use.

Comments

1. Testing for thrombophilias in a patient with unprovoked VTE: the two-step method. After 3 mo of anticoagulation, FVL, PGM, cardiolipin, and beta-2 glycoprotein-I antibodies are ordered. If negative, anticoagulation is stopped and 2–4 wk later a D-dimer, lupus anticoagulant, PC, PS, and AT are ordered. A final decision on anticoagulation can then be made on the basis of results.
2. FVL is the most common inherited thrombophilia, with estimated carrier frequency in the United States in Caucasians 5%, Hispanics 2%, Blacks 1%, Asians 0.5%, and Native Americans 1%.
3. PGM in the United States is present in approximately 4% of Caucasians, 4% in Hispanics, 1% of Blacks, and 0.3% in Native Americans.
4. The prevalence of Protein C (PC) deficiency heterozygosity depends on the cutoff used, but may be as high as 1.5%.

5. The prevalence of protein S deficiency is unknown, but in one case-control study it accounted for 1% of VTEs. Pregnancy, female sex, and estrogen use reduce the levels of protein S. Use of sex-specific reference intervals and testing prior to pregnancy or while not receiving estrogen preparations is preferred.

6. Antithrombin deficiency heterozygosity prevalence is approximately 1 per 2500 people or 0.04%.

7. **The presence of hereditary thrombophilia does not affect survival in patients with a history of VTE or the risk of post-thrombotic syndrome.**

8. Patients with an unprovoked DVT and negative thrombophilia evaluation have the same recurrence rate for VTE as patients with an unprovoked DVT and positive thrombophilia evaluation.

9. **Heterozygosity for FVL or PGM does not increase the predicted risk of recurrence to a clinically significant degree after an unprovoked VTE.**

10. **Family history alone of thrombosis alone carries an increased risk of thrombosis, even with a negative thrombophilia evaluation.**

11. **Degree of post-thrombotic symptoms, D-dimer levels after a minimum of 3 mo of anticoagulation, and residual vein thrombosis do modify the risk of recurrence in unprovoked VTE.**

MULTIPLE MYELOMA/MONOCLONAL GAMMOPATHY OF UNDETERMINED SIGNIFICANCE

Population
–Adults.

Recommendations
▶ NICE 2016, EMN 2014, EMN 2018, ASCO 2019

–Classic findings of multiple myeloma are CRAB: hyperCalcemia, Renal failure, Anemia, and Bony lesions/pain, in addition to clonal bone marrow plasma cells.

–Serum protein electrophoresis (SPEP) and serum-free light-chain assays confirm the presence of a paraprotein indicating possible myeloma (MM) or monoclonal gammopathy of undetermined significance (MGUS).

–If SPEP is abnormal, order immunofixation to confirm the presence of a paraprotein indicating possible myeloma or MGUS.

–Do not use SPEP, immunofixation, serum-free light-chain assay, or urine electrophoresis (UPEP) alone to exclude a diagnosis of myeloma.

−Order whole-body MRI as first-line imaging for all people with a plasma cell disorder suspected to be myeloma.
- Whole-body low-dose CT can be considered if whole-body MRI is unsuitable or the patient declines.
- Only consider skeletal survey if whole-body MRI and low-dose CT are unsuitable or the person declines them.
- Do not use isotope bone scans to identify myeloma-related bone disease.

−Bone marrow aspirate and trephine biopsy confirm the diagnosis based on plasma cell percentage and flow cytometry morphology.
- Perform FISH on CD138-selected bone marrow cells to identify t(4;14), t(14;16), 1q gain, del(1p), and del(17p)*TP53 deletion.
- Perform immunophenotyping of bone marrow to inform subsequent monitoring.
- Perform immunohistochemistry (including Ki-67 and p53 expression) on the trephine biopsy to identify plasma cell phenotypes and guide prognostic information.

−New diagnostic criteria for MM are:
- Involved/uninvolved serum-free light-chain ratio ≥100 and the involved serum-free light-chain level >100 mg/dL.
- Clonal bone marrow plasma cells ≥60%.
- Two or more focal lesions on MRI.

−MGUS is differentiated from MM by the absence of end organ damage (ie, hypercalcemia, renal insufficiency, anemia, and bone lesions), decreased amount of serum monoclonal protein (<30 g/L in MGUS), and decreased amount of bone marrow plasma cells (<10% in MGUS).
- 1% annual risk of progression to other lymphoproliferative disorder.
- Typically, IgG or IgA MGUS progresses to MM while IgG MGUS progresses to Waldenstrom macroglobulinemia (WM).
- WM is defined by the presence of an IgM monoclonal gammopathy and ≥10% clonal plasma cells in the bone marrow, as opposed to <10% in IgM MGUS.

−Test for hepatitis B, hepatitis C, and HIV before starting myeloma treatment.

−Bortezomib with dexamethasone +/− thalidomide is considered first line for induction of adults with previously untreated MM who are eligible for high-dose chemotherapy with hematopoietic stem cell transplantation (HSCT).
- Only a small portion of patients are suitable for HSCT.

−Thalidomide with an alkylating agent and dexamethasone is recommended for treatment of MM in patients for whom high-dose chemotherapy with SHCT is not appropriate.

–Do not perform plasma exchange for myeloma-induced acute renal disease.

–Treat with zolendronic acid to prevent bone disease in patients with MM.
  - Disodium pamidronate or, less desirably, sodium clodronate may be used if zolendronic acid is contraindication or not tolerated.
  - Refer for dental assessment and treatment ideally before but at least immediately after starting bisphosphonates.

–Consider surgical stabilization followed by radiotherapy for nonspinal bones that have fractures or are at high risk of fractures.
  - Consider radiotherapy alone for nonspinal bones that have fractured or are at high risk of fracture if surgical intervention is unsuitable or not immediately needed.

–Consider radiotherapy for patients with nonspinal bone diseases in whom chemotherapy and initial pain management have not led to prompt improvement in pain control or in whom chemotherapy is unsuitable and current pain medications are not working.
  - Consider palliative care or pain medicine consults for patients with complex nonspinal bone disease pain.

–For patients with myeloma-related spinal bone disease without instability, consider cement augmentation with or without radiotherapy or radiotherapy alone.

–For patients with radiological evidence of myeloma-related spinal instability, consider intervention with spinal surgery, with or without radiotherapy; cement augmentation, with or without radiotherapy; or radiotherapy alone.

–Ensure seasonal influenza vaccination and pneumococcal vaccination.

–Consider IVIG replacement therapy for patients with hypogammaglobulinemia and recurrent infections.

–Consider acyclovir prophylaxis during and after treatment with bortezomib and high-dose steroids.

–Smoldering myeloma should be monitored every 3 mo for the first 5 y with CBC, CMP, bone profile, SPEP, serum-free light-chain assay.
  - Do not routinely offer skeletal surveys.

–Any new bone symptoms should receive symptom-directed imaging (MRI, CT FDG PET-CT).

Comments

1. Myeloma is still an incurable disease, although the spectrum of disease is highly variable.
2. MGUS is present in approximately 3.5% of the population over age 50 y.

Infectious Diseases

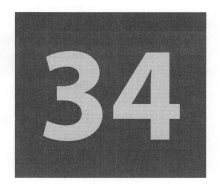

ASYMPTOMATIC BACTERIURIA

Population
–Nonpregnant women.

Recommendations
▶ IDSA 2019
–Do not treat asymptomatic bacteriuria with antibiotics.
–Only screen pregnant women and patients undergoing urologic procedures.

Source
–https://doi.org/10.1093/cid/ciy1121

COMMON COLD

Population
–Healthy adults (those without chronic lung disease or immunocompromising conditions).

Recommendation
▶ *Annals of Internal Medicine* 2016
–Do not prescribe antibiotics for the common cold.

Source
–http://annals.org/aim/fullarticle/2481815/appropriate-antibiotic-use-acute-respiratory-tract-infection-adults-advice-high

Comment
1. Harm from antibiotics outweighs benefits, as all causes of common cold are viral.

DIABETIC FOOT INFECTIONS, INPATIENT MANAGEMENT

Population
–Hospitalized adults older than 18 y with diabetic foot problems.

Recommendations

▶ IDF 2017

–Assess arterial perfusion and need for revascularization.
–Debride callus and necrotic tissue to fully visualize wound, measure depth and extent.
–Obtain cultures: tissue or bone specimen preferred; deep swab only after debriding wound.
–Obtain x-ray of all new diabetic foot infections. Obtain MRI if osteomyelitis suspected and plain film is not diagnostic.
–Request surgical consult for deep abscesses, compartment syndrome, and necrotizing soft tissue infection.
–Treat clinically infected wounds with antibiotics:
  • 1–2 wk for mild-to-moderate infections.
  • 3 wk for more serious skin and soft tissue infections.
  • 6 wk for osteomyelitis.

Source
–https://www.idf.org/e-library/guidelines/119-idf-clinical-practice-recommendations-on-diabetic-foot-2017.html

Comment
1. A deep space infection may have deceptively few superficial signs.

▶ NICE 2016

–Every hospital should have a multidisciplinary foot care team to assess and treat any diabetic patient with foot problems.
–Every patient with a diabetic foot problem should undergo an assessment for:
  • Need for debridement, pressure off-loading.
  • Vascular inflow.
  • Infection of the foot.
  • Glycemic control.
  • Neuropathy.
–If diabetic foot infection is suspected, obtain culture (soft tissue or bone sample preferred, or deep swab after debriding wound).
–If osteomyelitis is suspected, obtain an x-ray; if x-ray is normal, obtain an MRI.

–Provide off-loading for diabetic foot ulcers.
–For mild diabetic foot infections, treat with empiric antibiotics that provide good coverage of gram-positive organisms.
–For moderate-to-severe diabetic foot infections, treat with empiric antibiotics that provide coverage of gram-positive, gram-negative, and anaerobic bacteria.

Source
–https://www.nice.org.uk/guidance/ng19

Comments
1. The diabetic foot care team should include:
   a. Diabetologist.
   b. Surgeon with expertise managing DM foot problems.
   c. DM nurse specialist.
   d. Podiatrist.
   e. Tissue viability nurse.
   f. Biomechanic and orthotic specialist.
2. Unless part of a clinical trial, do *not* treat diabetic foot ulcers with:
   a. Electrical stimulation therapy, autologous platelet-rich plasma gel, regenerative wound matrices, dalteparin,
   b. Growth factors,
   c. Hyperbaric oxygen therapy.

HUMAN IMMUNODEFICIENCY VIRUS (HIV)

Population
–HIV-infected adults and children.

Recommendations
▶ IDSA 2018
–Obtain a comprehensive present and past medical history, physical examination, medication/social/family history, and review of systems, including HIV-related information upon initiation of care.
–Educate patient on high-risk behaviors to minimize risk of HIV transmission.
–Assess for the presence of depression, substance abuse, or domestic violence.
–Baseline labs upon initiation of care: HIV serostatus; CD4 count; quantitative HIV RNA by PCR (viral load); HIV genotyping; CBCD, chemistry panel, G6PD testing; fasting lipid profile; HLA B5701 test

(if abacavir will be used); tropism testing (if the use of a CCR5 antagonist is being considered); urinalysis; Pap smear in women.[a]

–Screening labs: *M. tuberculosis* testing (PPD or interferon-γ release assay); Toxoplasma antibodies; Hepatitis B panel, HCV antibodies; VDRL; urine NAAT for gonorrhea; and urine NAAT for chlamydia (except in men age <25 y); anti-CMV IgG in lower risk groups (populations other than men who have sex with men or IV drug users), trichomoniasis in all women, *Chlamydia trachomatis* in all women ≤25 y of age.

–Monitoring labs:
  • CD4 counts and HIV viral load every 3–4 mo.
  • STD screening and TB screening tests should be repeated periodically depending on symptoms and signs, behavioral risk, and possible exposures.
  • Fasting glucose and lipid panel 4–6 wk after initiation of therapy.

–Vaccination for pneumococcal infection, influenza, varicella, hepatitis A, HPV, and HBV according to standard immunization charts.

–All HIV-infected women of childbearing age should be asked about their plans and desires regarding pregnancy upon initiation of care and routinely thereafter.

–Pap smear with HPV or reflex to HPV based on age in women every 6 mo and annually thereafter if results are normal. For ASC-US Pap result, if reflex HPV testing is negative, a repeat Pap test in 6–12 mo or repeat co-testing in 12 mo is recommended. For any result ≥ASC-US on repeat cytology, referral to colposcopy is recommended.

–Perform individualized assessment of risk for breast cancer and inform them of the potential benefits and risks of screening mammography for women ages 40–49 y. Perform mammogram annually for age >50 y.

–Hormone replacement therapy is not recommended.

Sources

–Aberg JA, Gallant JE, Ghanem KG, Emmanuel P, Zingman BS, Horberg MA. Primary care guidelines for the management of persons infected with HIV: 2013 update by the HIV Medicine Association of the Infectious Diseases Society of America. *Clin Infect Dis.* 2014;58(1):e1-e34, http://academic.oup.com/cid/article/58/1/e1/374007#74163693

–https://www.idsociety.org/globalassets/idsa/practice-guidelines/guidelines-for-prevention-and-treatment-of-opportunistic-infections-in-hiv-infected-adults-and-adolescents.pdf

[a]CBCD, complete blood count with differential; G6PD, glucose-6-phosphate dehydrogenase; HLA, human leukocyte antigen; NAAT, nucleic acid amplification test; PCR, polymerase chain reaction; PPD, purified protein derivative; VDRL, Venereal Disease Research Laboratory.

Comments

1. Screen for anogenital human papilloma virus (HPV) with anal Pap testing for men who have sex with men, women with abnormal cervical Pap smear results, and persons with a history of genital warts.
2. Test for serum testosterone level in men complaining of fatigue, ED, or decreased libido.
3. Chest x-ray should be obtained in persons with pulmonary symptoms or who have a positive PPD test result.

HUMAN IMMUNODEFICIENCY VIRUS (HIV), ANTIRETROVIRAL THERAPY (ART) IN PEDIATRICS

Population

–HIV-infected children.

Recommendations

▶ HHS 2018

–ART is recommended for all children, regardless of symptoms or CD4 count.
–HIV genotypic resistance testing is recommended:
  • At the time of diagnosis.
  • Prior to initiation of therapy.
  • For all treatment-naive children.
–Evaluate for possible side effects and evaluate response to therapy in all children 1–2 wk after initiation of ART or changing ART regimen.
–Recommends laboratory testing for toxicity and viral load response at 2–4 wk after treatment initiation.
–Check absolute CD4 T lymphocyte (CD4) cell count and plasma HIV RNA (viral load) and evaluate therapy adherence, effectiveness, and toxicities every 3–4 mo. CD4 count can be monitored every 6–12 mo in children who are adherent to therapy and have had CD4 counts well above threshold for opportunistic infections, sustained viral suppression, and stable clinical status for 2–3 y.

Sources

–Panel on Antiretroviral Therapy and Medical Management of Children Living with HIV. Guidelines for the use of antiretroviral agents in pediatric HIV infection.
–http://aidsinfo.nih.gov/contentfiles/lvguidelines/pediatricguidelines.pdf.

Comment

1. Specific ART recommendations are beyond the scope of this book.

HUMAN IMMUNODEFICIENCY VIRUS, ANTIRETROVIRAL USE IN ADULTS

Population
–Adults and adolescents.

Recommendations

▶ HHS 2018

–Recommends one of these antiretroviral regimen for most patients with HIV:
- Dolutegravir/abacavir/lamivudinea—only for patients who are HLA-B*5701-negative.
- Dolutegravir plus tenofovir/emtricitabine.
- Elvitegravir/cobicistat/tenofovir/emtricitabine.
- Raltegravir plus tenofovir/emtricitabine.

–Selection of a regimen should be individualized.
- Efavirenz is teratogenic.
- Tenofovir should be used cautiously with renal insufficiency.
- Ritonavir-boosted atazanavir and rilpivirine should not be used with high-dose proton pump inhibitors.

–Recommend coreceptor tropism assay whenever a CCR5 coreceptor antagonist is considered.

–Screen for HLA-B*5701 before starting abacavir.

–Interruption of HAART is recommended for drug toxicity, intercurrent illness, or operations that precludes oral intake.

–Management of a patient with prior antiretroviral exposure is complex and should be managed by an HIV specialist if changing regimens.

Source

–http://aidsinfo.nih.gov/guidelines/html/1/adult-and-adolescent-arv-guidelines/0

Comments

1. This guideline focuses on antiretroviral management in HIV-1-infected individuals.
2. Alternative regimens for specific clinical scenarios or patient characteristics are beyond the scope of this book.
3. Baseline evaluation should include:
   a. Patient's readiness for ART.
   b. Psychosocial assessment.
   c. Substance abuse screening.
   d. Mental illness screening.
   e. HIV risk behavior screening.

f. Health insurance and coverage status.
g. Discussion of risk reduction and disclosure to sexual and/or needle-sharing partners.
h. Initial labs:
    i. CD4 T-cell count.
    ii. HIV-1 antibody testing.
    iii. HIV RNA viral load.
    iv. Genotypic drug-resistance testing.
    v. CBCD, chemistry panel, LFTs, urinalysis.
    vi. Serologies for HBV and HCV screening antibody.
    vii. Fasting glucose or A1c and lipid panel.
    viii. Pregnancy test.
    ix. STD screening.

IDENTIFYING RISK OF SERIOUS ILLNESS IN CHILDREN UNDER 5 Y

TRAFFIC LIGHT SYSTEM FOR IDENTIFYING RISK OF SERIOUS ILLNESS IN CHILDREN UNDER 5 Y

Category	Green—Low Risk	Yellow—Intermediate Risk	Red—High Risk
Color of skin, lips, or tongue	Normal color	Pallor	Mottled, ashen, or blue
Activity	• Responds normally to social cues • Smiles • Awakens easily • Strong cry	• Abnormal response to social cues • No smile • Wakes only with prolonged stimulation • Decreased activity	• No response to social cues • Appears toxic • Stuporous • Weak, high-pitched cry

Respiratory	• Normal breathing	• Nasal flaring
		• Tachypnea
		  ○ >50 breaths/min (6–12 mo)
		  ○ >40 breaths/min (>1 y)
		• SpO_2 ≤95%
		• Pulmonary rales
			• Grunting
			• Marked tachypnea
			  ○ >60 breaths/min
			• Moderate-to-severe chest retractions

TRAFFIC LIGHT SYSTEM FOR IDENTIFYING RISK OF SERIOUS ILLNESS IN CHILDREN UNDER 5 Y   (Continued)

Category	Green—Low Risk	Yellow—Intermediate Risk	Red—High Risk

Circulation	• Normal skin and eyes
	• Moist mucous membranes
		• Tachycardia
		  ○ >160 beats/min (<12 mo)
		  ○ >150 beats/min (12–24 mo)
		  ○ >140 beats/min (2–5 y)
		• Capillary refill ≥3 s
		• Dry mucous membranes
		• Poor feeding
		• Decreased urine output
			• Findings in yellow zone PLUS
			• Reduced skin turgor

Other	• Nontoxic appearance	• Temperature ≥39°C (age 3–6 mo) • Fever ≥5 d • Rigors • Swelling of a limb or joint • Non-weight bearing on one extremity	• Temperature ≥38°C (<3 mo) • Non-blanching rash • Bulging fontanelle • Neck stiffness • Status epilepticus • Focal neurological signs • Focal seizures

Source: Adapted from National Institute for Health and Care Excellence (NICE). Guideline on feverish illness in children: assessment and initial management in children younger than 5 years; 2013 May (Clinical Guideline no. 160).

INFLUENZA

Population
–Adults.

Recommendations

▶ CDC 2018

–Antiviral treatment is recommended for:
- Lab-confirmed cases of influenza within 48 h of symptom onset.
- Strongly suspected influenza within 48 h of symptom onset.
- Hospitalized patients with severe, complicated, or progressive lab-confirmed influenza or influenza-like illness with high likelihood of complications even if >48 h from symptom onset.
  - Children aged younger than 2 y or adults aged 65 y and older.
  - Persons with chronic pulmonary (including asthma), cardiovascular (except hypertension alone), renal, hepatic, hematological (including sickle cell disease), metabolic (including diabetes mellitus) or neurologic disorders (including disorders of the brain, spinal cord, peripheral nerve, and muscle, such as cerebral palsy, epilepsy [seizure disorders], stroke, intellectual disability, moderate-to-severe developmental delay, muscular dystrophy, or spinal cord injury).
  - Persons with immunosuppression, including that caused by medications or by HIV infection.
  - Women who are pregnant or postpartum (within 2 wk after delivery).
  - Persons aged younger than 19 y who are receiving long-term aspirin therapy.
  - American Indians/Alaska Natives.
  - Persons who are extremely obese (ie, body mass index is equal to or greater than 40).
  - Residents of nursing homes and other chronic care facilities.

–Antiviral chemoprophylaxis after exposure to a person with influenza is recommended for:
- Prevention of influenza in persons at high risk of influenza complications during the first 2 wk following vaccination.
- Patients at high risk for complications from influenza who have contraindications to the influenza vaccine.
- Patients with severe immune deficiencies or others who might not respond to influenza vaccination, such as persons receiving immunosuppressive medications.

- NOT recommended if more than 48 h have elapsed since first exposure to a person with influenza.

–Antiviral treatment options include oseltamivir, zanamivir, and peramivir.

- Oseltamivir for influenza A or B:
  - Treatment dose: 75 mg by mouth (PO) twice daily (bid) × 5 d.
  - Chemoprophylaxis dose: 75 mg by mouth (PO) once daily × 7 d.
  - Will need to be renally dosed for patients with decreased GFR.
- Zanamivir for influenza A or B:
  - Treatment dose: 10 mg (two 5-mg inhalations) twice daily × 5 d.
  - Chemoprophylaxis dose: 10 mg (two 5-mg inhalations) once daily × 7 d.
  - Avoid in patients with underlying respiratory disease (eg, asthma, COPD).
- Peramivir for influenza A or B:
  - Treatment dose: 600 mg IV once for creatinine clearance ≥50 mL/min.
  - 200 mg IV once for creatinine clearance 30–49 mL/min.
  - 100 mg IV once for creatinine clearance 10–29 mL/min.
  - ESRD patients on dialysis should receive a dose after dialysis at a dose adjusted based on creatinine clearance.

Source
–http://www.cdc.gov/mmwr/preview/mmwrhtml/rr6001a1.htm

Population
–Children.

Recommendations
▶ ACIP 2011

–Treatment indicated if symptom onset within 48 h and:
- Any child hospitalized with presumed influenza or with severe, complicated, or progressive illness attributable to influenza, regardless of influenza immunization status.
- Influenza infection of any severity in children at high risk of complications of influenza infection.
- Children aged <2 y.

–Chemoprophylaxis indicated as above for adults.

–Antiviral treatment options include oseltamivir and zanamivir.
- Oseltamivir for influenza A or B treatment dose (5 d):
  - If <1-y-old: 3 mg/kg/dose twice daily.
  - If 1 y or older, dose varies by child's weight:
    - 15 kg or less, the dose is 30 mg twice a day.

- >15 to 23 kg, the dose is 45 mg twice a day.
- >23 to 40 kg, the dose is 60 mg twice a day.
- >40 kg, the dose is 75 mg twice a day.
- Oseltamivir chemoprophylaxis dose (7 d):
  - Not recommended for <3 mo of age.
  - If child is 3 mo or older and younger than 1 y: 3 mg/kg/dose once daily.
  - If 1 y or older, dose varies by child's weight:
    - 15 kg or less, the dose is 30 mg once a day.
    - >15 to 23 kg, the dose is 45 mg once a day.
    - >23 to 40 kg, the dose is 60 mg once a day.
    - >40 kg, the dose is 75 mg once a day.
- Zanamivir for influenza A or B:
  - Treatment dose (7 y or older): 10 mg (two 5-mg inhalations) twice daily × 5 d.
  - Chemoprophylaxis dose (5 y or older): 10 mg (two 5-mg inhalations) once daily × 7 d.
  - Avoid in patients with underlying respiratory disease (eg, asthma, COPD).

Source
–http://www.cdc.gov/mmwr/preview/mmwrhtml/rr6001a1.htm

Comments

1. Consider an influenza nasal swab for diagnosis during influenza season in:
   a. Persons with acute onset of fever and respiratory illness.
   b. Persons with fever and acute exacerbation of chronic lung disease.
   c. Infants and children with fever of unclear etiology.
   d. Severely ill persons with fever or hypothermia.
2. Rapid influenza antigen tests have 70%–90% sensitivity in children and 40%–60% sensitivity in adults.
3. Direct or indirect fluorescent antibody staining is useful in screening tests.
4. Influenza PCR may be used as a confirmatory test.

NEUTROPENIA, FEBRILE (FN)

Population

–Patients with single temperature >100.9°F (38.3°C) or ≥100.4°F (38.0°C) sustained for >1 h in the setting of neutropenia (absolute neutrophil count including granulocytes and bands <1000/mm³).

Recommendations

▶ Infectious Disease Society of America 2018

–Evaluation and Therapy

- Two sets of blood cultures (1 from each lumen of central venous catheter [CVC] if present + 1 peripherally drawn)/urine culture/chemistries. CXR/ancillary studies based on clinical evaluation. Begin antibiotics as rapidly as possible, ideally within 60 min.
- Stratify into **LOW RISK**[b] (absence of comorbidity, no cardiovascular compromise, expected duration of neutropenia <7 d, compliant) vs. **HIGH RISK**[b] (absolute neutrophil count [ANC] <100 comorbidity, cardiovascular compromise, unreliable, expected duration of neutropenia >7 d).
- High-risk patients must be admitted to hospital with rapid initiation of single-agent antibiotic (cefepime, imipenem, ceftazidime) or combination therapy (extended spectrum beta-lactam plus either aminoglycoside or fluoroquinolone) depending on clinical features within 1 h of triage. Add antifungal agent if continued fever and negative cultures after 4–7 d.
- Low-risk patients can be treated as an outpatient with oral fluoroquinalone and amoxicillin/clavulanate (or clindamycin for penicillin allergy), with <5% requiring hospitalization for worsening symptoms. If patient does not defervesce in 2–3 d on empiric antibiotics, consider inpatient treatment.
- Continue broad-spectrum antibiotics in both low- and high-risk groups until ANC >500. Adjust antibiotics based on positive cultures and switch to oral to complete a 10–14 d course of antibiotics.

Sources

–*Clin Infect Dis.* 2011;52:e56-e93.
–*J Clin Oncol.* 2018;36:1443-1453.
–*J Oncol Pract.* 2015;11:450.

---

[b]Multinational Association for Supportive Care in Cancer (MASCC)
- Symptoms no or mild = 5, moderate = 3, severe = 0
- No hypotension:5
- No COPD:4
- No previous fungal infection:4
- No dehydration requiring parenteral fluids:3
- Outpatient status:3
- Age <60–2
- High risk ≤21; Low risk ≥21

Comments

1. **Clinical Concerns**

   a. Prophylactic granulocyte colony-stimulating factor (GCSF) should be used in patients on chemotherapy with an expected rate of FN ≥20%. Secondary use of GCSF after FN shortens hospital stay by 1 d but has no impact on survival.

   b. Vancomycin should not be given empirically unless history of MRSA, catheter tunnel infection, presence of pneumonia, soft tissue infection, or hemodynamic instability.

   c. Unique organisms requiring antibiotic adjustment:

      i. Vancomycin-resistant enterococci (VRE)—use linezolid or daptomycin or ceftarolin.

      ii. Extended-spectrum beta-lactamase (ESBL) producing gram-negative bacteria—use imipenem, meropenem, or ertapenem.

      iii. Carbapenemase-producing organism (*Klebsiella*)—use polymyxin-colistin or tigecycline; meropenem can be added.

   d. If CVC line infection is suspected, draw blood cultures from each lumen of CVC and peripheral vein. If CVC culture grows out >120 min before peripheral blood cultures, then CVC is the source of infection.

   e. CVC must be removed if infected with *Staphylococcus aureus*, *Pseudomonas*, other gram-negative bacteria, fungi, or mycobacteria, as well as for tunnel or port pocket infection. If the organism is coagulation-negative *Staphylococcus*, retain CVC and treat with an antibiotic for 4–6 wk with 85% cure rate.

   f. In afebrile patients with ANC <100, give oral fluoroquinolone as prophylaxis to lower risk of severe infection.

   g. With ANC <100, risk of serious infection is 10% per day.

MENINGITIS, BACTERIAL

Population

–Children and adults.

Recommendations

▶ Cochrane Database of Systematic Reviews 2013; IDSA 2004

–Recommends corticosteroids prior to or when antibiotics are administered for presumed bacterial meningitis in high-income countries.

–If bacterial meningitis is suspected, blood cultures should be obtained immediately.

–Perform lumbar puncture (LP). If patient is immunocompromised, has a history of CNS disease, or has papilledema or neurological deficit, administer empiric antibiotics and dexamethasone. Obtain immediate CT scan of the head. If CT head is negative, perform LP.

–Give dexamethasone and empiric antibiotics as soon as possible.

–Discontinue antibiotics when CSF fluid analysis result is obtained if negative.

- CSF analysis suggests bacterial etiology if:
- CSF glucose <34 mg/dL.
- Ratio CSF to serum glucose <0.23.
- CSF protein concentration >220 mg/dL.
- CSF leukocyte count >2000 leukocytes/mm^3.
- CSF neutrophil count >1180 neutrophils/mm^3.

–Empiric antibiotics: vancomycin + ceftriaxone or cefotaxime. Target antibiotics to identified pathogens.

Sources

–http://onlinelibrary.wiley.com/doi/10.1002/14651858.CD004405.pub4/pdf/abstract

–https://academic.oup.com/cid/article/39/9/1267/402080

Comments

1. Corticosteroids significantly reduced the incidence of hearing loss and neurological sequelae in bacterial meningitis.
2. Corticosteroids reduced mortality in meningitis from *Streptococcus pneumoniae*, but not with *Haemophilus influenzae* or *Neisseria meningitidis* infections.
3. No beneficial effect of corticosteroids in low-income countries.

METHICILLIN-RESISTANT *STAPHYLOCOCCUS AUREUS* INFECTIONS

TREATMENT OF METHICILLIN-RESISTANT *STAPHYLOCOCCUS AUREUS* INFECTIONS (MRSA) IN ADULTS AND CHILDREN

Infection	Primary Therapy	Alternative Therapy	Comments

Abscess associated with extensive involvement; cellulitis; systemic illness; immunosuppression; extremes of age; involvement of face, hands, or genitalia; septic phlebitis; trauma; infected ulcer or burn; or poor response to incision and drainage	1. Incision and drainage
	2. Antibiotics
	  a. Outpatient
	    i. Clindamycin
	    ii. Trimethoprim-sulfamethoxazole (TMP-SMX)
	  b. Inpatient
	    i. Vancomycin
	    ii. Linezolid
	    iii. Daptomycin
		1. Outpatient antibiotics
		  a. Tetracycline
		  b. Linezolid
		2. Inpatient antibiotics
		  a. Telavancin
		  b. Clindamycin
			1. Tetracyclines should not be used in children age <8 y.
			2. Vancomycin is recommended for hospitalized children.
			3. Clindamycin and linezolid are alternative choices for children.

Recurrent skin and soft-tissue infections (SSTIs)	1. Cover draining wounds
	2. Maintain good hygiene
	3. Avoid reusing or sharing personal toiletries
	4. Use oral antibiotics only for active infections
		1. Decolonization only if recurrent SSTI despite good hygiene
		  a. Mupirocin per nares bid × 5–10 d
		  b. Chlorhexidine or dilute bleach baths twice weekly (BIW) × 1–2 wk
			Screening cultures prior to decolonization or surveillance cultures after decolonization are not recommended.

NEUROCYSTICERCOSIS (NCC)

Population
–Adults and children with intraparenchymal neurocysticercosis.

Recommendations
▶ AAN 2013, IDSA 2017
–Obtain MRI and noncontrast CT of the brain for classification.
–Perform enzyme-linked immunotransfer blot (EITB) if suspected NCC.
–Screen for tuberculosis and treat for *Strongyloides stercoralis* if prolonged steroids are planned.
–Perform ocular fundoscopic exam prior to initiation of anthelmintic therapy.
–For symptomatic intraparenchymal neurocysticercosis, use albendazole plus either dexamethasone or prednisolone to decrease the number of active lesions and reduce the long-term seizure frequency.
–No evidence to support steroids alone in patients with intraparenchymal neurocysticercosis.
–It is reasonable to treat these patients with anti-epileptic drugs until the active lesions have subsided (expert opinion).
–Screen household members for tapeworm carriage if in a nonendemic area.

Sources
–Baird RA, Wiebe S, Zunt JR, Halperin JJ, Gronseth G, Roos KL. Evidence-based guideline: treatment of parenchymal neurocysticercosis. Report of the Guideline Development Subcommittee of the American Academy of Neurology. *Neurology*. 2013;80(15):1424-1429.
–http://www.ajtmh.org/content/journals/10.4269/ajtmh.18-88751

RESPIRATORY TRACT INFECTIONS, LOWER (COMMUNITY ACQUIRED PNEUMONIA)

Population
–Adults.

Recommendations
▶ ESCMID 2011, IDSA 2007
–Use severity-of-illness score to determine if inpatient treatment is appropriate:

- CURB-65: Confusion, uremia, respiratory rage, low blood pressure, age ≥65.
- Pneumonia severity index (PSI).

–Obtain chest radiograph or other imaging. Other diagnostic tests are optional for outpatient treatment.

–Empiric therapy:

- Previously health, no risk for drug-resistant *S. pneumonia*: macrolide (azithromycin, clarithromycin, or erythromycin) or doxycycline.
- Comorbidities (chronic heart, lung, liver, or renal disease; diabetes; alcoholism; malignancy; asplenia; immune suppression; antimicrobials in past 3 mo):
  ○ Respiratory fluoroquinalone (moxifloxacin, gemifloxacin, or levofloxacin).
  ○ Beta-lactam + macrolide.
  ○ High-dose amoxicillin 1 g tid or amoxicillin-clavulanate 2 g bid.
  ○ Alternatives: ceftriaxone, cefpodoxime, and cefuroxime; doxycycline.
- If high rate of *S. pneumonia* macrolide-resistance (MIC ≥16 µg/mL), then consider alternative agent to a macrolide.

–For *Streptococcus* pneumonia:

- Erythromycin MIC >0.5 mg/L predicts clinical failure.
- Penicillin MIC ≤8 mg/L predicts IV penicillin susceptibility.

–A C-reactive protein (CRP) <2 mg/dL at presentation with symptoms >24 h makes pneumonia highly unlikely; a CRP >10 mg/dL makes pneumonia likely.

–Indications for antibiotics in lower respiratory tract infections (LRTIs):

- Suspected pneumonia.
- Acute exacerbation of COPD with increased dyspnea, sputum volume, and sputum purulence.

Sources

–https://academic.oup.com/cid/article/44/Supplement_2/S27/372079

–http://www.escmid.org/fileadmin/src/media/PDFs/4ESCMID_Library/2Medical _Guidelines/ESCMID_Guidelines/Woodhead_et_al_CMI_Sep_2011_LRTI_GL_fulltext.pdf

Comment

1. Consider aspiration pneumonia in patients with pneumonia and dysphagia.

RESPIRATORY TRACT INFECTIONS, UPPER

Population
- Adults.

Recommendation

▶ IDSA 2015
- Do not prescribe antibiotics for upper respiratory tract infections.

Source
- http://www.choosingwisely.org/societies/infectious-diseases-society-of-america/

Comment
1. None.

SEXUALLY TRANSMITTED DISEASES

SEXUALLY TRANSMITTED DISEASES TREATMENT GUIDELINES

Infection	Recommended Treatment	Alternative Treatment
Chancroid	• Azithromycin 1 g PO × 1 • Ceftriaxone 250 mg IM × 1	• Ciprofloxacin 500 mg PO bid for 3 d • Erythromycin base 500 mg PO tid for 7 d
Genital HSV, first episode	• Acyclovir 400 mg PO tid × 7–10 d[a] • Famciclovir 250 mg PO tid × 7–10 d[a] • Valacyclovir 1 g PO bid × 7–10 d[a]	• Acyclovir 200 mg PO 5 times a day for 7–10 d[a]
Genital HSV, suppressive therapy	• Acyclovir 400 mg PO bid • Valacyclovir 1 g PO daily	• Famciclovir 250 mg PO bid
Genital HSV, episodic therapy for recurrent disease	• Acyclovir 400 mg PO tid × 5 d • Acyclovir 800 mg PO bid × 5 d • Acyclovir 800 mg PO tid × 2 d	• Valacyclovir 500 mg PO bid × 3 d • Valacyclovir 1 g PO daily × 5 d • Famciclovir 125 mg PO bid × 5 d • Famciclovir 1000 mg PO bid × 1 d • Famciclovir 500 mg PO × 1 then 250 mg bid × 2 d

SEXUALLY TRANSMITTED DISEASES TREATMENT GUIDELINES

Infection	Recommended Treatment	Alternative Treatment
Genital HSV, suppressive therapy for HIV-positive patients	Acyclovir 400–800 mg PO bid–tid Famciclovir 500 mg PO bid Valacyclovir 500 mg PO bid	
Genital HSV, episodic therapy for recurrent genital HSV in HIV-positive patients	• Acyclovir 400 mg PO tid × 5–10 d • Famciclovir 500 mg PO bid × 5–10 d • Valacyclovir 1 g PO bid × 5–10 d	
Granuloma inguinale (Donovanosis)	• Azithromycin 1 g orally once per week or 500 mg daily for at least 3 wk and until all lesions have completely healed	• Doxycycline 100 mg PO bid × ≥3 wk • Ciprofloxacin 750 mg PO bid × ≥3 wk
		• Erythromycin base 500 mg PO qid × ≥3 wk • TMP-SMX 1 double-strength (160/800 mg) tablet PO bid × ≥3 wk • Continue all of these treatments until all lesions have completely healed
Lymphogranuloma venereum	• Doxycycline 100 mg PO bid for × 21 d	• Erythromycin base 500 mg PO qid × 21 d
Primary and secondary syphilis in adults	• Benzathine penicillin G 2.4 million units IM × 1	• Doxycycline 100 mg PO bid × 14 d • Tetracycline 500 mg PO qid × 14 d • Amoxicillin 3 g + probenecid 500 mg, both PO bid × 14 d
Primary and secondary syphilis in infants and children	• Benzathine penicillin G 50,000 units/kg IM, up to the adult dose of 2.4 million units × 1	
Early latent syphilis in adults	• Benzathine penicillin G 2.4 million units IM × 1	

SEXUALLY TRANSMITTED DISEASES TREATMENT GUIDELINES

Infection	Recommended Treatment	Alternative Treatment
Early latent syphilis in children	• Benzathine penicillin G 50,000 units/kg IM, up to the adult dose of 2.4 million units × 1	
Late latent syphilis or latent syphilis of unknown duration in adults	• Benzathine penicillin G 2.4 million units IM weekly × 3 doses	• Doxycycline 100 mg PO bid × 4 wk
Late latent syphilis or latent syphilis of unknown duration in children	• Benzathine penicillin G 50,000 units/kg, up to the adult dose of 2.4 million units, IM weekly × 3 doses	
Tertiary syphilis	• Benzathine penicillin G 2.4 million units IM weekly × 3 doses	• Doxycycline 100 mg PO bid × 4 wk
Neurosyphilis	• Aqueous crystalline penicillin G 3–4 million units IV q4h × 10–14 d	• Procaine penicillin 2.4 million units IM daily × 10–14 d **PLUS** • Probenecid 500 mg PO qid × 10–14 d
Syphilis, pregnant women	• Pregnant women should be treated with the penicillin regimen appropriate for their stage of infection	• No good alternatives. Recommend penicillin allergy test and desensitization if patient has reported penicillin allergy
Congenital syphilis	• Aqueous crystalline penicillin G 50,000 units/kg/dose IV q12h × 7 d; then q8h × 3 more days	• Procaine penicillin G 50,000 units/kg/dose IM daily × 10 d • Benzathine penicillin G 50,000 units/kg/dose IM × 1
Older children with syphilis	• Aqueous crystalline penicillin G 50,000 units/kg IV q4–6h × 10 d	

SEXUALLY TRANSMITTED DISEASES TREATMENT GUIDELINES

Infection	Recommended Treatment	Alternative Treatment
Nongonococcal urethritis	• Azithromycin 1 g PO × 1 • Doxycycline 100 mg PO bid × 7 d	• Erythromycin base 500 mg PO qid × 7 d • Erythromycin ethylsuccinate 800 mg PO qid × 7 d • Levofloxacin 500 mg PO daily × 7 d • Ofloxacin 300 mg PO bid × 7 d
Recurrent or persistent urethritis	• Metronidazole 2 g PO × 1 • Tinidazole 2 g PO × 1 • Azithromycin 1 g PO × 1	
Cervicitis[b]	• Azithromycin 1 g PO × 1 • Doxycycline 100 mg PO bid × 7 d	
Chlamydia infections in adolescents, adults[b]	• Azithromycin 1 g PO × 1 • Doxycycline 100 mg PO bid × 7 d	• Erythromycin base 500 mg PO qid × 7 d • Erythromycin ethylsuccinate 800 mg PO qid × 7 d • Levofloxacin 500 mg PO daily × 7 d • Ofloxacin 300 mg PO bid × 7 d
Chlamydia infections in pregnancy[b]	• Azithromycin 1 g PO × 1 • Amoxicillin 500 mg PO tid × 7 d	• Erythromycin base 500 mg PO qid × 7 d • Erythromycin ethylsuccinate 800 mg PO qid × 7 d
Ophthalmia neonatorum from Chlamydia	• Erythromycin base or ethylsuccinate 50 mg/kg/d PO qid × 14 d	
Chlamydia trachomatis pneumonia in infants	• Erythromycin base or ethylsuccinate 50 mg/kg/d PO qid × 14 d	
Chlamydia infections in children <45 kg	• Erythromycin base or ethylsuccinate 50 mg/kg/d PO qid × 14 d	
Chlamydia infections in children ≥45 kg and age <8 y	• Azithromycin 1 g PO × 1	

SEXUALLY TRANSMITTED DISEASES TREATMENT GUIDELINES

Infection	Recommended Treatment	Alternative Treatment
Chlamydia infections in children age ≥8 y	• Azithromycin 1 g PO × 1 • Doxycycline 100 mg PO bid × 7 d	
Uncomplicated gonococcal infections of the cervix, urethra, pharynx, or rectum in adults or children >45 kg	• Ceftriaxone 250 mg IM × 1 **PLUS** • Azithromycin 1 g PO × 1 **OR** • Doxycycline 100 mg daily × 7 d	
Gonococcal conjunctivitis in adults or children >45 kg	• Ceftriaxone 1 g IM × 1	
Gonococcal meningitis or endocarditis in adults or children >45 kg	• Ceftriaxone 1 g IV q12h	
Disseminated gonococcal infection in adults or children >45 kg	• Ceftriaxone 1 g IV/IM daily	• Cefotaxime 1 g IV q8h • Ceftizoxime 1 g IV q8h
Ophthalmia neonatorum caused by gonococcus	• Ceftriaxone 25–50 mg/kg, not to exceed 125 mg, IV/IM × 1	
Prophylactic treatment of infants born to mothers with gonococcal infection	• Ceftriaxone 25–50 mg/kg, not to exceed 125 mg, IV/IM × 1	
Uncomplicated gonococcal infections of the cervix, urethra, pharynx, or rectum in children ≤45 kg	Ceftriaxone 125 mg IM × 1	

SEXUALLY TRANSMITTED DISEASES TREATMENT GUIDELINES

Infection	Recommended Treatment	Alternative Treatment
Gonococcal infections with bacteremia or arthritis in children or adults	• Ceftriaxone 50 mg/kg (maximum dose 1 g) IM/IV daily × 7 d	
Ophthalmia neonatorum prophylaxis	• Erythromycin (0.5%) ophthalmic ointment in each eye × 1	
Bacterial vaginosis	• Metronidazole 500 mg PO bid × 7 d[c] • Metronidazole gel 0.75%, 1 applicator (5 g) IVag daily × 5 d • Clindamycin cream 2%, 1 applicator (5 g) IVag qhs × 7 d[d]	• Tinidazole 2 g PO daily × 3 d • Clindamycin 300 mg PO bid × 7 d • Clindamycin ovules 100 mg IVag qhs × 3 d
Bacterial vaginosis in pregnancy	• Metronidazole 500 mg PO bid × 7 d • Metronidazole 250 mg PO tid × 7 d • Clindamycin 300 mg PO bid × 7 d	
Trichomoniasis	• Metronidazole 2 g PO × 1[c] • Tinidazole 2 g PO × 1	• Metronidazole 500 mg PO bid × 7 d[c]
Candida vaginitis	• Butoconazole 2% cream 5 g IVag × 3 d • Clotrimazole 1% cream 5 g IVag × 7–14 d • Clotrimazole 2% cream 5 g IVag × 3 d • Nystatin 100,000-unit vaginal tablet, 1 tablet IVag × 14 d • Miconazole 2% cream 5 g IVag × 7 d • Miconazole 4% cream 5 g IVag × 3 d • Miconazole 100-mg vaginal suppository, 1 suppository IVag × 7 d	• Fluconazole 150-mg oral tablet, 1 tablet in single dose

SEXUALLY TRANSMITTED DISEASES TREATMENT GUIDELINES

Infection	Recommended Treatment	Alternative Treatment
	• Miconazole 200-mg vaginal suppository, 1 suppository IVag × 3 d • Miconazole 1200-mg vaginal suppository, 1 suppository IVag × 1 • Tioconazole 6.5% ointment 5 g IVag × 1 • Terconazole 0.4% cream 5 g IVag × 7 d • Terconazole 0.8% cream 5 g IVag × 3 d • Terconazole 80-mg vaginal suppository, 1 suppository IVag × 3 d	
Severe pelvic inflammatory disease	• Cefotetan 2 g IV q12h **PLUS** • Doxycycline 100 mg PO/IV q12h **OR** • Cefoxitin 2 g IV q6h **OR** 1. Clindamycin 900 mg IV q8h **PLUS** 1. Gentamicin loading dose IV or IM (2 mg/kg of body weight), followed by a maintenance dose (1.5 mg/kg) q8h. Single daily dosing (3–5 mg/kg) can be substituted	• Ampicillin/sulbactam 3 g IV q6h **PLUS** • Doxycycline 100 mg PO/IV bid

SEXUALLY TRANSMITTED DISEASES TREATMENT GUIDELINES

Infection	Recommended Treatment	Alternative Treatment
Mild-to-moderate pelvic inflammatory disease	• Ceftriaxone 250 mg IM × 1 **PLUS** • Doxycycline 100 mg PO bid × 14 d ± metronidazole 500 mg PO bid × 14 d **OR** • Cefoxitin 2 g IM × 1 and probenecid 1 g PO × 1 **PLUS** • Doxycycline 100 mg PO bid × 14 d ± metronidazole 500 mg PO bid × 14 d^c	
Epididymitis	• Ceftriaxone 250 mg IM × 1 **PLUS** • Doxycycline 100 mg PO bid × 10 d For men who practice insertive anal sex: 1. Ceftriaxone 250 mg IM × 1 **PLUS** 1. Levofloxacin 500 mg PO daily × 10 d **OR** 1. Ofloxacin 300 mg PO bid × 10 d	• Levofloxacin 500 mg PO daily × 10 d • Ofloxacin 300 mg PO bid × 10 d
External genital warts	**Provider-Administered:** • Cryotherapy liquid nitrogen or cryoprobe • TCA or BCA 80%–90% • Surgical removal by tangential scissor excision, tangential shave excision, curettage, or electrosurgery	**Patient-Applied:** • Podofilox 0.5% solution or gel • Imiquimod 5% cream • Sinecatechins 15% ointment

SEXUALLY TRANSMITTED DISEASES TREATMENT GUIDELINES

Infection	Recommended Treatment	Alternative Treatment
Cervical warts	• Cryotherapy with liquid nitrogen • Surgical removal by tangential scissor excision, tangential shave excision, curettage, or electrosurgery • TCA or BCA 80%–90% applied only to warts • Recommend consulting with specialist in management • Biopsy to exclude high-grade SIL must be performed before treatment is initiated	
Vaginal warts	• Cryotherapy with liquid nitrogen • Surgical removal by tangential scissor excision, tangential shave excision, curettage, or electrosurgery • TCA or BCA 80%–90% applied only to warts	
Urethral meatal warts	• Cryotherapy with liquid nitrogen • Surgical removal by tangential scissor excision, tangential shave excision, curettage, or electrosurgery	
Anal warts	• Cryotherapy with liquid nitrogen • Surgical removal by tangential scissor excision, tangential shave excision, curettage, or electrosurgery • TCA or BCA 80%–90% applied only to warts	• Surgical removal by tangential scissor excision, tangential shave excision, curettage, or electrosurgery

SEXUALLY TRANSMITTED DISEASES TREATMENT GUIDELINES

Infection	Recommended Treatment	Alternative Treatment
Proctitis	• Ceftriaxone 250 mg IM × 1 **PLUS** • Doxycycline 100 mg PO bid × 7 d	
Pediculosis pubis	• Permethrin 1% cream rinse applied to affected areas and washed off after 10 min • Pyrethrins with piperonyl butoxide applied to the affected area and washed off after 10 min	• Malathion 0.5% lotion applied for 8–12 h and then washed off • Ivermectin 250 μg/kg PO, repeated in 2 wk
Scabies	• Permethrin cream (5%) applied to all areas of the body from the neck down and washed off after 8–14 h • Ivermectin 200 μg/kg PO, repeat in 2 wk	• Lindane (1%) 1 oz of lotion (or 30 g of cream) applied in a thin layer to all areas of the body from the neck down and thoroughly washed off after 8 h

BCA, bichloroacetic acid; bid, twice a day; h, hour(s); HIV, human immunodeficiency virus; HSV, herpes simplex virus; IM, intramuscular; IV, intravenous; IVag, intravaginally; PO, by mouth; q, every; qhs, at bedtime; qid, 4 times a day; SIL, squamous intraepithelial lesion; TCA, trichloroacetic acid; tid, 3 times a day; TMP-SMX, trimethoprim-sulfamethoxazole.

[a] Treatment can be extended if healing is incomplete after 10 d of therapy.

[b] Consider concomitant treatment of gonorrhea.

[c] Avoid alcohol during treatment and for 24 h after treatment is completed.

[d] Clindamycin cream may weaken latex condoms and diaphragms during treatment and for 5 d thereafter.

Source: Adapted from CDC Guidelines. *MMWR Recomm Rep.* 2015;64(RR3):1-137.

SINUSITIS

Population
–Adults and children.

Recommendations

▶ **IDSA 2012, CDC 2017, NICE 2017**

–Usually viral etiology and self-limited lasting for 2–3 wk.
–Sinus radiographs are not recommended.
–If persistent symptoms (>10 d) or if severe (>3–4 d + fever or purulent discharge) or change in symptoms (eg, "double sickening"), consider no antibiotic or back-up antibiotic and/or nasal corticosteroid (off label) (NICE 2017).
–If systemic symptoms or high-risk comorbidity or signs of more serious illness, offer antibiotics.
–Antibiotics (CDC 2017):
  - Adult >18-y-old:
    ○ Amoxicillin or amoxicillin-clavulanate.
    ○ Macrolides not recommended due to resistance.
    ○ PCN allergy: Doxycycline or respiratory fluoroquinolone (levofloxacin or moxifloxacin).
  - Children <18-y-old:
    ○ Amoxicillin or amoxicillin-clavulanate.
    ○ Intractable vomiting: ceftriaxone IM × 1, then oral antibiotics.

Sources
–https://academic.oup.com/cid/article/54/8/1041/364141
–https://www.cdc.gov/antibiotic-use/community/for-hcp/outpatient-hcp/adult-treatment-rec.html
–https://www.nice.org.uk/guidance/ng79

SKIN AND SOFT TISSUE INFECTIONS

Population
–Adults and children.

Recommendations

▶ **CDC 2007**

–Suspect skin infection: redness, swelling warmth, induration, pain, "spider bite":
  - No evidence of abscess, treat for *Streptococcus spp.*, provide close follow up, then add MRSA coverage if not improving.

- Fluctuant or evidence of abscess: drain lesion, send for culture, and advise on wound care. Prescribe antibiotics if failure or systemic symptoms.
-Empiric antibiotics for *Streptococcus spp.*:
  - Penicillin VK 500 mg PO qid.
  - Amoxicillin 500 mg PO q 8.
  - PCN rash: Cephalexin 500 mg PO qid × 7–10 d.
  - PCN allergy: azithromycin, linezolid, delafloxacin.
-Empiric antibiotics for MSSA:
  - Dicloxacillin 500 mg PO tid.
  - Cephalexin 500 PO tid to qid.
-Empiric antibiotics for MRSA:
  - Trimethoprim-sulfamethoxazole:
    ○ 160/800 PO bid (2 tab bid, if BMI >40)
    ○ May not cover group A streptococcus, not recommended in third trimester of pregnancy nor age <2 mo.
  - Clindamycin:
    ○ 300–450 mg PO tid (higher dose, if BMI >40).
    ○ Perform D-zone testing.
  - Doxycycline or minocycline (not for use in pregnancy or age <8 y; may not be effective for *Streptococcus spp.*)
  - Rifampin (use with other agents, many drug interactions).
  - Linezolid (consult infectious disease specialist, many severe side effects).

Sources
-https://www.cdc.gov/mrsa/pdf/flowchart_pstr.pdf
-https://www.sanfordguide.com/products/digital-subscriptions/sanford-guide-to-antimicrobial-therapy-mobile/

SYPHILIS

Population
-Adults, pregnancy, infants, and children.

Recommendations
▶ IDSA 2011, CDC 2015
-Penicillin G 2.4 million units IM is drug of choice for early syphilis.
-Cerebrospinal fluid (CSF) analysis is indicated if:
  - Early syphilis infection and neurologic symptoms.
  - Late latent syphilis

–Obtain CSF examination for patients with early syphilis do not achieve a ≥4-fold decline in RPR titers within 12 mo.

–Doxycycline is second-line therapy for early syphilis in penicillin-allergic patients.

–Ceftriaxone is second-line therapy for neurosyphilis in penicillin-allergic patients.

–Sexual partners within preceding 90 d should be evaluated and treated.

Sources

–http://cid.oxfordjournals.org/content/53/suppl_3/S110.abstract

–https://www.cdc.gov/std/tg2015/syphilis.htm

Comments

1. Penicillin (PCN) G is the only treatment in pregnancy. If PCN allergy, patient should be desensitized.
2. Avoid doxycycline in pregnancy.
3. Infants and children: Benzathine PCN G 50,000 U/kg IM up to adult dose 2.4 million units. If secondary syphilis is suspected, consult infectious disease specialist.

TUBERCULOSIS (TB), DIAGNOSIS

Population

–Adults suspected of having active TB.

Recommendations

▶ NICE 2016

–Perform a chest x-ray in all patients.

–Obtain 3 early-morning sputum samples for AFB smear and culture.

Source

–https://guidelines.gov/summaries/summary/49964

Comment

1. Consider sputum for nucleic acid amplification for mycobacterium TB complex if the person has HIV disease, need for a large contact tracing, or need for rapid diagnosis.

TUBERCULOSIS (TB), EXTRAPULMONARY DIAGNOSIS

Population

–Adults suspected of having extrapulmonary TB.

Recommendations

▶ NICE 2016

–To diagnose TB send fluid for adenosine deaminase and nucleic acid amplification for mycobacterium TB complex (pleural fluid, cerebrospinal fluid, ascitic fluid, pericardial fluid, synovial fluid).
–Option for TB diagnosis is tissue biopsy.
  • If suspicion for osteomyelitis, perform biopsy.
  • Perform pleural biopsy if suspicion for pleural TB.
  • Perform peritoneal biopsy if suspicion for peritoneal TB.
  • Perform pericardial biopsy if suspicion for pericardial TB.
  • Perform synovial biopsy if suspicion for synovial TB.

Source
–https://guidelines.gov/summaries/summary/49964

TUBERCULOSIS (TB), EXTRAPULMONARY

Population

–Adults suspected of having extrapulmonary TB.

Recommendations

▶ NICE 2016

–Refer the patient to a clinician with expertise in TB management.
–Report suspect to local public health office for case management and contact screening.
–Start patients on RIPE (rifampin, isoniazid, pyrazinamide, and ethambutol) therapy.
–Consider adjunctive corticosteroids for TB with CNS or pericardial involvement.

Source
–https://guidelines.gov/summaries/summary/49964

Comments

1. TB treatment regimens are modified based on TB sensitivities.
2. Typical duration of treatment for TB with CNS involvement is 12 mo.

TUBERCULOSIS (TB), MANAGEMENT

Population
–Adults suspected of having active TB.

Recommendations
▶ ATS/CDC/IDSA 2016

WHEN TO INITIATE ANTI-TUBERCULOSIS MEDICATION

		Favors Treatment Initiation	Favors Delayed or No Treatment
Patient		Risk for progression/dissemination (eg, HIV, TNF alpha inhibitor)	Elevated concern for adverse treatment events (eg, severe liver disease, pregnancy)
		Age <2 y / TB exposure risk (eg, contact, born in higher TB incidence country)	No TB exposure risk
Laboratory/ Radiographic		Radiographic imaging consistent with TB / Evidence of Mtb infection (ie, positive TST or IGRA)	Radiographic imaging not consistent with TB
		Extended time to microbiologic confirmation (eg, rapid molecular test not available)	
		Pathologic findings consistent with TB	
		AFB smear positive / Rapid molecular test positive	AFB smear positive, Rapid molecular test negative
		AFB smear negative, Rapid molecular test positive	AFB smear negative, Rapid molecular test negative
Clinical Status/ Suspicion		Life-threatening disease / Symptoms typical for TB	Clinically stable / Symptoms not typical for TB
		Alternative diagnosis less likely	Alternative diagnosis
Public Health		Concern for loss to follow-up / High transmission risk (eg, congregate setting, corrections)	Low transmission risk

TREATMENT OF DRUG-SUSCEPTIBLE TUBERCULOSIS

Table 2. Drug Regimens for Microbiologically Confirmed Pulmonary Tuberculosis Caused by Drug-Susceptible Organisms

| | | Intensive Phase | | Continuation Phase | | | |
Regimen	Drug[a]	Interval and Dose[b] (Minimum Duration)	Drugs	Interval and Dose[b,c] (Minimum Duration)	Range of Total Doses	Comments[c,d]	Regimen Effectiveness
1	INH RIF PZA EMB	7 d/wk for 56 doses (8 wk), or 5 d/wk for 40 doses (8 wk)	INH RIF	7 d/wk for 126 doses (18 wk), or 5 d/wk for 90 doses (18 wk)	182–130	This is the preferred regimen for patients with newly diagnosed pulmonary tuberculosis.	Greater
2	INH RIF PZA EMB	7 d/wk for 56 doses (8 wk), or 5 d/wk for 40 doses (8 wk)	INH RIF	3 times weekly for 54 doses (18 wk)	110–94	Preferred alternative regimen in situations in which more frequent DOT during continuation phase is difficult to achieve.	
3	INH RIF PZA EMB	3 times weekly for 24 doses (8 wk)	INH RIF	3 times weekly for 54 doses (18 wk)	78	Use regimen with caution in patients with HIV and/or cavitary disease. Missed doses can lead to treatment failure, relapse, and acquired drug resistance.	
4	INH RIF PZA EMB	7 d/wk for 14 doses then twice weekly for 12 doses[e]	INH RIF	Twice weekly for 36 doses (18 wk)	62	Do not use twice-weekly regimens in HIV-infected patients or patients with smear-positive and/or cavitary disease. If doses are missed, then therapy is equivalent to once weekly, which is inferior.	Lesser

Abbreviations: DOT, directly observed therapy; EMB, ethambutol; HIV, human immunodeficiency virus; INH, isoniazid; PZA, pyrazinamide; RIF, rifampin.

[a] Other combinations may be appropriate in certain circumstances; additional details are provided in the section "Recommended Treatment Regimens."

[b] When DOT is used, drugs may be given 5 d/wk and the necessary number of doses adjusted accordingly. Although there are no studies that compare 5 with 7 daily doses, extensive experience indicates this would be an effective practice. DOT should be used when drugs are administered <7 d/wk.

[c] Based on expert opinion, patients with cavitation on initial chest radiograph and positive cultures at completion of 2 mo of therapy should receive a 7-mo (31-wk) continuation phase.

[d] Pyridoxine (vitamin B6), 25–50 mg/d, is given with INH to all persons at risk of neuropathy (eg, pregnant women; breastfeeding infants; persons with HIV; patients with diabetes, alcoholism, malnutrition, or chronic renal failure; or patients with advanced age). For patients with peripheral neuropathy, experts recommend increasing pyridoxine dose to 100 mg/day.

Alternatively, some US tuberculosis control programs have administered intensive-phase regimens 5 d/wk for 15 doses (3 wk), then twice weekly for 12 doses.

Source
- Official American Thoracic Society/Centers for Disease Control and Prevention/Infectious Diseases Society of America. Clinical practice guidelines: treatment of drug-susceptible TB. *Clin Infect Dis.* 2016;63(7):853-867.

▶ NICE 2016
- Refer the patient to a clinician with expertise in TB management.
- Report suspect to local public health office for case management and contact screening.
- Isolate patients in negative pressure rooms within the hospital.
- Start patients on RIPE therapy (rifampin, isoniazid, pyrazinamide, and ethambutol).

Source
- https://guidelines.gov/summaries/summary/49964

Comments
1. TB treatment regimens are modified based on TB sensitivities.
2. Typical duration of treatment for pulmonary TB is 6 mo.
3. Consider de-escalation of hospital isolation after 2 wk of therapy if:
   a. Resolution of cough.
   b. Afebrile for a week.
   c. Immunocompetent patient.
   d. No extensive disease by x-ray.
   e. Initial smear grade was 2+ or less.

TUBERCULOSIS (TB), MANAGEMENT OF LATENT TB

Population
- Adults and children who have latent TB.

Recommendations
▶ NICE 2016
- High-risk individuals younger than 35 y with latent TB should be offered:
  - 3 mo of rifampin and isoniazid (with pyridoxine).
  - 6 mo of isoniazid (with pyridoxine).
- Offer adults HIV, HBV, and HCV testing before starting treatment for latent TB.
- Offer high-risk individuals between 35 and 65 y latent TB therapy if hepatotoxicity is not a concern.

Source
–https://guidelines.gov/summaries/summary/49964

Comment

1. **High-risk patients with latent TB:**
   a. HIV-positive.
   b. Younger than 5 y.
   c. Excessive alcohol intake.
   d. Injection drug users.
   e. Solid organ transplant recipients.
   f. Hematologic malignancies.
   g. Undergoing chemotherapy.
   h. Prior jejunoileal bypass.
   i. Diabetes.
   j. Chronic kidney disease.
   k. Prior gastrectomy.
   l. Receiving treatment with anti-tumor necrosis factor med or other biologic agents.

TUBERCULOSIS (TB), MULTIDRUG-RESISTANT (MDR-TB)

Population

–Patients with suspected or proven drug-resistant TB.

Recommendations

▶ WHO 2011

–Rapid drug susceptibility testing of isoniazid and rifampicin is recommended at the time of TB diagnosis.

–Recommends sputum smear microscopy and culture to monitor patients with MDR-TB.

–Recommends addition of a later-generation fluoroquinolone, ethionamide, pyrazinamide, and a parenteral agent ± cycloserine for ≥8 mo.

–Recommends total treatment duration of 20 mo.

Source

–http://whqlibdoc.who.int/publications/2011/9789241501583_eng.pdf

URINARY TRACT INFECTIONS (UTI)

Population
–Adult women.

Recommendations

▶ ACOG 2008, EAU 2010, IDSA 2011, NICE 2018
–Screening or treating asymptomatic bacteriuria is not recommended except in pregnancy or if undergoing urologic procedures.
–Perform a urinalysis or dipstick testing for symptoms of a UTI: dysuria, urinary frequency, suprapubic pain, or hematuria.
–Pyelonephritis: Obtain midstream urine sample prior to initiating antibiotics.
–Send urine culture in men, pregnant women, children or those with history of resistant bacteria.
–Pain control with acetaminophen recommended over NSAIDs in both UTI and pyelonephritis.
–No evidence for cranberry products or urine alkalization for treatment.
–Duration of antibiotics (consider any previous culture results and sensitivities):
  • Uncomplicated cystitis: 3–7 days (nitrofurantoin requires 5–7 d).
  • Uncomplicated pyelonephritis: 7–10 d.
  • Complicated pyelonephritis or UTI: 3–5 d after control/elimination of complicating factors and defervescence.
–Empiric antibiotics for uncomplicated cystitis[c]:
  • Trimethoprim-sulfamethoxazole 800 mg/160 mg bid × 3 d (not recommended if local resistance rate >20%).
  • Nitrofurantoin monohydrate 100 mg bid × 5–7 d.
  • Fosfomycin 3 g PO × 1 (second line)
  • Beta-lactam antibiotics are alternative agents.[d]
–Empiric antibiotics for complicated UTI or uncomplicated pyelonephritis:
  • Fluoroquinolones.
  • Ceftriaxone or cefuroxime.
  • Aminoglycosides.
–Empiric antibiotics for complicated pyelonephritis:
  • Fluoroquinolones.

[c]TMP-SMX only if regional *Escherichia coli* resistance is <20%; fluoroquinolones include ciprofloxacin, ofloxacin, or levofloxacin.
[d]Amoxicillin-clavulanate, cefdinir, cefaclor, or cefpodoxime-proxetil. Cephalexin may be appropriate in certain settings.

- Piperacillin-tazobactam.
- Carbapenem.
- Aminoglycosides.

–Consider a fluoroquinolone for symptoms of pyelonephritis or for refractory UTI.

–Special circumstances (NICE 2018):

- Children (age- and weight-specific dosing): cephalexin, amoxicillin-clavulanate (if sensitivities known).
- Pregnant women: cephalexin 500 mg bid or tid × 7–10 d.
- Men: nitrofurantoin, trimethoprim-sulfamethoxazole, ciprofloxacin or levofloxacin.

Sources

–http://www.guidelines.gov/content.aspx?id=12628
–http://www.uroweb.org/gls/pdf/Urological%20Infections%202010.pdf
–http://www.guidelines.gov/content.aspx?id=25652
–http://guidelines.gov/content.aspx?id=12628
–http://cid.oxfordjournals.org/content/52/5/e103.full.pdf+html
–http://nice.org.uk/guidance/ng111
–http://nice.org.uk/guidance/ng109
–https://www.sanfordguide.com/products/digital-subscriptions/sanford-guide-to-antimicrobial-therapy-mobile/

Comments

1. EAU recommends 7 d of antibiotics for men with otherwise uncomplicated cystitis.
2. EAU suggests the following options for antimicrobial prophylaxis of recurrent uncomplicated UTIs in nonpregnant women:
   a. Nitrofurantoin 50 mg PO daily.
   b. TMP-SMX 40/200 mg daily.
3. EAU suggests the following options for antimicrobial prophylaxis of recurrent uncomplicated UTIs in pregnant women:
   a. Cephalexin 125 mg PO daily.
4. Once urine culture and sensitivity results are known, antibiotics can be adjusted to the narrowest spectrum antibiotic.

Population

–Febrile children 2–24 mo.

Recommendations

▶ AAP 2016, NICE 2019

–Diagnose a UTI if patient has pyuria, abnormal urinalysis and ≥50,000 colonies/mL single uropathogenic organism.

–Obtain midstream sample for urine dipstick and culture prior to antibiotics. Bagged specimens can be used for urinalysis, but not for culture.

–Obtain blood cultures if toxic appearing.

–Recommend a renal and bladder ultrasound in all infants 2–24 mo with a febrile UTI.

–Treat febrile UTIs with 7–14 d of antibiotics and tailor antibiotics to culture result.

–Antibiotic prophylaxis is not indicated for a history of febrile UTI.

–A voiding cystourethrogram (VCUG) is indicated if ultrasound reveals hydronephrosis, renal scarring, or other findings of high-grade vesicoureteral reflux, and for recurrent febrile UTIs.

Sources

–http://pediatrics.aappublications.org/content/early/2016/11/24/peds.2016-3026

–http:// nice.org.uk/guidance/ng109

–https://www.sanfordguide.com/products/digital-subscriptions/sanford-guide-to-antimicrobial-therapy-mobile/

Comments

1. Urine obtained through catheterization has a 95% sensitivity and 99% specificity for UTI.
2. Bag urine cultures have a specificity of approximately 63% with an unacceptably high false-positive rate. Only useful if the cultures are negative.
3. Increased rate of false positives if the renal ultrasound is performed during acute phase of illness. Consider delaying until illness has defervesced.

Neurologic Disorders

BELL'S PALSY

Population
–Adults with Bell's palsy.

Recommendation

▶ AAN 2012, Reaffirmed in 2014

–For patients with recent-onset Bell's palsy (<72 h of symptoms):
- Give steroids (prednisone 1 mg/kg PO daily × 7 d) to increase the probability of facial nerve recovery.
- Consider antivirals (eg, acyclovir or valacyclovir) × 7 d, which given with steroids marginally improve outcomes.

Source
–www.guideline.gov/content.aspx?id=38700

Comment

1. Antivirals are thought to have a marginal effect at best of facial nerve recovery when added to steroids. The benefit is <7%.

Population
–Adult and children with Bell's palsy.

Recommendations

▶ AAO 2013, Cochrane Database of Systematic Reviews 2015

–Do not routinely obtain lab studies for unequivocal Bell's palsy. Consider Lyme disease (neuroborreliosis) testing in children <15 y.
–Recommend against routine diagnostic imaging for straightforward Bell's palsy.
–Recommend oral steroids for Bell's palsy with or without antiviral medications if initiated within 72 h of symptom onset in patients 16 y and older.

–Recommend against antiviral monotherapy for Bell's palsy.

–Recommend eye protection for patients with incomplete eye closure.

–Inadequate evidence to support surgical decompression with Bell's palsy.

–Recommend against electrodiagnostic testing for Bell's palsy with incomplete facial paralysis.

–Recommend against physical therapy or acupuncture for Bell's palsy.

Sources

–http://www.guideline.gov/content.aspx?id=47483

–http://www.cochrane.org/CD001869/NEUROMUSC_antiviral-treatment-for-bells-palsy

Comment

1. Cochrane analysis found no benefit of adding antivirals to corticosteroids vs. corticosteroid monotherapy.

CONCUSSIONS

Population

–Children and young adults.

Recommendations

▶ CDC 2016, ACEP 2016

–Obtain noncontrast CT indicated for loss of consciousness or post-traumatic amnesia. There is no evidence to prefer MRI over CT.

–Mild TBI with negative intracranial process is low risk.

–All patients must be educated and given materials about concussions and postconcussive syndrome. Use of tools such as the Acute Concussion Evaluation (ACE) care plan developed by Gioia and Collins for follow-up management.

Sources

–https://www.cdc.gov/traumaticbraininjury/pdf/tbi_clinicians_factsheet-a.pdf

–https://www.cdc.gov/headsup/pdfs/providers/ACE_care_plan_returning_to_work-a.pdf

▶ AAN 2013

–Standardized sideline assessment tools should be used to assess athletes with suspected concussions.

–Teams should immediately remove from play any athlete with a suspected concussion.

–Teams should not permit an athlete to return to play until he/she has been cleared to play by a licensed health care professional.

Source

–http://www.guideline.gov/content.aspx?id=43947

EPILEPSY

Population

–Children and adults.

Recommendations

▶ NICE 2018

–Educate adults about all aspects of epilepsy.

–Diagnosis of epilepsy should be made by a specialist in epilepsy.

–Evaluation of epilepsy

- Electroencephalogram.
- Sleep-deprived EEG if standard EEG is inconclusive.
- Neuroimaging to evaluate for any structural brain abnormalities.
  - MRI is preferred for children <2 y, adults, refractory seizures, and focal seizures.
- Measurement of prolactin is not recommended.
- Chemistry panel.
- ECG in adults.
- Urine toxicology screen.

–Antiepileptic drugs (AED)

- Start AED only after the diagnosis of epilepsy is made.

–Do not use valproate in pregnancy. If used in girls and women of childbearing potential, a pregnancy prevention plan must be in place.

- Focal seizures:
  - Carbamazepine.
  - Lamotrigine.
  - Adjunctive AED: levetiracetam, oxcarbazepine, or sodium valproate.
- Generalized tonic–clonic seizures:
  - Sodium valproate.
  - Lamotrigine.
  - Carbamazepine.
  - Oxcarbazepine.
  - Adjunctive AED: levetiracetam or topiramate.

- Absence seizures:
  - Ethosuximide.
  - Sodium valproate.
  - Alternative: lamotrigine.
- Myoclonic seizures:
  - Sodium valproate.
  - Alternatives: levetiracetam or topiramate.

Sources
–http://www.guidelines.gov/content.aspx?id=36082
–https://www.nice.org.uk/guidance/cg137

Comment
1. AED can decrease the efficacy of combined oral contraceptive pills.

MALIGNANT SPINAL CORD COMPRESSION (MSCC)

Population
–Adults with MSCC.

Recommendations

▶ American College of Radiology Appropriateness Criteria
–Motor deficits are prognostic of ultimate functional outcome.
–Surgical intervention should be considered in high Spinal Instability Neoplasticism Score (SINS) or retropulsion of bone fragments in the spinal cord.

Source
–*J Palliat Med.* 2015;18:7.

▶ Scottish Palliative Care Guidelines 2014, National Collaborating Centre for Cancer—Metastatic Spinal Cord Compression (MSCC) 2012
–**Stratify Patient for Therapy**
  - In patients presenting with paraplegia >48 h, offer radiation for pain control and surgery only if spine is unstable. The chance for neurological recovery is zero. (*Lancet Oncol.* 2005;6:15)
  - In patients presenting with significant or progressing weakness of lower extremities with no previous history of cancer, biopsy non-neural cancer if accessible. If biopsy not possible and lymphoma or myeloma unlikely, give dexamethasone 40–100 mg daily and take to surgery to make tissue diagnosis and relieve compression of spinal cord. (*Neurology.* 1989;39:1255. *Lancet Neurol.* 2008;7:459) If unstable, the spine should be stabilized. Taper steroids (decrease by

½ every 3 d) and begin radiation in 2–3 wk. If tumor is lymphoma or myeloma, consider initiating chemotherapy and high-dose dexamethasone. Recovery of lower extremity strength is dependent on degree of paraparesis initially.

- In patients presenting with back pain but mild neurologic symptoms, if no previous cancer, find site to biopsy, check PSA, serum protein electrophoresis, beta-2 microglobulin, and alfa-fetoprotein. Begin moderate-dose dexamethasone (16 mg/d) with radiation therapy initially. Surgery reserved for progression of symptoms after starting radiation especially in radioinsensitive cancers (renal cell, sarcoma, melanoma). Recovery of neurologic function in 80%–90% range.

- In patients presenting with back pain but no neurologic symptoms with no previous diagnosis of cancer, search for site to biopsy (physical exam, PET CT scan, tumor markers) and consult radiation therapy. If myeloma or lymphoma, treat with systemic chemotherapy. Radiation is primary treatment with surgery only on progression. Low dose or no steroids is acceptable. Chance of continued lower extremity strength approaches 100%.

Sources
–*Int J Radiat Oncol Bio/Phys.* 2012;84:312.
–*Quart J Med.* 2014;107:277-282.
–*N Engl J Med.* 2017;376:1358.

Comments

1. **Clinical Considerations**
   a. MRI with and without gadolinium of the entire spine is mandatory. Thirty percent of patients will have cord compression in more than 1 area.
   b. Twenty percent of patients presenting with MSCC have not had a previous diagnosis of cancer.
   c. Five to eight percent of patients with known cancer will develop MSCC during their course of disease.
   d. Most common tumors associated with MSCC are lung, breast, prostate, myeloma, and lymphoma.
   e. Most common site of MSCC is the thoracic spine (70%) and least common is cervical spine (10%).
   f. Back pain presents in 95% of patients, with average time to MSCC being 6–7 wk. Once motor, sensory, or autonomic dysfunction occur—time to total paraplegia is rapid (hours to days).
   g. Indications for surgery in MSCC include lack of diagnosis, progression on radiation, unstable fracture or bone in spinal canal, and previous radiation to site of MSCC. (*Int J Oncol.* 2011;38:5) (*J Clin Oncol.* 2011;29:3072)

h. Posterior decompression laminectomy was standard surgery for MSCC, but now resection of tumor with bone reconstruction and stabilization is done most commonly at centers of excellence.

i. Stereotactic body radiation therapy is being used more commonly with improved results especially in radiation-resistant cancers. (*Cancer.* 2010;116:2258)

NORMAL PRESSURE HYDROCEPHALUS (NPH)

Population
–Patients with normal pressure hydrocephalus.

Recommendations

▶ AAN 2015
–Consider shunting for NPH with gait abnormalities.
–A positive response to a therapeutic lumbar puncture increases the chance of success with shunting.
–Patients with an impaired cerebral blood flow reactivity to acetazolamide, measured by SPECT, are more likely to respond to shunting.

Source
–https://guidelines.gov/summaries/summary/49957

PAIN, CHRONIC, CANCER RELATED

Management of Chronic Pain in Survivors of Adult Cancers: ASCO Clinical Practice Guideline

Population
–Women treated for ovarian cancer with complete response (Stages I–IV).

Recommendations

▶ A. SCREENING AND COMPREHENSIVE ASSESSMENT
–Screen for pain at each encounter, document using quantitative or semi-quantitative tool (strength of recommendation [SOR]: strong).
–Conduct comprehensive pain assessment.
–Explore multidimensional nature of pain (pain descriptors, distress, impact on function and related physical, psychological, social, and spiritual factors)—explore information about cancer treatment history, comorbid conditions, and psychiatric history, including substance abuse as well as prior treatment for pain.

–The assessment should characterize the pain and clarify probable cause. A physical exam and diagnostic testing (if appropriate) should be done (SOR: moderate).

–Clinicians should be aware of chronic pain syndromes resulting from cancer treatment, the prevalence of the syndrome, risk factors for an individual patient, and appropriate treatment options.

–Common cancer pain syndromes.

–Evaluate and monitor for recurrent disease, second cancer or late-onset treatment effects in patients with new-onset pain (SOR: moderate).

▶ **B. TREATMENT AND CARE OPTIONS**

–Clinicians should aim to enhance, comfort, improve function, limit adverse events, and ensure safety in the management of pain in cancer survivors (SOR: moderate).

–Clinicians should engage patient and family/caregivers in all aspects of pain assessment and management including physical, psychological, social, and emotional domains of pain (SOR: moderate).

–Clinicians should decide if other health professionals can provide further care for patients with complex needs. If necessary, a referral should be made (SOR: moderate).

–Clinicians should directly refer selected patients to other professionals with expertise in hospice and palliative medicine, physical medicine and rehabilitation, integrative therapies, interventional therapies, psychological approaches, and neurostimulation therapies (SOR: moderate).

▶ **C. PHARMACOLOGICAL INTERVENTIONS**

Miscellaneous analgesics

–Clinicians may prescribe nonopioid analgesics to relieve chronic pain or improve function in cancer survivors. This includes nonsteroidal anti-inflammatory drugs, acetaminophen, and adjuvant analgesics including antidepressants and selected anticonvulsants with evidence of analgesic efficacy (antidepressant duloxetine and anticonvulsants gabapentin and pregabalin) for neuropathic pain (SOR: moderate).

–Clinicians may prescribe topical analgesics (nonsteroidal anti-inflammatory drugs, local anesthetics, or compounded creams/gels containing baclofen, amitriptyline, and ketamine) (SOR: moderate).

–Long-term corticosteroids are not recommended solely to relieve chronic pain (SOR: moderate).

–Clinicians may follow specific state regulations that allow access to medical cannabis for patients with chronic pain after consideration of benefits and risk (SOR: moderate).

▶ D. OPIOIDS

–Clinicians may prescribe a trial of opioids in carefully selected cancer survivors with chronic pain who do not respond to more conservative management and who continue to experience pain-related distress or functional impairment. Nonopioid analgesics and/or adjuvants can be added as clinically necessary (SOR: moderate).

–Clinicians should assess risks of adverse effects of opioids used for pain management.

▶ E. RISK ASSESSMENT, MITIGATION, AND UNIVERSAL PRECAUTIONS WITH OPIOID USE

–Clinicians should assess the potential risks and benefits when initiating treatment that will incorporate long-term use of opioids (SOR: moderate).

–Clinicians should clearly understand terminology such as tolerance, incomplete cross-tolerance, dependence, abuse, and addiction as it relates to the use of opioids for pain control (SOR: moderate).

–Clinicians should incorporate a universal precautions approach to minimize abuse, addiction, and adverse consequences of opioid use such as opioid-related deaths. Clinicians should be cautious in co-prescribing other centrally acting drugs especially benzodiazepines (SOR: moderate).

–Clinicians should educate patients and their family regarding risk and benefits of long-term opioid therapy and the safe storage use and disposal of controlled substances.

–If opioids are no longer warranted, clinicians should taper the dose to avoid withdrawal symptoms (SOR: moderate).

▶ F. ADVERSE EFFECTS ASSOCIATED WITH LONG-TERM OPIOID USE

–Persistent common adverse effects.

  • Constipation, mental clouding, upper GI symptoms.

–Endocrinopathy (hypogonadism, hyperprolactinemia).

  • Fatigue, infertility, reduced libido.

  • Osteoporosis/osteopenia, reduced or absence of menses.

–Neurotoxicity.

  • Myoclonus, changes in mental status.

  • Risk of opioid-induced hyperalgesia.

  • New onset or worsening of sleep apnea syndrome.

Sources

–*J Clin Oncol.* 2016;34:3325-3345.
–*J Pain Symptom Manage.* 2016;51:1070-1090.
–*J Clin Oncol.* 2014;32:1739-1747.
–*JAMA.* 2016;315:1624-1645.

PAIN, CHRONIC

Population
–Adults with chronic noncancer pain outside of palliative and end-of-life care.

Recommendations
▶ **CDC 2016**
–This guideline is focused on opioid use for chronic pain management.

When to initiate or continue opioids for chronic pain
–Nonpharmacologic therapy and nonopioid medications are preferred for chronic pain.
–Opioid therapy should be used for both pain and function only if the anticipated benefits outweigh the risks.
–Treatment goals, including goals for pain and function, should be established before starting opioid therapy for chronic pain. This plan should also address how opioid therapy will be discontinued if benefits do not outweigh the risks.
–Clinicians must discuss with patients the risks and benefits of opioid therapy before starting opioids and periodically during therapy.

Opioid selection, follow-up, and discontinuation
–When starting opioid therapy, use immediate-release opioids, and prescribe the lowest effective dose.
–Carefully reassess benefits and risks when increasing daily dosage to >50 morphine milligram equivalents.
–Avoid increasing daily dosage to >90 morphine milligram equivalents or carefully justify such large doses.
–Reassess efficacy within 4 wk of starting opioid therapy for chronic pain and consider discontinuing opioids if benefits do not outweigh risks.

Assessing risk of opioid use
–Clinicians should evaluate risks of opioid-related harms.
–Prescribe naloxone emergency kit when patients have an increased risk of opioid overdose especially in patients who are taking ≥50 morphine milligram equivalents per day or concurrently using a BZD.
–Frequent review of prescription drug monitoring program data.
–Recommend periodic urine drug testing to monitor diversion.
–Avoid concurrent opioid and benzodiazepine therapy whenever possible.
–Offer or arrange for medication-assisted treatment for patients with opioid use disorders (eg, buprenorphine or methadone).

Sources

–Dowell D, Haegerich TM, Chou R. CDC guideline for prescribing opioids for chronic pain—United States, 2016. *MMWR Recomm Rep.* 2016;65(1):1-49.

–https://www.cdc.gov/drugoverdose/pdf/guidelines_at-a-glance-a.pdf

▶ ICSI 2017

–Use validated tools to assess patient's functional status, pain, and quality of life.

–Assess for current or prior exposure to opioids and consider checking prescription drug monitoring program data before prescribing opioids.

–Prescribe NSAIDs and acetaminophen for dental pain.

–Assess for mental health comorbidities in patients with chronic pain.

–Screen all patients with chronic pain for substance use disorders.

–Recommend a multidisciplinary approach to patients with chronic pain.

–Recommend incorporating cognitive behavioral therapy or mindfulness-based stress reduction and exercise/physical therapy to pharmacologic therapy in chronic pain patients.

–Minimize benzodiazepine or carisoprodol use for chronic pain. If used, limit duration of therapy to 1 wk.

–Before initiating opioids for chronic pain, providers should seek a diagnostic cause of the pain and document objective findings on physical exam.

–Opioid risk assessment tools and knowledge of patient's risk of opioid-related harm should guide decision about initiation or continuation of opioids.

–Geriatric patients should be assessed for their fall risk, cognitive impairment, respiratory function, and renal/hepatic impairment prior to initiation of opioids.

–Patients who are initiating opioids or who have their opioid dose increased should be advised not to operate heavy machinery, drive a car, or participate in any activity that may be affected by the sedating effect of opioids.

–Long-acting opioids should be reserved for patients with opioid tolerance and in whom prescriber is confident of medication adherence.

–Avoid daily opioid doses of >100 morphine milligram equivalents.

–Avoid opioid use for patients with substance use disorders.

–Urine drug screening should be done at least annually.

–If an opioid use disorder is suspected, refer patient to an addiction specialist.

Sources
  –Hooten M, Thorson D, Bianco J, et al. *Pain: Assessment, Non-opioid Treatment Approaches and Opioid Management.* Bloomington, MN: Institute for Clinical Systems Improvement (ICSI); 2016, 160 pp.
  –https://www.icsi.org/wp-content/uploads/2019/01/Pain.pdf

DELIRIUM

Population
  –Adults age ≥18 y in the hospital or in long-term care facilities.

Recommendations
▶ NICE 2019
  –Older adults and people with dementia, severe illness, or a hip fracture are more at risk for developing delirium.
  –The prevalence of delirium in people on medical wards in hospital is about 20%–30%, and 10%–50% of people having surgery develop delirium. In long-term care the prevalence is under 20%.
  –Perform a short Confusion Assessment Method (CAM) screen to confirm the diagnosis of delirium.
  –Recommended approach to the management of delirium:
  • Treat the underlying cause.
  • Provide frequent reorientation and reassurance to patients and their families.
  • Provide cognitively stimulating activities.
  • Ensure adequate hydration.
  • Provide adequate oxygenation.
  • Prevent constipation.
  • Early mobilization.
  • Treat pain if present.
  • Provide hearing aids or corrective lenses if sensory impairment is present.
  • Promote good sleep hygiene.
  –Avoid Foley catheter.
  –Avoid drugs with anticholinergic side effect profiles.
  • Consider short-term antipsychotic use (<1 wk) for patients who are distressed or considered at risk to themselves or others.
  • Use antipsychotic drugs with caution or not at all for people with conditions such as Parkinson's disease or dementia with Lewy bodies.

Sources
- http://www.nice.org.uk/nicemedia/live/13060/49909/49909.pdf
- https://www.hospitalelderlifeprogram.org/uploads/disclaimers/Long_CAM_Training_Manual_10-9-14.pdf

▶ American Geriatrics Society 2015
- Do not use physical restraints for behavioral control in elderly patients with delirium.

Source
- http://www.choosingwisely.org/societies/american-geriatrics-society/

PAIN, NEUROPATHIC

Population
- Adults with neuropathic pain.

Recommendations
NICE 2013; Updated July 2019
- Offer a choice of amitriptyline, duloxetine, gabapentin, or pregabalin as initial treatment for neuropathic pain (except trigeminal neuralgia).
- Consider tramadol only as acute rescue therapy.
- Offer carbamazepine as initial treatment for trigeminal neuralgia.
- Consider capsaicin cream for localized neuropathic pain.
- Pregabalin and gabapentin carry a risk of dependence and abuse; schedule III.
- Consider the following agents with expert supervision:
  - Cannabidiol (CBD).
  - Capsaicin patch.
  - Lacosamide.
  - Lamotrigine.
  - Levetiracetam.
  - Morphine.
  - Methadone.
  - Tapentadol.
  - Oxcarbazepine.
  - Topiramate.
  - Tramadol (for long-term use).
  - Venlafaxine.
- Spinal cord stimulation (SCS).

Sources
- http://www.guideline.gov/content.aspx?id=47701

–Neuropathic Pain in Adults: Pharmacological Management in Non-specialist Settings (2013 updated 2019). NICE guideline CG173.

PROCEDURAL SEDATION

▶ ACEP 2014

Population
–Adults or children.

Recommendations
–No preprocedural fasting needed prior to procedural sedation.
–Recommends continuous capnometry and oximetry to detect hypoventilation.
–During procedural sedation, a nurse or other qualified individual must be present for continuous monitoring in addition to the procedural operator.
–Safe options for procedural sedation in children and adults include ketamine, propofol, and etomidate.

Source
–http://www.guideline.gov/content.aspx?id=47772

Comments
1. The combination of ketamine and propofol is also deemed to be safe for procedural sedation in children and adults.
2. Alfentanil can be safely administered to adults for procedural sedation.

RESTLESS LEGS SYNDROME AND PERIODIC LIMB MOVEMENT DISORDERS

Population
–Adults.

Recommendations
▶ American Academy of Neurology 2016, American Academy of Sleep Medicine 2012
–Nonpharmacologic:
  • Avoid or reduce caffeine, nicotine, and EtOH.
  • Perform evening stretches, massage, warm or cool baths, light exercise.

–Recommends for moderate-to-severe restless legs syndrome (RLS).
- Strong evidence for following meds:
  ◦ Pramipexole.
  ◦ Rotigotine.
  ◦ Cabergoline.
  ◦ Gabapentin.
- Moderate evidence for:
  ◦ Ropinirole.
  ◦ Pregabalin.
  ◦ IV ferric carboxymaltose.
- For primary RLS with periodic limb movements of sleep:
  ◦ Ropinirole.
- For primary RLS with concomitant anxiety or depression:
  ◦ Ropinirole.
  ◦ Pramipexole.
  ◦ Gabapentin.
- For RLS and ferritin <75 mcg/mL:
  ◦ Ferrous sulfate with vitamin C.
- For RLS with ESRD on hemodialysis:
  ◦ Vitamin C and E supplementation.
  ◦ Consider adding ropinirole, levodopa, or exercise.

Sources
–Winkelman JW, Armstrong MJ, Allen RP, et al. Practice guideline summary: treatment of restless legs syndrome in adults: report of the Guideline Development, Dissemination, and Implementation Subcommittee of the American Academy of Neurology. *Neurology*. 2016;87(24):2585-2593. (http://guidelines.gov/summaries/summary/50689/)
–www.guidelines.gov/content.aspx?id=38320

Comments
1. Potential for heart valve damage with pergolide and cabergoline.
2. Insufficient evidence to support any pharmacological treatment for periodic limb movement disorder.

SCIATICA

Population
–People age ≥16 y with suspected sciatica.

Recommendations

▶ NICE 2016

For low-back pain with sciatica

–Do not routinely offer imaging in a primary care setting to patient with low-back pain with or without sciatica.

–Continue aerobic exercise program.

–Consider spinal manipulation or soft tissue massage as part of treatment for sciatica.

–Consider cognitive behavioral therapy as part of treatment for sciatica.

–Promote return to work and normal activities.

–Consider NSAIDs and low-dose opioids for acute sciatica.

–For acute, severe sciatica can consider epidural steroid injection.

–Recommend against opioids and anticonvulsants for chronic low-back pain with sciatica.

–Consider spinal decompression for people with disabling sciatica for neurological deficits or chronic symptoms refractory to medical management, and spine imaging is consistent with sciatica symptoms.

–No proven benefit for belts, corsets, foot orthotics, rocker sole shoes, spine traction, acupuncture, ultrasound, transcutaneous electrical nerve stimulation (TENS), and interferential therapy for patients with sciatica.

Source

–National Guideline Centre. *Low Back Pain and Sciatica in Over 16s: Assessment and Management.* London (UK): National Institute for Health and Care Excellence (NICE); 2016, 18 pp.

SEIZURES

Population

–Adults.

Recommendations

▶ ACEP 2014

–For first generalized convulsive seizure, ED physicians need not initiate chronic antiepileptic therapy.

- A precipitating medical condition should be sought.
- Need not admit patients who have returned to their clinical baseline.

–If known seizure disorder, antiepileptic therapy in ED can be administered orally or by IV.

–For status epilepticus:

- First-line therapy is benzodiazepines.
- Options for second-line therapy: phenytoin, fosphenytoin, valproic acid, levetiracetam.

Source

–http://www.guideline.gov/content.aspx?id=47921

Comment

1. For refractory status epilepticus, consider intubation and use of a propofol infusion.

Population

–Adults with first unprovoked seizure.

Recommendations

▶ AAN 2015

–Patient education.

- Recurrent seizures occur most frequently in the first 2 y.
- Over the long term (>3 y), immediate antiepileptic drug (AED) therapy is unlikely to improve the prognosis for sustained seizure remission.

–Indications for immediate antiepileptic therapy are based on clinical risk of a recurrent seizure.

–Risk factors for a recurrent seizure include:

- Brain injury.
- Prior stroke.
- Abnormal EEG with epileptiform activity.
- Structural abnormality on brain imaging.
- Nocturnal seizure.

Source

–https://guidelines.gov/summaries/summary/49218

SEIZURES, FEBRILE

Population
–Children age 6 mo to 5 y.

Recommendations
▶ AAP 2011

–A lumbar puncture should be performed in any child who presents with a fever and seizure and has meningeal signs or whose history is concerning for meningitis.

–Lumbar puncture is an option in children 6–12 mo of age who present with a fever and seizure and are not up to date with their *Haemophilus influenzae* or *Streptococcus pneumoniae* vaccinations.

–Lumbar puncture is an option in a child presenting with a fever and a seizure who has been pretreated with antibiotics.

–Studies that should not be performed for a simple febrile seizure:
  • An EEG.
  • Routine labs including a basic metabolic panel, calcium, phosphorus, magnesium, glucose, or CBC.
  • Neuroimaging.

Source
–http://pediatrics.aappublications.org/content/127/2/389.full.pdf+html

Comment
1. A febrile seizure is a seizure accompanied by fever ($T \geq 100.4°F$ [38°C]) without CNS infection in a child age 6 mo to 5 y.

STROKE, ACUTE ISCHEMIC

Population
–Adults age 18 y and older presenting to the emergency department with an acute ischemic stroke.

Recommendations
–In the field, EMS first responders should use quick assessment tools such as FAST (face, arm, speech test), Los Angeles Prehospital Stroke Screen, or Cincinnati Prehospital Stroke Scale.

–Transport patients with a positive stroke screen and/or a strong suspicion of stroke rapidly to the closest health care facilities that can capably administer IV alteplase.

–When assessing new stroke, ED/Hospital teams should use the National Institutes of Health Stroke Scale (NIHSS) scoring system.

NATIONAL INSTITUTES OF HEALTH STROKE SCALE SCORE

1a. Level of consciousness	0 = Alert; keenly responsive 1 = Not alert, but arousable by minor stimulation 2 = Not alert; requires repeated stimulation 3 = Unresponsive or responds only with reflex
1b. Level of consciousness questions: What is the month? What is your age?	0 = Answers two questions correctly 1 = Answers one question correctly 2 = Answers neither question correctly
1c. Level of consciousness commands: Open and close your eyes. Grip and release your hand.	0 = Performs both tasks correctly 1 = Performs one task correctly 2 = Performs neither task correctly
2. Best gaze	0 = Normal 1 = Partial gaze palsy 2 = Forced deviation
3. Visual	0 = No visual loss 1 = Partial hemianopia 2 = Complete hemianopia 3 = Bilateral hemianopia
4. Facial palsy	0 = Normal symmetric movements 1 = Minor paralysis 2 = Partial paralysis 3 = Complete paralysis of one or both sides
5. Motor arm 5a. Left arm 5b. Right arm	0 = No drift 1 = Drift 2 = Some effort against gravity 3 = No effort against gravity; limb falls 4 = No movement
6. Motor leg 6a. Left leg 6b. Right leg	0 = No drift 1 = Drift 2 = Some effort against gravity 3 = No effort against gravity 4 = No movement

7. Limb ataxia	0 = Absent
	1 = Present in one limb
	2 = Present in two limbs
8. Sensory	0 = Normal; no sensory loss
	1 = Mild-to-moderate sensory loss
	2 = Severe to total sensory loss
9. Best language	0 = No aphasia; normal
	1 = Mild-to-moderate aphasia
	2 = Severe aphasia
	3 = Mute, global aphasia
10. Dysarthria	0 = Normal
	1 = Mild-to-moderate dysarthria
	2 = Severe dysarthria
11. Extinction and inattention	0 = No abnormality
	1 = Visual, tactile, auditory, spatial, or personal inattention
	2 = Profound hemi-inattention or extinction

Total score = 0–42.

▶ AHA/ASA 2018

–Obtain brain imaging evaluation upon arrival to hospital for all patients admitted to the hospital with suspected acute. Noncontrast CT (NCCT) will provide the necessary information to make decisions about acute management.

–Establish systems so that brain imaging studies can be performed within 20 min of arrival in the ED in at least 50% of patients who may be candidates for IV alteplase and/or mechanical thrombectomy.

–Do not routinely use magnetic resonance imaging (MRI) to exclude cerebral microbleeds (CMBs) before administration of IV alteplase.

–For patients who otherwise meet criteria for endovascular treatment (EVT), obtain a noninvasive intracranial vascular study during the initial imaging evaluation of the acute stroke patient but do not delay IV alteplase if indicated.

–For patients who otherwise meet criteria for EVT, proceed with CTA if indicated in patients with suspected intracranial large vessel occlusion (LVO) before obtaining a serum creatinine concentration in patients without a history of renal impairment.

–In patients who are potential candidates for mechanical thrombectomy, consider imaging the extracranial carotid and vertebral arteries, in addition to the intracranial circulation, to provide useful information on patient eligibility and endovascular procedural planning.

–Establish door-to-needle (DTN) time goals with a primary goal of achieving DTN times within 60 min in ≥50% of AIS patients treated with IV alteplase.

–For otherwise medically eligible patients ≥18 y of age, intravenous alteplase administration within 3 h is equally recommended for patients <80 y of age AND >80 y of age.

–For severe stroke symptoms, give IV alteplase within 3 h from symptom onset of ischemic stroke. Despite increased risk of hemorrhagic transformation, there is still proven clinical benefit for patients with severe stroke symptoms.

–Give IV alteplase in patients whose BP can be lowered safely (to <185/110 mm Hg) with antihypertensive agents, with the physician assessing the stability of the BP before starting IV alteplase (see Table I).

–Give IV alteplase in otherwise eligible patients with initial glucose levels >50 mg/dL.

–Give IV alteplase for patients taking antiplatelet drug monotherapy before stroke on the basis of evidence that the benefit of alteplase outweighs a possible small increased risk of symptomatic intracerebral hemorrhage (sICH).

–Give IV alteplase for patients taking antiplatelet drug combination therapy (eg, aspirin and clopidogrel) before stroke on the basis of evidence that the benefit of alteplase outweighs a probable increased risk of sICH.

–In patients with end-stage renal disease on hemodialysis and normal aPTT, IV alteplase is recommended. However, those with elevated aPTT may have elevated risk for hemorrhagic complications.

–Do not give IV alteplase in the following scenarios:

- Ischemic stroke patients who have an unclear time and/or unwitnessed symptom onset and in whom last known normal (LKN) is >3 or 4.5 h.
- Ischemic stroke patients who awoke with stroke with time LKN >3 or 4.5 h.
- Patients who have had a prior ischemic stroke within 3 mo.
- Recent severe head trauma (within 3 mo).
- Patients who have a history of intracranial hemorrhage.
- Patients with platelets <100,000/mm^3, INR >1.7, aPTT >40 s, or PT >15 s (safety and efficacy are unknown). In patients without history of thrombocytopenia, treatment with IV alteplase can be initiated before availability of platelet count but should be discontinued if platelet count is <100,000/mm^3.

- Patients who have received a treatment dose of LMWH within the previous 24 h. The use of IV alteplase in patients taking direct thrombin inhibitors or direct factor Xa inhibitors has not been firmly established but may be harmful.
- Patients with symptoms consistent with infective endocarditis, treatment with IV alteplase should not be administered because of the increased risk of intracranial hemorrhage.

–For patients >80 y of age presenting in the 3- to 4.5-h window, IV alteplase is safe and can be as effective as in younger patients.

–For patients taking warfarin and with an INR ≤1.7 who present in the 3- to 4.5-h window, IV alteplase appears safe and may be beneficial.

–In AIS patients with prior stroke and diabetes mellitus presenting in the 3- to 4.5-h window, IV alteplase may be as effective as treatment in the 0- to 3-h window and may be a reasonable option.

–Within 3 h from symptom onset, treatment of patients with mild ischemic stroke symptoms that are judged as nondisabling may be considered. Treatment risks should be weighed against possible benefits; however, more study is needed to further define the risk-to-benefit ratio.

–For otherwise eligible patients with mild stroke presenting in the 3- to 4.5-h window, IV alteplase may be as effective as treatment in the 0- to 3-h window and may be a reasonable option.

–The benefit of IV alteplase between 3 and 4.5 h from symptom onset for patients with very severe stroke symptoms (NIHSS >25) is uncertain.

–IV alteplase treatment is reasonable for patients who present with moderate-to-severe ischemic stroke and demonstrate early improvement but remain moderately impaired and potentially disabled in the judgment of the examiner.

–IV alteplase is reasonable in patients with a seizure at the time of onset of acute stroke if evidence suggests that residual impairments are secondary to stroke and not a postictal phenomenon.

–IV alteplase may be reasonable in patients who have a history of warfarin use and an INR ≤1.7 and/or a PT <15 s.

–IV alteplase may be considered for patients who present with AIS, even in instances when they may have undergone a lumbar dural puncture in the preceding 7 d.

–Use of IV alteplase in carefully selected patients presenting with AIS who have undergone a major surgery in the preceding 14 d may be considered, but the potential increased risk of surgical-site hemorrhage should be weighed against the anticipated benefits of reduced stroke-related neurological deficits.

–There is a low bleeding risk with IV alteplase administration in the setting of past GI/genitourinary bleeding; however, IV alteplase administration within 21 d of a GI bleeding event is not recommended.

–For patients presenting with AIS who are known to harbor a small or moderate-sized (<10 mm) unruptured and unsecured intracranial aneurysm, administration of IV alteplase is reasonable and probably recommended.

–In otherwise eligible patients who have previously had a high burden (>10) of CMBs demonstrated on MRI, treatment with IV alteplase may be associated with an increased risk of sICH and the benefits of treatment are uncertain. Treatment may be reasonable if there is the potential for substantial benefit.

–IV alteplase is reasonable for patients with AIS who harbor an extra-axial intracranial neoplasm.

–For patients presenting with concurrent AIS and acute MI, treatment with IV alteplase at the dose appropriate for cerebral ischemia, followed by percutaneous coronary angioplasty and stenting, is reasonable.

–For patients presenting with AIS and a history of recent MI in the past 3 mo, treating the ischemic stroke with IV alteplase is reasonable if the recent MI was non-STEMI.

–The safety and efficacy of IV alteplase in patients with current malignancy are not well established. Patients with systemic malignancy and reasonable (>6 mo) life expectancy may benefit from IV alteplase if other contraindications such as coagulation abnormalities, recent surgery, or systemic bleeding do not coexist.

–IV alteplase administration may be considered in pregnancy when the anticipated benefits of treating moderate or severe stroke outweigh the anticipated increased risks of uterine bleeding.

–The safety and efficacy of IV alteplase in the early postpartum period (<14 d after delivery) have not been well established.

–Use of IV alteplase in patients presenting with AIS who have a history of diabetic hemorrhagic retinopathy or other hemorrhagic ophthalmic conditions is reasonable to recommend, but the potential increased risk of visual loss should be weighed against the anticipated benefits of reduced stroke-related neurological deficits.

–Delay placement of nasogastric tubes, indwelling bladder catheters, or intraarterial pressure catheters if the patient can be safely managed without them.

–Obtain a follow-up CT or MRI scan at 24 h after IV alteplase before starting anticoagulants or antiplatelet agents.

–IV alteplase treatment in the 3- to 4.5-h time window is recommended for those patients ≤80 y of age, without a history of both diabetes mellitus and prior stroke, NIHSS score ≤25, not taking any OACs, and without imaging evidence of ischemic injury involving more than one-third of the MCA territory.

–In patients with end-stage renal disease on hemodialysis and normal aPTT, intravenous alteplase is recommended.

–It is mandatory to measure blood glucose prior to the initiation of IV alteplase in all patients.

–Hypoglycemia (blood glucose <60 mg/dL) should be treated in patients with AIS.

–Baseline ECG assessment is recommended in patients presenting with AIS but should not delay initiation of IV alteplase.

–Supplemental oxygen should be provided to maintain oxygen saturation >94%.

–Baseline troponin is recommended in patients presenting with AIS but should not delay initiation of IV alteplase.

–Sources of hyperthermia (temperature >38°C) should be identified and treated; antipyretic medications should be administered to lower temperature in hyperthermic patients with stroke.

–Hypotension and hypovolemia should be corrected to maintain systemic perfusion levels necessary to support organ function.

–Patients who have elevated BP and are otherwise eligible for treatment with IV alteplase should have their BP carefully lowered so that their systolic BP is <185 mm Hg and their diastolic BP is <110 mm Hg.

–Patients otherwise eligible for acute reperfusion therapy but exhibit BP >185/110 mm Hg should have their blood pressure lowered with any of the following agents:

  • Labetalol 10–20 mg IV over 1–2 min, may repeat 1 time.
  • Nicardipine 5 mg/h IV, titrate up by 2.5 mg/h every 5–15 min, maximum 15 mg/h; when desired BP reached, adjust to maintain proper BP limits.
  • Clevidipine 1–2 mg/h IV, titrate by doubling the dose every 2–5 min until desired BP reached; maximum 21 mg/h.
  • Other agents including hydralazine and enalaprilat may also be considered.
  • If BP is not maintained ≤185/110 mm Hg, do not administer alteplase.
  • Management of BP during and after alteplase is to maintain BP ≤180/105 mm Hg.
  • Monitor BP every 15 min for 2 h from the start of alteplase therapy, then every 30 min for 6 h, and then every hour for 16 h.

–If systolic BP >180–230 mm Hg or diastolic BP >105–120 mm Hg:

  • Labetalol 10 mg IV followed by continuous IV infusion 2–8 mg/min.

- Nicardipine 5 mg/h IV, titrate up to desired effect by 2.5 mg/h every 5–15 min, maximum 15 mg/h.
- Clevidipine 1–2 mg/h IV, titrate by doubling the dose every 2–5 min until desired BP reached; maximum 21 mg/h.
- If BP not controlled or diastolic BP >140 mm Hg, consider IV sodium nitroprusside.
- Evidence indicates that persistent in-hospital hyperglycemia during the first 24 h after AIS is associated with worse outcomes than normoglycemia, and thus, it is reasonable to treat hyperglycemia to achieve blood glucose levels in a range of 140–180 mg/dL and to closely monitor to prevent hypoglycemia in patients with AIS.

IV Alteplase Dosing

–IV alteplase, 0.9 mg/kg, maximum dose 90 mg over 60 min with initial 10% of dose given as bolus over 1 min is recommended for selected patients who may be treated within 3 h of ischemic stroke symptom onset or patient LKN.

–IV alteplase 0.9 mg/kg, maximum dose 90 mg over 60 min with initial 10% of dose given as bolus over 1 min is also recommended for selected patients who can be treated within 3 and 4.5 h of ischemic stroke symptom onset or patient LKN.

–For otherwise eligible patients with mild stroke presenting in the 3- to 4.5-h window, treatment with IV alteplase may be reasonable.

–In otherwise eligible patients who have had a previously demonstrated small number (1–10) of CMBs on MRI, administration of IV alteplase is reasonable.

–In otherwise eligible patients who have had a previously demonstrated high burden of CMBs (>10) on MRI, treatment with IV alteplase may be associated with an increased risk of symptomatic intracerebral hemorrhage (sICH), and the benefits of treatment are uncertain. Treatment may be reasonable if there is the potential for substantial benefit.

–Abciximab should not be administered concurrently with IV alteplase.

–IV alteplase should not be administered to patients who have received a treatment dose of low-molecular-weight heparin (LMWH) within the previous 24 h.

–BP should be maintained <180/105 mm Hg for at least the first 24 h after IV alteplase treatment.

–Tenecteplase administered as a 0.4-mg/kg single IV bolus has not been proven to be superior or noninferior to alteplase but might be considered as an alternative to alteplase in patients with minor neurological impairment and no major intracranial occlusion.

–In selected patients with AIS within 6–16 h of LKN who have LVO in the anterior circulation and meet other DAWN or DEFUSE 3 eligibility criteria, mechanical thrombectomy is recommended.

–In selected patients with AIS within 16–24 h of LKN who have LVO in the anterior circulation and meet other DAWN eligibility criteria, mechanical thrombectomy is reasonable.

–Patients ≥18 y should undergo mechanical thrombectomy with a stent retriever if they have minimal prestroke disability, have a causative occlusion of the internal carotid artery or proximal middle cerebral artery, have a NIHSS score of ≥6, have a reassuring noncontrast head CT (ASPECT score of ≥6), and if they can be treated within 6 h of last known normal. No perfusion imaging (CT-P or MR-P) is required in these patients.

–The CT hyperdense MCA sign should not be used as a criterion to withhold IV alteplase from patients who otherwise qualify.

–Routine use of MRI to exclude CMBs before administration of IV alteplase is not recommended.

–In patients who are potential candidates for mechanical thrombectomy, imaging of the extracranial carotid and vertebral arteries, in addition to the intracranial circulation, is reasonable to provide useful information on patient eligibility and endovascular procedural planning.

–In selected patients with AIS within 6–24 h of LKN who have LVO in the anterior circulation, obtaining CTP, DW-MRI, or MRI perfusion is recommended to aid in patient selection for mechanical thrombectomy, but only when imaging and other eligibility criteria from RCTs showing benefit are being strictly applied in selecting patients for mechanical thrombectomy.

–Administration of aspirin is recommended in patients with AIS within 24–48 h after onset. For those treated with IV alteplase, aspirin administration is generally delayed until 24 h.

–In patients presenting with minor stroke, treatment for 21 d with dual antiplatelet therapy (aspirin and clopidogrel) begun within 24 h can be beneficial for early secondary stroke prevention for a period of up to 90 d from symptom onset.

–In patients >60 y of age with unilateral MCA infarctions who deteriorate neurologically within 48 h despite medical therapy, decompressive craniectomy with epidural expansion may be considered because it reduces mortality close to 50%, with 11% of the surgical survivors achieving moderate disability (able to walk [mRS score 3]) and none achieving independence (mRS score ≤2) at 12 mo.

Post-Ischemic Stroke Blood Pressure Management

–In patients with AIS, early treatment of hypertension is indicated when required by comorbid conditions (eg, concomitant acute coronary event, acute heart failure, aortic dissection, post-thrombolysis, sICH, or preeclampsia/eclampsia). Lowering BP initially by 15% is probably safe.

–In patients with BP ≥220/120 mm Hg who did not receive IV alteplase or EVT and have no comorbid conditions requiring acute antihypertensive treatment, the benefit of initiating or reinitiating treatment of hypertension within the first 48–72 h is uncertain. It might be reasonable to lower BP by 15% during the first 24 h after onset of stroke.

–Starting or restarting antihypertensive therapy during hospitalization in patients with BP >140/90 mm Hg who are neurologically stable is safe and is reasonable to improve long-term BP control unless contraindicated.

–Hypotension and hypovolemia should be corrected to maintain systemic perfusion levels necessary to support organ function.

–BP should be maintained <180/105 mm Hg for at least the first 24 h after IV alteplase treatment.

TABLE I: BLOOD PRESSURE MEDICATIONS FROM 2018 AHA GUIDELINES

For patients with AIS and otherwise eligible for acute reperfusion therapy except that BP is >185/110 mm Hg, first lower blood pressure with one of the following therapies:

- Labetalol 10–20 mg IV over 1–2 min, may repeat 1 time
- Nicardipine 5 mg/h IV, titrate up by 2.5 mg/h every 5–15 min, maximum 15 mg/h
- Clevidipine 1–2 mg/h IV, titrate by doubling the dose every 2–5 min until desired BP reached; maximum 21 mg/h
- Other agents such as hydralazine and enalaprilat may also be considered
- If BP is not maintained ≤185/110 mm Hg, do not administer alteplase
- Goal BP during and after IV alteplase is ≤180/105 mm Hg
- Monitor BP every 15 min for 2 h from the start of IV alteplase therapy, then every 30 min for 6 h, and then every hour for 16 h

If systolic BP >180–230 mm Hg or diastolic BP >105–120 mm Hg:

- Labetalol 10 mg IV followed by continuous IV infusion 2–8 mg/min
- Nicardipine 5 mg/h IV, titrate up to desired effect by 2.5 mg/h every 5–15 min, maximum 15 mg/h
- Clevidipine 1–2 mg/h IV, titrate by doubling the dose every 2–5 min until desired BP reached; maximum 21 mg/h
- If BP not controlled or diastolic BP >140 mm Hg, consider IV sodium nitroprusside

Stroke Rehabilitation

–Provide rehabilitation to stroke survivors at an intensity commensurate with anticipated benefit and tolerance.

–During hospitalization and inpatient rehabilitation, perform regular skin assessments with objective scales of risk such as the Braden scale.

–Continue regular turning, good skin hygiene, and use of specialized mattresses, wheelchair cushions, and seating until mobility returns.

–Consider resting ankle splints used at night and during assisted standing for prevention of ankle contracture in the hemiplegic limb.

–In ischemic stroke, use prophylactic-dose subcutaneous heparin (UFH or LMWH) for the duration of the acute and rehabilitation hospital stay or until the stroke survivor regains mobility.

–Remove a Foley catheter within 24 h of hospitalization if possible.

–Assessment of urinary retention through bladder scanning or intermittent catheterizations after voiding while recording volumes is recommended for patients with urinary incontinence or retention.

–Refer individuals with stroke discharged to the community to participate in exercise programs with balance training to reduce falls.

–Provide individuals with stroke a formal fall prevention program during hospitalization.

–Administer a structured depression inventory such as the Patient Health Questionnaire-2 to routinely screen for poststroke depression. Prescribe antidepressants to all patients with depression.

–Evaluate individuals with stroke residing in long-term care facilities be evaluated for calcium and vitamin D supplementation.

–Provide individuals with stroke a formal assessment of their ADLs and IADLs, communication abilities, and functional mobility before discharge from acute care hospitalization and incorporate the findings into the care transition and the discharge planning process.

–Assess speech, language, cognitive communication, pragmatics, reading, and writing; identify communicative strengths and weaknesses; and identify helpful compensatory strategies.

–Start enteral diet within 7 d of admission after an acute stroke.

–For patients with dysphagia, consider using nasogastric tubes initially for feeding in the early phase of stroke (starting within the first 7 d) and to place percutaneous gastrostomy tubes in patients with longer anticipated persistent inability to swallow safely ($>$2–3 wk).

–Consider directing patients and families with stroke to palliative care resources as appropriate. Caregivers should ascertain and include patient-centered preferences in decision making, especially during prognosis formation and considering interventions or limitations in care.

Sources
- –2018 Guidelines for the Early Management of Patients with Acute Ischemic Stroke: A Guideline for Healthcare Professionals from the American Heart Association/American Stroke Association. *Stroke.* 2018;49:e46-e99.
- –Scientific rationale for the inclusion and exclusion criteria for intravenous alteplase in acute ischemic stroke: a statement for healthcare professionals from the American Heart Association/American Stroke Association. *Stroke.* 2016;47:581-641.
- –Guidelines for Adult Stroke Rehabilitation and Recovery: a guideline for healthcare professionals from the American Heart Association/American Stroke Association. *Stroke.* 2016;47:e98-e169.

STROKE, RECURRENCE

Population
- –Adults with atrial fibrillation.

Recommendations

▶ AHA/ASA 2014

- –For most patients with a stroke or TIA in the setting of AF, initiate oral anticoagulation within 14 d after the onset of neurological symptoms. In the presence of high risk for hemorrhagic conversion (ie, large infarct, hemorrhagic transformation on initial imaging, uncontrolled hypertension, or hemorrhage tendency), consider delaying initiation of oral anticoagulation beyond 14 d.
- –VKA therapy (Class I; Level of Evidence A), apixaban (Class I; Level of Evidence A), and dabigatran (Class I; Level of Evidence B) are all indicated for the prevention of recurrent stroke in patients with nonvalvular AF, whether paroxysmal or permanent. Rivaroxaban is reasonable for the prevention of recurrent stroke in patients with nonvalvular AF.
- –For patients with ischemic stroke or TIA and AF who are unable to take oral anticoagulants, aspirin alone is recommended. The addition of clopidogrel to aspirin therapy might be reasonable.
- –The usefulness of closure of the left atrial appendage with the WATCHMAN device in patients with ischemic stroke or TIA and AF is uncertain.

Population
- –Hypertension.

Recommendation

▶ AHA/ASA 2018

–Initiation of BP therapy is indicated for previously untreated patients with ischemic stroke or TIA who after the first several days have an established SBP ≥140 mm Hg or DBP ≥90 mm Hg. In patients previously treated for HTN, resumption of BP therapy is indicated beyond the first several days for both prevention of recurrent stroke and other vascular events. Goals: <140/90 mm Hg; for recent lacunar stroke reasonable SBP target <130 mm Hg.

Population

–Dyslipidemia.

Recommendation

▶ AHA/ASA 2014

–Intensive lipid-lowering effects are recommended in patients with ischemic stroke or TIA presumed to be of atherosclerotic origin, an LDL-C ≥100 mg/dL and with/without evidence of other clinical ASCVD.

Population

–Glucose disorders.

Recommendation

▶ AHA/ASA 2018

–All patients should be screened for DM (HgbA1c).

Population

–Obesity.

Recommendation

▶ AHA/ASA 2014

–Calculate BMI for all patients and start weight-loss management when necessary.

Population

–Sleep apnea.

Recommendation

▶ AHA/ASA 2014

–A sleep study might be considered for patients with history of CVA or TIA on the basis of very high prevalence in this population.

Population

–MI and thrombus.

Recommendation

▶ AHA/ASA 2014

–VKA therapy (INR: 2–3) for 3 mo may be considered in patients with ischemic stroke or TIA in the setting of acute anterior STEMI.

Population

–Cardiomyopathy.

Recommendation

▶ AHA/ASA 2014

–In patients with ischemic stroke or TIA in sinus rhythm who have left atrial or left ventricular thrombus demonstrated by echocardiography or other imaging modality, anticoagulant therapy with a VKA is recommended for ≥3 mo.

Population

–Valvular heart disease.

Recommendations

▶ AHA/ASA 2014

–For patients with ischemic stroke or TIA who have rheumatic mitral valve disease and AF, long-term VKA therapy with an INR target of 2.5 (range 2.0–3.0) is recommended.

–For patients with ischemic stroke or TIA and native aortic or nonrheumatic mitral valve disease who do not have AF or another indication for anticoagulation, antiplatelet therapy is recommended.

Population

–Prosthetic heart valve.

Recommendations

▶ AHA/ASA 2014

–For patients with a mechanical aortic valve and a history of ischemic stroke or TIA before its insertion, VKA therapy is recommended with an INR target of 2.5 (range 2.0–3.0).

–For patients with a mechanical mitral valve and a history of ischemic stroke or TIA before its insertion, VKA therapy is recommended with an INR target of 3.0 (range 2.5–3.5).

–For patients with a mechanical mitral or aortic valve who have a history of ischemic stroke or TIA before its insertion and who are at low risk for bleeding, the addition of aspirin 75–100 mg/d to VKA therapy is recommended.

–For patients with a bioprosthetic aortic or mitral valve, a history of ischemic stroke or TIA before its insertion, and no other indication for anticoagulation therapy beyond 3–6 mo from the valve placement, long-term therapy with aspirin 75–100 mg/d is recommended in preference to long-term anticoagulation.

Population

–Aortic arch atheroma.

Recommendation

▶ AHA/ASA 2014

–For patients with an ischemic stroke or TIA and evidence of aortic arch atheroma, antiplatelet therapy is recommended.

Population

–PFO.

Recommendations

▶ AHA/ASA 2014

–For patients with an ischemic stroke or TIA and a PFO who are not undergoing anticoagulation therapy, antiplatelet therapy is recommended.

–For patients with an ischemic stroke or TIA and both a PFO and a venous source of embolism, anticoagulation is indicated, depending on stroke characteristics. When anticoagulation is contraindicated, an inferior vena cava filter is reasonable.

–For patients with a cryptogenic ischemic stroke or TIA and a PFO without evidence for DVT, available data do not support a benefit for PFO closure.

–In the setting of PFO and DVT, PFO closure by a transcatheter device might be considered, depending on the risk of recurrent DVT.

Population

–<30 y, stroke, and homocysteinemia.

Recommendation

▶ AHA

–Screening for hyperhomocysteinemia among young patients with a recent ischemic stroke or TIA may be of benefit in an effort to prevent future cardiovascular and cerebrovascular disease. Most common concern is mutation in MTHFR gene.

Source
–*Circulation*. 2015;132:e6-e9.

Population

–Hypercoagulation.

Recommendations

▶ AHA/ASA 2014

–The usefulness of screening for thrombophilic states in patients with ischemic stroke or TIA is unknown.

–Antiplatelet therapy is recommended in patients who are found to have abnormal findings on coagulation testing after an initial ischemic stroke or TIA if anticoagulation therapy is not administered.

Population

–Sickle cell disease.

Recommendations

▶ AHA/ASA 2014

–For patients with sickle cell disease and prior ischemic stroke or TIA, chronic blood transfusions to reduce hemoglobin S to <30% of total hemoglobin are recommended.

–IV alteplase for adults presenting with an AIS with known sickle cell disease can be beneficial.

Population

–Pregnancy.

Recommendations

▶ AHA/ASA 2014

–In the presence of a high-risk condition that would require anticoagulation outside of pregnancy, the following options are reasonable:

- LMWH twice daily throughout pregnancy, with dose adjusted to achieve the LMWH manufacturer's recommended peak anti-Xa level 4 h after injection, **OR**
- Adjusted-dose UFH throughout pregnancy, administered subcutaneously every 12 h in doses adjusted to keep the mid-interval aPTT at least twice control or to maintain an anti-Xa heparin level of 0.35–0.70 U/mL, **OR**
- UFH or LMWH (as above) until the 13th wk, followed by substitution of a VKA until close to delivery, when UFH or LMWH is resumed.

–For pregnant women receiving adjusted-dose LMWH therapy for
a high-risk condition that would require anticoagulation outside of
pregnancy, and when delivery is planned, it is reasonable to discontinue
LMWH ≥24 h before induction of labor or cesarean section.

–In the presence of a low-risk situation in which antiplatelet therapy
would be the treatment recommendation outside of pregnancy, UFH or
LMWH, or no treatment may be considered during the first trimester
of pregnancy depending on the clinical situation.

Population
–Breast-feeding.

Recommendations
▶ AHA/ASA 2014

–In the presence of a high-risk condition that would require
anticoagulation outside of pregnancy, it is reasonable to use warfarin,
UFH, or LMWH.

–In the presence of a low-risk situation in which antiplatelet therapy
would be the treatment recommendation outside of pregnancy, low-
dose aspirin use may be considered.

Sources
–Guidelines for the prevention of stroke in patients with stroke and
transient ischemic attack: a guideline for healthcare professionals from
the American Heart Association/American Stroke Association. *Stroke.*
2014;45.

–http://stroke.ahajournals.org

–2018 Guidelines for the early management of patients with acute
ischemic stroke: a guideline for healthcare professionals from the
American Heart Association/American Stroke Association. *Stroke.*
2018;49:e46–e99. doi: 10.1161/STR.0000000000000158.

SYNCOPE

Population
–Adults presenting with syncope.

Recommendations
▶ ACC/AHA 2017

ADDITIONAL EVALUATION AND DIAGNOSIS FOR SYNCOPE

Initial Evaluation of Syncope

HISTORICAL CHARACTERISTICS ASSOCIATED WITH INCREASED PROBABILITY OF CARDIAC AND NONCARDIAC CAUSES OF SYNCOPE
More Often Associated with Cardiac Causes of Syncope
• Older age (>60 y)
• Male sex
• Presence of known ischemic heart disease, structural heart disease, previous arrhythmias, or reduced ventricular function
• Brief prodrome, such as palpitations, or sudden loss of consciousness without prodrome
• Syncope during exertion
• Syncope in the supine position
• Low number of syncope episodes (1 or 2)
• Abnormal cardiac examination
• Family history of inheritable conditions or premature SCD (<50 y of age)
• Presence of known congenital heart disease
More Often Associated with Noncardiac Causes of Syncope
• Younger age
• No known cardiac disease
• Syncope only in the standing position
• Positional change from supine or sitting to standing
• Presence of prodrome: nausea, vomiting, feeling warmth
• Situational triggers: cough, laugh, micturition, defecation, deglutition
• Frequent recurrence and prolonged history of syncope with similar characteristics

SCD, sudden cardiac death.

Historical Features of Cardiac vs. Noncardiac Syncope

EXAMPLE OF SERIOUS MEDICAL CONDITIONS THAT MIGHT WARRANT CONSIDERATION OF FURTHER EVALUTION AND THERAPY IN HOSPITAL SETTING		
Cardiac Arrhythmic Conditions	**Cardiac or Vascular Nonarrhythmic Conditions**	**Noncardiac Conditions**
• Sustained or symptomatic VT • Symptomatic conduction system disease or Mobitz II or third-degree heart block • Symptomatic bradycardia or sinus pauses not related to neurally mediated syncope • Symptomatic SVT • Pacemaker, ICD malfunction • Inheritable cardiovascular conditions predisposing to arrhythmias	• Cardiac ischemia • Severe aortic stenosis • Cardiac tamponade • HCM • Severe prosthetic valve dysfunction • Pulmonary embolism • Aortic dissection • Acute HF • Moderate-to-severe LV dysfunction	• Severe anemia/gastrointestinal bleeding • Major traumatic injury due to syncope • Persistent vital sign abnormalities

Serious Medical Conditions Associated with Syncope

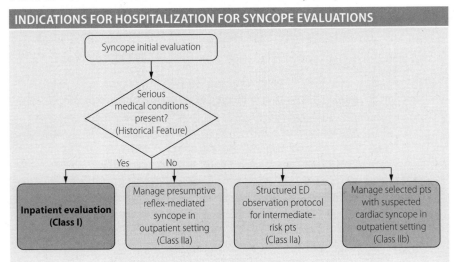

Source: Circulation. 2017;136(5):e25-e59. Reprinted with permission. ©2017, American Heart Association, Inc.

Recommended Tests for Syncope

–EKG.

–Complete blood count, basic metabolic panel, and other targeted labs based on clinical assessment.

–Echocardiogram if structural heart disease is suspected.

–Stress test if exertional syncope of unclear etiology.

–Continuous telemetry monitoring for patients admitted to hospital.

–Prolonged cardiac monitoring if arrhythmic syncope is suspected.

–Electrophysiologic study if syncope of suspected arrhythmic etiology with negative cardiac monitoring.

Other Interventions for Syncope

–Implantable cardioverter-defibrillator (ICD) implantation is recommended in patients with arrhythmogenic right ventricular cardiomyopathy who present with syncope and have a documented sustained ventricular arrhythmia.

▶ ESC 2018

–Diagnosis of syncope requires transient loss of consciousness without other explanation (epilepsy, psychogenic).

–If syncope, evaluate with history and physical exam, EKG, and orthostatic blood pressure. Include echocardiogram if history of heart disease or if the exam suggests structural heart disease. Consider carotid sinus massage in patients greater than 40 y. Consider tilt testing if reflex syncope or orthostatic hypertension is suspected. Consider lab testing including hemoglobin if hemorrhage is suspected, blood gas if hypoxia is suspected, troponin if ischemia is suspected, and D-dimer if pulmonary embolism is suspected.

–If diagnosis remains uncertain, stratify risk of serious sequela and recurrence as high or low. Presume the patient with exclusively low-risk features has had reflex, situational, or orthostatic syncope and pursue outpatient follow-up. Others should be observed in an emergency department or inpatient setting for further workup.

- Low-risk features include an event with a typical prodrome or with specific trigger, a long history of similar syncopal episodes, absence of structural heart disease, normal physical examination, and normal EKG.
- High-risk features include chest discomfort, dyspnea, abdominal pain, headache, relation to exertion, preceding palpitation, structural or coronary heart disease, unexplained hypotension, signs of GI bleeding, persistent bradycardia, undiagnosed murmur, or concerning EKG changes.

–Treatment reflex and orthostatic syncope with education and lifestyle modification. For patients with persistent symptoms, consider fludrocortisone or midodrine if blood pressure is low, counter pressure maneuvers if the prodrome exists, de-escalating therapy if on hypotensive drugs, and perhaps cardiac pacing if severe carotid sinus sensitivity.

Source
  –2017 AHA/ACC focused update of the 2014 AHA/ACC guideline for the management of patients with valvular heart disease: a report of the American College of Cardiology/American Heart Association Task Force on clinical practice guidelines. *Circulation.* 2017;135:e1159–e1195.

TRAUMATIC BRAIN INJURY

Recommendation
▶ ACEP 2013
  –Avoid CT scan of head for minor head trauma in patients who are low risk based on validated decision rules.

Source
  –http://www.choosingwisely.org/societies/american-college-of-emergency-physicians/

TREMOR, ESSENTIAL

Population
  –Adults.

Recommendations
▶ AAN 2011
  –Recommends treatment with propranolol or primidone.
  –Alternative treatment options include alprazolam, atenolol, gabapentin, sotalol, or topiramate.
  –Recommends against treatment with levetiracetam, pindolol, trazodone, acetazolamide, or 3,4-diaminopyridine.

Source
  –http://www.neurology.org/content/77/19/1752.full.pdf+html

Comment
  1. Unilateral thalamotomy may be effective for severe refractory essential tremors.

Prenatal and Obstetric Care

ABORTION

Population
–Women with incomplete abortion.

Recommendations
▶ WHO 2018

–Offer surgical or medical management vs. watchful waiting.

–If patient <13-wk gestation elects medical management, give misoprostol 600 μg orally or 400 μg sublingually. Do not use vaginal misoprostol.

–If patient ≥13-wk gestation elects medical management, give repeated doses of misoprostol 400 μg every 3 h sublingually, vaginally, or buccally.

Population
–Women with intrauterine fetal demise between 14- and 28-wk gestation.

Recommendation
▶ WHO 2018

–Offer surgical or medical management vs. watchful waiting.

–If patient elects medical management, give 200-mg mifepristone orally; 1–2 d later, give 400-μg misoprostol sublingually or vaginally, and repeat every 4–6 h. If mifepristone is not available or not preferred by the patient, give misoprostol 400 μg every 4–6 h as the initial treatment.

Population
–Women who elect to induce an abortion.

Recommendations

WHO 2018

–Options include vacuum aspiration (manual or electric), dilation, and evacuation or medical management.

–For medical abortion, give mifepristone 200 mg once as initial dose. At least 24 h later, give misoprostol vaginally, sublingually, or buccally. If <12-wk gestation, use 800 µg. If ≥12-wk gestation give 400 µg. If mifepristone is not available, use misoprostol as initial dose.

Source

–*Medical Management of Abortion.* Geneva: World Health Organization; 2018. License: CC BY-NC-SA 3.0 IGO.

CONTRACEPTION

PERCENTAGE OF WOMEN EXPERIENCING AN UNINTENDED PREGNANCY WITHIN THE FIRST YEAR OF TYPICAL USE AND THE FIRST YEAR OF PERFECT USE AND THE PERCENTAGE CONTINUING USE AT THE END OF THE FIRST YEAR: UNITED STATES

% of Women Experiencing an Unintended Pregnancy Within the First Year of Use

Method	Typical Use[a]	Perfect Use[b]	Women Continuing Use at 1 Y[c]
Male sterilization	0.15	0.10	100
Female sterilization	0.5	0.5	100
Implanon	0.05	0.05	84
Intrauterine contraceptives			
ParaGard (copper T)	0.8	0.6	78
Mirena (LNG-IUS)	0.2	0.2	80
Depo-Provera	3	0.3	56
NuvaRing	8	0.3	68
Evra patch	8	0.3	68
Combined pill and Progestin-only pill	8	0.3	68
Diaphragm	12	6	57
Condom			
Female (fc)	21	5	49
Male	15	2	53

PERCENTAGE OF WOMEN EXPERIENCING AN UNINTENDED PREGNANCY WITHIN THE FIRST YEAR OF TYPICAL USE AND THE FIRST YEAR OF PERFECT USE AND THE PERCENTAGE CONTINUING USE AT THE END OF THE FIRST YEAR: UNITED STATES *(Continued)*

% of Women Experiencing an Unintended Pregnancy Within the First Year of Use

Method	Typical Use[a]	Perfect Use[b]	Women Continuing Use at 1 Y[c]
Sponge			
Parous women	24	20	
Nulliparous women	16	9	
Withdrawal	22	4	46
Fertility awareness-based methods	24		47
Standard Days method[e]		5	
Two-Day method[e]		4	
Ovulation method[e]		3	
Symptothermal method[e]		0.4	
Spermicides[f]	28	18	42
No method[g]	85	85	

Emergency Contraceptive Pills: Treatment with COCs initiated within 120 h after unprotected intercourse reduces the risk of pregnancy by at least 60%–75%.[h] Pregnancy rates are lower if initiated in first 12 h. Progestin-only EC reduces pregnancy risk by 89%.

Lactational Amenorrhea Method: LAM is a highly effective, temporary method of contraception.[i]

[a]Among typical couples who initiate use of a method (not necessarily for the first time), the percentage who experience an accidental pregnancy during the first year if they do not stop use for any other reason. Estimates of the probability of pregnancy during the first year of typical use for spermicides, withdrawal, fertility awareness-based methods, the diaphragm, the male condom, the oral contraceptive pill, and Depo-Provera are taken from the 1995 National Survey of Family Growth corrected for underreporting of abortion; see the text for the derivation of estimates for the other methods.

[b]Among couples who initiate use of a method (not necessarily for the first time) and who use it perfectly (both consistently and correctly), the percentage who experience an accidental pregnancy during the first year if they do not stop use for any other reason. See the text for the derivation of the estimate for each method.

[c]Among couples attempting to avoid pregnancy, the percentage who continue to use a method for 1 y.

[e]The Ovulation and Two-Day methods are based on evaluation of cervical mucus. The Standard-Days method avoids intercourse on cycle days 8 through 19. The Symptothermal method is a double-check method based on evaluation of cervical mucus to determine the first fertile day and evaluation of cervical mucus and temperature to determine the last fertile day.

[f]Foams, creams, gels, vaginal suppositories, and vaginal film.

[g]The percentages becoming pregnant in columns (2) and (3) are based on data from populations where contraception is not used and from women who cease using contraception in order to become pregnant. Among such populations, about 89% become pregnant within 1 y. This estimate was lowered slightly (to 85%) to represent the percentage who would become pregnant within 1 y among women now relying on reversible methods of contraception if they abandoned contraception altogether.

ʰella, Plan B One-Step, and Next Choice are the only dedicated products specifically marketed for emergency contraception. The label for Plan B One-Step (1 dose is 1 white pill) says to take the pill within 72 h after unprotected intercourse. Research has shown that all of the brands listed here are effective when used within 120 h after unprotected sex. The label for Next Choice (1 dose is 1 peach pill) says to take 1 pill within 72 h after unprotected intercourse and another pill 12 h later. Research has shown that both pills can be taken at the same time with no decrease in efficacy or increase in side effects and that they are effective when used within 120 h after unprotected sex. The Food and Drug Administration has in addition declared the following 19 brands of oral contraceptives to be safe and effective for emergency contraception: Ogestrel (1 dose is 2 white pills), Nordette (1 dose is 4 light-orange pills), Cryselle, Levora, Low-Ogestrel, Lo/Ovral, or Quasence (1 dose is 4 white pills), Jolessa, Portia, Seasonale, or Trivora (1 dose is 4 pink pills), Seasonique (1 dose is 4 light-blue-green pills), Enpresse (1 dose is 4 orange pills), Lessina (1 dose is 5 pink pills), Aviane or LoSeasonique (1 dose is 5 orange pills), Lutera or Sronyx (1 dose is 5 white pills), and Lybrel (1 dose is 6 yellow pills).

ⁱHowever, to maintain effective protection against pregnancy, another method of contraception must be used as soon as menstruation resumes, the frequency or duration of breastfeeds is reduced, bottle feeds are introduced, or the baby reaches 6 mo of age.

Source: Hatcher RA, Zieman M, Allen AZ, Lathrop E, Haddad L. *Managing Contraception 2017-2018.* Tiger, Georgia: Bridging the Gap Foundation, 2017.

CONTRACEPTION, EMERGENCY

Population

- –Women of childbearing age who had unprotected or inadequately protected sexual intercourse within the last 5 d and who do not desire pregnancy.

Recommendations

▶ ACOG 2015

- –Emergency contraception should be offered to women who have had unprotected or inadequately protected sexual intercourse and who do not desire pregnancy.
- –Emergency contraceptive pills or copper IUD should be made available to patients who request it up to 5 days after unprotected or inadequately protected sexual intercourse.
- –Women should begin using barrier contraceptives to prevent pregnancy after using emergency contraception or abstain from sexual intercourse for 14 days or until her next menses.

Source

- –*Obstet Gynecol.* 2015;126:e1-e1.

Condition	Sub-Condition	Cu-IUD		LNG-IUD		Implant		DMPA		POP		CHC	
		I	C	I	C	I	C	I	C	I	C	I	C
Age		Menarche to <20 yrs:**2**		Menarche to <20 yrs:**2**		Menarche to <18 yrs:**1**		Menarche to <18 yrs:**2**		Menarche to <18 yrs:**1**		Menarche to <40 yrs:**1**	
		≥20 yrs:**1**		≥20 yrs:**1**		18-45 yrs:**1**		18-45 yrs:**1**		18-45 yrs:**1**		≥40 yrs:**2**	
						>45 yrs:**1**		>45 yrs:**2**		>45 yrs:**1**			
Anatomical abnormalities	a) Distorted uterine cavity	4		4									
	b) Other abnormalities	2		2									
Anemias	a) Thalassemia	2		1		1		1		1		1	
	b) Sickle cell disease[s]	2		1		1		1		1		2	
	c) Iron-deficiency anemia	2		1		1		1		1		1	
Benign ovarian tumors	(including cysts)	1		1		1		1		1		1	
Breast disease	a) Undiagnosed mass	1		2		2*		2*		2*		2*	
	b) Benign breast disease	1		1		1		1		1		1	
	c) Family history of cancer	1		1		1		1		1		1	
	d) Breast cancer[s]												
	i) Current	1		4		4		4		4		4	
	ii) Past and no evidence of current disease for 5 years	1		3		3		3		3		3	
Breastfeeding	a) <21 days postpartum					2*		2*		2*		4*	
	b) 21 to <30 days postpartum												
	i) With other risk factors for VTE					2*		2*		2*		3*	
	ii) Without other risk factors for VTE					2*		2*		2*		3*	
	c) 30-42 days postpartum												
	i) With other risk factors for VTE					1*		1*		1*		3*	
	ii) Without other risk factors for VTE					1*		1*		1*		2*	
	d) >42 days postpartum					1*		1*		1*		2*	
Cervical cancer	Awaiting treatment	4	2	4	2	2		2		1		2	
Cervical ectropion		1		1		1		1		1		1	
Cervical intraepithelial neoplasia		1		2		2		2		1		2	
Cirrhosis	a) Mild (compensated)	1		1		1		1		1		1	
	b) Severe[s] (decompensated)	1		3		3		3		3		4	
Cystic fibrosis[s]		1*		1*		1*		2*		1*		1*	
Deep venous thrombosis (DVT)/Pulmonary embolism (PE)	a) History of DVT/PE, not receiving anticoagulant therapy												
	i) Higher risk for recurrent DVT/PE	1		2		2		2		2		4	
	ii) Lower risk for recurrent DVT/PE	1		2		2		2		2		3	
	b) Acute DVT/PE	2		2		2		2		2		4	
	c) DVT/PE and established anticoagulant therapy for at least 3 months												
	i) Higher risk for recurrent DVT/PE	2		2		2		2		2		4*	
	ii) Lower risk for recurrent DVT/PE	2		2		2		2		2		3*	
	d) Family history (first-degree relatives)	1		1		1		1		1		2	
	e) Major surgery												
	i) With prolonged immobilization	1		2		2		2		2		4	
	ii) Without prolonged immobilization	1		1		1		1		1		2	
	f) Minor surgery without immobilization	1		1		1		1		1		1	
Depressive disorders		1*		1*		1*		1*		1*		1*	

Key:	
1 No restriction (method can be used)	**3** Theoretical or proven risks usually outweigh the advantages
2 Advantages generally outweigh theoretical or proven risks	**4** Unacceptable health risk (method not to be used)

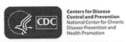

Condition	Sub-Condition	Cu-IUD I	Cu-IUD C	LNG-IUD I	LNG-IUD C	Implant I	Implant C	DMPA I	DMPA C	POP I	POP C	CHC I	CHC C
Diabetes	a) History of gestational disease	1	1	1	1	1	1	1	1	1	1	1	1
	b) Nonvascular disease												
	i) Non-insulin dependent	1	1	2	2	2	2	2	2	2	2	2	2
	ii) Insulin dependent	1	1	2	2	2	2	2	2	2	2	2	2
	c) Nephropathy/retinopathy/neuropathy‡	1	1	2	2	2	2	3	3	2	2	3/4*	3/4*
	d) Other vascular disease or diabetes of >20 years' duration‡	1	1	2	2	2	2	3	3	2	2	3/4*	3/4*
Dysmenorrhea	Severe	2	2	1	1	1	1	1	1	1	1	1	1
Endometrial cancer‡		4	2	4	2	1	1	1	1	1	1	1	1
Endometrial hyperplasia		1	1	1	1	1	1	1	1	1	1	1	1
Endometriosis		2	2	1	1	1	1	1	1	1	1	1	1
Epilepsy‡	(see also Drug Interactions)	1	1	1	1	1*	1*	1*	1*	1*	1*	1*	1*
Gallbladder disease	a) Symptomatic												
	i) Treated by cholecystectomy	1	1	2	2	2	2	2	2	2	2	2	2
	ii) Medically treated	1	1	2	2	2	2	2	2	2	2	3	3
	iii) Current	1	1	2	2	2	2	2	2	2	2	3	3
	b) Asymptomatic	1	1	2	2	2	2	2	2	2	2	2	2
Gestational trophoblastic disease‡	a) Suspected GTD (immediate postevacuation)												
	i) Uterine size first trimester	1*	1*	1*	1*	1*	1*	1*	1*	1*	1*	1*	1*
	ii) Uterine size second trimester	2*	2*	2*	2*	1*	1*	1*	1*	1*	1*	1*	1*
	b) Confirmed GTD												
	i) Undetectable/non-pregnant ß-hCG levels	1*	1*	1*	1*	1*	1*	1*	1*	1*	1*	1*	1*
	ii) Decreasing ß-hCG levels	2*	1*	2*	1*	1*	1*	1*	1*	1*	1*	1*	1*
	iii) Persistently elevated ß-hCG levels or malignant disease, with no evidence or suspicion of intrauterine disease	2*	1*	2*	1*	1*	1*	1*	1*	1*	1*	1*	1*
	iv) Persistently elevated ß-hCG levels or malignant disease, with evidence or suspicion of intrauterine disease	4*	2*	4*	2*	1*	1*	1*	1*	1*	1*	1*	1*
Headaches	a) Nonmigraine (mild or severe)	1	1	1	1	1	1	1	1	1	1	1*	1*
	b) Migraine												
	i) Without aura (includes menstrual migraine)	1	1	1	1	1	1	1	1	1	1	2*	2*
	ii) With aura	1	1	1	1	1	1	1	1	1	1	4*	4*
History of bariatric surgery‡	a) Restrictive procedures	1	1	1	1	1	1	1	1	1	1	1	1
	b) Malabsorptive procedures	1	1	1	1	1	1	1	1	3	3	COCs: 3 P/R: 1	COCs: 3 P/R: 1
History of cholestasis	a) Pregnancy related	1	1	1	1	1	1	1	1	1	1	2	2
	b) Past COC related	1	1	2	2	2	2	2	2	2	2	3	3
History of high blood pressure during pregnancy		1	1	1	1	1	1	1	1	1	1	2	2
History of Pelvic surgery		1	1	1	1	1	1	1	1	1	1	1	1
HIV	a) High risk for HIV	2	2	2	2	1	1	1*	1*	1	1	1	1
	b) HIV infection					1*	1*	1*	1*	1*	1*	1*	1*
	i) Clinically well receiving ARV therapy	1	1	1	1	If on treatment, see Drug Interactions							
	ii) Not clinically well or not receiving ARV therapy‡	2	1	2	1	If on treatment, see Drug Interactions							

Abbreviations: C=continuation of contraceptive method; CHC=combined hormonal contraception (pill, patch, and, ring); COC=combined oral contraceptive; Cu-IUD=copper-containing intrauterine device; DMPA = depot medroxyprogesterone acetate; I=initiation of contraceptive method; LNG-IUD=levonorgestrel-releasing intrauterine device; NA=not applicable; POP=progestin-only pill; P/R=patch/ring ‡ Condition that exposes a woman to increased risk as a result of pregnancy. *Please see the complete guidance for a clarification to this classification: www.cdc.gov/reproductivehealth/unintendedpregnancy/USMEC.htm.

Condition	Sub-Condition	Cu-IUD I	Cu-IUD C	LNG-IUD I	LNG-IUD C	Implant I	Implant C	DMPA I	DMPA C	POP I	POP C	CHC I	CHC C
Hypertension	a) Adequately controlled hypertension	1*		1*		1*		2*		1*		3*	
	b) Elevated blood pressure levels (*properly taken measurements*)												
	i) Systolic 140-159 or diastolic 90-99	1*		1*		1*		2*		1*		3*	
	ii) Systolic ≥160 or diastolic ≥100‡	1*		2*		2*		3*		2*		4*	
	c) Vascular disease	1*		2*		2*		3*		2*		4*	
Inflammatory bowel disease	(*Ulcerative colitis, Crohn's disease*)	1		1		1		2		2		2/3*	
Ischemic heart disease‡	Current and history of	1		2	3	2	3	3		2	3	4	
Known thrombogenic mutations‡		1*		2*		2*		2*		2*		4*	
Liver tumors	a) Benign												
	i) Focal nodular hyperplasia	1		2		2		2		2		2	
	ii) Hepatocellular adenoma‡	1		3		3		3		3		4	
	b) Malignant‡ (hepatoma)	1		3		3		3		3		4	
Malaria		1		1		1		1		1		1	
Multiple risk factors for atherosclerotic cardiovascular disease	(e.g., older age, smoking, diabetes, hypertension, low HDL, high LDL, or high triglyceride levels)	1		2		2*		3*		2*		3/4*	
Multiple sclerosis	a) With prolonged immobility	1		1		1		2		1		3	
	b) Without prolonged immobility	1		1		1		2		1		1	
Obesity	a) Body mass index (BMI) ≥30 kg/m²	1		1		1		1		1		2	
	b) Menarche to <18 years and BMI ≥ 30 kg/m²	1		1		1		2		1		2	
Ovarian cancer‡		1		1		1		1		1		1	
Parity	a) Nulliparous	2		2		1		1		1		1	
	b) Parous	1		1		1		1		1		1	
Past ectopic pregnancy		1		1		1		1		2		1	
Pelvic inflammatory disease	a) Past												
	i) With subsequent pregnancy	1	1	1	1	1		1		1		1	
	ii) Without subsequent pregnancy	2	2	2	2	1		1		1		1	
	b) Current	4	2*	4	2*	1		1		1		1	
Peripartum cardiomyopathy‡	a) Normal or mildly impaired cardiac function												
	i) <6 months	2		2		1		1		1		4	
	ii) ≥6 months	2		2		1		1		1		3	
	b) Moderately or severely impaired cardiac function	2		2		2		2		2		4	
Postabortion	a) First trimester	1*		1*		1*		1*		1*		1*	
	b) Second trimester	2*		2*		1*		1*		1*		1*	
	c) Immediate postseptic abortion	4		4		1*		1*		1*		1*	
Postpartum (*nonbreastfeeding women*)	a) <21 days					1		1		1		4	
	b) 21 days to 42 days												
	i) With other risk factors for VTE					1		1		1		3*	
	ii) Without other risk factors for VTE					1		1		1		2	
	c) >42 days					1		1		1		1	
Postpartum (*in breastfeeding or non-breastfeeding women, including cesarean delivery*)	a) <10 minutes after delivery of the placenta												
	i) Breastfeeding	1*		2*									
	ii) Nonbreastfeeding	1*		1*									
	b) 10 minutes after delivery of the placenta to <4 weeks	2*		2*									
	c) ≥4 weeks	1*		1*									
	d) Postpartum sepsis	4		4									

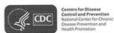

Condition	Sub-Condition	Cu-IUD I	Cu-IUD C	LNG-IUD I	LNG-IUD C	Implant I	Implant C	DMPA I	DMPA C	POP I	POP C	CHC I	CHC C
Pregnancy		4*		4*		NA*		NA*		NA*		NA*	
Rheumatoid arthritis	a) On immunosuppressive therapy	2	1	2	1	1		2/3*		1		2	
	b) Not on immunosuppressive therapy	1		1		1		2		1		2	
Schistosomiasis	a) Uncomplicated	1		1		1		1		1		1	
	b) Fibrosis of the liver[‡]	1		1		1		1		1		1	
Sexually transmitted diseases (STDs)	a) Current purulent cervicitis or chlamydial infection or gonococcal infection	4	2*	4	2*	1		1		1		1	
	b) Vaginitis (including trichomonas vaginalis and bacterial vaginosis)	2	2	2	2	1		1		1		1	
	c) Other factors relating to STDs	2*	2	2*	2	1		1		1		1	
Smoking	a) Age <35	1		1		1		1		1		2	
	b) Age ≥35, <15 cigarettes/day	1		1		1		1		1		3	
	c) Age ≥35, ≥15 cigarettes/day	1		1		1		1		1		4	
Solid organ transplantation[‡]	a) Complicated	3	2	3	2	2		2		2		4	
	b) Uncomplicated	2		2		2		2		2		2*	
Stroke[‡]	History of cerebrovascular accident	1		2		2	3	3		2	3	4	
Superficial venous disorders	a) Varicose veins	1		1		1		1		1		1	
	b) Superficial venous thrombosis (acute or history)	1		1		1		1		1		3*	
Systemic lupus erythematosus[‡]	a) Positive (or unknown) antiphospholipid antibodies	1*	1*	3*		3*		3*	3*	3*		4*	
	b) Severe thrombocytopenia	3*	2*	2*		2*		3*	2*	2*		2*	
	c) Immunosuppressive therapy	2*	1*	2*		2*		2*	2*	2*		2*	
	d) None of the above	1*	1*	2*		2*		2*	2*	2*		2*	
Thyroid disorders	Simple goiter/ hyperthyroid/hypothyroid	1		1		1		1		1		1	
Tuberculosis[‡] (see also Drug Interactions)	a) Nonpelvic	1	1	1	1	1*		1*		1*		1*	
	b) Pelvic	4	3	4	3	1*		1*		1*		1*	
Unexplained vaginal bleeding	(suspicious for serious condition) before evaluation	4*	2*	4*	2*	3*		3*		2*		2*	
Uterine fibroids		2		2		1		1		1		1	
Valvular heart disease	a) Uncomplicated	1		1		1		1		1		2	
	b) Complicated[‡]	1		1		1		1		1		4	
Vaginal bleeding patterns	a) Irregular pattern without heavy bleeding	1		1	1	2		2		2		1	
	b) Heavy or prolonged bleeding	2*		1*	2*	2*		2*		2*		1*	
Viral hepatitis	a) Acute or flare	1		1		1		1		1		3/4*	2
	b) Carrier/Chronic	1		1		1		1		1		1	1
Drug Interactions													
Antiretroviral therapy All other ARV's are 1 or 2 for all methods.	Fosamprenavir (FPV)	1/2*	1*	1/2*	1*	2*		2*		2*		3*	
Anticonvulsant therapy	a) Certain anticonvulsants (phenytoin, carbamazepine, barbiturates, primidone, topiramate, oxcarbazepine)	1		1		2*		1*		3*		3*	
	b) Lamotrigine	1		1		1		1		1		3*	
Antimicrobial therapy	a) Broad spectrum antibiotics	1		1		1		1		1		1	
	b) Antifungals	1		1		1		1		1		1	
	c) Antiparasitics	1		1		1		1		1		1	
	d) Rifampin or rifabutin therapy	1		1		2*		1*		3*		3*	
SSRIs		1		1		1		1		1		1	
St. John's wort		1		1		2		1		2		2	

Updated July 2016. This summary sheet only contains a subset of the recommendations from the U.S. MEC. For complete guidance, see: http://www.cdc.gov/reproductivehealth/unintendedpregnancy/USMEC.htm. Most contraceptive methods do not protect against sexually transmitted diseases (STDs). Consistent and correct use of the male latex condom reduces the risk of STDs and HIV.

CS266008-A

SUMMARY OF CHANGES IN CLASSIFICATIONS FROM WHO MEDICAL ELIGIBILITY CRITERIA FOR CONTRACEPTIVE USE, 4TH EDITION[a,b]

Condition	COC/P/R	POP	DMPA	Implants	LNG-IUD	Cu-IUD	Clarification
Breast-feeding							The US Department of Health and Human Services recommends that infants be exclusively breast-fed during the first 4–6 mo of life, preferably for a full 6 mo. Ideally, breast-feeding should continue through the first year of life (1). {Not included in WHO MEC}
a. <1 mo postpartum {WHO: <6 wk postpartum}	3[b] {4}	2[b] {3}	2[b] {3}	2[b] {3}			
b. 21 mo to <6 mo {WHO: ≥6 wk to <6 mo postpartum}	2[b] {3}						
Postpartum (in breast-feeding or non-breast-feeding women), including postcesarean section							
a. <10 min after delivery of the placenta {WHO: <48 h, including insertion immediately after delivery of the placenta}					2 {1 if not breast-feeding and 3 if breast-feeding}	2 {3}	
b. 10 min after delivery of the placenta to <4 wk {WHO: ≥48 h to <4 wk}					2 {3}		

SUMMARY OF CHANGES IN CLASSIFICATIONS FROM WHO MEDICAL ELIGIBILITY CRITERIA FOR CONTRACEPTIVE USE, 4TH EDITION[a,b]

Condition	COC/P/R	POP	DMPA	Implants	LNG-IUD	Cu-IUD	Clarification
Deep venous thrombosis (DVT)/pulmonary embolism (PE)							Women on anticoagulant therapy are at risk for gynecologic complications of therapy such as hemorrhagic ovarian cysts and severe menorrhagia. Hormonal contraceptive methods can be of benefit in preventing or treating these complications. When a contraceptive method is used as a therapy, rather than solely to prevent pregnancy, the risk/benefit ratio may be different and should be considered on a case-by-case basis. {Not included in WHO MEC}
a. History of DVT/PE, not on anticoagulant therapy							
i. Lower risk for recurrent DVT/PE (no risk factors)	3 {4}						
b. Acute DVT/PE		2 {3}	2 {3}	2 {3}	2 {3}	2 {1}	
c. DVT/PE and established on anticoagulant therapy for at least 3 mo							
i. Higher risk for recurrent DVT/PE (≥1 risk factors)						2 {1}	
• Known thrombophilia, including antiphospholipid syndrome							
• Active cancer (metastatic, on therapy, or within 6 mo after clinical remission), excluding nonmelanoma skin cancer							
• History of recurrent DVT/PE	3[b] {4}						
ii. Lower risk for recurrent DVT/PE (no risk factors)						2 {1}	

SUMMARY OF CHANGES IN CLASSIFICATIONS FROM WHO MEDICAL ELIGIBILITY CRITERIA FOR CONTRACEPTIVE USE, 4TH EDITION[a,b]

Condition	COC/P/R	POP	DMPA	Implants	LNG-IUD	Cu-IUD	Clarification
Valvular heart disease							
a. Complicated (pulmonary hypertension, risk for atrial fibrillation, history of subacute bacterial endocarditis)						1 {2}	1 {2}
Ovarian cancer[c]						1 {Initiation = 3, Continuation = 2}	1 {Initiation = 3, Continuation = 2}
Uterine fibroids						2 {1 if no uterine distortion and 4 if uterine distortion is present}	2 {1 if no uterine distortion and 4 if uterine distortion is present}

COC, combined oral contraceptive; Cu-IUD, copper intrauterine device; DMPA, depot medroxyprogesterone acetate; DVT, deep venous thrombosis; LNG-IUD, levonorgestrel-releasing intrauterine device; P, combined hormonal contraceptive patch; PE, pulmonary embolism; POP, progestin-only pill; R, combined hormonal vaginal ring; VTE, venous thromboembolism; WHO, World Health Organization.

[a]For conditions for which classification changed for ≥1 methods or the condition description underwent a major modification, WHO conditions and recommendations appear in curly brackets.

[b]Consult the clarification column for this classification.

[c]Condition that exposes a woman to increased risk as a result of unintended pregnancy.

SUMMARY OF RECOMMENDATIONS FOR MEDICAL CONDITIONS ADDED TO THE US MEDICAL ELIGIBILITY CRITERIA FOR CONTRACEPTIVE USE

Condition	COC/P/R	POP	DMPA	Implants	LNG-IUD	Cu-IUD	Clarification
History of bariatric surgery[a]							
a. Restrictive procedures: decrease storage capacity of the stomach (vertical banded gastroplasty, laparoscopic adjustable gastric band, laparoscopic sleeve gastrectomy)	1	1	1	1	1	1	
b. Malabsorptive procedures: decrease absorption of nutrients and calories by shortening the functional length of the small intestine (Roux-en-Y gastric bypass, biliopancreatic diversion)	COCs: 3 P/R: 1	3	1	1	1	1	

SUMMARY OF RECOMMENDATIONS FOR MEDICAL CONDITIONS ADDED TO THE US MEDICAL ELIGIBILITY CRITERIA FOR CONTRACEPTIVE USE

Condition	COC/P/R	POP	DMPA	Implants	LNG-IUD	Cu-IUD	Clarification
Peripartum cardiomyopathy[b]							
a. Normal or mildly impaired cardiac function (New York Heart Association Functional Class I or II: patients with no limitation of activities or patients with slight, mild limitation of activity) (2)							
i. <6 mo	4	1	1	1	2	2	
ii. ≥6 mo	3	1	1	1	2	2	
b. Moderately or severely impaired cardiac function (New York Heart Association Functional Class III or IV: patients with marked limitation of activity or patients who should be at complete rest) (2)	4	2	2	2	2	2	

SUMMARY OF RECOMMENDATIONS FOR MEDICAL CONDITIONS ADDED TO THE US MEDICAL ELIGIBILITY CRITERIA FOR CONTRACEPTIVE USE *(Continued)*

Condition	COC/P/R	POP	DMPA	Implants	LNG-IUD Initiation	LNG-IUD Continuation	Cu-IUD Initiation	Cu-IUD Continuation	Clarification
Rheumatoid arthritis									
a. On immunosuppressive therapy	2	1	2/3c	1	2	1	2	1	DMPA use among women on long-term corticosteroid therapy with a history of, or risk factors for, nontraumatic fractures is classified as Category 3. Otherwise, DMPA use for women with rheumatoid arthritis is classified as Category 2.
b. Not on immunosuppressive therapy	2	1	2	1	1			1	
Endometrial hyperplasia	1	1	1	1	1		1		
Inflammatory bowel disease (IBD) (ulcerative colitis, Crohn's disease)	2/3c	2	2	1	1		1		For women with mild IBD, with no other risk factors for VTE, the benefits of COC/P/R use generally outweigh the risks (Category 2). However, for women with IBD with increased risk for VTE (eg, those with active or extensive disease, surgery, immobilization, corticosteroid use, vitamin deficiencies, fluid depletion), the risks for COC/P/R use generally outweigh the benefits (Category 3).

SUMMARY OF RECOMMENDATIONS FOR MEDICAL CONDITIONS ADDED TO THE US MEDICAL ELIGIBILITY CRITERIA FOR CONTRACEPTIVE USE

Condition	COC/P/R	POP	DMPA	Implants	LNG-IUD Initiation	LNG-IUD Continuation	Cu-IUD Initiation	Cu-IUD Continuation	Clarification
Solid organ transplantation[a]									
a. Complicated: graft failure (acute or chronic), rejection, cardiac allograft vasculopathy	4	2	2	2	3	2	3	2	
b. Uncomplicated	2[d]	2	2	2	2		2		Women with Budd–Chiari syndrome should not use COC/P/R because of the increased risk for thrombosis.

COC, combined oral contraceptive; Cu-IUD, copper intrauterine device; DMPA, depot medroxyprogesterone acetate; IBD, inflammatory bowel disease; LNG-IUD, levonorgestrel-releasing intrauterine device; P, combined hormonal contraceptive patch; POP, progestin-only pill; R, combined hormonal vaginal ring; VTE, venous thromboembolism.

[a]History of bariatric surgery. *Contraception.* 2010;82(1):86-94.

[b]Condition that exposes a woman to increased risk as a result of unintended pregnancy.

[c]Consult the clarification column for this classification.

[d]History of solid organ transplantation. *Transplantation.* 2013;95(10):1183-1186.

Comments

1. No clinician examination or pregnancy testing is necessary before provision or prescription of emergency contraception.
2. The copper intrauterine device (IUD) is appropriate for use as emergency contraception for women who desire long-acting contraception.
3. Information regarding effective long-term contraceptive methods should be made available whenever a woman requests emergency contraception.

SUMMARY OF ADDITIONAL CHANGES TO THE US MEDICAL ELIGIBILITY CRITERIA FOR CONTRACEPTIVE USE	
Condition/ Contraceptive Method	**Change**
Emergency contraceptive pills	History of bariatric surgery, rheumatoid arthritis, inflammatory bowel disease, and solid organ transplantation was given a Category 1.
Barrier methods	For six conditions—history of bariatric surgery, peripartum cardiomyopathy, rheumatoid arthritis, endometrial hyperplasia, IBD, and solid organ transplantation—the barrier methods are classified as Category 1.
Sterilization	In general, no medical conditions would absolutely restrict a person's eligibility for sterilization. Recommendations from the WHO Medical Eligibility criteria for contraceptive use about specific settings and surgical procedures for sterilization are not included here. The guidance has been replaced with general text on sterilization.
Other deleted items	Guidance for combined injectables, levonorgestrel implants, and norethisterone enanthate has been removed because these methods are not currently available in the United States. Guidance for "blood pressure measurement unavailable" and "history of hypertension, where blood pressure *cannot* be evaluated (including hypertension in pregnancy)" has been removed.
Unintended pregnancy and increased health risk	The following conditions have been added to the WHO list of conditions that expose a woman to increased risk as a result of unintended pregnancy: history of bariatric surgery within the past 2 y, peripartum cardiomyopathy, and receiving a solid organ transplant within 2 y.

4. Ulipristal acetate is more effective than levonorgestrel-only regimen and maintains its efficacy for up to 5 days.
5. The levonorgestrel-only regimen is more effective than combined hormonal regimen and is associated with less nausea and vomiting compared with the combined estrogen–progestin regimen.
6. Insertion of copper IUD is the most effective method of emergency contraception.

DELIVERY: TRIAL OF LABOR AFTER CESAREAN (TOLAC)

Population
–Pregnant women with history of one previous cesarean delivery with a low-transverse incision.

Recommendations
–Most women with one previous cesarean delivery and a low-transverse incision should be counseled about and offered TOLAC.
–In patients who have had a cesarean delivery or major uterine surgery, misoprostol should not be used for cervical ripening.
–Epidural analgesia may be used as a part of TOLAC during labor.

Source
–ACOG Practice Bulletin No. 205: Vaginal birth after cesarean delivery. *Obstet Gynecol.* 2019;133(2):e110-e127.

Comment
1. The benefits of a vaginal birth after cesarean (VBAC) include avoiding major abdominal surgery, lower rates of hemorrhage, thromboembolism, infection, and a shorter recovery period. VBAC may also decrease maternal risks associated with cesarean sections, including hysterectomy, bowel/bladder injury, and future abnormal placentation.

DELIVERY: VAGINAL LACERATIONS

Population
–Women delivering vaginally.

Recommendations
–Insufficient evidence to recommend specific mode of manual perineal support at delivery:
  • Consider applying warm perineal compresses during pushing to help reduce incidence of third-degree and fourth-degree lacerations.

- There is insufficient evidence to definitively recommend perineal massage during the second stage of labor, though some studies indicate a reduction in third-degree and fourth-degree lacerations.
- Restrictive episiotomy[a] use is recommended over routine episiotomy.
- For full-thickness external anal sphincter lacerations, either end-to-end repair or overlap repair is acceptable. There is limited data to support a single dose of antibiotic at the time of anal sphincter repair.

Source
  –ACOG Practice Bulletin No. 198: Prevention and management of obstetric lacerations at vaginal delivery. *Obstet Gynecol.* 2018;132(3):e87-e102.

ECTOPIC PREGNANCY

Population
  –Pregnant women.

Recommendations
▶ NICE 2012
  –Recommended evaluation for stable women with an early pregnancy.
- Transvaginal ultrasound (TVUS) with a crown-rump length ≥7 mm but no cardiac activity.
  ○ Repeat ultrasound in 7 d.
  ○ Quantitative beta-hCG q48h × 2 levels.
- TVUS with gestational sac ≥25 mm and no fetal pole.
  ○ Repeat ultrasound in 7 d.
  ○ Quantitative beta-hCG q48h × 2 levels.

  –Management of ectopic pregnancies.
- Differentiating early intrauterine pregnancy loss from ectopic pregnancy:
  ○ Uterine aspiration to identify presence of chorionic villi (indicate intrauterine pregnancy).
  ○ If chorionic villi not confirmed, monitor hCG levels:
    . Take first level 12–24 h after aspiration.
    . Plateau/increase in hCG suggests incomplete evacuation or nonvisualized ectopic warranting further treatment.

---

[a]Restrictive episiotomy denotes episiotomies performed in high-risk cases only, eg, shoulder dystocia, vaginal breech, instrumental deliveries.

- Decrease in hCG suggests failed intrauterine pregnancy; monitor with serial hCG measurements.
- Methotrexate candidates[b].
  - No significant pain.
  - Adnexal mass <3.5 cm.
  - No cardiac activity on TVUS.
  - Beta-hCG <5000 IU/L.
  - Dose is 50 mg/m² IM.
- Laparoscopy if:
  - Unstable patient.
  - Severe pain.
  - Adnexal mass >3.5 cm.
  - Cardiac activity seen.
  - Beta-hCG >5000 IU/L.
- Rhogam 250 IU to all Rh-negative women who undergo surgery for an ectopic.

Sources
- –www.guidelines.gov/content.aspx?id=39274
- –Practice Bulletin No. 191: Tubal ectopic pregnancy. *Obstet Gynecol.* 2017. doi: 10.1097/AOG.0000000000002464

Comments

1. Ectopic pregnancy can present with:
   a. Abdominal or pelvic pain.
   b. Vaginal bleeding.
   c. Amenorrhea.
   d. Breast tenderness.
   e. GI symptoms.
   f. Dizziness.
   g. Urinary symptoms.
   h. Rectal pressure.
   i. Dyschezia.
2. Most normal intrauterine pregnancies will show an increase in beta-hCG level by at least 63% in 48 h.
3. Intrauterine pregnancies are usually apparent by TVUS if beta-hCG >1500 IU/L.

---

[b]Contraindications to methotrexate use include renal or hepatic disease, bone marrow dysfunction, active gastrointestinal or respiratory disease. Asthma is not a contraindication.

DIABETES MELLITUS, GESTATIONAL (GDM)

Population
–Pregnant women.

Recommendations

▶ ACOG 2018

- –Treat all women with gestational diabetes with nutrition therapy and exercise.
- –For pharmacologic therapy of GDM, insulin is preferred (start at 0.7–1.0 U/kg/d); metformin may be a reasonable alternative.
- –Counsel women with GDM and estimated fetal weight of 4500 g or more regarding the option of scheduled cesarean delivery vs. vaginal trial of labor.
- –Instruct women with GDM to follow fasting and 1-h postprandial glucose levels. Target fasting blood glucose of 95 mg/dL and 1-h postprandial of 140 mg/dL.
- –Start antepartum fetal testing at 32-wk gestational age in women with GDM requiring medication or under poor control and without other comorbidities. Consider starting surveillance earlier if other comorbidities are present.
- –Unless otherwise indicated, do not induce women with GDM who are well-controlled by diet and exercise (A1GDM) before 39 wk. Expectant management until 40-6/7 wk is appropriate; antepartum fetal testing may not be necessary unless other comorbidities are present.
- –Screen all women with GDM with a 75-g 2-h GTT 4–12 wk after delivery.

Source

- –https://www.scribd.com/document/371228843/190-Gestational-Diabetes-Mellitus-Agog

HUMAN IMMUNODEFICIENCY VIRUS (HIV), PREGNANCY

Population
–Pregnant women.

Recommendations

▶ AAFP 2010, USPSTF 2013, ACOG 2015, CDC 2015

- –Clinicians should screen all pregnant women for HIV as early as possible during each pregnancy using opt-out approach.

–Repeat HIV testing in 3rd trimester for women in areas with high HIV incidence or prevalence.

–Women who were not tested earlier in pregnancy or whose HIV is undocumented should be offered rapid screening. If rapid HIV test result in labor is reactive, antiretroviral prophylaxis should be immediately initiated while waiting for supplemental test results.

Sources

–AAFP. *Clinical Recommendation: HIV Infection, Adolescents and Adults.* 2013.

–USPSTF. *HIV Infection: Screening.* 2013.

–CDC. *Sexually Transmitted Diseases Treatment Guidelines.* 2015.

–*Obstet Gynecol.* 2015;125:1544-1547.

Population

–HIV-infected pregnant women.

Recommendations

–Recommends combination ART regimens during the antepartum period.

–Women who were taking ART prior to conception should have their regimen reviewed (ie, teratogenic potential of drugs), but continue combination ART throughout the pregnancy.

–Initial prenatal labs should include a CD4 count, HIV viral load, and HCV antibody.

  • If HIV RNA is detectable (>500–1000 copies/mL), perform HIV genotypic resistance testing to help guide antepartum therapy.

–Women who do not require ART for their own health should initiate combination ART between 14 and 28 gestational weeks and continue until delivery.

  • Zidovudine should be a component of the regimen when feasible.

  • Recommend against single-dose intrapartum/newborn nevirapine in addition to antepartum ART.

–Antepartum monitoring:

  • Monitor CD4 count every 3 mo.

  • HIV viral load should be assessed 2–4 wk after initiating or changing ART, monthly until undetectable, and then at 34–36 wk.

  • Recommend a first-trimester ultrasound to confirm dating.

  • Screen for gestational diabetes at 24–28 wk.

–Scheduled cesarean delivery is recommended for HIV-infected women who have HIV RNA levels >1000 copies/mL and intact membranes near term.

–Intrapartum IV zidovudine is recommended for all HIV-infected pregnant women.

–Avoid artificial rupture of membranes.

–Avoid routine use of fetal scalp electrodes.

–Breast-feeding is not recommended.

Source
–http://www.guideline.gov/content.aspx?id=38253

Comments
1. Avoid Methergine for postpartum hemorrhage in women receiving a protease inhibitor or efavirenz.
2. If women do not receive antepartum/intrapartum ART prophylaxis, infants should receive zidovudine for 6 wk.
3. Infants born to HIV-infected women should have an HIV viral load checked at 14 d, at 1–2 mo, and at 4–6 mo.

HYPERTENSION, CHRONIC IN PREGNANCY

Population
–Pregnant women with hypertension diagnosed or present before pregnancy or before 20 wk of gestation.

Recommendations
–Obtain baseline evaluation of LFTs, serum creatinine, serum electrolytes, BUN, CBC, spot urine protein/creatinine ratio or 24-h urine for total protein and creatinine, EKG should be done upon entry to prenatal care or prior to conception.

–Evaluating chronic hypertension in the beginning of pregnancy can help differentiate transient blood pressure increases in chronic hypertension from superimposed preeclampsia later on in pregnancy.

–In cases of diagnostic uncertainty between chronic HTN and superimposed preeclampsia, admit patient for inpatient surveillance with assessment of hematocrit, platelets, creatinine, LFTs, and new-onset proteinuria.

–In chronic hypertension with preexisting end organ damage and renal disease, superimposed preeclampsia may be impossible to differentiate later in pregnancy.

–Initiate low-dose aspirin (81 mg) between 12 and 28 wk of gestation and continue through delivery.

–Consider initiation of antihypertensive medications when SBP >160 mm Hg or DBP >110 mm Hg.

–For long-term treatment of pregnant women requiring antihypertension medications, use labetalol and nifedipine as first line.

–There is no clear optimal delivery date for women with chronic hypertension. For women with chronic hypertension but no complicating factors, do not deliver before 38 0/7 wk of gestation. For women requiring antihypertension maintenance medications, do not deliver before 37 0/7 wk unless there are additional maternal or fetal complications. For women with difficult to control blood pressures or other complicating factors, consider earlier delivery on a case-by-case basis.

–For women who develop superimposed preeclampsia with severe features, do not employ expectant management past 34 0/7 wk.

Source

–ACOG Practice Bulletin No. 203: Chronic hypertension in pregnancy. *Obstet Gynecol.* 2019;133(1):e26-e50.

Comments

1. Risks of chronic hypertension in pregnancy include maternal death, stroke, pulmonary edema, renal insufficiency/failure, myocardial infarction, preeclampsia, placental abruption, GDM, postpartum hemorrhage, cesarean delivery.

2. Risks of chronic hypertension in pregnancy also include stillbirth/perinatal death, growth restriction, preterm birth, congenital anomalies.

PREGNANCY, POSTPARTUM HEMORRHAGE (PPH)

Population

–Pregnant women.

Recommendations

▶ WHO 2012, ACOG 2017

–Uterotonics for the treatment of PPH.
- Intravenous oxytocin is the recommended agent.
- Alternative uterotonics:
  ◦ Misoprostol 800 μg sublingual.
  ◦ Methylergonovine 0.2 mg IM.
  ◦ Carboprost 0.25 mg IM.

–Additional interventions for PPH.
- Isotonic crystalloid resuscitation.
- Bimanual uterine massage.

–Therapeutic options for persistent PPH.
- Tranexamic acid is recommended for persistent PPH refractory to oxytocin.

- Uterine artery embolization.
- Balloon tamponade.

–Therapeutic options for a retained placenta.

- Controlled cord traction with oxytocin 10 IU IM/IV.
- Manual removal of placenta.
  ◦ Give single dose of first-generation antibiotic for prophylaxis against endometritis.
- Recommend against methylergonovine, misoprostol, or carboprost (Hemabate) for retained placenta.

Sources

–*Obstet Gynecol*. 2017;130:e168-e186.

–http://www.guidelines.gov/content.aspx?id=39383

Comment

1. Misoprostol 800–1000 µg can also be administered as a rectal suppository for PPH related to uterine atony.

PREMATURE RUPTURE OF MEMBRANES

Population

–Pregnant women.

Recommendations

▶ ACOG 2018, Cochrane Database of Systematic Reviews 2013

–Diagnose PROM based on history and physical exam. Per ACOG, digital examinations should be avoided unless patient appears to be in active labor or delivery seems imminent. Prefer sterile speculum exam.

–In all patients with PROM, initial period of electronic fetal heart monitoring and uterine activity monitoring should be done. Nonreassuring fetal status and clinical chorioamnionitis are indications for delivery.

–Women with preterm premature rupture of membranes before 24 gestational weeks at risk for imminent delivery:

- Expectant management or induction of labor.
- Antibiotics may be considered.
- GBS prophylaxis is not recommended before viability.
- Tocolysis is not recommended before viability.
- Magnesium sulfate for neuroprotection is not recommended before viability.

–Women with preterm premature rupture of membranes before 34 gestational weeks at risk for imminent delivery should be considered for intravenous magnesium sulfate treatment for its fetal neuroprotective effect.

- Can trial expectant management.
- Antibiotics are recommended to prolong latency if there are no contraindications.
- Single course of corticosteroids is recommended between 24 0/7 weeks and 34 0/7 wk gestation.
- Therapeutic tocolysis is not recommended as it has not been shown to prolong latency or improve neonatal outcomes.

–For women with premature rupture of membranes at 37 gestational weeks or more, labor should be induced if spontaneous labor does not occur near the time of presentation.

- Induction of labor with prostaglandins has been shown to be equally effective for labor induction compared with oxytocin but was associated with higher rates of chorioamnionitis.
- GBS prophylaxis as indicated.

–At 34 gestational weeks or greater, delivery is recommended for all women with ruptured membranes.

–Not enough evidence to show that removal of cerclage after preterm PROM diagnosis has been made. If cerclage remains in place with preterm PROM, prolonged antibiotics prophylaxis beyond 7 days is not recommended.

–Outpatient management of preterm premature rupture of membranes is not recommended.

Sources

–*Obstet Gynecol.* 2018;131:e1-e14.

–http://www.cochrane.org/CD001058/PREG_antibiotics-for-preterm-rupture-of-membranes

Comment

1. Twenty-two studies involving over 6800 pregnant women with PROM prior to 37 gestational weeks were analyzed. Routine antibiotics decreased the incidence of chorioamnionitis (RR 0.66), prolonged pregnancy by at least 7 d (RR 0.79), and decreased neonatal infection (RR 0.67), but had no effect on perinatal mortality compared with placebo.

PRETERM LABOR

Population
–Pregnant women.

Recommendations

▶ ACOG 2016, Cochrane Database of Systematic Reviews 2013

–Utility of fetal fibronectin testing and/or the cervical length measurement can improve clinical ability to diagnose preterm labor and predict preterm birth in symptomatic women, but the positive predictive value of these tests is poor and should not be used exclusively to direct management in a setting of acute symptoms.

–Single dose of corticosteroids for pregnant women between 24 and 34 gestational weeks or women with ROM or multiple gestations who may deliver within 7 d.

  • Consider single course of corticosteroids at 23 wk gestation for pregnant women who are at risk of delivery within 7 d.
  • Betamethasone or Dexamethasone IM are most widely studied corticosteroids.

–Magnesium sulfate for possible preterm delivery prior to 32 wk for neuroprotection.

  • Indomethacin is a potential option for use in conjunction with magnesium sulfate.

–Tocolytic options for up to 48 h. Upper limit for use of tocolytic agents to prevent preterm birth is 34 wk gestation. Do not recommend maintenance therapy.

  • Beta-agonists.
  • Nifedipine.
  • Indomethacin.

–Women with preterm contractions without cervical change, especially if <2 cm, should not be treated with tocolytics.

–No role for antibiotics in preterm labor and intact membranes.

–Bedrest and hydration have not been shown to prevent preterm birth and should not be routinely recommended.

Sources
–*Obstet Gynecol.* 2016;128:e155-e164.
–http://www.cochrane.org/CD003096/PREG_hydration-for-treatment-of-preterm-labour

Comments
1. Magnesium sulfate administered prior to 32 wk reduces the severity and risk of cerebral palsy.

2. Cochrane analysis found no difference in the incidence of preterm delivery comparing hydration and bedrest with bedrest alone.

PREGNANCY, PRETERM LABOR, TOCOLYSIS

Population
–Pregnant women in preterm labor.

Recommendation

▶ ACOG 2016

–Tocolytic options for up to 48 h. Upper limit for use of tocolytic agents to prevent preterm birth is 34 wk gestation. Do not recommend maintenance therapy.
- Beta-agonists.
- Nifedipine.
- Indomethacin.

Source
–*Obstet Gynecol.* 2016;128:e155-e164.

ROUTINE PRENATAL CARE

ROUTINE PRENATAL CARE

Preconception Visit
1. Measure height, weight, blood pressure, and total and HDL cholesterol.
2. Determine rubella, rubeola, and varicella immunity status.
3. Assess all patients for pregnancy risk: substance abuse, domestic violence, sexual abuse, psychiatric disorders, risk factors for preterm labor, exposure to chemicals or infectious agents, hereditary disorders, gestational diabetes, or chronic medical problems.
4. Educate patients about proper nutrition; offer weight reduction strategies for obese patients.
5. Immunize if not current on the following: Tdap (combined tetanus, diphtheria, and pertussis vaccine), MMR (measles, mumps, rubella), varicella, or hepatitis B vaccine.
6. Initiate folic acid 400–800 μg/d; 4 mg/d for a history of a child affected by a neural tube defect.

Initial Prenatal Visit
1. Medical, surgical, social, family, and obstetrical history, and do complete examination.
2. Pap smear, urine NAAT for gonorrhea and *Chlamydia*, and assess for history of genital herpes.
3. Consider a varicella antibody test if the patient unsure about prior varicella infection.
4. Urinalysis for proteinuria and glucosuria, and urine culture for asymptomatic bacteriuria (between 11 and 16 wk gestation).

5. Order prenatal labs to include a complete blood count, blood type, antibody screen, rubella titer, VDRL, hepatitis B surface antigen, and an HIV test.
6. Order an obstetrical ultrasound for dating if any of the following: beyond 16-wk gestational age, unsure of last menstrual period, size/date discrepancy on examination, or for inability to hear fetal heart tones by 12 gestational weeks.
7. Discuss fetal aneuploidy screening and counseling regardless of maternal age.
8. Prenatal testing offered for sickle cell anemia (African descent), thalassemia (African, Mediterranean, Middle Eastern, Southeast Asians), Canavan disease and Tay-Sachs (Jewish patients), cystic fibrosis (whites and Ashkenazi Jews), and fragile X syndrome (family history of nonspecified mental retardation).
9. Place a tuberculosis skin test for all medium- to high-risk patients.[a]
10. Consider a 1-h 50-g glucose tolerance test for certain high-risk groups.[b]
11. Obtain an operative report in all women who have had a prior cesarean section.
12. Psychosocial risk assessment for mood disorders, substance abuse, or domestic violence.

Frequency of Visits for Uncomplicated Pregnancies
1. Every 4 wk until 28 gestational weeks; q 2 wk from 28 to 36 wk; weekly >36 wk.
2. It is standard of care in most US communities to offer a single ultrasound examination at 18–20 wk gestation, even if dating confirmation not needed. There is no evidence to support routine ultrasonography in uncomplicated pregnancies.

Routine Checks at Follow-up Prenatal Visits
1. Assess weight, blood pressure, and urine for glucose and protein.
2. Exam: edema, fundal height, and fetal heart tones at all visits; fetal presentation starting at 36 wk.
3. Ask about regular uterine contractions, leakage of fluid, vaginal bleeding, or decreased fetal movement.
4. Discuss labor precautions.

Antepartum Lab Testing
1. All women should be offered first trimester, second trimester, or combined testing to screen for fetal aneuploidy; invasive diagnostic testing for fetal aneuploidy should be available to all women regardless of maternal age.
   a. First trimester.
   b. Second trimester screening options: amniocentesis at 14 wk; a Quad Marker Screen at 16–18 wk; and/or a screening ultrasound with nuchal translucency assessment.
2. Consider serial transvaginal sonography of the cervix every 2–3 wk to assess cervical length for patients at high risk for preterm delivery starting at 16 wk.
3. No role for routine bacterial vaginosis screening.
4. 1-h 50-g glucose tolerance test in all women between 24 and 28 wk.
5. Rectovaginal swab for group B streptococcal (GBS) testing between 35 and 37 wk.
6. Recommend weekly amniotic fluid assessments and twice weekly nonstress testing starting at 41 wk.

Prenatal Counseling

1. Cessation of smoking, drinking alcohol, or use of any illicit drugs.
2. Avoid cat litter boxes, hot tubs, certain foods (ie, raw fish or unpasteurized cheese).
3. Proper nutrition and expected weight gain: National Academy of Sciences advises weight gain 28–40 lb (prepregnancy BMI <20), 25–35 lb (BMI 20–26), 15–25 lb (BMI 26–29), and 15–20 lb (BMI ≥30).
4. Inquire about domestic violence and depression at initial visit, at 28 wk, and at postpartum visit.
5. Recommend regular mild-to-moderate exercise 3 or more times a week.
6. Avoid high-altitude activities, scuba diving, and contact sports during pregnancy.
7. Benefits of breast-feeding vs. bottle-feeding.
8. Discuss postpartum contraceptive options (including tubal sterilization) during third trimester.
9. Discuss analgesia and anesthesia options and offer prenatal classes at 24 wk.
10. Discuss repeat C-section vs. vaginal birth after cesarean (if applicable).
11. Discuss the option of circumcision if a boy is delivered.
12. Avoid air travel and long train or car trips beyond 36 wk.

Prenatal Interventions

1. Suppressive antiviral medications starting at 36 wk for women with a history of genital herpes.
2. Cesarean delivery is indicated for women who are HIV positive or have active genital herpes and are in labor.
3. For patients who report a history of abuse, offer interventions and resources to increase their safety during and after pregnancy.
4. For patients with severe depression, consider treatment with an SSRI (avoid paroxetine if possible).
5. Rh immune globulin 300 μg IM for all Rh-negative women with negative antibody screens between 26 and 28 wk.
6. Refer for nutrition counseling at 10–12 wk for BMI <20 kg/m^2 or at any time during pregnancy for inadequate weight gain.

7. Start prenatal vitamins with iron and folic acid 400–800 µg/d and 1200 mg elemental calcium/d starting at 4 wk preconception (or as early as possible during pregnancy) and continued until 6 wk postpartum.
8. Give inactivated influenza vaccine IM to all pregnant women during influenza season.
9. Give Tdap vaccine during each pregnancy between 27 and 36 wk gestation.
10. Consider progesterone therapy IM weekly or intravaginally daily to women at high risk for preterm birth.
11. Recommend an external cephalic version at 37 wk for all noncephalic presentations.
12. Offer labor induction to women at 41 wk by good dates.
13. Treat all women with confirmed syphilis with penicillin G during pregnancy.
14. Treat all women with gonorrhea with ceftriaxone; follow treatment with a test of cure.
15. Treat all women with *Chlamydia* with azithromycin; follow treatment with a test of cure.
16. Treat all GBS-positive women with penicillin G when in labor or with spontaneous rupture of membranes.

Postpartum Interventions

1. Treat all infants born to HBV-positive women with hepatitis B immunoglobulin (HBIG) and initiate HBV vaccine series within 12 h of life.
2. All women with a positive tuberculosis skin test and no evidence of active disease should receive a postpartum chest x-ray; treat with isoniazid 300 mg PO daily for 9 mo if chest x-ray is negative.
3. Administer a Tdap booster if tetanus status is unknown or the last Td (tetanus-diphtheria) vaccine was >10 y ago.
4. Administer an MMR vaccine to all rubella nonimmune women.
5. Offer HPV vaccine to all women ≤26 wk who have not been immunized.
6. Initiate contraception.
7. Repeat Pap smear at 6-wk postpartum check.

---

[a]Postgastrectomy, gastric bypass, immunosuppressed (HIV-positive, diabetes, renal failure, chronic steroid/immunosuppressive therapy, head/neck or hematologic malignancies), silicosis, organ transplant recipients, malabsorptive syndromes, alcoholics, intravenous drug users, close contacts of persons with active pulmonary tuberculosis, medically underserved, low socioeconomic class, residents/employees of long-term care facilities and jails, health care workers, and immigrants from endemic areas.
[b]Overweight (BMI ≥25 kg/m²) and an additional risk factor: physical inactivity; first-degree relative with DM; high-risk ethnicity (eg, African American, Latino, Native American, Asian American, Pacific Islander); history of gestational diabetes mellitus (GDM); prior baby with birthweight >9 lb; unexplained stillbirth or malformed infant; HTN on therapy or with BP ≥140/90 mm Hg; HDL cholesterol level <35 mg/dL (0.90 mmol/L) and/or a triglyceride level >250 mg/dL (2.82 mmol/L); polycystic ovary syndrome; history of impaired glucose tolerance or HgbA1c ≥5.7%; acanthosis nigricans; cardiovascular disease; or ≥2+ glucosuria.
Source: Adapted from ACOG ICSI Guideline on Routine Prenatal Care, July 2010. (http://www.icsi.org/prenatal_care_4/prenatal_care_routine_full_version_2.html) *Am Fam Physician.* 2014;89(3):199-208.

AAP AND AFP PERINATAL AND POSTNATAL GUIDELINES	
Breast-feeding	Strongly recommends education and counseling to promote breast-feeding.
Hemoglobinopathies	Strongly recommends ordering screening tests for hemoglobinopathies in neonates.
Hyperbilirubinemia	Perform ongoing systematic assessments during the neonatal period for the risk of an infant developing severe hyperbilirubinemia.
Phenylketonuria	Strongly recommends ordering screening tests for phenylketonuria in neonates.
Thyroid function abnormalities	Strongly recommends ordering screening tests for thyroid function abnormalities in neonates.

Sources: Pediatrics. 2004;114:297-316. *Pediatrics.* 2005;115:496-506.

THYROID DISEASE, PREGNANCY AND POSTPARTUM

Population
–Women during and immediately after pregnancy.

Recommendations
▶ ATA 2011, ATA 2017

–Hypothyroidism in pregnancy is defined as:
- An elevated TSH (>2.5 mIU/L) and a suppressed free thyroxine (FT_4).
- TSH ≥10 mIU/L (irrespective of FT_4).
- Subclinical hypothyroidism is defined as a TSH (2.5–9.9 mIU/L) and a normal FT_4.

–Insufficient evidence to support treatment of subclinical hypothyroidism in pregnancy.

–Goal therapy is to normalize TSH levels.

–PTU is the preferred antithyroid drug (ATD) in pregnancy.

–Monitor TSH levels every 4 wk when treating thyroid disease in pregnancy.

–Measure a TSH receptor antibody level at 20–24 wk for any history of Graves' disease (GD).

–All pregnant and lactating women should ingest at least 250-μg iodine daily.

–All pregnant women with thyroid nodules should undergo thyroid ultrasound and TSH testing.

–Patients found to have thyroid cancer during pregnancy would ideally undergo surgery during second trimester.

–Transient hCG-mediated TSH suppression in early pregnancy should not be treated with ATD therapy.

–GD during pregnancy should be treated with the lowest possible dose of ATD needed to keep the mother's thyroid hormone levels at or slightly above the reference range for total T4 and T3 values in pregnancy (1.5 times above nonpregnant reference ranges in the second and third trimesters), and the TSH below the reference range for pregnancy.

–Pregnancy is a relative contraindication to thyroidectomy and should only be used when medical management has been unsuccessful or ATDs cannot be used.

Sources

–2016 American Thyroid Association guidelines for diagnosis and management of hyperthyroidism and other causes of thyrotoxicosis. *Thyroid.* 2016;26(10):1343-1421.

–2017 Guidelines of the American Thyroid Association for the diagnosis and management of thyroid disease during pregnancy and the postpartum. *Thyroid.* 2017;27(3):315-390.

–http://thyroidguidelines.net/sites/thyroidguidelines.net/files/file/thy.2011.0087.pdf

Comment

1. Surgery for well-differentiated thyroid carcinoma can often be deferred until postpartum period.

Pulmonary Disorders

37

APNEA, CENTRAL SLEEP (CSAS)

Population
–Adults.

Recommendations
▶ American Academy of Sleep Medicine 2012

–**Primary CSAS**
- Use positive airway pressure therapy.
- Limited evidence to support the use of acetazolamide for CSAS.
- Consider zolpidem or triazolam if patients are not at high risk for respiratory depression.

–**CSAS related to CHF**
- Nocturnal oxygen therapy.
- CPAP therapy targeted to normalize the apnea-hypopnea index.

–**CSAS related to ESRD**
- Options for therapy include CPAP, nocturnal oxygen, and bicarbonate buffer use during dialysis.

Source
–http://www.guideline.gov/content.aspx?id=35175

APNEA, OBSTRUCTIVE SLEEP (OSA)

Population
–Adults.

Recommendations
▶ AASM 2017

–Recommends that diagnostic testing for OSA be performed in conjunction with a comprehensive sleep evaluation.

–Recommends that a polysomnogram, or home sleep apnea testing with a technically adequate device, be used for the diagnosis of OSA in uncomplicated adult patients presenting with signs and symptoms that indicate an increased risk of moderate-to-severe OSA.

–Recommends that a polysomnogram, rather than home sleep apnea testing, be used for the diagnosis of OSA in patients with significant cardiorespiratory disease, potential respiratory muscle weakness due to neuromuscular condition, awake hypoventilation or suspicion of sleep-related hypoventilation, chronic opioid medication use, and history of stroke or severe insomnia.

–Recommends that if a single home sleep apnea testing is negative, inconclusive, or technically inadequate, a polysomnogram be performed for the diagnosis or exclusion of OSA.

Sources

–http://guidelines.gov/summaries/summary/50887/

–Kapur VK, Auckley DH, Chowdhuri S, et al. Clinical practice guideline for diagnostic testing for adult obstructive sleep apnea: an American Academy of Sleep Medicine clinical practice guideline. *J Clin Sleep Med.* 2017;13(3):479-504.

▶ ACP 2013

–Encourage all overweight adults diagnosed with OSA to lose weight.

–Use nocturnal CPAP (continuous positive airway pressure) therapy as first-line therapy for OSA.

–Option to use mandibular advancement devices for those patients intolerant of CPAP.

Source

–http://www.guideline.gov/content.aspx?id=47136

ASTHMA, EXACERBATIONS

Population

–Children >5 y and adults.

Recommendations

▶ GINA 2018

–Assess severity of asthma exacerbation while starting SABA and supplemental oxygen as needed.

–Consider alternative causes for the patient's respiratory symptoms. Consider anaphylaxis.

–Arrange for transfer of patient to acute care facility if there are signs of severe exacerbation, altered mentation, or silent chest. Give inhaled SABA, inhaled ipratropium bromide, oxygen, and systemic corticosteroids as soon as possible while awaiting/arranging for transfer.

–Start treatment with repeated doses of inhaled SABA, early oral corticosteroids, and supplemental oxygen. Titrate oxygen to maintain oxygen saturation 93%–95% in adults, and 94%–98% in children ages 6–12 y.

–For severe exacerbations, add ipratropium bromide, consider inhaled nebulized SABA. Consider IV magnesium if patient is not responding to initial treatment.

–No role for routine antibiotics, chest x-ray, or blood gases in asthma exacerbation. Use antibiotics only for suspected bacterial infections.

–Follow up and assess response of symptoms frequently.

–Use the exacerbation as an opportunity to review the patient's chronic medication regimen, identify misunderstanding, and review the asthma action plan.

–Arrange for early follow-up of an exacerbation, within 2–7 d. All patients should be followed until their symptoms return to normal.

Comment

1. Corticosteroids dosing:
   a. Prednisolone 1 mg/kg PO daily (up to 50 mg) or equivalent $\times$ 7 d for mild-to-moderate exacerbations.
   b. Methylprednisolone 1 mg/kg IV q6h initially for severe exacerbations.
   c. Magnesium dosing: Magnesium sulfate 2 g IV.
   d. Rapid-acting beta-agonists (SABA) dosing: 4–10 puffs albuterol pMDI with spacer or 2.5–5 mg nebulized every 20 min for 1 h.

Source

–*Pocket Guide for Asthma Management and Prevention.* 2018 Global Initiative for Asthma. http://www.ginasthma.org.

▼ ASTHMA, STABLE

Population

–Children age >5 y and adults.

Recommendations

▶ GINA 2018

–**Basic Principles:**
- Diagnosis of asthma by history: typical symptoms are a combination of shortness of breath, cough, wheezing, and chest tightness; variability over time and in intensity; frequent triggers; FEV_1 and FEV_1/FVC ratio are reduced and increase by more than 12% after a bronchodilator challenge.

- Classify asthma by level of symptom control.
- Obtain a chest radiograph at the initial visit to exclude alternative diagnoses.
- Assess for tobacco use and strongly advise smokers to quit.
- Recommend spirometry with bronchodilators to determine the severity of airflow limitation and its reversibility. Repeat spirometry at least every 1–2 y for asthma monitoring.
- Consider allergy testing for history of atopy, rhinitis, rhinorrhea, and seasonal variation or specific extrinsic triggers.
- Recommend an asthma action plan based on peak expiratory flow (PEF) monitoring for all patients.
- Encourage allergen and environmental or occupational trigger avoidance.
- Physicians should help educate patients, assist them in self-management, develop goals of treatment, create an asthma action plan, and regularly monitor asthma control.

STEPWISE APPROACH TO ASTHMA MANAGEMENT

Stepwise approach to asthma treatment

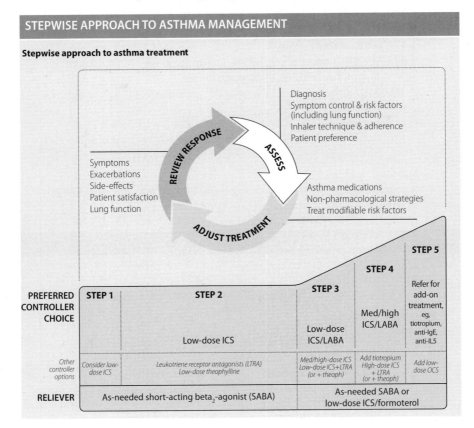

–Achieving asthma control:

- Controlled asthma is defined by:
  - Daytime symptoms $\leq 2\times$/wk.
  - No limitations of daily activities.
  - No nocturnal symptoms.
  - Need for reliever medicines $\leq 2\times$/wk.
  - Normal or near-normal lung function.
  - No exacerbations.
- Partially controlled asthma if:
  - Daytime symptoms $>2\times$/wk.
  - Any limitations of daily activities or any nocturnal symptoms.
  - Need for reliever medicines $\leq 2\times$/wk.
  - $<80\%$ predicted PEF or forced expiratory volume at 1 s (FEV_1).
  - Any exacerbations.
- Uncontrolled asthma if there are ≥ 3 features of partially controlled asthma in any week.
- Risk factors for asthma exacerbations:
  - Poor clinical control/uncontrolled symptoms.
  - High SABA use, ≥ 3 canisters per year.
  - Frequent asthma exacerbations, ≥ 1 in the past 12 mo.
  - History of ICU admission or intubation for asthma exacerbation.
  - FEV_1 $<60\%$ predicted or high bronchodilator reversibility.
  - Exposure to cigarette smoke.
  - Need for high-dose medications.
  - Incorrect inhaler technique and/or poor adherence.
  - Obesity, chronic rhinosinusitis, pregnancy, blood eosinophilia.
- Recommend at least a low-dose inhaled corticosteroid for almost all patients with asthma to reduce risk of exacerbations and death. Consider SABA-only treatment for patients with symptoms $<2\times$/mo, no nighttime symptoms, and no risk factors for exacerbations.
- Add a long-acting beta-agonist or leukotriene inhibitor for incomplete control with inhaled corticosteroid alone.
- Short-acting beta$_2$-agonists should be used as needed for relief of acute asthma symptoms or 20 min prior to planned exercise in exercise-induced asthma. Alternatives for exercise-induced asthma include a leukotriene inhibitor or cromolyn.
- For difficult-to-control asthma:
  - Treat potentially aggravating conditions: rhinitis, gastroesophageal reflux disease (GERD), nasal polyps.
  - Consider alternative diagnoses: chronic obstructive pulmonary disease (COPD) or vocal cord dysfunction.
- Continue inhaled corticosteroid as this reduces the risk of exacerbation in pregnancy.

Sources
  –*Pocket Guide for Asthma Management and Prevention.* 2018 Global
    Initiative for Asthma. http://www.ginasthma.org
  –*Global Initiative for Asthma: What's new in GINA 2018?* 2018 Global
    Initiative for Asthma. http://www.ginasthma.org

CHRONIC OBSTRUCTIVE PULMONARY DISEASE (COPD), EXACERBATIONS

Population
  –Adults.

ERS/ATS RECOMMENDATIONS FOR COPD EXACERBATIONS

TABLE I: RECOMMENDATIONS FOR THE TREATMENT OF CHRONIC OBSTRUCTIVE PULMONARY DISEASE [COPD] EXACERBATIONS

	Recommendation	Strength	Quality of Evidence
1	For ambulatory patients with an exacerbation of COPD, we suggest a short course (≤14 d) of oral corticosteroids	Conditional	Very low
2	For ambulatory patients with an exacerbation of COPD, we suggest the administration of antibiotics	Conditional	Moderate
3	For patients who are hospitalized with a COPD exacerbation, we suggest the administration of oral corticosteroids rather than intravenous corticosteroids if gastrointestinal access and function are intact	Conditional	Low
4	For patients who are hospitalized with a COPD exacerbation associated with acute or acute-on-chronic respiratory failure, we recommend the use of noninvasive mechanical ventilation	Strong	Low
5	For patients with a COPD exacerbation who present to the emergency department or hospital, we suggest a home-based management program (hospital-at-home)	Conditional	Moderate
6	For patients who are hospitalized with a COPD exacerbation, we suggest the initiation of pulmonary rehabilitation within 3 wk after hospital discharge	Conditional	Very low
7	For patients who are hospitalized with a COPD exacerbation, we suggest not initiating pulmonary rehabilitation during hospitalization	Conditional	Very low

Recommendations

▶ ERS/ATS 2017

Source
–Management of COPD exacerbations: a European Respiratory Society/ American Thoracic Society guideline. *Eur Respir J.* 2017;49(3):1600791.

▶ NICE 2018, GOLD 2018

–Recommend noninvasive positive pressure ventilation for moderate-to-severe hypercapnic respiratory failure.
–Prednisolone 30 mg orally, or its equivalent IV, should be prescribed for 5–7 d.
–Treat with antibiotics for 5–7 d for COPD exacerbations associated with sputum color change, increases in volume or thickness beyond the person's normal day-to-day variation.
–Bronchodilators can be delivered by either nebulizers or meter-dosed inhalers depending on the patient's ability to use the device during a COPD exacerbation. Bi-level positive airway pressure (Bi-PAP) is indicated for moderate-to-severe COPD exacerbations.
–Noninvasive mechanical ventilation improves survival, and decreases need for mechanical ventilation, infectious complications, and hospital length of stay.
–Consider subcutaneous heparin or low-molecular-weight heparin for DVT prophylaxis.
–Monitor fluid balance.
–Methylxanthines are not recommended due to side-effect profiles.

Sources
–Global Initiative for Chronic Obstructive Lung Disease: Pocket Guide to COPD Diagnosis, Management, and Prevention. 2018 Report. https://goldcopd.org/
–GOLD 2017 Global Strategy for the Diagnosis, Management and Prevention of COPD. https://goldcopd.org
–https://www.nice.org.uk/guidance/ng115

▶ Cochrane Database of Systematic Reviews 2018

–There was no difference in treatment failure or time to next exacerbation between patients treated with 7 or fewer days of systemic corticosteroid compared to treatment longer than 7 d.

Source
–Walters JAE, Tan DJ, White CJ, Wood-Baker R. Different durations of corticosteroid therapy for exacerbations of chronic obstructive pulmonary disease. Cochrane Database of Systematic Reviews 2018, Issue 3. Art. No.: CD006897.

Comment

1. Initial empiric antibiotics should be an aminopenicillin, macrolide, or a tetracycline and should be given for 5–10 d.

CHRONIC OBSTRUCTIVE PULMONARY DISEASE (COPD), STABLE

Population

–Adults.

Recommendations

▶ NICE 2018, GOLD 2018

–Confirm suspected COPD with postbronchodilator spirometry.

–Obtain spirometry in all persons age >35 y who are current or ex-smokers and have a chronic cough to evaluate for early-stage COPD.

–Counsel for smoking cessation. Smoking cessation has the greatest capacity to influence the natural history of COPD.

–Administer annual influenza vaccination, and pneumococcal vaccination including PPSV23 for adults with COPD and PCV13 for adults age ≥65 y.

–GOLD: assess severity of COPD by GOLD Grades 1–4 based on spirometry and GOLD Stages A–D based on symptoms and exacerbation history.

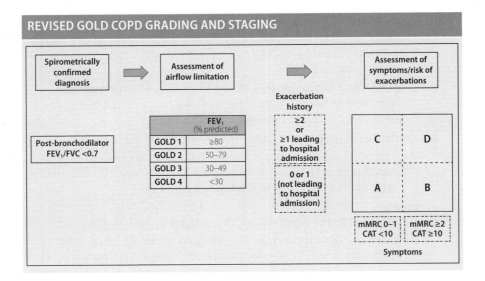

REVISED GOLD COPD GRADING AND STAGING

–The main treatment goals are reduction in symptoms and decreasing risk of future exacerbations.

–Stepwise medication approach[a]:

- Short-acting beta-agonist (SABA) and short-acting muscarinic agonist (SAMA) as needed (PRN).
- If persistent symptoms, add:
  - FEV_1 ≥50% of predicted, add either a long-acting beta-agonist (LABA) or long-acting muscarinic agonist (LAMA).
  - FEV_1 <50% of predicted, add either LABA + inhaled corticosteroid (ICS), or LAMA.
- If persistent symptoms, add:
  - LAMA to LABA + ICS.
  - Roflumilast, a phosphodiesterase-4 inhibitor, improves lung function and reduces moderate-to-severe exacerbations for patients with severe COPD.
  - In refractory cases, consider extended course (up to 1 y) azithromycin 250 mg/d for severe COPD to prevent exacerbations.

–Recommend pulmonary rehabilitation for symptomatic patients with moderate-to-severe COPD (FEV_1 <50% of predicted).

–Continuous oxygen therapy should be prescribed for COPD patients with room air hypoxemia (PaO_2 ≤55 mm Hg or SpO_2 ≤88%).

–Recommend screening COPD patients for osteoporosis and depression.

–Recommend against regular mucolytic therapy.

–Nutritional support indicated for patients with severe COPD with malnutrition.

–Recommend calculating the BODE index (BMI, airflow obstruction, dyspnea, and exercise capacity on a 6-min walk test) to calculate the risk of death in severe COPD.[b]

Sources

–Global Initiative for Chronic Obstructive Lung Disease: Pocket Guide to COPD Diagnosis, Management, and Prevention. 2018 Report. https://goldcopd.org/

–*GOLD 2017 Global Strategy for the Diagnosis, Management and Prevention of COPD.* http://goldcopd.org

–http://www.nice.org.uk/nicemedia/live/13029/49397/49397.pdf

---

[a]ICS: beclomethasone, budesonide, ciclesonide, flunisolide, fluticasone, mometasone, and triamcinolone; LABA: arformoterol, formoterol, or salmeterol; LAMA: tiotropium; SABA: albuterol, fenoterol, levalbuterol, metaproterenol, pirbuterol, and terbutaline.
[b]See http://www.nejm.org/doi/full/10.1056/NEJMoa021322#t=article

COMMON MEDICATIONS FOR THE MANAGEMENT OF COPD

Drug	Inhaler (µg/dose)	Nebulizer (mg/mL)	Drug	Inhaler (µg/dose)	Nebulizer (mg/mL)
Short-acting Beta$_2$-agonists			**Combination beta$_2$-agonist-anticholinergics**		
Albuterol	100–200$^{M/D}$	5	Albuterol-ipratropium	100/20^{SMI}	1 vial
Levalbuterol	45–90^M	0.21, 0.42	**Methylxanthines**		
Long-acting beta$_2$-agonists			**Aminophylline**	**200–600 mg pill PO**	
Arformoterol		0.0075	Theophylline SR	100–600 mg pill PO	
Formoterol	4.5–12$^{M/D}$	0.01	**Inhaled corticosteroids**		
Indacaterol	75–300^D		Beclomethasone	50–400$^{M/D}$	0.2–0.4
Salmeterol	25–50$^{M/D}$		Budesonide	100,200,400^D	0.2,0.25,0.5
Short-acting anticholinergics			Fluticasone	50–500$^{M/D}$	
Ipratropium bromide	20, 40^M	0.25–0.5	**Combination beta$_2$-agonist-corticosteroids**		
Long-acting anticholinergics			Formoterol-budesonide	4.5/160^M; 9/320^D	
Aclidinium bromide	322^D		Formoterol-mometasone	10/200^M or 10/400^M	
Tiotropium	18^D, 5^{SMI}		Salmeterol-fluticasone	50/100, 50/250, 50/500^D 25/50, 25/125, 25/250^M	
Phosphodiesterase-4 inhibitors			Vilanterol-fluticasone	25/100^D	
Roflumilast	500 µg PO daily				

M = metered dose inhalers.
D = dry powder inhalers.
SMI = soft mist inhalers.
Source: Data from *GOLD Guide to COPD Diagnosis, Management and Prevention.* http://goldcopd.org

Comments

1. $FEV_1/FVC < 0.7$ confirms the presence of airflow obstruction and COPD.
2. Classification of COPD by spirometry:
   a. Mild COPD = $FEV_1 \geq 80\%$ of predicted.
   b. Moderate COPD = FEV_1 50%–79% of predicted.
   c. Severe COPD = FEV_1 30%–49% of predicted.
   d. Very severe COPD = $FEV_1 < 30\%$ of predicted.

3. Can consider lung volume reduction surgery in patients with severe upper lobe emphysema and low post-pulmonary rehab exercise capacity.
4. Consider roflumilast, a phosphodiesterase-4 inhibitor, to reduce exacerbations for patients with severe chronic bronchitis and frequent exacerbations.

COUGH, CHRONIC

Population
–Adults with cough >8-wk duration.

Recommendations
▶ ACCP 2006, 2018
–To identify the etiology of the cough, determine the duration of the cough as acute (<3 wk), subacute (3–8 wk), or chronic (>8 wk), as this can limit the differential diagnosis.
–Evaluation to include—Review of red flag symptoms, occupational/environmental exposures, travel exposures, physical exam, and chest x-ray.
–The most common causes of chronic cough with a normal chest x-ray include smoking, ACE inhibitor use, upper airway cough syndrome (formerly known as postnasal drip syndrome), asthma, GERD, and nonasthmatic eosinophilic bronchitis.
–Evaluate chronic cough using a guideline/protocol-based approach that includes objective testing for bronchial hyperresponsiveness and eosinophilic bronchitis, or a therapeutic corticosteroid trial.
–If history and physical suggest no cause and there is no exposure to cigarette smoke or ace inhibitor, the Chest guideline offers a protocol suggesting the following steps:
  • Empiric treatment of upper airway cough syndrome
  • Empiric therapy for GERD
  • Evaluation or empiric therapy for asthma
  • Evaluation for sputum eosinophilia
–Unexplained chronic cough is defined as chronic cough lasting >8 wk without an identifiable cause after investigation and supervised therapeutic trials.
–For unexplained chronic cough, consider treatment with speech therapy or gabapentin.

Comments
1. Red flag symptoms for cough:
   a. Hemoptysis

b. Smoker age >45 with new cough, change in cough or coexisting voice disturbance

c. Adults age 55–80 with a 30-pack year history or who have quit less than 15 y ago

d. Dyspnea, especially at rest or at night

e. Hoarseness

f. Systemic symptoms: fever, weight loss, peripheral edema with weight gain

g. Dysphagia

h. Vomiting

i. Recurrent pneumonia

j. Abnormal physical exam or chest x-ray

Sources
–CHEST Guideline and Expert Panel Report. *CHEST*. 2018;153(1):196-209.
–CHEST Guideline and Expert Panel Report. *CHEST*. 2016;149(1):27-44.

NON-SMALL CELL LUNG CANCER (NSCLC) FOLLOW-UP CARE

Population
–Non-small cell lung cancer patients treated with curative intent.

Recommendation

▶ American College of Chest Physicians (ACCP) 2013

–**Follow-up Program**

• Chest CT scan should be performed every 6 mo for first 2 y after resection then once a year thereafter out to 10 y (second primary in 10% who survive first lung cancer).

• Routine imaging with PET scanning is not recommended.

• Patients should be seen every 3–4 mo for 2 y then less frequently. Health-related quality of life should be assessed with each visit.

• Surveillance biomarker testing should not be done outside of clinical trials.

• Offer smoking cessation interventions, annual influenza vaccine, and every 5 y pneumococcal vaccinations.

• Any headache or neurologic symptoms should prompt MRI brain with gadolinium, as lung cancer is the most common cancer to have brain metastases.

Source
–*JAMA*. 2010;303:1070.

Comments

Lung Cancer Facts

1. Only 30%–35% of patients diagnosed with NSCLC are candidates for surgery with curative intent. Lung CA is responsible for 165,000 deaths/y.
2. Cure rates are reflective of stage:
   a. Stage I—65%–70%
   b. Stage II—40%
   c. Stage IIIA—25%
   d. Stage IIIB—18%
3. Platinum-based chemotherapy is standard of care for NSCLC resected for cure. This adjuvant therapy reduces recurrence risk by 5%–10%.
4. Symptoms of local recurrence include increase or change in cough, dyspnea, and chest pain.
5. In older, compromised patients with a Stage I lung cancer, less than 3 cm in size, treatment with radiosteriotactic body radiation has a 70%–75% chance of prolonged disease-free survival.

PLEURAL EFFUSION, NEW

Population

–Adults with undiagnosed unilateral pleural effusion.

Recommendations

▶ BTS 2010

–A posteroanterior chest x-ray (CXR) should be used to detect the presence of a pleural effusion. A lateral decubitus CXR may be used to differentiate pleural liquid from pleural thickening. Pleural ultrasonography is preferred for investigation, however, and is generally available.

–CT scans can detect very small effusions (less than 10 mL of fluid). CT scan should be performed in the investigation of undiagnosed exudative pleural effusions prior to complete pleural fluid drainage. CT scan should be performed in the setting of pleural infection which has not responded to initial chest tube drainage.

–Thoracic ultrasound is more sensitive than CT scan to distinguish loculations.

–During thoracentesis, bedside ultrasound guidance improves the likelihood of successful pleural fluid aspiration and reduces risk of organ puncture.

–Undiagnosed effusions of more than 1 cm from the chest wall on lateral decubitus CXR should be diagnostically evaluated by ultrasound-assisted thoracentesis. Thoracentesis should not be performed on bilateral pleural effusions in a setting which is strongly suggestive of a transudative process, unless there are atypical features or a failure to respond to therapy. In patients with advanced cancer, thoracentesis for small effusions is unnecessary.

–All patients with a pleural effusion in the setting of sepsis or pneumonic illness should have diagnostic thoracentesis.

–Pleural fluid should be sent for: cell count and differential, gram stain and culture, protein, lactate dehydrogenase (LDH), and cytology. A minimum of 50–60 mL of pleural fluid should be withdrawn for analysis. Pleural fluid pH should be assessed in nonpurulent effusions when pleural infection is suspected. Check pleural fluid glucose when pleural fluid pH is not available and pleural infection is suspected.

–A chest physician or thoracic surgeon should be involved in the care of all patients who require chest tube drainage for pleural infection.

Sources
–*BTS Pleural Disease Guideline.* 2010
–*Thorax.* 2010;65(suppl 2):ii1-76.

PLEURAL EFFUSION, MALIGNANT (MPE)

Population
–Adult men and women with lung cancer or metastatic malignancy to the lung with a malignant pleural effusion.

Recommendations
▶ BTS 2010, ACCP 2014

–Diagnosis and baseline investigations:
- All effusions should be sent for cytology if a patient does not have a diagnosis of an MPE. Diagnosis can be made of MPE with pleural fluid cytology in about 60% of cases. A minimum of 50–60 mL of fluid should be sent. Increased amounts of fluid (100–200 cc) can be sent for a cell block and molecular testing (eg, epidermal growth factor receptor mutation, *Alk* gene rearrangement, and ROS 1 rearrangement).
- All patients with a diagnosis of significant MPE should be referred to pulmonologist and/or thoracic surgery for treatment options.
- Chest ultrasound is recommended at point of care for any thoracentesis or percutaneous chest drain placement (including indwelling pleural catheter [IPC]).
- Treatment is not required in asymptomatic patients but follow-up should be frequent especially if large MPE present.

–Symptomatic patients:

- Patients with symptoms should have initial therapeutic thoracentesis to relieve symptoms. The recommended amount of fluid removed per session is 1000–1500 mL. The rate of reaccumulation of the pleural effusion, and the patient's clinical and symptomatic response and prognosis will help to guide the subsequent choice of therapy.
- Outpatient therapeutic thoracentesis alone may be indicated for patients with survival expected to be less than 1 mo and/or poor performance status (PS) and/or slow reaccumulation of the pleural effusion (ie, more than 1 mo).
- Patients should be considered for more definitive intervention after the first or second thoracentesis.
- All treatment decisions should be guided by patient preferences.
- Selection of a treatment approach is largely dependent on projected duration of survival and availability of adequate resources. The management of a malignant pleural effusion (MPE) should be individualized and these patients should be commonly presented to a multidisciplinary Tumor Board for advice. (*JAMA.* 2012;307:2432).
- Management of MPE is palliative, and treatment decisions should focus on type of malignancy, patient's symptoms, life expectancy, functional status, quality of life, and goals of therapy. Palliative therapy goals should improve patient's quality of life through (1) relief of dyspnea and (2) less need for reintervention and reduced hospitalizations and length of stay.

–Treatment options:

- Indwelling (tunneled) pleural catheter (considered for patients with trapped lung who experience some relief following thoracentesis) for patients who want to avoid hospitalization or discomfort of pleurodesis.
- Talc pleurodesis (Talc poudrage) via thoracoscopy consider for patients with longer projected survival and those who don't want an indwelling catheter. This approach is contraindicated for patients with trapped lung.
- Talc pleurodesis (slurry) via chest tube—Indicated for patients with longer projected survival or contraindication to thoracoscopy. Contraindicated for patients with trapped lung.
- Chemotherapy may be considered as an adjunct treatment option. In particular, patients undergoing first-line systemic therapy for tumors with high response rates (small cell lung cancer and lymphoma) may avoid the previously discussed definitive treatments.

Comment

1. Indwelling pleural catheter (IPC-pleurex catheter) requires a regular outpatient drainage schedule that may be a burden for the patient or caregiver. This issue needs to be addressed. Complications from IPCs are uncommon. The infection rate is 5% with more than half the patients responding to antibiotics without removing the catheter. (*Chest.* 2013;144:1597) Other problems with IPCs include pneumothorax (5.9%), cellulitis (3.4%), obstruction/clogging (3.7%), and unspecified catheter malfunction (9.1%). The most common adverse events with talc pleurodesis include fever, pain, and GI symptoms. Less common are cardiac arrhythmia, dyspnea, systemic inflammatory response, empyema, and talc dissemination.

Sources

–https://www.guideline.gov/summaries/summary/49355/management-of-malignant-pleural-effusion
–*Chest.* 2012;142:394
–*Chest.* 2013;143(5):e4555-e4975.
–*J Natl Compr Canc Netw.* 2012;10:975.
–*Thoracic Society Pleural Disease Guideline.* 2010.
–*Thorax.* 2010;65(suppl 2):132.

PNEUMONIA

PNEUMONIA, COMMUNITY-ACQUIRED: EVALUATION

Diagnostic Testing
- CXR or other chest imaging required for diagnosis
- Sputum Gram stain and culture
  - Outpatients: optional
  - Inpatients: if unusual or antibiotic resistance suspected

Admission Decision
- Severity of illness (eg, CURB-65) and prognostic indices (eg, PSI) support decision
- One must still recognize social and individual factors

CURB-65
(*Thorax.* 2003;58:337-382)

Pneumonia Severity Index
(*N Engl J Med.* 1997;336:243-250)

Clinical Factor	Points	Demographic Factor	Points
Confusion	1		
BUN >19 mg/dL	1	Men age	Age in years
Respiratory rate ≥30 breaths/min	1	Women age	Age in years − 10

Systolic BP <90 mm Hg **OR** Diastolic BP ≤60 mm Hg	1	Nursing home resident	+10
		Coexisting illnesses	
Age >65 y	1	Neoplastic disease	+30
Total Points		Liver disease	+20
• CURB-65 ≥2 suggests need for hospitalization		Congestive heart failure	+10
		Cerebrovascular disease	+10

Score	In-hospital Mortality
0	
1	0.7%
2	3.2%
3	3.0%
4	17%
5	42%
	57%

Renal disease	+10
Physical exam findings	
Altered mental status	+20
Respiratory rate 30 breaths/min	+20
Systolic BP <90 mm Hg	+20
Temperature <95°F (35°C)	+15
Temperature >104°F (40°C)	+15
Pulse >125 beats/min	+10
Laboratory and radiographic findings	
Arterial blood pH <7.35	+30
BUN >30 mg/dL	+20
Sodium level <130 mmol/L	+20
Glucose level >250 mg/dL	+10
Hematocrit <30%	+10
PaO_2 <60 mm Hg or O_2 saturation <90%	+10
Pleural effusion	+10

Add up total points to estimate mortality risk

Class	Points	Overall Mortality
I	<51	0.1%
II	51–70	0.6%
III	71–90	0.9%
IV	91–130	9.5%
V	>130	26.7%

BP, blood pressure; BUN, blood urea nitrogen; CURB-65, confusion, urea nitrogen, respiratory rate, blood pressure, 65 of age and older; CXR, chest x-ray; PSI, pneumonia severity index.
Sources: Mandell LA, Wunderink RG, Anzueto A, et al; Infectious Diseases Society of America; American Thoracic Society. Infectious Diseases Society of America/American Thoracic Society consensus guidelines on the management of community-acquired pneumonia in adults. *Clin Infect Dis*. 2007;44(suppl 2):S27-S72. Fine MJ, Auble TE, Yealy DM, et al. A prediction rule to identify low-risk patients with community-acquired pneumonia. *N Engl J Med*. 1997;336:243-250.

PNEUMONIA, COMMUNITY-ACQUIRED: SUSPECTED PATHOGENS

Condition and Risk Factors	Commonly Encountered Pathogens
Alcoholism	*Streptococcus pneumoniae*, oral anaerobes, *Klebsiella pneumoniae*, *Acinetobacter* species, *Mycobacterium tuberculosis*
COPD and/or smoking	*Haemophilus influenzae*, *Pseudomonas aeruginosa*, *Legionella* species, *S. pneumoniae*, *Moraxella catarrhalis*, *Chlamydia pneumoniae*
Aspiration	Gram-negative enteric pathogens, oral anaerobes
Lung abscess	CA-MRSA, oral anaerobes, endemic fungal pneumonia, *M. tuberculosis*, and atypical mycobacteria
Exposure to bat or bird droppings	Histoplasma capsulatum
Exposure to birds	*Chlamydophila psittaci* (if poultry: avian influenza)
Exposure to rabbits	*Francisella tularensis*
Exposure to farm animals or parturient cats	*Coxiella burnetii* (Q fever)
HIV infection (early)	*S. pneumoniae*, *H. influenzae*, and *M. tuberculosis*
HIV infection (late)	The pathogens listed for early infection plus *Pneumocystis jirovecii*, *Cryptococcus*, *Histoplasma*, *Aspergillus*, atypical mycobacteria (especially *Mycobacterium kansasii*), *P. aeruginosa*, *H. influenzae*
Hotel or cruise ship stay in previous 2 wk	*Legionella* species
Travel to or residence in southwestern United States	*Coccidioides* species, *Hantavirus*
Travel to or residence in Southeast and East Asia	*Burkholderia pseudomallei*, avian influenza, SARS
Influenza active in community	Influenza, *S. pneumoniae*, *Staphylococcus aureus*, *H. influenzae*
Cough ≥2 wk with whoop or posttussive vomiting	*Bordetella pertussis*
Structural lung disease (eg, bronchiectasis)	*P. aeruginosa*, *Burkholderia cepacia*, and *S. aureus*
Injection drug use	*S. aureus*, anaerobes, *M. tuberculosis*, and *S. pneumoniae*
Endobronchial obstruction	Anaerobes, *S. pneumoniae*, *H. influenzae*, *S. aureus*
In context of bioterrorism	*Bacillus anthracis* (anthrax), *Yersinia pestis* (plague), *F. tularensis* (tularemia)

CA-MRSA, community-acquired methicillin-resistant *S. aureus*; COPD, chronic obstructive pulmonary disease; SARS, severe acute respiratory syndrome.
Sources: IDSA 2007, ATS 2007.

PNEUMONIA, COMMUNITY ACQUIRED: TREATMENT

Population
–Adults with diagnosis of community-acquired pneumonia.

Recommendations

▶ IDSA/ATS 2007

–Initial antimicrobial treatment:
- For previously healthy patients with no risk factors for drug resistant pathogens, choose a macrolide or doxycycline.
- For patients with comorbidities (including CHF, COPD, CKD, liver disease, DM, asplenia, or immunosuppression), IV antibiotic treatment within the last 3 mo, or other risk factors for drug-resistant pathogens, choose a respiratory fluoroquinolone or beta-lactam plus a macrolide. For penicillin-allergic patients, choose a respiratory fluoroquinolone.

Source
–The IDSA/ATS consensus guidelines on the management of CAP in adults. *Breathe*. 2007;4(2):110-115.

PNEUMOTHORAX, SPONTANEOUS

Population
–Adults with diagnosis of spontaneous pneumothorax.

Recommendations

▶ BTS 2010

–Use standard standing chest x-ray for the initial diagnosis; expiratory films are not necessary. CT scan is recommended for uncertain or complex cases.
–Tension pneumothorax is a medical emergency, which should be suspected in the setting of respiratory distress or hypotension. Treatment includes oxygen supplementation and needle decompression.
–Symptoms including dyspnea are more important than the size of pneumothorax in determining the management strategy.
–If the patient has pneumothorax size <2 cm and minimal symptoms, consider discharge with outpatient follow-up and return precautions.
–If the patient has significant dyspnea or pneumothorax size >2 cm, recommend needle aspiration with 16–18 G needle. If pneumothorax is then <2 cm and symptoms improved, consider discharge with outpatient follow-up. For pneumothorax >2 cm with minimal

symptoms, consider conservative management/observation. If after
needle aspiration, the patient is still symptomatic, or size still >2 cm,
recommend chest drain size 8–14 French and admission.
- Needle aspiration and small bore chest drains (<20 Fr) are preferred
over large bore chest drains, and may be associated with reduced
hospitalization and length of stay.
- If there is a persistent air leak at 48 h, recommend consultation with
Chest Physician.
- Smoking cessation counseling is recommended to prevent recurrence.

Notes:

These recommendations do not apply for secondary pneumothorax,
or pneumothorax in the setting of underlying lung disease. For these
patients, admission is recommended at a minimum for observation and
oxygen, even if not actively managed.

Sources
- *Thoracic Society Pleural Disease Guideline*. 2010.
- *Thorax*. 2010;65(suppl 2):ii18-31.
- Wilkerson RG, et al. Sensitivity of bedside ultrasound and
supine anteroposterior chest radiographs for the identification of
pneumothorax after blunt trauma. *Acad Emerg Med*. 2010. PMID:
20078434.

Comment

1. Ultrasound with attention to pleural interface for lung sliding (sea
shore sign on M-mode) is highly sensitive for pneumothorax. While
the guidelines are yet to be updated, ultrasound has proven more
sensitive than chest x-ray for pneumothorax (*Acad Emerg Med*.
2010;17(1):11-17) (*Am J Emerg Med*. 2019. https://doi.org/10.1016/j.
ajem.2019.02.028)

PULMONARY NODULES

Population
- Adults with incidental pulmonary nodules. These guidelines do not
apply to immunocompromised patients, patients with cancer, or for
lung cancer screening.

Recommendations

▶ Fleischer Society 2017
- Fleischner Society Guidelines recommend:
  • Categorize nodules by size, solid or subsolid, single or multiple, low
or high risk.
- Do not follow up solid nodules 6 mm or less in diameter in low-risk
adults >35-y-old, even if multiple nodules are present.

- Provide thin-slice CT surveillance for solid nodules 6–8 mm at 6–12 mo, and consider a third CT at 18–24 mo. "Suspicious morphology, upper lobe location, or both can increase cancer risk into the 1%–5% range; therefore, follow-up at 12 mo may be considered, depending on comorbidity and patient preferences."
  - Use the Brock model for initial risk assessment of pulmonary nodules larger than 8 mm in patients who have ever smoked.
  - Do not follow up diffuse, central, or laminated pattern of calcification or fat.
  - Consider a PET-CT scan for patients with a pulmonary nodule and an initial risk of malignancy >5%.
  - Suggestions for pulmonary nodules management:
    - Serial CT scans when the malignancy risk is <5%.
    - CT-guided biopsy when the risk of malignancy is 5%–65%.
    - Video-assisted thoracoscopic surgery when the chance of malignancy exceeds 65%.
    - Consider bronchoscopy when a bronchus sign is present on CT scan.

Source
  - Guidelines for Management of Incidental Pulmonary Nodules Detected from CT Images: From the Fleischner Society 2017. *Radiology*. 2017;284(1):228-243.

FLEISCHNER SOCIETY 2017 GUIDELINES FOR MANAGEMENT OF INCIDENTALLY DETECTED PULMONARY NODULES IN ADULTS

A: Solid Nodules[a]

Nodule Type	Size			Comments
	<6 mm (<100 mm³)	6–8 mm (100–250 mm³)	>8 mm (>250 mm³)	
Single				
Low risk[b]	No routine follow-up	CT at 6–12 mo, then consider CT at 18–24 mo	Consider CT at 3 mo, PET/CT, or tissue sampling	Nodules <6 mm do not require routine follow-up in low-risk patients (recommendation 1A).
High risk[b]	Optional CT at 12 mo	CT at 6–12 mo, then CT at 18–24 mo	Consider CT at 3 mo, PET/CT, or tissue sampling	Certain patients at high risk with suspicious nodule morphology, upper lobe location, or both may warrant 12-mo follow-up (recommendation 1A).

FLEISCHNER SOCIETY 2017 GUIDELINES FOR MANAGEMENT OF INCIDENTALLY DETECTED PULMONARY NODULES IN ADULTS *(Continued)*

Multiple				
Low risk[b]	No routine follow-up	CT at 3–6 mo, then consider CT at 18–24 mo	CT at 3–6 mo, then consider CT at 18–24 mo	Use most suspicious nodule as guide to management. Follow-up intervals may vary according to size and risk (recommendation 2A).
High risk[b]	Optional CT at 12 mo	CT at 3–6 mo, then at 18–24 mo	CT at 3–6 mo, then at 18–24 mo	Use most suspicious nodule as guide to management. Follow-up intervals may vary according to size and risk (recommendation 2A).

B: Subsolid Nodules[a]

Nodule Type	Size		Comments
	<6 mm (<100 mm³)	≥6 mm (>100 mm³)	
Single			
Ground glass	No routine follow-up	CT at 6–12 mo to confirm persistence, then CT every 2 y until 5 y	In certain suspicious nodules <6 mm, consider follow-up at 2 and 4 y. If solid component(s) or growth develops, consider resection (recommendations 3A and 4A).
Part solid	No routine follow-up	CT at 3–6 mo to confirm persistence. If unchanged and solid component remains <6 mm, annual CT should be performed for 5 y.	In practice, part-solid nodules cannot be defined as such until ≥6 mm, and nodules <6 mm do not usually require follow-up. Persistent part-solid nodules with solid components ≥6 mm should be considered highly suspicious (recommendations 4A–4C).

FLEISCHNER SOCIETY 2017 GUIDELINES FOR MANAGEMENT OF INCIDENTALLY DETECTED PULMONARY NODULES IN ADULTS *(Continued)*			
Multiple	CT at 3–6 mo. If stable, consider CT at 2 and 4 y.	CT at 3–6 mo. Subsequent management based on the most suspicious nodule(s).	Multiple <6 mm pure ground-glass nodules are usually benign, but consider follow-up in selected patients at high risk at 2 and 4 y (recommendation 5A).

[a]Dimensions are average of long and short axes, rounded to the nearest millimeter.
[b]Consider all relevant risk factors (see Risk Factors).
Note—These recommendations do not apply to lung cancer screening, patients with immunosuppression, or patients with known primary cancer.

Renal Disorders

KIDNEY DISEASE, CHRONIC—MINERAL AND BONE DISORDERS (CKD-MBDs)

Population
–Adults and children.

Recommendations

▶ 2017 KDIGO CKD-MBD Guidelines

–Monitor serum calcium, phosphorus, immunoreactive parathyroid hormone (iPTH), and alkaline phosphatase levels:
- Beginning with Stage G3a CKD (adults).
- Beginning with Stage G2 CKD (children).

–Measure 25-OH vitamin D levels beginning in stage G3a CKD.

–Treat all vitamin D deficiency with vitamin D supplementation with standard recommended dosing. Decisions to treat should be based on trends of vitamin D levels, not a single level.

–In Stages G3–5 CKD, consider a bone biopsy before bisphosphonate therapy if a dynamic bone disease is a possibility.

–In Stages G3–5 CKD, aim to normalize calcium and phosphorus levels.

–In Stage G5 CKD, seek to maintain a parathyroid hormone (PTH) level of approximately 2–9 times the upper normal limit for the assay.

Source
–https://kdigo.org/wp-content/uploads/2017/02/KDIGO_CKD_MBD_Guideline_r6.pdf

Comment

1. Options for oral phosphate binders:
   a. Calcium acetate.
   b. Calcium carbonate.
   c. Calcium citrate.

   d. Sevelamer carbonate.
   e. Lanthanum carbonate.

KIDNEY DISEASE, CHRONIC

Population
–Adults.

Recommendations

▶2012 KDIGO, 2014 NKF-KDOQI

–Stage CKD based on cause, GFR category and albuminuria category with abnormalities being present for at least 3 mo.
  • Cause: Assign cause of CKD based on absence or presence of systemic disease and the location within the kidney of observed or presumed pathologic-anatomic abnormalities.
  • GFR category
    ○ G1: GFR >90 (mL/min/1.73 m^2)
    ○ G2: GFR 60–89
    ○ G3a: GFR 45–59
    ○ G3b: GFR 30–44
    ○ G4: GFR 15–29
    ○ G5: GFR <15
  • Albuminuria category
    ○ A1: ACR (urine albumin-to-creatinine ratio) <3
    ○ A2: ACR 3–30
    ○ A3: ACR >30
–Use creatinine and GFR estimating equation for initial assessment.
–Evaluation for chronicity.
  • In those with GFR <60 mL/min/1.73 m^2 (GFR categories G3a–5), evaluate history of prior indicators for kidney disease and prior measurements.
  • If duration is >3 mo then CKD is confirmed. If not >3 mo CKS is not confirmed or is unclear.
–Assess GFR and albuminuria at least annually for people with CKD. Assess more frequently for those at higher risk for progression. For people with CKD G3a measure serum cystatin C and calculate GFR using a GFR estimating equation and cystatin C if the confirmation of CKD is required.
–Management of disease progression.
  • Control BP and individualize BP targets based on age, coexisting comorbidities, presence of retinopathy, and tolerance of treatment.

- Recommend that an ACE-I or ARB be used in diabetic patients with CKD and urine albumin excretion of 30–300 mg/24 h (or equivalent).
- Suggest lowering protein intake to 0.8 g/kg/d in adults with diabetes and nondiabetics with GFR categories G4–5.
- Recommend a large hemoglobin A1C of approximately 7% in people with diabetes and CKD.
- Recommend a salt intake of <2 g/24 h in people with CKD.
  –Check at least once serum calcium, phosphate, intact parathyroid hormone, 25-OH vitamin D, and hemoglobin levels for Stages G3a–5 CKD to inform future clinical decisions.

Source
  –https://www.ajkd.org/article/S0272-6386(14)00491-0/pdf

▶Va/DoD 2014
  –Restrict dietary sodium to reduce hypertension and proteinuria.
  –Restrict protein 0.6–0.8 g/kg/d for patients with Stage 3–4 CKD.
  –Vaccinate against influenza, Tdap, 13-valent pneumococcal conjugate vaccine, hepatitis B virus, Zoster, and MMR vaccines.
  –Give ACEI or ARB therapy for patients with diabetes, hypertension, or albuminuria.
  –Supplement bicarbonate in CKD with metabolic acidosis.
  –Give oral iron therapy for Stage 3 or worse CKD.
  –Use erythropoietic-stimulating agents if hemoglobin <10 g/dL.

Source
  –http://www.guideline.gov/content.aspx?id=48951

KIDNEY INJURY, ACUTE

Population
  –Children and adults.

Recommendations
▶NICE 2013
  –Perform a urinalysis in all patients with AKI. Consider checking urine electrolytes (ie, urine sodium, urine creatine, urine urea, and urine osmolarity) to calculate a FENa or FEUrea.
  –Do not routinely obtain a renal ultrasound when the cause of the AKI has been identified.
  –Detect AKI with any of the following criteria:
    - Rise in serum creatinine ≥0.3 mg/dL in 48 h.
    - 50% or more rise in creatinine in last 7 d.
    - Urine output <0.5 mL/kg/h.

–Refer for renal replacement therapy patients with any of the following refractory to medical management:
- Hyperkalemia.
- Metabolic acidosis.
- Uremia.
- Fluid overload.

Sources
–https://doi.org/10.1016/0002-9343(84)90368-1
–http://www.guideline.gov/content.aspx?id=47080

RENAL CANCER (RCC) FOLLOW-UP CARE

Recommendations
▶ NCCN 2016
–**Stage I—Follow-up after a partial or radical nephrectomy**
- History and physical (H&P) every 6 mo for 2 y then annually up to 5 y after surgery.
- Comprehensive metabolic panel or other blood tests as indicated every 6 mo for 2 y then annually until 5 y.

–**Abdominal imaging after partial nephrectomy**
- Baseline abdominal CT, MRI, or US within 3–9 mo of surgery. If initial scan-negative abdominal imaging may be considered annually for 3 y based on overall risk factors.

–**After radical nephrectomy**
- Abdominal CT, MRI, or US within 3–12 mo of surgery.
- If initial post-op imaging is negative, abdominal imaging beyond 12 mo may be done at the discretion of the physician.
- Chest x-ray or CT annually for 3 y then as indicated clinically.

–**Stage II or III—follow-up after radical nephrectomy**
- H&P every 3–6 mo for 3 y then annually up to 5 y after radical nephrectomy, then as clinically indicated.
- Comprehensive metabolic panel, LDH, and C-reactive protein every 6 mo for 2 y then annually up to 5 y.

–**Abdominal imaging after radical nephrectomy**
- Baseline abdominal CT or MRI within 3–6 mo then CT, MRI, or US every 3–6 mo for 3 y then annually up to 5 y.
- Chest imaging—baseline chest CT within 3–6 mo.
- Pelvic, brain, or spinal imaging as clinically indicated. Nuclear bone scan as clinically indicated.

Source

−*J Clin Oncol.* 2014; j32:4059.

Comments

1. **RCC staging**
   a. Stage I—Tumor <7 cm N0M0.
   b. Stage II—Tumor >7 cm limited to kidney N0M0.
   c. Stage III—Any tumor size with regional node metastasis.
   d. Stage IV—T4 (spread beyond Gerota's fascia—any T, any N, M [systemic metastases]).

2. **Features of high risk for relapse**
   a. Stage III, size of tumor, high grade (Fuhrman 3 or 4), coagulative tumor necrosis (5 times increase in risk of death). (*Br J Urol.* 2009; 103:165)

3. **Paraneoplastic syndromes in RCC and clinical caveats**
   a. Anemia, hepatic dysfunction, fever, hypercalcemia, cachexia, erythrocytosis, thrombocytosis, polymyalgia rheumatica. (*Lancet.* 1998;352:1691)
   b. Chemotherapy no longer used in treatment of RCC. Multi-targeted tyrosine kinase inhibitors and checkpoint immune blockade are treatments of choice. High-dose interleukin-2 is used occasionally in young, fit patients. (*NEJM.* 2015;373:1803) (*NEJM.* 2013;369:722)
   c. In patients with small-volume metastasis a nephrectomy to remove the primary mass has resulted in a prolongation of survival. (*N Engl J Med.* 2001;345:1655)
   d. In selected patients with low-volume, limited, resectable metastatic disease, surgical removal of the metastasis increases overall survival with occasional long-term remission. (*Cancer.* 2011;117:2873)
   e. The use of adjuvant therapy with multi-targeted tyrosine kinase inhibitors does not extend progression-free or overall survival in a placebo-controlled trial. (*Lancet.* 2016; published online March 14, 2016). A second trial in higher risk patients did show a survival benefit with adjuvant TKI inhibitors. (*N Engl J Med.* 2016; 375:2246)

CANCER SURVIVORSHIP: LATE EFFECTS OF CANCER TREATMENTS

CA Treatment History	Late Effects	Periodic Evaluation
Any CA experience	Psychosocial disorders[b]	
Any chemotherapy	Oral and dental abnormalities	Dental examination and cleaning (every 6 mo)
Chemotherapy—alkylating agents (cyclophosphamide, melphelan, ifosfamide, chlorambucil, nitrosoureas)[a]	Gonadal dysfunction Hematologic disorders[c] Ocular toxicity[d] Pulmonary toxicity Renal toxicity[f] Urinary tract toxicity[g]	Pubertal assessment (yearly) in adults if symptoms of hypogonadism present History, examination for bleeding disorder; CBC/differential (yearly) Visual acuity, funduscopic examination, evaluation by ophthalmologist (yearly if ocular tumors, TBI, or $\geq$ 30 Gy; otherwise, every 3 y) CXR, PFTs (at entry into long-term follow-up, then as clinically indicated)
		Blood pressure (yearly); electrolytes, BUN, creatinine, Ca^{++}, Mg^{++}, PO_4^- urinalysis (at entry into long-term follow-up, then clinically as indicated) Bone marrow injury with myelodysplasia
Chemotherapy—antitumor antibiotics (anthracycline, epirubicin)[a]	Cardiac toxicity[h]	ECHO or MUGA; ECG at entry into long-term follow-up, periodic thereafter ($\uparrow$ frequency if chest radiation); fasting glucose, lipid panel (every 3–5 y)
	Hematologic disorders[c]	See "Chemotherapy—Alkylating agents"—risk of acute myelocytic leukemia
Chemotherapy—antitumor antibiotics (mitomycin C[f], bleomycin[e])	Pulmonary toxicity[e] Renal injury[f]	Chest x-ray and pulmonary function tests at end of exposure to bleomycin, with re-evaluation as clinically indicated Monitor urinalysis and creatinine (mito C)

Chemotherapy—antimetabolites (cytarabine, MTX) (high-dose IV, intrathecal)[b]	Clinical leukoencephalopathy[i] Neurocognitive deficits	Full neurologic examination (yearly) Neuropsychological evaluation (at entry into long-term follow-up, then as clinically indicated)
Chemotherapy—epipodophyllotoxins (Ixabepilone)[a]	Hematologic disorders (causes AML with specific 11q 23 translocation[c])	See "Chemotherapy—alkylating agents" Hematologic disorders, AML gonadal dysfunction
Chemotherapy heavy metals (cis-platinum, carboplatin)	Dyslipidemia/hypertension and increased risk of cardiovascular disease Gonadal dysfunction Hematologic disorders[c] Ototoxicity[j] Peripheral sensory neuropathy Renal toxicity[f]	See "Chemotherapy—alkylating agents" Fasting lipid panel at entry Complete pure tone audiogram or brainstem auditory-evoked response (yearly × 2 then as indicated by symptoms) Examination yearly for at least 5 y Increased risk of renal insufficiency, neuropathy and cardiac events—lab work and careful F/U at least yearly
Chemotherapy—microtubular inhibitors (taxanes, eribulin)	Peripheral neuropathy	Examination yearly for 2–3 y If neuropathy persistent—duloxetine or venlafaxine may help
Chemotherapy—nonclassical alkylators (dacarbazine and temazolomide)	Gonadal dysfunction Reduced CD4 count Hematologic disorders[c]	See "Chemotherapy—alkylating agents" Monitor for opportunistic infections (CD_4 count at 6 and 12 mo)
Chemotherapy—plant alkaloids (vincristine, vinorelbine, vinblastin)	Peripheral sensory neuropathy Raynaud phenomenon	Yearly history/examination. May have persistent neuropathy—duloxetine may help
Chemotherapy—purine agonists (fludarabine, pentostatin)	Hematologic disorders[c] Reduction in CD4 count	See "Chemotherapy—alkylating agents" Monitor for infection
Corticosteroids (dexamethasone, prednisone)	Ocular toxicity[d] Avascular osteonecrosis Osteopenia/osteoporosis	Musculoskeletal examination (yearly)

CANCER SURVIVORSHIP: LATE EFFECTS OF CANCER TREATMENTS (*Continued*)		
CA Treatment History	**Late Effects**	**Periodic Evaluation**
Targeted biologic therapy • Monoclonal antibodies • Trastuzumab (anti–HER-2) • Rituximab (anti-CD20 antibody to B lymphocyte receptor) • Panitumumab, cetuximab (anti-EGFR)	Cardiac dysfunction is usually reversible Reduction in immunoglobulins and increased risk of infection	Monitor 2D echo for ejection fraction every 3 mo during therapy and as needed for symptoms Monitor quantitative immunoglobulins if increased frequency of infection
Multi-targeted tyrosine kinase inhibitors (TKIs) • Erlotinib • Carbozantinib • Regorafenib • Sunitinib • Sorafenib • Axitinib • Pazopanib • Imatinib • Lenvatinib • Dasatinib • Nilotinib • Lapatinib	Fatigue, diarrhea, hypertension, liver injury while on drug but little long-term toxicity Hand and foot syndrome (palmar–plantar, erythrodysethesia) Vascular injury, fluid retention, renal dysfunction	Routine monitoring for end-organ damage after completion of therapy not indicated
Immune-mediated therapy (checkpoint inhibitors) • Pembrolizumab • Ipilimumab • Nivolumab	Autoimmunity—colitis, hepatitis, dermatitis, thyroiditis, hypophysitis, rare myocardial injury Adrenal insufficiency, pneumonitis—often reversible but not always Gonadal dysfunction Growth hormone deficiency (children and adolescents) Hyperthyroidism Hyperprolactinemia Hypothyroidism	Check hormone levels every 4–6 mo Cortisol and ACTH stimulation testing based on clinical symptoms TSH, free thyroxine (T_4) yearly Prolactin level (as clinically indicated) Monitor for pituitary insufficiency based on clinical findings Major activity in lung cancer, Hodgkin's lymphoma, and renal cell cancer

Chemotherapy drugs with minimal long-term toxicity effects • Topoisomerase I inhibitors (Camptosar, topotecan) • Antibiotics (actinomycin) • Antimetabolites (L-asparaginase, 5-fluorouracil [5-FU], capecitabine, gemcitabine, 6-mercaptopurine)	Mild reduction in bone marrow and renal reserve Neuropathy Mild bone marrow suppression	Routine monitoring for end-organ dysfunction is not indicated Monitor neuropathy and platelet count. These problems are largely reversed when treatment stops
Drug–Antibody Conjugates • Bretuximb vedotin (anti-CD30 antibody—in Hodgkin lymphoma and T-cell lymphoma) • TDM1 (Kadcyla®) Her2-directed Herceptin linked to chemo for Her2 positive breast cancer		
Radiation therapy (field- and dose-dependent)	Cardiac toxicity[h] (chest radiation) Central adrenal insufficiency (pediatric brain tumors) Cerebrovascular complications[i] Pulmonary injury with symptoms[e] Functional asplenia Bowel injury and obstruction	8 AM serum cortisol (yearly × 15 y, and as clinically indicated) Neurologic examination (yearly) Head/neck examination (yearly)—persistent dry mouth Blood culture when temperature ≥101°F (38.3°C), rapid institution of empiric antibiotics—increased infection risk with poor spleen function Increased risk of breast cancer with mediastinal radiation in women 15–35 y—breast MRI yearly Surveillance for second cancers related to therapeutic radiation

CANCER SURVIVORSHIP: LATE EFFECTS OF CANCER TREATMENTS

CA Treatment History	Late Effects	Periodic Evaluation

AML, acute myelocytic leukemia; BMI, body mass index; BUN, blood urea nitrogen; CBC, complete blood count; CXR, chest x-ray; ECG, electrocardiogram; ECHO, echocardiogram; IV, intravenous; MTX, methotrexate; MUGA, multiple-gated acquisition scan; PFTs, pulmonary function tests; TBI, total-body irradiation; TSH, thyroid-stimulating hormone.

[a]Chemotherapeutic agents, by mechanism of action:

• Alkylating agents: busulfan, carmustine (BCNU), chlorambucil, cyclophosphamide, ifosfamide, lomustine (CCNU), mechlorethamine, melphalan, procarbazine, thiotepa.

• Antimetabolites: MTX, cytosine arabinoside, gemcitabine.

• Heavy metals: carboplatin, cisplatin, oxaliplatin.

• Nonclassical alkylators: dacarbazine (DTIC), temozolomide.

• Anthracycline antibiotics: daunorubicin, doxorubicin, epirubicin, idarubicin, mitoxantrone.

• Antitumor antibiotics: bleomycin, mitomycin C.

• Plant alkaloids: vinblastine, vincristine, vinorelbine.

• Purine agonists: fludarabine, pentostatin, cladribine.

• Microtubular inhibitors: docetaxel, paclitaxel, cabazitaxel, ixabepilone.

• Epipodophyllotoxins: etoposide (VP16), teniposide (VM26).

[b]Psychosocial disorders: mental health disorders, risky behaviors, psychosocial disability because of pain, fatigue, limitations in health care/insurance access, "chemo brain" syndrome.
[c]Hematologic disorders: acute myeloid leukemia, myelodysplasia.
[d]Ocular toxicity: cataracts, orbital hypoplasia, lacrimal duct atrophy, xerophthalmia, keratitis, telangiectasias, retinopathy, optic chiasm neuropathy, endophthalmos, chronic painful eye, maculopathy, glaucoma.
[e]Pulmonary toxicity: pulmonary fibrosis, interstitial pneumonitis, restrictive lung disease, obstructive lung disease. Increased sensitivity to oxygen toxicity—keep FiO_2 ≤28% in patients with previous bleomycin exposure.
[f]Renal toxicity: glomerular and tubular renal insufficiency, hypertension, hemolytic uremic syndrome.
[g]Urinary tract toxicity: hemorrhagic cystitis, bladder fibrosis, dysfunctional voiding, vesicoureteral reflux, hydronephrosis, bladder malignancy.
[h]Cardiac toxicity: cardiomyopathy, arrhythmias, left ventricular dysfunction, congestive heart failure, pericarditis, pericardial fibrosis, valvular disease, myocardial infarction, atherosclerotic heart disease.
[i]Clinical leukoencephalopathy: spasticity, ataxia, dysarthria, dysphagia, hemiparesis, seizures.
[j]Ototoxicity: sensorineural hearing loss, tinnitus, vertigo, tympanosclerosis, otosclerosis, eustachian tube dysfunction, conductive hearing loss.
[k]Oncologic disorders: secondary benign or malignant neoplasm, especially breast CA after mantle radiation, gastrointestinal malignancy after paraaortic radiation for seminoma of the testis.
[l]Cerebrovascular complications: stroke and occlusive cerebral vasculopathy.
Note: Guidelines for surveillance and monitoring for late effects after treatment for adult CAs, available via the National Comprehensive Cancer Network, Inc. (NCCN). (http://www.nccn.org/professionals/physician_gls).
Source: Long-Term Follow-Up Guidelines for Survivors of Childhood, Adolescent, and Young Adult Cancers. Children's Oncology Group, Version 3.0, October 2008. (For full guidelines and references, see http://www. survivorshipguidelines.org). See also: *N Engl J Med.* 2006;355:1722-1782; *J Clin Oncol.* 2007;25:3991-4008; *JAMA.* 2011;305:2311.

RENAL MASSES, SMALL

Population
–Adults with small renal masses SRM (<4 cm).

Recommendations
▶ ASCO Guidelines (*J Clin Oncol*. 2017;35:668-680)

–Based on tumor-specific findings and competing risks of mortality, all patients with an SRM (<4 cm in size) should be considered for renal tumor biopsy (RTB) when the results may alter management (strength of recommendation: strong).

–Active surveillance should be an initial management option for patients who have significant comorbidities and limited life expectancy (end-stage renal disease, SRM <1 cm, life expectancy <5 y).

–Partial nephrectomy (PN) for SRM is the standard treatment that should be offered to all patients for whom an intervention is indicated and who possess a tumor that is amenable to this approach (recommendation: strong).

–Percutaneous thermal ablation should be considered an option for patients who possess tumors such that complete ablation will be achieved. A biopsy should be obtained before or at the time of ablation (recommendation: moderate).

–Radical nephrectomy for SRM should be reserved only for patients who possess a tumor of significant complexity that is not amenable to PN or where PN may result in unacceptable morbidity even when performed at centers of excellence. Referral to experienced surgeon and a center with experience should be considered (recommendation: strong).

–Referral to a nephrologist should be considered if CKD (GFR<45 mL/min) or progressive CKD develops after treatment, especially if associated with proteinuria (recommendation: moderate).

Sources
–*N Engl J Med*. 2010;362:624.
–*Eur Urol*. 2016;69:116.
–*JAMA*. 2015;150:664.
–*Eur Urol*. 2015;67.

Comments
1. SRM are commonly discovered incidentally during diagnostic evaluation for other medical conditions. A significant number of SRM are benign. As the size increases (especially >4 cm), the likelihood of malignancy increases. Imaging with MRI, CT scans, and ultrasound cannot make an absolute diagnosis of malignancy, necessitating

a core biopsy if possible. About 10%–15% of patients will have a nondiagnostic biopsy and must be followed closely and rebiopsied if the mass is growing. Radiofrequency ablation (RFA) is commonly used to ablate small cancers but should have a biopsy done first to document malignancy.

2. Decision regarding therapy in patients with significant comorbidities is difficult. The Charleston Comorbidity Index (CCI) is a tool that can predict 1-y mortality. In patients with a short life expectancy, surveillance and supportive care is the best approach for this population. Partial nephrectomy is the treatment of choice for SRM that are amenable to nephron-sparing surgery. Radical nephrectomy in the past has been the procedure of choice in managing small RCC. Today partial nephrectomy is preferred and radical nephrectomy now is the treatment of choice in <30% of patients with SRM.

Appendices

ESTIMATE OF 10-Y CARDIAC RISK FOR MEN

ESTIMATE OF 10-Y CARDIAC RISK FOR MEN[a]

Age (y)	Points
20–34	–9
35–39	–4
40–44	0
45–49	3
50–54	6
55–59	8
60–64	10
65–69	11
70–74	12
75–79	13

Total Cholesterol	Points				
	Age 20–39	Age 40–49	Age 50–59	Age 60–69	Age 70–79
<160	0	0	0	0	0
160–199	4	3	2	1	0
200–239	7	5	3	1	0
240–279	9	6	4	2	1
≥280	11	8	5	3	1

	Age 20–39	Age 40–49	Points Age 50–59	Age 60–69	Age 70–79
Nonsmoker	0	0	0	0	0
Smoker	8	5	3	1	1

High-Density Lipoprotein (mg/dL)	Points
≥60	−1
50–59	0
40–49	1
<40	2

Systolic Blood Pressure (mm Hg)	If Untreated	If Treated
<120	0	0
120–129	0	1
130–139	1	2
140–159	1	2
≥160	2	3

Point Total	10-y Risk %
<0	<1
0	1
1	1

Point Total	10-y Risk %
9	5
10	6
11	8

ESTIMATE OF 10-Y CARDIAC RISK FOR MEN[a] (Continued)

Age (y)		Points	
2	1	12	10
3	1	13	12
4	1	14	16
5	2	15	20
6	2	16	25
7	3	≥17	≥30
8	4		

10-y Risk _____ %

[a]Framingham point scores.

Source: U.S. Department of Health and Human Services, Public Health Service, National Institutes of Health, National Heart, Lung, and Blood Institute. NIH Publication No. 01-3305, May 2001. https://www.nhlbi.nih.gov/files/docs/guidelines/atglance.pdf

ESTIMATE OF 10-Y CARDIAC RISK FOR WOMEN

ESTIMATE OF 10-Y CARDIAC RISK FOR WOMEN[a]

Age (y)	Points
20–34	–7
35–39	–3
40–44	0
45–49	3
50–54	6
55–59	8
60–64	10
65–69	12
70–74	14
75–79	16

Total Cholesterol	Points				
	Age 20–39	Age 40–49	Age 50–59	Age 60–69	Age 70–79
<160	0	0	0	0	0
160–199	4	3	2	1	1
200–239	8	6	4	2	1
240–279	11	8	5	3	2
≥280	13	10	7	4	2

ESTIMATE OF 10-Y CARDIAC RISK FOR WOMEN[a] (Continued)

Age (y)

	Points				
	Age 20–39	Age 40–49	Age 50–59	Age 60–69	Age 70–79
Nonsmoker	0	0	0	0	0
Smoker	9	7	4	2	1

High-Density Lipoprotein (mg/dL)

	Points
≥60	−1
50–59	0
40–49	1
<40	2

Systolic Blood Pressure (mm Hg)

	If Untreated	If Treated
<120	0	0
120–129	1	3
130–139	2	4
140–159	3	5
≥160	4	6

Point Total

Point Total	10-y Risk %	Point Total	10-y Risk %
<9	<1	17	5
9	1	18	6

10	1	19	8
11	1	20	11
12	1	21	14
13	2	22	17
14	2	23	22
15	3	24	27
16	4	≥25	≥30

10-y Risk _____ **%**

[a] Framingham point scores.

Source: U.S. Department of Health and Human Services, Public Health Service, National Institutes of Health, National Heart, Lung, and Blood Institute. NIH Publication No. 01-3305, May 2001. https://www.nhlbi.nih.gov/files/docs/guidelines/atglance.pdf

ESTIMATE OF 10-Y STROKE RISK FOR MEN

ESTIMATE OF 10-Y STROKE RISK FOR MEN

Age (y)	Points	Untreated Systolic Blood Pressure (mm Hg)	Points
54–56	0	97–105	0
57–59	1	106–115	1
60–62	2	116–125	2
63–65	3	126–135	3
66–68	4	136–145	4
69–72	5	146–155	5
73–75	6	156–165	6
76–78	7	166–175	7
79–81	8	176–185	8
82–84	9	186–195	9
85	10	196–205	10

Treated Systolic Blood Pressure (mm Hg)	Points	History of Diabetes	Points
97–105	0	No	0
106–112	1	Yes	2
113–117	2		
118–123	3		
124–129	4		

	Points
130–135	5
136–142	6
143–150	7
151–161	8
162–176	9
177–205	10

Cigarette Smoking	Points
No	0
Yes	3

Atrial Fibrillation	Points
No	0
Yes	4

Cardiovascular Disease	Points
No	0
Yes	4

Left Ventricular Hypertrophy on Electrocardiogram	Points
No	0
Yes	5

Point Total	10-y Risk %
1	3
2	3
3	4
4	4
5	5
16	22
17	26
18	29
19	33
20	37

ESTIMATE OF 10-Y STROKE RISK FOR MEN (*Continued*)

Age (y)	Points	Untreated Systolic Blood Pressure (mm Hg)	Points
6	5	42	21
7	6	47	22
8	7	52	23
9	8	57	24
10	10	63	25
11	11	68	26
12	13	74	27
13	15	79	28
14	17	84	29
15	20	88	30

10-y Risk _____ **%**

Source: Modified Framingham Stroke Risk Profile. *Circulation.* 2006;113:e873-e923.

ESTIMATE OF 10-Y STROKE RISK FOR WOMEN

ESTIMATE OF 10-Y STROKE RISK FOR WOMEN

Age (y)	Points	Untreated Systolic Blood Pressure (mm Hg)	Points
54–56	0	95–106	1
57–59	1	107–118	2
60–62	2	119–130	3
63–64	3	131–143	4
65–67	4	144–155	5
68–70	5	156–167	6
71–73	6	168–180	7
74–76	7	181–192	8
77–78	8	193–204	9
79–81	9	205–216	10
82–84	10		

Treated Systolic Blood Pressure (mm Hg)	Points	History of Diabetes	Points
95–106	1	No	0
107–113	2	Yes	3
114–119	3		
120–125	4		
126–131	5		
132–139	6		

ESTIMATE OF 10-Y STROKE RISK FOR WOMEN (Continued)

Age (y)	Points	Untreated Systolic Blood Pressure (mm Hg)	Points
		140–148	7
		149–160	8
		161–204	9
		205–216	10

Cigarette Smoking	Points	Cardiovascular Disease	Points
No	0	No	0
Yes	3	Yes	2

Atrial Fibrillation	Points	Left Ventricular Hypertrophy on Electrocardiogram	Points
No	0	No	0
Yes	6	Yes	4

Point Total	10-y Risk %	Point Total	10-y Risk %
1	1	16	19
2	1	17	23
3	2	18	27
4	2	19	32
5	2	20	37
6	3	21	43
7	4	22	50

	10-y Risk %
8	4
9	5
10	6
11	8
12	9
13	11
14	13
15	16
23	57
24	64
25	71
26	78
27	84
28	
29	
30	

Source: Modified Framingham Stroke Risk Profile. *Circulation.* 2006;113:e873–e923.

95TH PERCENTILE OF BLOOD PRESSURE FOR BOYS

95TH PERCENTILE OF BLOOD PRESSURE FOR BOYS

Age (y)	Systolic Blood Pressure (mm Hg) by Percentile of Height							Diastolic Blood Pressure (mm Hg) by Percentile of Height						
	5%	10%	25%	50%	75%	90%	95%	5%	10%	25%	50%	75%	90%	95%
3	104	105	107	109	110	112	113	63	63	64	65	66	67	67
4	106	107	109	111	112	114	115	66	67	68	69	70	71	71
5	108	109	110	112	114	115	116	69	70	71	72	73	74	74
6	109	110	112	114	115	117	117	72	72	73	74	75	76	76
7	110	111	113	115	117	118	119	74	74	75	76	77	78	78
8	111	112	114	116	118	119	120	75	76	77	78	79	79	80
9	113	114	116	118	119	121	121	76	77	78	79	80	81	81
10	115	116	117	119	121	122	123	77	78	79	80	81	81	82
11	117	118	119	121	123	124	125	78	78	79	80	81	82	82
12	119	120	122	123	125	127	127	78	79	80	81	82	82	83
13	121	122	124	126	128	129	130	79	79	80	81	82	83	83
14	124	125	127	128	130	132	132	80	80	81	82	83	84	84
15	126	127	129	131	133	134	135	81	81	82	83	84	85	85
16	129	130	132	134	135	137	137	82	83	83	84	85	86	87
17	131	132	134	136	138	139	140	84	85	86	87	87	88	89

95TH PERCENTILE OF BLOOD PRESSURE FOR GIRLS

95TH PERCENTILE OF BLOOD PRESSURE FOR GIRLS

Age (y)	Systolic Blood Pressure (mm Hg) by Percentile of Height							Diastolic Blood Pressure (mm Hg) by Percentile of Height						
	5%	10%	25%	50%	75%	90%	95%	5%	10%	25%	50%	75%	90%	95%
3	104	104	105	107	108	109	110	65	66	66	67	68	68	69
4	105	106	107	108	110	111	112	68	68	69	70	71	71	72
5	107	107	108	110	111	112	113	70	71	71	72	73	73	74
6	108	109	110	111	113	114	115	72	72	73	74	74	75	76
7	110	111	112	113	115	116	116	73	74	74	75	76	76	77
8	112	112	114	115	116	118	118	75	75	75	76	77	78	78
9	114	114	115	117	118	119	120	76	76	76	77	78	79	79
10	116	116	117	119	120	121	122	77	77	77	78	79	80	80
11	118	118	119	121	122	123	124	78	78	78	79	80	81	81
12	119	120	121	123	124	125	126	79	79	79	80	81	82	82
13	121	122	123	124	126	127	128	80	80	80	81	82	83	83
14	123	123	125	126	127	129	129	81	81	81	82	83	84	84
15	124	125	126	127	129	130	131	82	82	82	83	84	85	85
16	125	126	127	128	130	131	132	82	82	83	84	85	85	86
17	125	126	127	129	130	131	132	82	83	83	84	85	85	86

Source: Blood Pressure Tables for Children and Adolescents from the Fourth Report on the Diagnosis, Evaluation, and Treatment of High Blood Pressure in Children and Adolescents. http://www.nhlbi.nih.gov/guidelines/hypertension/child_tbl.htm. Accessed June 3, 2008.

BODY MASS INDEX (BMI) CONVERSION TABLE

BODY MASS INDEX (BMI) CONVERSION TABLE

Height in inches (cm)	BMI 25 kg/m²	BMI 27 kg/m²	BMI 30 kg/m²
	Body weight in pounds (kg)		
58 (147.32)	119 (53.98)	129 (58.51)	143 (64.86)
59 (149.86)	124 (56.25)	133 (60.33)	148 (67.13)
60 (152.40)	128 (58.06)	138 (62.60)	153 (69.40)
61 (154.94)	132 (59.87)	143 (64.86)	158 (71.67)
62 (157.48)	136 (61.69)	147 (66.68)	164 (74.39)
63 (160.02)	141 (63.96)	152 (68.95)	169 (76.66)
64 (162.56)	145 (65.77)	157 (71.22)	174 (78.93)
65 (165.10)	150 (68.04)	162 (73.48)	180 (81.65)
66 (167.64)	155 (70.31)	167 (75.75)	186 (84.37)
67 (170.18)	159 (72.12)	172 (78.02)	191 (86.64)
68 (172.72)	164 (74.39)	177 (80.29)	197 (89.36)
69 (175.26)	169 (76.66)	182 (82.56)	203 (92.08)
70 (177.80)	174 (78.93)	188 (85.28)	207 (93.90)
71 (180.34)	179 (81.19)	193 (87.54)	215 (97.52)
72 (182.88)	184 (83.46)	199 (90.27)	221 (100.25)
73 (185.42)	189 (85.73)	204 (92.53)	227 (102.97)
74 (187.96)	194 (88.00)	210 (95.26)	233 (105.69)
75 (190.50)	200 (90.72)	216 (97.98)	240 (108.86)
76 (193.04)	205 (92.99)	221 (100.25)	246 (111.59)

Metric conversion formula = weight (kg)/ height (m²)

Example of BMI calculation:

A person who weighs 78.93 kg and is 177 cm tall has a BMI of 25:

weight (78.93 kg)/height (1.77 m²) = **25**

BMI categories:

Underweight = <18.5

Normal weight = 18.5–24.9

Overweight = 25–29.9

Obesity = ≥30

Nonmetric conversion formula = [weight (lb)/height (in.²)] × 704.5

Example of BMI calculation:

A person who weighs 164 lb and is 68 in. (or 5'8") tall has a BMI of 25:

[weight (164 lb)/height (68 in.²)] × 704.5 = 25

Source: Adapted from NHLBI Obesity Guidelines in Adults. http://www.nhlbi.nih.gov/guidelines/obesity/bmi_tbl.htm. Accessed October 13, 2011.

BMI online calculator. http://www.nhlbisupport.com/bmi/bmicalc.htm. Accessed October 13, 2011.

FUNCTIONAL ASSESSMENT SCREENING IN THE ELDERLY

FUNCTIONAL ASSESSMENT SCREENING IN THE ELDERLY

Target Area	Assessment Procedure	Abnormal Result	Suggested Intervention
Vision	Inquire about vision changes, Snellen chart testing.	Presence of vision changes; inability to read >20/40	Refer to ophthalmologist.
Hearing	Whisper a short, easily answered question such as "What is your name?" in each ear while the examiner's face is out of direct view. Use audioscope set at 40 dB; test using 1000 and 2000 Hz. Brief hearing loss screener.	Inability to answer question Inability to hear 1000 or 2000 Hz in both ears or inability to hear frequencies in either ear Brief hearing loss screen score ≥3	Examine auditory canals for cerumen and clean if necessary. Repeat test; if still abnormal in either ear, refer for audiometry and possible prosthesis.
Balance and gait	Observe the patient after instructing as follows: "Rise from your chair, walk 10 ft, return, and sit down." Check orthostatic blood pressure and heart rate.	Inability to complete task in 15 s	Performance-Oriented Mobility Assessment (POMA). Consider referral for physical therapy.
Continence of urine	Ask, "Do you ever lose your urine and get wet?" If yes, then ask, "Have you lost urine on at least 6 separate days?"	"Yes" to both questions	Ascertain frequency and amount. Search for remediable causes, including local irritations, polyuric states, and medications. Consider urologic referral.
Nutrition	Ask, "Without trying, have you lost 10 lb or more in the last 6 mo?" Weigh the patient. Measure height.	"Yes" or weight is below acceptable range for height	Do appropriate medical evaluation.

FUNCTIONAL ASSESSMENT SCREENING IN THE ELDERLY

Target Area	Assessment Procedure	Abnormal Result	Suggested Intervention
Mental status	Instruct as follows: "I am going to name three objects (pencil, truck, and book). I will ask you to repeat their names now and then again a few minutes from now."	Inability to recall all three objects after 1 min	Administer Folstein Mini-Mental State Examination. If score is <24, search for causes of cognitive impairment. Ascertain onset, duration, and fluctuation of overt symptoms. Review medications. Assess consciousness and affect. Do appropriate laboratory tests.
Depression	Ask, "Do you often feel sad or depressed?" or "How are your spirits?"	"Yes" or "Not very good, I guess"	Administer Geriatric Depression Scale or PHQ-9. If positive, check for antihypertensive, psychotropic, or other pertinent medications. Consider appropriate pharmacologic or psychiatric treatment.
ADL-IADL[a]	Ask, "Can you get out of bed yourself?" "Can you dress yourself?" "Can you make your own meals?" "Can you do your own shopping?"	"No" to any question	Corroborate responses with patient's appearance; question family members if accuracy is uncertain. Determine reasons for the inability (motivation compared with physical limitation). Institute appropriate medical, social, or environmental interventions.
Home environment	Ask, "Do you have trouble with stairs inside or outside of your home?" Ask about potential hazards inside the home with bathtubs, rugs, or lighting.	"Yes"	Evaluate home safety and institute appropriate countermeasures.

Social support	Ask, "Who would be able to help you in case of illness or emergency?"	—	List identified persons in the medical record. Become familiar with available resources for the elderly in the community.
Pain	Inquire about pain.	Presence of pain	Pain inventory.
Dentition	Oral examination.	Poor dentition	Dentistry referral.
Falls	Inquire about falls in past year and difficulty with walking or balance.	Presence of falls or gait/ balance problems	Falls evaluation.

[a]Activities of Daily Living–Instrumental Activities of Daily Living.

Source: Modified from Fleming KC, Evans JM, Weber DC, Chutka DS. Practical functional assessment of elderly persons: a primary-care approach. *Mayo Clin Proc.* 1995;70(9):890-910.

GERIATRIC DEPRESSION SCALE

GERIATRIC DEPRESSION SCALE

Choose the best answer for how you felt over the past week

1. Are you basically satisfied with your life?	yes/no
2. Have you dropped many of your activities and interests?	yes/no
3. Do you feel that your life is empty?	yes/no
4. Do you often get bored?	yes/no
5. Are you hopeful about the future?	yes/no
6. Are you bothered by thoughts you can't get out of your head?	yes/no
7. Are you in good spirits most of the time?	yes/no
8. Are you afraid that something bad is going to happen to you?	yes/no
9. Do you feel happy most of the time?	yes/no
10. Do you often feel helpless?	yes/no
11. Do you often get restless and fidgety?	yes/no
12. Do you prefer to stay at home, rather than going out and doing new things?	yes/no
13. Do you frequently worry about the future?	yes/no
14. Do you feel you have more problems with memory than most?	yes/no
15. Do you think it is wonderful to be alive now?	yes/no
16. Do you often feel downhearted and blue?	yes/no
17. Do you feel pretty worthless the way you are now?	yes/no
18. Do you worry a lot about the past?	yes/no
19. Do you find life very exciting?	yes/no
20. Is it hard for you to get started on new projects?	yes/no
21. Do you feel full of energy?	yes/no
22. Do you feel that your situation is hopeless?	yes/no
23. Do you think that most people are better off than you are?	yes/no
24. Do you frequently get upset over little things?	yes/no
25. Do you frequently feel like crying?	yes/no
26. Do you have trouble concentrating?	yes/no
27. Do you enjoy getting up in the morning?	yes/no
28. Do you prefer to avoid social gatherings?	yes/no
29. Is it easy for you to make decisions?	yes/no
30. Is your mind as clear as it used to be?	yes/no

One point for each is response suggestive of depression. (Specifically "no" responses to questions 1, 5, 7, 9, 15, 19, 21, 27, 29, and 30, and "yes" responses to the remaining questions are suggestive of depression.)

A score of ≥15 yields a sensitivity of 80% and a specificity of 100%, as a screening test for geriatric depression. *Clin Gerontol.* 1982;1:37.

Source: Reproduced with permission from Yesavage JA, Brink TL, Rose TL, et al. Development and validation of a geriatric depression screening scale: a preliminary report. *J Psychiatr Res.* 1982-1983;17:37.

IMMUNIZATION SCHEDULE

CDC VACCINE SCHEDULES FOR CHILDREN AND ADOLESCENTS

Figure 1. Recommended immunization schedule for children and adolescents aged 18 y or younger—United States, 2018. (FOR THOSE WHO FALL BEHIND OR START LATE, SEE THE CATCH-UP SCHEDULE [FIGURE 2]).

These recommendations must be read with the notes that follow. For those who fall behind or start late, provide catch-up vaccination at the earliest opportunity as indicated by the dark grey bars. To determine minimum intervals between doses, see the catch-up schedule (Table 2). School entry and adolescent vaccine age groups are shaded in gray.

Vaccine	Birth	1 mo	2 mos	4 mos	6 mos	9 mos	12 mos	15 mos	18 mos	19–23 mos	2–3 yrs	4–6 yrs	7–10 yrs	11–12 yrs	13–15 yrs	16 yrs	17–18 yrs
Hepatitis B (HepB)	1st dose	2nd dose			←—— 3rd dose ——→												
Rotavirus (RV): RV1 (2-dose series), RV5 (3-dose series)			1st dose	2nd dose	See Notes												
Diphtheria, tetanus, acellular pertussis (DTaP <7 yrs)			1st dose	2nd dose	3rd dose		←—— 4th dose ——→					5th dose					
Haemophilus influenzae type b (Hib)			1st dose	2nd dose	See Notes		3rd or 4th dose, See Notes										
Pneumococcal conjugate (PCV13)			1st dose	2nd dose	3rd dose		←—— 4th dose ——→										
Inactivated poliovirus (IPV <18 yrs)			1st dose	2nd dose	←—— 3rd dose ——→							4th dose					
Influenza (IIV)							Annual vaccination 1 or 2 doses				Annual vaccination 1 or 2 doses					
Influenza (LAIV)												Annual vaccination 1 dose only		Annual vaccination 1 dose only		
Measles, mumps, rubella (MMR)					See Notes		←—— 1st dose ——→					2nd dose					
Varicella (VAR)					See Notes		←—— 1st dose ——→					2nd dose					
Hepatitis A (HepA)					See Notes		2-dose series, See Notes										
Tetanus, diphtheria, acellular pertussis (Tdap ≥7 yrs)														Tdap			
Human papillomavirus (HPV)														See Notes			
Meningococcal (MenACWY-D ≥9 mos, MenACWY-CRM ≥2 mos)										See Notes				1st dose		2nd dose	
Meningococcal B														See Notes			
Pneumococcal polysaccharide (PPSV23)												See Notes					

Range of recommended ages for all children

Range of recommended ages for catch-up immunization

Range of recommended ages for certain high-risk groups

Recommended based on shared clinical decision-making or *can be used in this age group

No recommendation/ not applicable

Figure 2. Catch-up immunization schedule for persons age 4 mo through 18 y who start late or who are more than 1 mo behind—United States, 2017.

The table below provides catch-up schedules and minimum intervals between doses for children whose vaccinations have been delayed. A vaccine series does not need to be restarted, regardless of the time that has elapsed between doses. **Always use this table in conjunction with Table 1 and the notes that follow.**

Children age 4 months through 6 years

Vaccine	Minimum Age for Dose 1	Dose 1 to Dose 2	Dose 2 to Dose 3	Minimum Interval Between Doses	Dose 3 to Dose 4	Dose 4 to Dose 5
Hepatitis B	Birth	4 weeks	8 weeks and at least 16 weeks after first dose. Minimum age for the final dose is 24 weeks.			
Rotavirus	6 weeks Maximum age for first dose is 14 weeks, 6 days	4 weeks	4 weeks Maximum age for final dose is 8 months, 0 days.			
Diphtheria, tetanus, and acellular pertussis	6 weeks	4 weeks	4 weeks	6 months	6 months	6 months
Haemophilus influenzae type b	6 weeks	**No further doses needed** if first dose was administered at age 15 months or older. **4 weeks** if first dose was administered before the 1st birthday. **8 weeks (as final dose)** if first dose was administered at age 12 through 14 months.	**No further doses needed** if previous dose was administered at age 15 months or older. **4 weeks** if current age is younger than 12 months **and** first dose was administered at younger than age 7 months **and** at least 1 previous dose was PRP-T (ActHib, Pentacel, Hiberix) or unknown. **8 weeks and age 12 through 59 months (as final dose)** if current age is younger than 12 months **and** first dose was administered at age 7 through 11 months; OR if current age is 12 through 59 months **and** first dose was administered before the 1st birthday **and** second dose administered at younger than 15 months; OR if both doses were PRP-OMP (PedvaxHIB, Comvax) **and** were administered before the 1st birthday.	**8 weeks (as final dose)** This dose only necessary for children age 12 through 59 months who received 3 doses before the 1st birthday.		
Pneumococcal conjugate	6 weeks	**No further doses needed** for healthy children if first dose was administered at age 24 months or older. **4 weeks** if first dose was administered before the 1st birthday. **8 weeks (as final dose for healthy children)** if first dose was administered at the 1st birthday or after.	**No further doses needed** for healthy children if previous dose was administered at age 24 months or older. **4 weeks** if current age is younger than 12 months and previous dose was administered at <7 months old. **8 weeks (as final dose for healthy children)** if previous dose was administered between 7–11 months (wait until at least 12 months old); OR if current age is 12 months or older and at least 1 dose was given before age 12 months.	**8 weeks (as final dose)** This dose only necessary for children age 12 through 59 months who received 3 doses before age 12 months or for children at high risk who received 3 doses at any age.		
Inactivated poliovirus	6 weeks	4 weeks	**4 weeks** if current age is <4 years. **6 months (as final dose)** if current age is 4 years or older.	**6 months (minimum age 4 years for final dose).**		
Measles, mumps, rubella	12 months	4 weeks				
Varicella	12 months	3 months				
Hepatitis A	12 months	6 months				
Meningococcal ACWY	2 months MenACWY-CRM 9 months MenACWY-D	8 weeks	See Notes	See Notes		

Children and adolescents age 7 through 18 years

Vaccine	Minimum Age for Dose 1	Dose 1 to Dose 2	Dose 2 to Dose 3	Minimum Interval Between Doses	Dose 3 to Dose 4	Dose 4 to Dose 5
Meningococcal ACWY	Not applicable (N/A)	8 weeks				
Tetanus, diphtheria; tetanus, diphtheria, and acellular pertussis	7 years	4 weeks	**4 weeks** if first dose of DTaP/DT was administered before the 1st birthday. **6 months (as final dose)** if first dose of DTaP/DT or Tdap/Td was administered at or after the 1st birthday.	**6 months** if first dose of DTaP/DT was administered before the 1st birthday.		
Human papillomavirus	9 years	Routine dosing intervals are recommended.				
Hepatitis A	N/A	6 months				
Hepatitis B	N/A	4 weeks	8 weeks and at least 16 weeks after first dose.			
Inactivated poliovirus	N/A	4 weeks	**6 months** A fourth dose is not necessary if the third dose was administered at age 4 years or older and at least 6 months after the previous dose.	A fourth dose of IPV is indicated if all previous doses were administered at <4 years or if the third dose was administered <6 months after the second dose.		
Measles, mumps, rubella	N/A	4 weeks				
Varicella	N/A	3 months if younger than age 13 years. 4 weeks if age 13 years or older.				

Figure 3. Vaccines that might be indicated for children and adolescents age 18 y or younger based on medical indications.

Always use this table in conjunction with Table 1 and the notes that follow.

VACCINE	Pregnancy	Immunocom-promised status (excluding HIV infection)	HIV infection CD4+ count[1] <15% and total CD4 cell count of <200/mm³	HIV infection CD4+ count[1] ≥15% and total CD4 cell count of ≥200/mm³	Kidney failure, end-stage renal disease, or on hemodialysis	Heart disease or chronic lung disease	CSF leaks or cochlear implants	Asplenia or persistent complement component deficiencies	Chronic liver disease	Diabetes
Hepatitis B										
Rotavirus		SCID[2]								
Diphtheria, tetanus, & acellular pertussis (DTaP)										
Haemophilus influenzae type b										
Pneumococcal conjugate										
Inactivated poliovirus										
Influenza (IIV) or										
Influenza (LAIV)					Asthma, wheezing 2–4 yrs[3]					
Measles, mumps, rubella										
Varicella										
Hepatitis A										
Tetanus, diphtheria, & acellular pertussis (Tdap)										
Human papillomavirus										
Meningococcal ACWY										
Meningococcal B										
Pneumococcal polysaccharide										

Vaccination according to the routine schedule recommended

Recommended for persons with an additional risk factor for which the vaccine would be indicated

Vaccination is recommended, and additional doses may be necessary based on medical condition. See Notes.

Not recommended/ contraindicated—vaccine should not be administered

Precaution—vaccine might be indicated if benefit of protection outweighs risk of adverse reaction

Delay vaccination until after pregnancy if vaccine indicated

No recommendation/ not applicable

1 For additional information regarding HIV laboratory parameters and use of live vaccines, see the General Best Practice Guidelines for Immunization, "Altered Immunocompetence," at www.cdc.gov/vaccines/hcp/acip-recs/general-recs/immunocompetence.html and Table 4-1 (footnote D) at www.cdc.gov/vaccines/hcp/acip-recs/general-recs/contraindications.html.
2 Severe Combined Immunodeficiency
3 LAIV contraindicated for children 2–4 years of age with asthma or wheezing during the preceding 12 months.

Notes Recommended Child and Adolescent Immunization Schedule for ages 18 years or younger, United States, 2020

For vaccine recommendations for persons 19 years of age or older, see the Recommended Adult Immunization Schedule.

Additional information

• Consult relevant ACIP statements for detailed recommendations at www.cdc.gov/vaccines/hcp/acip-recs/index.html.

• For information on contraindications and precautions for the use of a vaccine, consult the General Best Practice Guidelines for Immunization at www.cdc.gov/vaccines/hcp/acip-recs/general-recs/contraindications.html and relevant ACIP statements at www.cdc.gov/vaccines/hcp/acip-recs/index.html.

• For calculating intervals between doses, 4 weeks = 28 days. Intervals of ≥4 months are determined by calendar months.

• Within a number range (e.g., 12–18), a dash (–) should be read as "through."

• Vaccine doses administered ≤4 days before the minimum age or interval are considered valid. Doses of any vaccine administered ≥5 days earlier than the minimum age or minimum interval should not be counted as valid and should be repeated as age-appropriate. The repeat dose should be spaced after the invalid dose by the recommended minimum interval. For further details, see Table 3-1, Recommended and minimum ages and intervals between vaccine doses, in General Best Practice Guidelines for Immunization at www.cdc.gov/vaccines/hcp/acip-recs/general-recs/timing.html.

• Information on travel vaccine requirements and recommendations is available at www.cdc.gov/travel/.

• For vaccination of persons with immunodeficiencies, see Table 8-1, Vaccination of persons with primary and secondary immunodeficiencies, in General Best Practice Guidelines for Immunization at www.cdc.gov/vaccines/hcp/acip-recs/general-recs/immunocompetence.html, and Immunization in Special Clinical Circumstances (In: Kimberlin DW, Brady MT, Jackson MA, Long SS, eds. Red Book: 2018 Report of the Committee on Infectious Diseases. 31st ed. Itasca, IL: American Academy of Pediatrics; 2018:67–111).

• For information regarding vaccination in the setting of a vaccine-preventable disease outbreak, contact your state or local health department.

• The National Vaccine Injury Compensation Program (VICP) is a no-fault alternative to the traditional legal system for resolving vaccine injury claims. All routine child and adolescent vaccines are covered by VICP except for pneumococcal polysaccharide vaccine (PPSV23). For more information, see www.hrsa.gov/vaccinecompensation/index.html.

Diphtheria, tetanus, and pertussis (DTaP) vaccination (minimum age: 6 weeks [4 years for Kinrix or Quadracel])

Routine vaccination

• 5-dose series at 2, 4, 6, 15–18 months, 4–6 years
 - Prospectively: Dose 4 may be administered as early as age 12 months if at least 6 months have elapsed since dose 3.
 - Retrospectively: A 4th dose that was inadvertently administered as early as 12 months may be counted if at least 4 months have elapsed since dose 3.

Catch-up vaccination

• Dose 5 is not necessary if dose 4 was administered at age 4 years or older and at least 6 months after dose 3.
• For other catch-up guidance, see Table 2.

Haemophilus influenzae type b vaccination (minimum age: 6 weeks)

Routine vaccination

• ActHIB, Hiberix, or Pentacel: 4-dose series at 2, 4, 6, 12–15 months
• PedvaxHIB: 3-dose series at 2, 4, 12–15 months

Catch-up vaccination

• Dose 1 at 7–11 months: Administer dose 2 at least 4 weeks later and dose 3 (final dose) at 12–15 months or 8 weeks after dose 2 (whichever is later).
• Dose 1 at 12–14 months: Administer dose 2 (final dose) at least 8 weeks after dose 1.
• Dose 1 before 12 months and dose 2 before 15 months: Administer dose 3 (final dose) 8 weeks after dose 2.
• 2 doses of PedvaxHIB before 12 months: Administer dose 3 (final dose) at 12–59 months and at least 8 weeks after dose 2.
• Unvaccinated at 15–59 months: 1 dose
• Previously unvaccinated children age 60 months or older who are not considered high risk do not require catch-up vaccination.
• For other catch-up guidance, see Table 2.

Special situations

• Chemotherapy or radiation treatment:
 12–59 months
 - Unvaccinated or only 1 dose before age 12 months: 2 doses, 8 weeks apart
 - 2 or more doses before age 12 months: 1 dose at least 8 weeks after previous dose
 Doses administered within 14 days of starting therapy or during therapy should be repeated at least 3 months after therapy completion.

• Hematopoietic stem cell transplant (HSCT):
 - 3-dose series 4 weeks apart starting 6 to 12 months after successful transplant, regardless of Hib vaccination history
• Anatomic or functional asplenia (including sickle cell disease):
 12–59 months
 - Unvaccinated or only 1 dose before age 12 months: 2 doses, 8 weeks apart
 - 2 or more doses before age 12 months: 1 dose at least 8 weeks after previous dose
 Unvaccinated* persons age 5 years or older
 - 1 dose
• Elective splenectomy:
 Unvaccinated* persons age 15 months or older
 - 1 dose (preferably at least 14 days before procedure)
• HIV infection:
 12–59 months
 - Unvaccinated or only 1 dose before age 12 months: 2 doses, 8 weeks apart
 - 2 or more doses before age 12 months: 1 dose at least 8 weeks after previous dose
 Unvaccinated* persons age 5–18 years
 - 1 dose
• Immunoglobulin deficiency, early component complement deficiency:
 12–59 months
 - Unvaccinated or only 1 dose before age 12 months: 2 doses, 8 weeks apart
 - 2 or more doses before age 12 months: 1 dose at least 8 weeks after previous dose

*Unvaccinated = Less than routine series (through 14 months) OR no doses (15 months or older)

Hepatitis A vaccination
(minimum age: 12 months for routine vaccination)

Routine vaccination
- 2-dose series (minimum interval: 6 months) beginning at age 12 months

Catch-up vaccination
- Unvaccinated persons through 18 years should complete a 2-dose series (minimum interval: 6 months).
- Persons who previously received 1 dose at age 12 months or older should receive dose 2 at least 6 months after dose 1.
- Adolescents 18 years and older may receive the combined HepA and HepB vaccine, **Twinrix**, as a 3-dose series (0, 1, and 6 months).

International travel
- Persons traveling to or working in countries with high or intermediate endemic hepatitis A (www.cdc.gov/travel/):
- **Infants age 6-11 months:** 1 dose before departure; revaccinate with 2 doses, separated by at least 6 months, between 12 and 23 months of age
- **Unvaccinated age 12 months and older:** Administer dose 1 as soon as travel is considered.

Hepatitis B vaccination
(minimum age: birth)

Birth dose (monovalent HepB vaccine only)
- **Mother is HBsAg-negative:** 1 dose within 24 hours of birth for all medically stable infants ≥2,000 grams. Infants <2,000 grams: Administer 1 dose at chronological age 1 month or hospital discharge.
- **Mother is HBsAg-positive:**
- Administer **HepB vaccine** and **hepatitis B immune globulin (HBIG)** (in separate limbs) within 12 hours of birth, regardless of birth weight. For infants <2,000 grams, administer 3 additional doses of vaccine (total of 4 doses) beginning at age 1 month.
- Test for HBsAg and anti-HBs at age 9-12 months. If HepB series is delayed, test 1-2 months after final dose.
- **Mother's HBsAg status is unknown:**
- Administer **HepB vaccine** within 12 hours of birth, regardless of birth weight.
- For infants <2,000 grams, administer **HBIG** in addition to HepB vaccine (in separate limbs) within 12 hours of birth. Administer 3 additional doses of vaccine (total of 4 doses) beginning at age 1 month.
- Determine mother's HBsAg status as soon as possible. If mother is HBsAg-positive, administer **HBIG** to infants ≥2,000 grams as soon as possible, but no later than 7 days of age.

Routine series
- 3-dose series at 0, 1-2, 6-18 months (use monovalent HepB vaccine for doses administered before age 6 weeks)

- Infants who did not receive a birth dose should begin the series as soon as feasible (see Table 2).
- Administration of **4 doses** is permitted when a combination vaccine containing HepB is used after the birth dose.
- **Minimum age** for the final (3rd or 4th) dose: 24 weeks.
- **Minimum intervals:** dose 1 to dose 2: 4 weeks / dose 2 to dose 3: 8 weeks / dose 1 to dose 3: 16 weeks (when 4 doses are administered, substitute "dose 4" for "dose 3" in these calculations)

Catch-up vaccination
- Unvaccinated persons should complete a 3-dose series at 0, 1-2, 6 months.
- Adolescents age 11-15 years may use an alternative 2-dose schedule with at least 4 months between doses (adult formulation **Recombivax HB** only).
- Adolescents 18 years and older may receive a 2-dose series of HepB (**Heplisav-B**†) at least 4 weeks apart.
- Adolescents 18 years and older may receive the combined HepA and HepB vaccine, **Twinrix**, as a 3-dose series (0, 1, and 6 months) or 4-dose series (0, 7, and 21-30 days, followed by a dose at 12 months).
- For other catch-up guidance, see Table 2.

Special situations
- Revaccination is not generally recommended for persons with a normal immune status who were vaccinated as infants, children, adolescents, or adults.
- **Revaccination** may be recommended for certain populations, including:
  - **Infants born to HBsAg-positive mothers**
  - **Hemodialysis patients**
  - **Other immunocompromised persons**
- For detailed revaccination recommendations, see www.cdc.gov/vaccines/hcp/acip-recs/vacc-specific/hepb.html.

Human papillomavirus vaccination
(minimum age: 9 years)

Routine and catch-up vaccination
- HPV vaccination routinely recommended at **age 11-12 years** (can start at age 9 years) and catch-up HPV vaccination recommended for all persons through age 18 years if not adequately vaccinated
- 2- or 3-dose series depending on age at initial vaccination:
  - **Age 9 through 14 years at initial vaccination:** 2-dose series at 0, 6-12 months (minimum interval: 5 months; repeat dose if administered too soon)
  - **Age 15 years or older at initial vaccination:** 3-dose series at 0, 1-2, 6 months (minimum intervals: dose 1 to dose 2: 4 weeks / dose 2 to dose 3: 12 weeks / dose 1 to dose 3: 5 months; repeat dose if administered too soon)
- If completed valid vaccination series with any HPV vaccine, no additional doses needed

Special situations
- **Immunocompromising conditions, including HIV infection:** 3-dose series as above
- **History of sexual abuse or assault:** Start at age 9 years.
- **Pregnancy:** HPV vaccination not recommended until after pregnancy; no intervention needed if vaccinated while pregnant; pregnancy testing not needed before vaccination

Influenza vaccination
(minimum age: 6 months [IIV], 2 years [LAIV], 18 years [recombinant influenza vaccine, RIV])

Routine vaccination
- Use any influenza vaccine appropriate for age and health status annually:
  - 2 doses, separated by at least 4 weeks, for children age 6 **months-8 years** who have received fewer than 2 influenza vaccine doses before July 1, 2019, or whose influenza vaccination history is unknown (administer dose 2 even if the child turns 9 between receipt of dose 1 and dose 2)
  - 1 dose for **children age 6 months-8 years** who have received at least 2 influenza vaccine doses before July 1, 2019
  - 1 dose for **all persons age 9 years and older**
- For the 2020-21 season, see the 2020-21 ACIP influenza vaccine recommendations.

Special situations
- **Egg allergy, hives only:** Any influenza vaccine appropriate for age and health status annually
- **Egg allergy with symptoms other than hives** (e.g., angioedema, respiratory distress, need for emergency medical services or epinephrine): Any influenza vaccine appropriate for age and health status annually in medical setting under supervision of health care provider who can recognize and manage severe allergic reactions
- **LAIV should not be used** in persons with the following conditions or situations:
  - History of severe allergic reaction to a previous dose of any influenza vaccine or to any vaccine component (excluding egg, see details above)
  - Receiving aspirin or salicylate-containing medications
  - Age 2-4 years with history of asthma or wheezing
  - Immunocompromised due to any cause (including medications and HIV infection)
  - Anatomic or functional asplenia
  - Cochlear implant
  - Cerebrospinal fluid-oropharyngeal communication
  - Close contacts or caregivers of severely immunosuppressed persons who require a protected environment
  - Pregnancy
  - Received influenza antiviral medications within the previous 48 hours

Measles, mumps, and rubella vaccination
(minimum age: 12 months for routine vaccination)

Routine vaccination
- 2-dose series at 12–15 months, 4–6 years
- Dose 2 may be administered as early as 4 weeks after dose 1.

Catch-up vaccination
- Unvaccinated children and adolescents: 2-dose series at least 4 weeks apart
- The maximum age for use of MMRV is 12 years.

Special situations

International travel
- **Infants age 6–11 months:** 1 dose before departure; revaccinate with 2-dose series with dose 1 at 12–15 months (12 months for children in high-risk areas) and dose 2 as early as 4 weeks later.
- **Unvaccinated children age 12 months and older:** 2-dose series at least 4 weeks apart before departure

Meningococcal serogroup A,C,W,Y vaccination
(minimum age: 2 months [MenACWY-CRM, MenVeo], 9 months [MenACWY-D, Menactra])

Routine vaccination
- 2-dose series at 11–12 years, 16 years

Catch-up vaccination
- Age 13–15 years: 1 dose now and booster at age 16–18 years (minimum interval: 8 weeks)
- Age 16–18 years: 1 dose

Special situations
Anatomic or functional asplenia (including sickle cell disease), HIV infection, persistent complement component deficiency, complement inhibitor (e.g., eculizumab, ravulizumab) use:
- **Menveo**
  - Dose 1 at age 8 weeks: 4-dose series at 2, 4, 6, 12 months
  - Dose 1 at age 7–23 months: 2-dose series (dose 2 at least 12 weeks after dose 1 and after age 12 months)
  - Dose 1 at age 24 months or older: 2-dose series at least 8 weeks apart
- **Menactra**
  - **Persistent complement component deficiency or complement inhibitor use:**
    - Age 9–23 months: 2-dose series at least 8 weeks apart
    - Age 24 months or older: 2-dose series at least 8 weeks apart
  - **Anatomic or functional asplenia, sickle cell disease, or HIV infection:**
    - Age 9–23 months: Not recommended
    - Age 24 months or older: 2-dose series at least 8 weeks apart
    - **Menactra** must be administered at least 4 weeks after completion of PCV13 series.

Travel in countries with hyperendemic or epidemic meningococcal disease, including countries in the African meningitis belt or during the Hajj (www.cdc.gov/travel/):
- Children less than age 24 months:
  - **Menveo (age 2–23 months):**
    - Dose 1 at 8 weeks: 4-dose series at 2, 4, 6, 12 months
    - Dose 1 at 7–23 months: 2-dose series (dose 2 at least 12 weeks after dose 1 and after age 12 months)
  - **Menactra (age 9–23 months):**
    - 2-dose series (dose 2 at least 12 weeks after dose 1; dose 2 may be administered as early as 8 weeks after dose 1 in travelers)
- Children age 2 years or older: 1 dose **Menveo or Menactra**

First-year college students who live in residential housing (if not previously vaccinated at age 16 years or older) or military recruits:
- 1 dose **Menveo or Menactra**

Adolescent vaccination of children who received MenACWY prior to age 10 years:
- **Children for whom boosters are recommended** because of an ongoing increased risk of meningococcal disease (e.g., those with complement deficiency, HIV, or asplenia): Follow the booster schedule for persons at increased risk (see below).
- **Children for whom boosters are not recommended** (e.g., those who received a single dose for travel to a country where meningococcal disease is endemic): Administer MenACWY according to the recommended adolescent schedule with dose 1 at age 11–12 years and dose 2 at age 16 years.

Note: Menactra should be administered either before or at the same time as DTaP. For MenACWY **booster dose** recommendations for groups listed under "Special situations" and in an outbreak setting and for additional meningococcal vaccination information, see www.cdc.gov/vaccines/hcp/acip-recs/vacc-specific/mening.html.

Meningococcal serogroup B vaccination
(minimum age: 10 years [MenB-4C, Bexsero; MenB-FHbp, Trumenba])

Shared clinical decision-making
- **Adolescents not at increased risk** age 16–23 years (preferred age 16–18 years) based on shared clinical decision-making:
  - **Bexsero:** 2-dose series at least 1 month apart
  - **Trumenba:** 2-dose series at least 6 months apart; if dose 2 is administered earlier than 6 months, administer a 3rd dose at least 4 months after dose 2.

Special situations
Anatomic or functional asplenia (including sickle cell disease), persistent complement component deficiency, complement inhibitor (e.g., eculizumab, ravulizumab) use:
- **Bexsero:** 2-dose series at least 1 month apart
- **Trumenba:** 3-dose series at 0, 1–2, 6 months

Bexsero and **Trumenba** are not interchangeable; the same product should be used for all doses in a series. For MenB **booster dose recommendations** for groups listed under "Special situations" and in an outbreak setting and for additional meningococcal vaccination information, see www. cdc.gov/vaccines/acip/recommendations.html and www.cdc.gov/vaccines/hcp/acip-recs/vacc-specific/mening.html.

Pneumococcal vaccination
(minimum age: 6 weeks [PCV13], 2 years [PPSV23])

Routine vaccination with PCV13
- 4-dose series at 2, 4, 6, 12–15 months

Catch-up vaccination with PCV13
- 1 dose for healthy children age 24–59 months with any incomplete* PCV13 series
- For other catch-up guidance, see Table 2.

Special situations
High-risk conditions below: When both PCV13 and PPSV23 are indicated, administer PCV13 first. PCV13 and PPSV23 should not be administered during the same visit.

Chronic heart disease (particularly cyanotic congenital heart disease and cardiac failure), chronic lung disease (including asthma treated with high-dose, oral corticosteroids), diabetes mellitus:

Age 2–5 years
- Any incomplete* series with:
  - 3 PCV13 doses: 1 dose PCV13 (at least 8 weeks after any prior PCV13 dose)
  - Less than 3 PCV13 doses: 2 doses PCV13 (8 weeks after the most recent dose and administered 8 weeks apart)
  - No history of PPSV23: 1 dose PPSV23 (at least 8 weeks after any prior PCV13 dose)

Age 6–18 years
- No history of PPSV23: 1 dose PPSV23 (at least 8 weeks after any prior PCV13 dose)

Cerebrospinal fluid leak, cochlear implant:

Age 2–5 years
- Any incomplete* series with:
  - 3 PCV13 doses: 1 dose PCV13 (at least 8 weeks after any prior PCV13 dose)
  - Less than 3 PCV13 doses: 2 doses PCV13 (8 weeks after the most recent dose and administered 8 weeks apart)
  - No history of PPSV23: 1 dose PPSV23 (at least 8 weeks after any prior PCV13 dose)

Age 6–18 years
- No history of either PCV13 or PPSV23: 1 dose PCV13, 1 dose PPSV23 at least 8 weeks later
- Any PCV13 but no PPSV23: 1 dose PPSV23 at least 8 weeks after the most recent dose of PCV13
- PPSV23 but no PCV13: 1 dose PCV13 at least 8 weeks after the most recent dose of PPSV23

Sickle cell disease and other hemoglobinopathies; anatomic or functional asplenia; congenital or acquired immunodeficiency; HIV infection; chronic renal failure; nephrotic syndrome; malignant neoplasms, leukemias, lymphomas, Hodgkin disease, and other diseases associated with treatment with immunosuppressive drugs or radiation therapy; solid organ transplantation; multiple myeloma:

Age 2–5 years

- Any incomplete* series with:
  - 3 PCV13 doses: 1 dose PCV13 (8 weeks after any prior PCV13 dose)
  - Less than 3 PCV13 doses: 2 doses PCV13 (8 weeks after the most recent dose and administered 8 weeks apart)
- No history of PPSV23: 1 dose PPSV23 (at least 8 weeks after any prior PCV13 dose) and a 2nd dose of PPSV23 5 years later

Age 6–18 years

- No history of either PCV13 or PPSV23: 1 dose PCV13, 2 doses PPSV23 (dose 1 of PPSV23 administered 8 weeks after PCV13 and dose 2 of PPSV23 administered at least 5 years after dose 1 of PPSV23)
- Any PCV13 but no PPSV23: 2 doses PPSV23 (dose 1 of PPSV23 administered 8 weeks after the most recent dose of PCV13 and dose 2 of PPSV23 administered at least 5 years after dose 1 of PPSV23)
- PPSV23 but no PCV13: 1 dose PCV13 (at least 8 weeks after the most recent PPSV23 dose and a 2nd dose of PPSV23 administered 5 years after dose 1 of PPSV23 and at least 8 weeks after a dose of PCV13

Chronic liver disease, alcoholism:

Age 6–18 years

- No history of PPSV23: 1 dose PPSV23 (at least 8 weeks after any prior PCV13 dose)

*Incomplete series = Not having received all doses in either the recommended series or an age-appropriate catch-up series. See Tables 8, 9, and 11 in the ACIP pneumococcal vaccine recommendations at www.cdc.gov/mmwr/pdf/rr/rr5911.pdf for complete schedule details.

Poliovirus vaccination
(minimum age: 6 weeks)

Routine vaccination

- 4-dose series at ages 2, 4, 6–18 months, 4–6 years; administer the final dose on or after age 4 years and at least 6 months after the previous dose.
- 4 or more doses of IPV can be administered before age 4 years when a combination vaccine containing IPV is used. However, a dose is still recommended at or after age 4 years and at least 6 months after the previous dose.

Catch-up vaccination

- In the first 6 months of life, use minimum ages and intervals only for travel to a polio-endemic region or during an outbreak.
- IPV is not routinely recommended for U.S. residents 18 years and older.

Series containing oral polio vaccine (OPV), either mixed OPV-IPV or OPV-only series:

- Total number of doses needed to complete the series is the same as that recommended for the U.S. IPV schedule. See www.cdc.gov/mmwr/volumes/66/wr/mm6601a6.htm?s_cid=mm6601a6_w.
- Only trivalent OPV (tOPV) counts toward the U.S. vaccination requirements.
  - Doses of OPV administered before April 1, 2016, should be counted (unless specifically noted as administered during a campaign).
  - Doses of OPV administered on or after April 1, 2016, should not be counted.
- For guidance to assess doses documented as "OPV," see www.cdc.gov/mmwr/volumes/66/wr/mm6606a7.htm?s_cid=mm6606a7_w.
- For other catch-up guidance, see Table 2.

Rotavirus vaccination
(minimum age: 6 weeks)

Routine vaccination

- **Rotarix:** 2-dose series at 2 and 4 months
- **RotaTeq:** 3-dose series at 2, 4, and 6 months
- If any dose in the series is either RotaTeq or unknown, default to 3-dose series.

Catch-up vaccination

- Do not start the series on or after age 15 weeks, 0 days.
- The maximum age for the final dose is 8 months, 0 days.
- For other catch-up guidance, see Table 2.

Tetanus, diphtheria, and pertussis (Tdap) vaccination
(minimum age: 11 years for routine vaccination, 7 years for catch-up vaccination)

Routine vaccination

- **Adolescents age 11–12 years:** 1 dose Tdap
- **Pregnancy:** 1 dose Tdap during each pregnancy, preferably in early part of gestational weeks 27–36
- Tdap may be administered regardless of the interval since the last tetanus- and diphtheria-toxoid-containing vaccine.

Catch-up vaccination

- **Adolescents age 13–18 years who have not received Tdap:** 1 dose Tdap, then Td or Tdap booster every 10 years
- **Persons age 7–18 years not fully vaccinated† with DTaP:** 1 dose Tdap as part of the catch-up series (preferably the first dose); if additional doses are needed, use Td or Tdap.
- **Tdap administered at 7–10 years:**
  - **Children age 7–9 years** who receive Tdap should receive the routine Tdap dose at age 11–12 years.
  - **Children age 10 years** who receive Tdap do not need to receive the routine Tdap dose at age 11–12 years.
- **DTaP inadvertently administered at or after age 7 years:**
  - **Children age 7–9 years:** DTaP may count as part of catch-up series. Routine Tdap dose at age 11–12 years should be administered.
  - **Children age 10–18 years:** Count dose of DTaP as the adolescent Tdap booster.
- For other catch-up guidance, see Table 2.
- For information on use of Tdap or Td as tetanus prophylaxis in wound management, see www.cdc.gov/mmwr/volumes/67/rr/rr6702a1.htm.

†Fully vaccinated = 5 valid doses of DTaP OR 4 valid doses of DTaP if dose 4 was administered at age 4 years or older

Varicella vaccination
(minimum age: 12 months)

Routine vaccination

- 2-dose series at 12–15 months, 4–6 years
- Dose 2 may be administered as early as 3 months after dose 1 (a dose administered after a 4-week interval may be counted).

Catch-up vaccination

- Ensure persons age 7–18 years without evidence of immunity (see www.cdc.gov/mmwr/pdf/rr/rr5604.pdf) have 2-dose series:
  - **Age 7–12 years:** routine interval: 3 months (a dose administered after a 4-week interval may be counted)
  - **Age 13 years and older:** routine interval: 4–8 weeks (minimum interval: 4 weeks)
- The maximum age for use of MMRV is 12 years.

CDC VACCINE SCHEDULES FOR ADULTS

Figure 4. Recommended immunization schedule for adults aged 19 y or older by age group, United States, 2017.

Vaccine	19–26 years	27–49 years	50–64 years	≥65 years
Influenza inactivated (IIV) or Influenza recombinant (RIV), **or**	1 dose annually			
Influenza live, attenuated (LAIV)	1 dose annually			
Tetanus, diphtheria, pertussis (Tdap or Td)	1 dose Tdap, then Td or Tdap booster every 10 years			
Measles, mumps, rubella (MMR)	1 or 2 doses depending on indication (if born in 1957 or later)			
Varicella (VAR)	2 doses			
Zoster recombinant (RZV) *(preferred)*, **or**			2 doses	
Zoster live (ZVL)			1 dose	
Human papillomavirus (HPV)	2 or 3 doses depending on age at initial vaccination or condition	27 through 45 years		
Pneumococcal conjugate (PCV13)		1 dose		65 years and older
Pneumococcal polysaccharide (PPSV23)	1 or 2 doses depending on indication			1 dose
Hepatitis A (HepA)	2 or 3 doses depending on vaccine			
Hepatitis B (HepB)	2 or 3 doses depending on vaccine			
Meningococcal A, C, W, Y (MenACWY)	1 or 2 doses depending on indication, see notes for booster recommendations			
Meningococcal B (MenB)	19 through 23 years	2 or 3 doses depending on vaccine and indication, see notes for booster recommendations		
Haemophilus influenzae type b (Hib)	1 or 3 doses depending on indication			

Recommended vaccination for adults who meet age requirement, lack documentation of vaccination, or lack evidence of past infection

Recommended vaccination for adults with an additional risk factor or another indication

Recommended vaccination based on shared clinical decision-making

No recommendation/Not applicable

Vaccine	Pregnancy	Immunocompromised (excluding HIV infection)	HIV infection CD4 count <200	HIV infection CD4 count ≥200	Asplenia, complement deficiencies	End-stage renal disease; or on hemodialysis	Heart or lung disease, alcoholism[1]	Chronic liver disease	Diabetes	Health care personnel[2]	Men who have sex with men
IIV or RIV	1 dose annually										
LAIV	1 dose annually (or)	NOT RECOMMENDED					PRECAUTION			1 dose annually (or)	1 dose annually
Tdap or Td	1 dose Tdap each pregnancy	1 dose Tdap, then Td or Tdap booster every 10 years									
MMR	NOT RECOMMENDED	NOT RECOMMENDED	NOT RECOMMENDED	1 or 2 doses depending on indication							
VAR	NOT RECOMMENDED	NOT RECOMMENDED	NOT RECOMMENDED	2 doses							
RZV (preferred) (or) ZVL	DELAY (or) NOT RECOMMENDED	NOT RECOMMENDED		2 doses at age ≥50 years (or) 1 dose at age ≥60 years							
HPV	DELAY	3 doses through age 26 years			2 or 3 doses through age 26 years						
PCV13					1 dose						
PPSV23					1, 2, or 3 doses depending on age and indication						
HepA					2 or 3 doses depending on vaccine						
HepB					2 or 3 doses depending on vaccine						
MenACWY	1 or 2 doses depending on indication, see notes for booster recommendations										
MenB	PRECAUTION	2 or 3 doses depending on vaccine and indication, see notes for booster recommendations									
Hib		3 doses HSCT[3] recipients only			1 dose						

Legend:
- Recommended vaccination for adults who meet age requirement, lack documentation of vaccination, or lack evidence of past infection
- Recommended vaccination for adults with an additional risk factor or another indication
- Precaution—vaccination might be indicated if benefit of protection outweighs risk of adverse reaction
- Delay vaccination until after pregnancy if vaccine is indicated
- Not recommended/contraindicated—vaccine should not be administered
- No recommendation/Not applicable

1. Precaution for LAIV does not apply to alcoholism. 2. See notes for influenza; hepatitis B; measles, mumps, and rubella; and varicella vaccinations. 3. Hematopoietic stem cell transplant.

Notes　Recommended Adult Immunization Schedule, United States, 2020

Haemophilus influenzae type b vaccination

Special situations

Anatomical or functional asplenia (including sickle cell disease): 1 dose if previously did not receive Hib; if elective splenectomy, 1 dose, preferably at least 14 days before splenectomy

• **Hematopoietic stem cell transplant (HSCT):** 3-dose series 4 weeks apart starting 6–12 months after successful transplant, regardless of Hib vaccination history

Hepatitis A vaccination

Routine vaccination

• **Not at risk but want protection from hepatitis A** (identification of risk factor not required): 2-dose series HepA (Havrix 6–12 months apart or Vaqta 6–18 months apart [minimum interval: 6 months]) or 3-dose series HepA-HepB (Twinrix at 0, 1, 6 months [minimum intervals: 4 weeks between doses 1 and 2/5 months between doses 2 and 3])

Special situations

• **At risk for hepatitis A virus infection:** 2-dose series HepA or 3-dose series HepA-HepB as above
• **Chronic liver disease** (e.g., persons with hepatitis B, hepatitis C, cirrhosis, fatty liver disease, alcoholic liver disease, autoimmune hepatitis, alanine aminotransferase [ALT] or aspartate aminotransferase [AST] level greater than twice the upper limit of normal)
• **HIV infection**
• **Men who have sex with men**
• **Injection or noninjection drug use**
• **Persons experiencing homelessness**
• **Work with hepatitis A virus** in research laboratory or with nonhuman primates with hepatitis A virus infection
• **Travel in countries with high or intermediate endemic hepatitis A**
• **Close, personal contact with international adoptee** (e.g., household or regular babysitting) in first 60 days after arrival from country with high or intermediate endemic hepatitis A (administer dose 1 as soon as adoption is planned, at least 2 weeks before adoptee's arrival)

Pregnancy if at risk for infection or severe outcome from infection during pregnancy

Settings for exposure, including health care settings targeting services to injection or noninjection drug users or group homes and nonresidential day care facilities for developmentally disabled persons (individual risk factor screening not required)

Hepatitis B vaccination

Routine vaccination

• **Not at risk but want protection from hepatitis B** (identification of risk factor not required): 2- or 3-dose series (2-dose series Heplisav-B at least 4 weeks apart [2-dose series HepB only applies when 2 doses of Heplisav-B are used at least 4 weeks apart] or 3-dose series Engerix-B or Recombivax HB at 0, 1, 6 months [minimum intervals: 4 weeks between doses 1 and 2/8 weeks between doses 2 and 3/16 weeks between doses 1 and 3]) or 3-dose series HepA-HepB (Twinrix at 0, 1, 6 months [minimum intervals: 4 weeks between doses 1 and 2/5 months between doses 2 and 3])

Special situations

• **At risk for hepatitis B virus infection:** 2-dose (Heplisav-B) or 3-dose (Engerix-B, Recombivax HB) series or 3-dose series HepA-HepB (Twinrix) as above
• **Chronic liver disease** (e.g., persons with hepatitis C, cirrhosis, fatty liver disease, alcoholic liver disease, autoimmune hepatitis, alanine aminotransferase [ALT] or aspartate aminotransferase [AST] level greater than twice upper limit of normal)
• **HIV infection**
• **Sexual exposure risk** (e.g., sex partners of hepatitis B surface antigen [HBsAg]-positive persons; sexually active persons not in mutually monogamous relationships; persons seeking evaluation or treatment for a sexually transmitted infection; men who have sex with men)
• **Current or recent injection drug use**
• **Percutaneous or mucosal risk for exposure to blood** (e.g., household contacts of HBsAg-positive persons; residents and staff of facilities for developmentally disabled persons; health care and public safety personnel with reasonably anticipated risk for

exposure to blood or blood-contaminated body fluids; hemodialysis, peritoneal dialysis, home dialysis, and predialysis patients; persons with diabetes mellitus age younger than 60 years and, at discretion of treating clinician, those age 60 years or older)

• **Incarcerated persons**
• **Travel in countries with high or intermediate endemic hepatitis B**

Pregnancy if at risk for infection or severe outcome from infection during pregnancy (Heplisav-B not currently recommended due to lack of safety data in pregnant women)

Human papillomavirus vaccination

Routine vaccination

• **HPV vaccination recommended for all adults through age 26 years:** 2- or 3-dose series depending on age at initial vaccination or condition:

• **Age 15 years or older at initial vaccination:** 3-dose series at 0, 1–2, 6 months (minimum intervals: 4 weeks between doses 1 and 2/12 weeks between doses 2 and 3/5 months between doses 1 and 3; repeat dose if administered too soon)

• **Age 9 through 14 years at initial vaccination and received 1 dose or 2 doses less than 5 months apart:** 1 dose

• **Age 9 through 14 years at initial vaccination and received 2 doses at least 5 months apart:** HPV vaccination complete, no additional dose needed.

• **If completed valid vaccination series with any HPV vaccine, no additional doses needed**

Shared clinical decision-making

• **Age 27 through 45 years based on shared clinical decision-making:**
  • 2- or 3-dose series as above

Special situations

• **Pregnancy through age 26 years:** HPV vaccination is not recommended until after pregnancy; no intervention needed if vaccinated while pregnant; pregnancy testing not needed before vaccination

Influenza vaccination

Routine vaccination

- **Persons age 6 months or older:** 1 dose any influenza vaccine appropriate for age and health status annually
- For additional guidance, see www.cdc.gov/flu/professionals/index.htm

Special situations

- **Egg allergy, hives only:** 1 dose any influenza vaccine appropriate for age and health status annually
- **Egg allergy more severe than hives** (e.g., angioedema, respiratory distress): 1 dose any influenza vaccine appropriate for age and health status annually in medical setting under supervision of health care provider who can recognize and manage severe allergic reactions
- **LAIV should not be used** in persons with the following conditions or situations:
  - History of severe allergic reaction to any vaccine component (excluding egg) or to a previous dose of any influenza vaccine
  - Immunocompromised due to any cause (including medications and HIV infection)
  - Anatomic or functional asplenia
  - Cochlear implant
  - Cerebrospinal fluid-oropharyngeal communication
  - Close contacts or caregivers of severely immunosuppressed persons who require a protected environment
  - Pregnancy
  - Received influenza antiviral medications within the previous 48 hours
- **History of Guillain-Barré syndrome within 6 weeks of previous dose of influenza vaccine:** Generally should not be vaccinated unless vaccination benefits outweigh risks for those at higher risk for severe complications from influenza

Measles, mumps, and rubella vaccination

Routine vaccination

- **No evidence of immunity to measles, mumps, or rubella:** 1 dose
  - **Evidence of immunity:** Born before 1957 (health care personnel, see below), documentation of receipt of MMR vaccine, laboratory evidence of immunity or disease (diagnosis of disease without laboratory confirmation is not evidence of immunity)

Special situations

- **Pregnancy with no evidence of immunity to rubella:** MMR contraindicated during pregnancy; after pregnancy (before discharge from health care facility), 1 dose
- **Nonpregnant women of childbearing age with no evidence of immunity to rubella:** 1 dose
- **HIV infection with CD4 count ≥200 cells/µL for at least 6 months and no evidence of immunity to measles, mumps, or rubella:** 2-dose series at least 4 weeks apart; MMR contraindicated in HIV infection with CD4 count <200 cells/µL
- **Severe immunocompromising conditions:** MMR contraindicated
- **Students in postsecondary educational institutions, international travelers, and household or close, personal contacts of immunocompromised persons with no evidence of immunity to measles, mumps, or rubella:** 2-dose series at least 4 weeks apart if previously did not receive any doses of MMR or 1 dose if previously received 1 dose MMR
- **Health care personnel:**
  - Born in 1957 or later with no evidence of immunity to measles, mumps, or rubella: 2-dose series at least 4 weeks apart for measles or mumps or at least 1 dose for rubella
  - Born before 1957 with no evidence of immunity to measles, mumps, or rubella: Consider 2-dose series at least 4 weeks apart for measles or mumps or 1 dose for rubella

Meningococcal vaccination

Special situations for MenACWY

- **Anatomical or functional asplenia (including sickle cell disease), HIV infection, persistent complement component deficiency, complement inhibitor (e.g., eculizumab, ravulizumab) use:** 2-dose series MenACWY (Menactra, Menveo) at least 8 weeks apart and revaccinate every 5 years if risk remains
- **Travel in countries with hyperendemic or epidemic meningococcal disease, microbiologists routinely exposed to *Neisseria meningitidis*:** 1 dose MenACWY (Menactra, Menveo) and revaccinate every 5 years if risk remains
- **First-year college students who live in residential housing (if not previously vaccinated at age 16 years or older) and military recruits:** 1 dose MenACWY (Menactra, Menveo)

Shared clinical decision-making for MenB

- **Adolescents and young adults age 16 through 23 years (age 16 through 18 years preferred) not at increased risk for meningococcal disease:** Based on shared clinical decision-making, 2-dose series

  MenB-4C at least 1 month apart or 2-dose series

  MenB-FHbp at 0, 6 months (if dose 2 was administered less than 6 months after dose 1, administer dose 3 at least 4 months after dose 2); MenB-4C and MenB-FHbp are not interchangeable (use same product for all doses in series)

Special situations for MenB

- **Anatomical or functional asplenia (including sickle cell disease), persistent complement component deficiency, complement inhibitor (e.g., eculizumab, ravulizumab) use, microbiologists routinely exposed to *Neisseria meningitidis*:** 2-dose primary series

  MenB-4C (Bexsero) at least 1 month apart or 3-dose primary series MenB-FHbp (Trumenba) at 0, 1–2, 6 months (if dose 2 was administered at least 6 months after dose 1, dose 3 not needed); MenB-4C and MenB-FHbp are not interchangeable (use same product for all doses in series); 1 dose MenB booster 1 year after primary series and revaccinate every 2–3 years if risk remains
- **Pregnancy:** Delay MenB until after pregnancy unless at increased risk and vaccination benefits outweigh potential risks

Figure 5. Recommended immunization schedule for adults aged 19 yr or older by medical condition and other indications, United States, 2017.

Pneumococcal vaccination

Routine vaccination

- **Age 65 years or older** (immunocompetent--see www.cdc.gov/mmwr/volumes/68/wr/mm6846a5.htm?s_cid=mm6846a5_w): 1 dose PPSV23
  - If PPSV23 was administered prior to age 65 years, administer 1 dose PPSV23 at least 5 years after previous dose

Shared clinical decision-making

- **Age 65 years and older** (immunocompetent): 1 dose PCV13 based on shared clinical decision-making
  - If both PCV13 and PPSV23 are to be administered, PCV13 should be administered first
  - PCV13 and PPSV23 should be administered at least 1 year apart
  - PCV13 and PPSV23 should not be administered during the same visit

Special situations
(see www.cdc.gov/mmwr/volumes/68/wr/mm6846a5.htm?s_cid=mm6846a5_w)

- **Age 19 through 64 years with chronic medical conditions** (chronic heart [excluding hypertension], lung, or liver disease, diabetes], alcoholism, or cigarette smoking): 1 dose PPSV23

- **Age 19 years or older with immunocompromising conditions** (congenital or acquired immunodeficiency [including B- and T-lymphocyte deficiency, complement deficiencies, phagocytic disorders, HIV infection], chronic renal failure, nephrotic syndrome, leukemia, lymphoma, Hodgkin disease, generalized malignancy, iatrogenic immunosuppression [e.g., drug or radiation therapy], solid organ transplant, multiple myeloma) or anatomical or functional asplenia (including sickle cell disease and other hemoglobinopathies): 1 dose PCV13 followed by 1 dose PPSV23 at least 8 weeks later, then another dose PPSV23 at least 5 years after previous PPSV23; at age 65 years or older, administer 1 dose PPSV23 at least 5 years after most recent PPSV23 (note: only 1 dose PPSV23 recommended at age 65 years or older)

- **Age 19 years or older with cerebrospinal fluid leak or cochlear implant:** 1 dose PCV13 followed by 1 dose PPSV23 at least 8 weeks later; at age 65 years or older, administer another dose PPSV23 at least 5 years after PPSV23 (note: only 1 dose PPSV23 recommended at age 65 years or older)

Tetanus, diphtheria, and pertussis vaccination

Routine vaccination

- **Previously did not receive Tdap at or after age 11 years:** 1 dose Tdap, then Td or Tdap every 10 years

Special situations

- **Previously did not receive primary vaccination series for tetanus, diphtheria, or pertussis:** At least 1 dose Tdap followed by 1 dose Td or Tdap at least 4 weeks after Tdap and another dose Td or Tdap 6-12 months after last Td or Tdap (Tdap can be substituted for any Td dose, but preferred as first dose); Td or Tdap every 10 years thereafter

- **Pregnancy:** 1 dose Tdap during each pregnancy, preferably in early part of gestational weeks 27-36

- For information on use of Td or Tdap as tetanus prophylaxis in wound management, see www.cdc.gov/mmwr/volumes/67/rr/rr6702a1.htm

Varicella vaccination

Routine vaccination

- **No evidence of immunity to varicella:** 2-dose series varicella-containing vaccine (VAR or MMRV [measles-mumps-rubella-varicella vaccine] for children); if previously received 1 dose varicella-containing vaccine, 1 dose at least 4 weeks after first dose
  - Evidence of immunity: U.S.-born before 1980 (except for pregnant women and health care personnel [see below]), documentation of 2 doses varicella-containing vaccine at least 4 weeks apart, diagnosis or verification of history of varicella or herpes zoster by a health care provider, laboratory evidence of immunity or disease

Special situations

- **Pregnancy with no evidence of immunity to varicella:** VAR contraindicated during pregnancy; after pregnancy (before discharge from health care facility) 1 dose if previously received 1 dose varicella-containing vaccine or dose 1 of 2-dose series (dose 2: 4-8 weeks later) if previously did not receive any varicella-containing vaccine, regardless of whether U.S.-born before 1980

- **Health care personnel with no evidence of immunity to varicella:** 1 dose if previously received 1 dose varicella-containing vaccine; 2-dose series 4-8 weeks apart if previously did not receive any varicella-containing vaccine, regardless of whether U.S.-born before 1980

- **HIV infection with CD4 count ≥200 cells/μL with no evidence of immunity:** Vaccination may be considered (2 doses, administered 3 months apart); VAR contraindicated in HIV infection with CD4 count <200 cells/μL

- **Severe immunocompromising conditions:** VAR contraindicated

Zoster vaccination

Routine vaccination

- **Age 50 years or older:** 2-dose series RZV (Shingrix) 2-6 months apart (minimum interval: 4 weeks; repeat dose if administered too soon), regardless of previous herpes zoster or history of ZVL (Zostavax) vaccination (administer RZV at least 2 months after ZVL)

- **Age 60 years or older:** 2-dose series RZV 2-6 months apart (minimum interval: 4 weeks; repeat if administered too soon) or 1 dose ZVL if not previously vaccinated. RZV preferred over ZVL (if previously received ZVL, administer RZV at least 2 months after ZVL)

Special situations

- **Pregnancy:** ZVL contraindicated; consider delaying RZV until after pregnancy if RZV is otherwise indicated

- **Severe immunocompromising conditions (including HIV infection with CD4 count <200 cells/μL):** ZVL contraindicated; recommended use of RZV under review

MODIFIED CHECKLIST FOR AUTISM IN TODDLERS, REVISED WITH FOLLOW-UP (M-CHAT-R/F)

MODIFIED CHECKLIST FOR AUTISM IN TODDLERS, REVISED WITH FOLLOW-UP (M-CHAT-R/F)

Instructions: Please answer these questions about your child. Keep in mind how your child usually behaves. If you have seen your child do the behavior a few times, but he or she does not usually do it, then please answer no. Please circle YES or NO for every question. Thank you very much!

1. If you point at something across the room, does your child look at it? (FOR EXAMPLE, if you point at a toy or an animal, does your child look at the toy or animal?)	YES or NO
2. Have you ever wondered if your child might be deaf?	YES or NO
3. Does your child play pretend or make-believe? (FOR EXAMPLE, pretend to drink from an empty cup, pretend to talk on a phone, or pretend to feed a doll or stuffed animal?)	YES or NO
4. Does your child like climbing on things? (FOR EXAMPLE, furniture, playground equipment, or stairs)	YES or NO
5. Does your child make unusual finger movements near his or her eyes? (FOR EXAMPLE, does your child wiggle his or her fingers close to his or her eyes?)	YES or NO
6. Does your child point with one finger to ask for something or to get help? (FOR EXAMPLE, pointing to a snack or a toy that is out of reach)	YES or NO
7. Does your child point with one finger to show you something interesting? (FOR EXAMPLE, pointing to an airplane in the sky or a big truck in the road)	YES or NO
8. Is your child interested in other children? (FOR EXAMPLE, does your child watch other children, smile at them, or go to them?)	YES or NO
9. Does your child show you things by bringing them to you or holding them up for you to see—not to get help, but just to share? (FOR EXAMPLE, showing you a flower, a stuffed animal, or a toy truck)	YES or NO
10. Does your child respond when you call his or her name? (FOR EXAMPLE, does he or she look up, talk or babble, or stop what he or she is doing when you call his or her name?)	YES or NO
11. When you smile at your child, does he or she smile back at you?	YES or NO
12. Does your child get upset by everyday noises? (FOR EXAMPLE, does your child scream or cry to noise such as a vacuum cleaner or loud music?)	YES or NO
13. Does your child walk?	YES or NO
14. Does your child look you in the eye when you are talking to him or her, playing with him or her, or dressing him or her?	YES or NO

MODIFIED CHECKLIST FOR AUTISM IN TODDLERS, REVISED WITH FOLLOW-UP (M-CHAT-R/F) (*Continued*)

15. Does your child try to copy what you do? (FOR EXAMPLE, wave bye-bye, clap, or make a funny noise when you do)	YES or NO
16. If you turn your head to look at something, does your child look around to see what you are looking at?	YES or NO
17. Does your child try to get you to watch him or her? (FOR EXAMPLE, does your child look at you for praise, or say "look" or "watch me"?)	YES or NO
18. Does your child understand when you tell him or her to do something? (FOR EXAMPLE, if you don't point, can your child understand "put the book on the chair" or "bring me the blanket"?)	YES or NO
19. If something new happens, does your child look at your face to see how you feel about it? (FOR EXAMPLE, if he or she hears a strange or funny noise, or sees a new toy, will he or she look at your face?)	YES or NO
20. Does your child like movement activities? (FOR EXAMPLE, being swung or bounced on your knee)	YES or NO

Scoring: For all items except 2, 5, and 12, "NO" response indicates autism spectrum disorder risk.
Low-risk: 0–2; no further action required.
Medium-risk: 3–7; administer the follow-up (M-CHAT-R/F); if score remains ≥2, screening is positive.
High-risk: ≥8; refer immediately for diagnostic evaluation and early intervention.
Source: © 2009 Diana Robins, Deborah Fein, & Marianne Barton. Follow-up questions and additional information can be found at www.mchatscreen.com.

PROFESSIONAL SOCIETIES AND GOVERNMENTAL AGENCIES

PROFESSIONAL SOCIETIES AND GOVERNMENTAL AGENCIES

Abbreviation	Full Name	Internet Address
AACE	American Association of Clinical Endocrinologists	http://www.aace.com
AAD	American Academy of Dermatology	http://www.aad.org
AAFP	American Academy of Family Physicians	http://www.aafp.org
AAHPM	American Academy of Hospice and Palliative Medicine	http://www.aahpm.org
AAN	American Academy of Neurology	http://www.aan.com
AAO	American Academy of Ophthalmology	http://www.aao.org
AAO-HNS	American Academy of Otolaryngology—Head and Neck Surgery	http://www.entnet.org

AAOS	American Academy of Orthopaedic Surgeons and American Association of Orthopaedic Surgeons	http://www.aaos.org
AAP	American Academy of Pediatrics	http://www.aap.org
ACC	American College of Cardiology	http://www.acc.org
ACCP	American College of Chest Physicians	http://www.chestnet.org
ACIP	Advisory Committee on Immunization Practices	http://www.cdc.gov/vaccines/acip/index.html
ACOG	American Congress of Obstetricians and Gynecologists	http://www.acog.com
ACP	American College of Physicians	http://www.acponline.org
ACR	American College of Radiology	http://www.acr.org
ACR	American College of Rheumatology	http://www.rheumatology.org
ACS	American Cancer Society	http://www.cancer.org
ACSM	American College of Sports Medicine	http://www.acsm.org
ADA	American Diabetes Association	http://www.diabetes.org
AGA	American Gastroenterological Association	http://www.gastro.org
AGS	American Geriatrics Society	http://www.americangeriatrics.org
AHA	American Heart Association	http://www.americanheart.org
ANA	American Nurses Association	http://www.nursingworld.org
AOA	American Optometric Association	http://www.aoa.org
ASA	American Stroke Association	http://www.strokeassociation.org
ASAM	American Society of Addiction Medicine	http://www.asam.org
ASCCP	American Society for Colposcopy and Cervical Pathology	http://www.asccp.org
ASCO	American Society of Clinical Oncology	http://www.asco.org
ASCRS	American Society of Colon and Rectal Surgeons	http://www.fascrs.org

PROFESSIONAL SOCIETIES AND GOVERNMENTAL AGENCIES   (Continued)

Abbreviation	Full Name	Internet Address
ASGE	American Society for Gastrointestinal Endoscopy	http://asge.org
ASHA	American Speech-Language-Hearing Association	http://www.asha.org
ASN	American Society of Neuroimaging	http://www.asnweb.org
ATA	American Thyroid Association	http://www.thyroid.org
ATS	American Thoracic Society	http://www.thoracic.org
AUA	American Urological Association	http://auanet.org
BASHH	British Association for Sexual Health and HIV	http://www.bashh.org
	Bright Futures	http://brightfutures.org
BGS	British Geriatrics Society	http://www.bgs.org.uk/
BSAC	British Society for Antimicrobial Chemotherapy	http://www.bsac.org.uk
CDC	Centers for Disease Control and Prevention	http://www.cdc.gov
COG	Children's Oncology Group	http://www.childrensoncologygroup.org
CSVS	Canadian Society for Vascular Surgery	http://canadianvascular.ca
CTF	Canadian Task Force on Preventive Health Care	http://canadiantaskforce.ca
EASD	European Association for the Study of Diabetes	http://www.easd.org
EAU	European Association of Urology	http://www.uroweb.org
ERS	European Respiratory Society	http://ersnet.org
ESC	European Society of Cardiology	http://www.escardio.org
ESH	European Society of Hypertension	http://www.eshonline.org
ARC	International Agency for Research on Cancer	http://screening.iarc.fr
ICSI	Institute for Clinical Systems Improvement	http://www.icsi.org
IDF	International Diabetes Federation	http://www.idf.org
NAPNAP	National Association of Pediatric Nurse Practitioners	http://www.napnap.org

NCCN	National Comprehensive Cancer Network	http://www.nccn.org/cancer-guidelines.html
NCI	National Cancer Institute	http://www.cancer.gov/cancerinformation
NEI	National Eye Institute	http://www.nei.nih.gov
NGC	National Guideline Clearinghouse	http://www.guidelines.gov
NHLBI	National Heart, Lung, and Blood Institute	http://www.nhlbi.nih.gov
NIAAA	National Institute on Alcohol Abuse and Alcoholism	http://www.niaaa.nih.gov
NICE	National Institute for Health and Clinical Excellence	http://www.nice.org.uk
NIDCR	National Institute of Dental and Craniofacial Research	http://www.nidr.nih.gov
NIHCDC	National Institutes of Health Consensus Development Program	http://www.consensus.nih.gov
NIP	National Immunization Program	http://www.cdc.gov/vaccines
NKF	National Kidney Foundation	http://www.kidney.org
NOF	National Osteoporosis Foundation	http://www.nof.org
NTSB	National Transportation Safety Board	http://www.ntsb.gov
SCF	Skin Cancer Foundation	http://www.skincancer.org
SGIM	Society of General Internal Medicine	http://www.sgim.org
SKI	Sloan-Kettering Institute	http://www.mskcc.org/mskcc/html/5804.cfm
SVU	Society for Vascular Ultrasound	http://www.svunet.org
UK-NHS	United Kingdom National Health Service	http://www.nhs.uk
USPSTF	United States Preventive Services Task Force	http://www.ahrq.gov/clinic/uspstfix.htm
WHO	World Health Organization	http://www.who.int/en

SCREENING INSTRUMENTS: ALCOHOL ABUSE

SENSITIVITY AND SPECIFICITY OF SCREENING TESTS FOR PROBLEM DRINKING

Instrument Name	Screening Questions/Scoring	Threshold Score	Sensitivity/ Specificity (%)	Source
CAGE[a]	See page 717	>1	77/58	*Am J Psychiatry.* 1974;131:1121
		>2	53/81	*J Gen Intern Med.* 1998;13:379
		>3	29/92	
AUDIT	See page 717	>4	87/70	*BMJ.* 1997;314:420
		>5	77/84	*J Gen Intern Med.* 1998;13:379
		>6	66/90	

[a]The CAGE may be less applicable to binge drinkers (eg, college students), the elderly, and minority populations.

SCREENING INSTRUMENTS: ALCOHOL ABUSE

SCREENING PROCEDURES FOR PROBLEM DRINKING

1. CAGE screening test[a]

Have you ever felt the need to	Cut down on drinking?
Have you ever felt	Annoyed by criticism of your drinking?
Have you ever felt	Guilty about your drinking?
Have you ever taken a morning	Eye opener?

INTERPRETATION: Two "yes" answers are considered a positive screen. One "yes" answer should arouse a suspicion of alcohol abuse.

2. The Alcohol Use Disorder Identification Test (AUDIT)[b] (Scores for response categories are given in parentheses. Scores range from 0 to 40, with a cutoff score of ≥5 indicating hazardous drinking, harmful drinking, or alcohol dependence.)

1. How often do you have a drink containing alcohol?
   Never   (1) Monthly or less   (2) Two to four times a month   (3) Two or three times a week   (4) Four or more times a week

2. How many drinks containing alcohol do you have on a typical day when you are drinking?
   (0) 1 or 2   (1) 3 or 4   (2) 5 or 6   (3) 7 to 9   (4) 10 or more

3. How often do you have 6 or more drinks on 1 occasion?
   Never   (1) Less than monthly   (2) Monthly   (3) Weekly   (4) Daily or almost daily

4. How often during the last year have you found that you were not able to stop drinking once you had started?
   Never   (1) Less than monthly   (2) Monthly   (3) Weekly   (4) Daily or almost daily

5. How often during the last year have you failed to do what was normally expected of you because of drinking?
   Never   (1) Less than monthly   (2) Monthly   (3) Weekly   (4) Daily or almost daily

6. How often during the last year have you needed a first drink in the morning to get yourself going after a heavy drinking session?
   Never   (1) Less than monthly   (2) Monthly   (3) Weekly   (4) Daily or almost daily

7. How often during the last year have you had a feeling of guilt or remorse after drinking?
   (0) Never   (1) Less than monthly   (2) Monthly   (3) Weekly   (4) Daily or almost daily

8. How often during the last year have you been unable to remember what happened the night before because you had been drinking?
   Never   (1) Less than monthly   (2) Monthly   (3) Weekly   (4) Daily or almost daily

SCREENING INSTRUMENTS: ALCOHOL ABUSE

SCREENING PROCEDURES FOR PROBLEM DRINKING (Continued)

9. Have you or has someone else been injured as a result of your drinking?

No   (2) Yes, but not in the last year   (4) Yes, during the last year

10. Has a relative or friend or a doctor or other health worker been concerned about your drinking or suggested you cut down?

(0) No   (2) Yes, but not in the last year   (4) Yes, during the last year

[a]Modified from Mayfield D, McLeod G, Hall P. The CAGE questionnaire: validation of a new alcoholism screening instrument. Am J Psychiatry. 1974;131:1121.
[b]From Piccinelli M, Tessari E, Bortolomasi M, et al. Efficacy of the alcohol use disorders identification test as a screening tool for hazardous alcohol intake and related disorders in primary care: a validity study. BMJ. 1997;314:420.

SCREENING TESTS FOR DEPRESSION

SCREENING INSTRUMENTS: DEPRESSION

Instrument Name	Screening Questions/Scoring	Threshold Score	Source
Beck Depression Inventory (short form)	See page 722	0–4: None or minimal depression 5–7: Mild depression 8–15: Moderate depression >15: Severe depression	*Postgrad Med.* 1972;81
Geriatric Depression Scale	See page 698	≥15: Depression	*J Psychiatr Res.* 1983;17:37
PRIME-MD© (mood questions)	1. During the last month, have you often been bothered by feeling down, depressed, or hopeless? 2. During the last month, have you often been bothered by little interest or pleasure in doing things?	"Yes" to either question[a]	*JAMA.* 1994;272:1749 *J Gen Intern Med.* 1997;12:439
Patient Health Questionnaire (PHQ-9)©	http://www.pfizer.com/phq-9/ See page 720	*Major depressive syndrome:* if answers to #1a or b and ≥5 of #1a–i are at least "More than half the days" (count #1i if present at all) *Other depressive syndrome:* if #1a or b and 2–4 of #1a–i are at least "More than half the days" (count #1i if present at all) 5–9: mild depression 10–14: moderate depression 15–19: moderately severe depression 20–27: severe depression	*JAMA.* 1999;282:1737 *J Gen Intern Med.* 2001;16:606

[a]Sensitivity 86%–96%; specificity 57%–75%.

Source: ©Pfizer Inc.

SCREENING INSTRUMENTS: DEPRESSION

PHQ-9 DEPRESSION SCREEN, ENGLISH

Over the past 2 wk, how often have you been bothered by any of the following problems?

	Not at all	Several days	>Half the days	Nearly every day
a. Little interest or pleasure in doing things	0	1	2	3
b. Feeling down, depressed, or hopeless	0	1	2	3
c. Trouble falling or staying asleep, or sleeping too much	0	1	2	3
d. Feeling tired or having little energy	0	1	2	3
e. Poor appetite or overeating	0	1	2	3
f. Feeling bad about yourself—or that you are a failure or that you have let yourself or your family down	0	1	2	3
g. Trouble concentrating on things, such as reading the newspaper or watching television	0	1	2	3
h. Moving or speaking so slowly that other people could have noticed? Or the opposite—being so fidgety or restless that you have been moving around a lot more than usual?	0	1	2	3
i. Thoughts that you would be better off dead or of hurting yourself in some way	0	1	2	3
For office coding: Total Score	=	+	+	+

Major depressive syndrome: If ≥5 items present scored ≥2 and one of the items is depressed mood (b) or anhedonia (a). If item "i" is present, then this counts, even if score = 1.

Depressive screen positive: If at least one item ≥2 (or item "i" is ≥1).

Source: From the Primary Care Evaluation of Mental Disorders Patient Health Questionnaire (PRIME-MD PHQ). The PHQ was developed by Drs. Robert L., et al. For research information, contact Dr. Spitzer at rls8@columbia.edu. PRIME-MD® is a trademark of Pfizer Inc. Copyright © 1999 Pfizer Inc. All rights reserved. Reproduced with permission. For office coding: Maj Dep Syn if answer to #2a or b and ≥5 of #2a–i are at least "More than half the days" (count #2i if present at all). Other Dep Syn if #2a or b and 2, 3, or 4 of #2a–i are at least "More than half the days" (count #2i if present at all).

SCREENING INSTRUMENTS: DEPRESSION

PHQ-9 DEPRESSION SCREEN, SPANISH

Durante las últimas 2 semanas, ¿con qué frecuencia le han molestado los siguientes problemas?

	Nunca	Varios días	>La mitad de los días	Casi todos los días
a. Tener poco interés o placer en hacer las cosas	0	1	2	3
b. Sentirse desanimada, deprimida, o sin esperanza	0	1	2	3
c. Con problemas en dormirse o en mantenerse dormida, o en dormir demasiado	0	1	2	3
d. Sentirse cansada o tener poca energía	0	1	2	3
e. Tener poco apetito o comer en exceso	0	1	2	3
f. Sentir falta de amor propio—o qe sea un fracaso o que decepcionara a sí misma o a su familia	0	1	2	3
g. Tener dificultad para concentrarse en cosas tales como leer el periódico o mirar la televisión	0	1	2	3
h. Se mueve o habla tan lentamente que otra gente se podría dar cuenta—o de lo contrario, está tan agitada o inquieta que se mueve mucho más de lo acostumbrado	0	1	2	3
i. Se le han ocurrido pensamientos de que se haría daño de alguna manera	0	1	2	3
For office coding: Total Store	=	+	+	

Source: From the Primary Care Evaluation of Mental Disorders Patient Health Questionnaire (PRIME-MD PHQ). The PHQ was developed by Drs. Robert L., et al. For research information, contact Dr. Spitzer at rls8@columbia.edu. PRIME-MD® is a trademark of Pfizer Inc. Copyright © 1999 Pfizer Inc. All rights reserved. Reproduced with permission. For office coding: Maj Dep Syn if answer to #2a or b and ≥5 of #2a–i are at least "More than half the days" (count #2i if present at all). Other Dep Syn if #2a or b and 2, 3, or 4 of #2a–i are at least "More than half the days" (count #2i if present at all).

SCREENING INSTRUMENTS: DEPRESSION

BECK DEPRESSION INVENTORY, SHORT FORM

Instructions: This is a questionnaire. On the questionnaire are groups of statements. Please read the entire group of statements in each category. Then pick out the one statement in that group that best describes the way you feel today, that is, right now! Circle the number beside the statement you have chosen. If several statements in the group seem to apply equally well, circle each one. Sum all numbers to calculate a score.

Be sure to read all the statements in each group before making your choice.

A. Sadness
3 I am so sad or unhappy that I can't stand it.
2 I am blue or sad all the time and I can't snap out of it.
1 I feel sad or blue.
0 I do not feel sad.

B. Pessimism
3 I feel that the future is hopeless and that things cannot improve.
2 I feel I have nothing to look forward to.
1 I feel discouraged about the future.
0 I am not particularly pessimistic or discouraged about the future.

C. Sense of failure
3 I feel I am a complete failure as a person (parent, husband, wife).
2 As I look back on my life, all I can see is a lot of failures.
1 I feel I have failed more than the average person.
0 I do not feel like a failure.

D. Dissatisfaction
3 I am dissatisfied with everything.
2 I don't get satisfaction out of anything anymore.
1 I don't enjoy things the way I used to.
0 I am not particularly dissatisfied.

E. Guilt
3 I feel as though I am very bad or worthless.
2 I feel quite guilty.
1 I feel bad or unworthy a good part of the time.
0 I don't feel particularly guilty.

F. Self-dislike
3 I hate myself.
2 I am disgusted with myself.
1 I am disappointed in myself.
0 I don't feel disappointed in myself.

G. Self-harm
3 I would kill myself if I had the chance.
2 I have definite plans about committing suicide.
1 I feel I would be better off dead.
0 I don't have any thoughts of harming myself.

H. Social withdrawal

3 I have lost all of my interest in other people and don't care about them at all.

2 I have lost most of my interest in other people and have little feeling for them.

1 I am less interested in other people than I used to be.

0 I have not lost interest in other people.

I. Indecisiveness

3 I can't make any decisions at all anymore.

2 I have great difficulty in making decisions.

1 I try to put off making decisions.

0 I make decisions about as well as ever.

J. Self-image change

3 I feel that I am ugly or repulsive looking.

2 I feel that there are permanent changes in my appearance and they make me look unattractive.

1 I am worried that I am looking old or unattractive.

0 I don't feel that I look worse than I used to.

K. Work difficulty

3 I can't do any work at all.

2 I have to push myself very hard to do anything.

1 It takes extra effort to get started at doing something.

0 I can work about as well as before.

L. Fatigability

3 I get too tired to do anything.

2 I get tired from doing anything.

1 I get tired more easily than I used to.

0 I don't get any more tired than usual.

M. Anorexia

3 I have no appetite at all anymore.

2 My appetite is much worse now.

1 My appetite is not as good as it used to be.

0 My appetite is no worse than usual.

Source: Reproduced with permission from Beck AT, Beck RW. Screening depressed patients in family practice: a rapid technic. *Postgrad Med.* 1972;52:81-85.

VULNERABLE SENIORS: PREVENTING ADVERSE DRUG EVENTS

For older adults, minimize exposure to potentially inappropriate medications. Below is a summary of the 2015 American Geriatric Society Beers Criteria to prevent adverse drug events in older patients.

SELECTED MEDICATIONS TO AVOID IN OLDER ADULTS

These medications carry risks specific to an older population and should be avoided except in specific situations.

Class of Medications	Reason to Avoid	Exceptions
First-Generation Antihistamines (ie, diphenhydramine, hydroxyzine, promethazine, etc.)	Clearance is reduced as age advances; risk of confusion and other anticholinergic effects	Diphenhydramine for acute allergic reaction may be appropriate
Antiparkinsonian agents (ie, benztropine, trihexyphenidyl)	More effective agents exist for Parkinson's disease	
Antispasmodics (ie, atropine, belladonna alkaloids, dicyclomine, etc.)	Risk of confusion and other anticholinergic effects	
Nitrofurantoin	Pulmonary, hepato-, and neurotoxicity with long-term use; safer alternatives exist for UTI ppx.	
Alpha-1 blockers, peripheral (ie, doxazosin, prazosin, terazosin)	High risk of orthostatic hypotension	
Alpha blockers, central (ie, clonidine, guanfacine, methyldopa)	Risk of CNS effect, bradycardia, orthostatic hypotension.	Clonidine may be appropriate in some cases as adjunctive agent in refractory HTN

Drug	Concern	Recommendation
Digoxin	AFib: more effective alternatives exist and mortality may increase Heart failure: Benefit is arguable; mortality may increase	May be appropriate in some cases as adjunctive agent for refractory symptomatic atrial fibrillation or heart failure. If used, avoid doses >0.125 mg/d
Nifedipine	Risk of hypotension, myocardial ischemia	
Amiodarone	Afib: More toxicity than other agents	May be appropriate for rhythm control if LVH or significant heart failure
Antidepressants with anticholinergic profile (ie, amitriptyline, nortriptyline, paroxetine)	Sedating; orthostatic hypotension; anticholinergic effects including confusion	
Antipsychotics, 1st & 2nd generation	Risk of CVA, cognitive decline	Schizophrenia, bipolar disorder Dementia/delirium: only appropriate if nonpharmacologic options fail and patient threatens significant harm to self or others
Barbiturates (ie, phenobarbital, butalbital)	Risk of overdose at low dosages, dependence, escalating dose due to tolerance	
Benzodiazepines	Increased sensitivity with age, slower metabolism of longer-acting agents. Risk of cognitive impairment, falls, delirium	Seizure disorders, alcohol withdrawal, severe generalized anxiety, anesthesia
Nonbenzodiazepine hypnotics (ie, zolpidem, zaleplon, eszopiclone)	Similar to benzodiazepine risk; minimal improvement in sleep	
Androgens (ie, testosterone, methyltestosterone)	Cardiac problems; contraindicated in prostate cancer	Lab-verified symptomatic hypogonadism

SELECTED MEDICATIONS TO AVOID IN OLDER ADULTS   (Continued)

Medication	Risk/Concern	Comments
Estrogen, +/− progestin	Risk of breast and endometrial cancer; no evidence for cardioprotection or cognitive protection in elderly.	Vaginal estrogens safe/effective for vaginal dryness
Insulin on a sliding scale	Hypoglycemia risk; no outcome benefit in outpatient or inpatient settings.	
Megestrol	Does not improve weight; higher risk of VTE and death.	
Sulfonylureas of longer duration (ie, glyburide, chlorpropamide)	Severe prolonged hypoglycemia	
Metoclopramide	Extrapyramidal effects	Gastroparesis
Proton pump inhibitors	Clostridium difficile infection; osteopenia/osteoporosis	Short-courses (ie, <8 wk). May be appropriate to treat severe conditions such as erosive esophagitis, Barrett's esophagus, or for prevention in high-risk patients (ie, NSAID or corticosteroid use)
NSAIDs (ie, high-dose aspirin, ibuprofen, naproxen, indomethacin, ketorolac, etc.)	GI bleed or peptic ulcer disease. Some (ie, indomethacin, ketorolac) carry higher risk of AKI.	Only use if alternative treatments are exhausted and patient can take PPI or misoprostol for gastroprotection (which reduces but does not eliminate risk)
Muscle relaxants (ie, cyclobenzaprine, methocarbamol, carisoprodol)	Anticholinergic effects, sedation, fracture risk; minimal efficacy	Urinary retention

Source: https://www.ncbi.nlm.nih.gov/pubmed/26446832

Index

Page numbers followed by *t.* denote tabular material, those followed by *f* denote figures, and page numbers followed by "n" denote notes.